Advances in Motor Neuroprostheses

Advances in Motor Neuroprostheses

Editor: Isaac Anderson

MURPHY & MOORE
www.murphy-moorepublishing.com

www.murphy-moorepublishing.com

MURPHY & MOORE

Cataloging-in-Publication Data

Advances in motor neuroprostheses / edited by Isaac Anderson.
p. cm.
Includes bibliographical references and index.
ISBN 978-1-63987-020-2
1. Neuroprostheses. 2. Prosthesis. 3. Biomedical engineering. 4. Neurotechnology (Bioengineering). I. Anderson, Isaac.
R856 .A38 2022
610.28--dc23

Murphy & Moore Publishing,
1 Rockefeller Plaza,
New York City, NY 10020, USA

ISBN 978-1-63987-020-2 (Hardback)

Contents

Preface

Neuroprotheses are the devices that are used to replace lost nervous system functions. They provide stimulated hand and arm function and are considered an effective method for restoring function. The discipline which relates biomedical engineering and neuroscience, and is concerned with the development of neural prostheses, is known as neuroprosthetics. Neuroprostheses include a series of devices that can replace sensory, motor or cognitive modality that has been damaged due to a disease or injury. Motor neuroprosthesis involves the usage of electrical stimulation of neural structures. It can be used for the patients suffering from a stroke. This book brings forth some of the most innovative concepts and elucidates the unexplored aspects of motor neuroprotheses. The readers would gain knowledge that would broaden their perspective about this field. This book will also provide interesting topics for research which interested readers can take up.

This book is a result of research of several months to collate the most relevant data in the field.

When I was approached with the idea of this book and the proposal to edit it, I was overwhelmed. It gave me an opportunity to reach out to all those who share a common interest with me in this field. I had 3 main parameters for editing this text:

1. Accuracy - The data and information provided in this book should be up-to-date and valuable to the readers.
2. Structure - The data must be presented in a structured format for easy understanding and better grasping of the readers.
3. Universal Approach - This book not only targets students but also experts and innovators in the field, thus my aim was to present topics which are of use to all.

Thus, it took me a couple of months to finish the editing of this book.

I would like to make a special mention of my publisher who considered me worthy of this opportunity and also supported me throughout the editing process. I would also like to thank the editing team at the back-end who extended their help whenever required.

Editor

1

Control of an Ambulatory Exoskeleton with a Brain–Machine Interface for Spinal Cord Injury Gait Rehabilitation

Eduardo López-Larraz[1,2], Fernando Trincado-Alonso[3], Vijaykumar Rajasekaran[4], Soraya Pérez-Nombela[3], Antonio J. del-Ama[3], Joan Aranda[4], Javier Minguez[1,2,5], Angel Gil-Agudo[3] and Luis Montesano[1,2]*

[1] Departamento de Informática e Ingeniería de Sistemas, University of Zaragoza, Zaragoza, Spain, [2] Instituto de Investigación en Ingeniería de Aragón (I3A), Zaragoza, Spain, [3] Biomechanics and Technical Aids Unit, National Hospital for Spinal Cord Injury, Toledo, Spain, [4] Institute for Bioengineering of Catalunya, Universitat Politécnica de Catalunya, Barcelona, Spain, [5] Bit & Brain Technologies, Zaragoza, Spain

Edited by:
*Timothée Levi,
University of Bordeaux 1, France*

Reviewed by:
*Jose Luis Contreras-Vidal,
University of Houston, USA
Ren Xu,
University of Göttingen, Germany*

***Correspondence:**
*Eduardo López-Larraz
edulop@unizar.es*

The closed-loop control of rehabilitative technologies by neural commands has shown a great potential to improve motor recovery in patients suffering from paralysis. Brain–machine interfaces (BMI) can be used as a natural control method for such technologies. BMI provides a continuous association between the brain activity and peripheral stimulation, with the potential to induce plastic changes in the nervous system. Paraplegic patients, and especially the ones with incomplete injuries, constitute a potential target population to be rehabilitated with brain-controlled robotic systems, as they may improve their gait function after the reinforcement of their spared intact neural pathways. This paper proposes a closed-loop BMI system to control an ambulatory exoskeleton—without any weight or balance support—for gait rehabilitation of incomplete spinal cord injury (SCI) patients. The integrated system was validated with three healthy subjects, and its viability in a clinical scenario was tested with four SCI patients. Using a cue-guided paradigm, the electroencephalographic signals of the subjects were used to decode their gait intention and to trigger the movements of the exoskeleton. We designed a protocol with a special emphasis on safety, as patients with poor balance were required to stand and walk. We continuously monitored their fatigue and exertion level, and conducted usability and user-satisfaction tests after the experiments. The results show that, for the three healthy subjects, 84.44 ± 14.56% of the trials were correctly decoded. Three out of four patients performed at least one successful BMI session, with an average performance of 77.6 1 ± 14.72%. The shared control strategy implemented (i.e., the exoskeleton could only move during specific periods of time) was effective in preventing unexpected movements during periods in which patients were asked to relax. On average, 55.22 ± 16.69% and 40.45 ± 16.98% of the trials (for healthy subjects and patients, respectively) would have suffered from unexpected activations (i.e., false positives) without the proposed control strategy. All the patients showed low exertion and fatigue levels during the performance of the experiments. This paper constitutes a proof-of-concept study to validate the feasibility of a BMI to control an ambulatory exoskeleton by patients with incomplete paraplegia (i.e., patients with good prognosis for gait rehabilitation).

Keywords: spinal cord injury (SCI), brain machine interfaces (BMI), ambulatory exoskeletons, gait rehabilitation, movement intention decoding, electroencephalography (EEG), event related desynchronization (ERD), movement related cortical potentials (MRCP)

1. INTRODUCTION

Recovery of lower-limb function in spinal cord injury (SCI) patients is crucial to enhance the independence and quality of life in this population (Ditunno et al., 2008). Two-third of SCI patients are reported as paraplegic (Wyndaele and Wyndaele, 2006), from which a considerable percentage is able to regain certain locomotion function, especially those with low and incomplete lesions (Nene et al., 1996; Scivoletto et al., 2014). Technological advances, such as robotic exoskeletons, have emerged as a valuable option to rehabilitate and restore gait in paraplegic patients beyond traditional means such as crutches, walkers, and orthoses. These robotic systems can range from clinical devices to bioinspired wearable ones. Firstly, weight-suspended robotic systems with a treadmill, such as the Lokomat (Hocoma Medical Engineering Inc, Zurich, Switzerland) and the Gait Trainer (GT II, Rehastim, Berlin, Germany), have demonstrated their rehabilitative efficacy, but they are generally expensive and cannot be used for motor substitution (Wirz et al., 2005). Secondly, robotic walking devices with balance control, such as the REX (REX Bionics Ltd), can be used by people with high SCI (up to C4/5 level), as they completely substitute their gait function, but it may be too bulky and inefficient for those patients who maintain certain balance control. Hence, these systems can be more appropriate for assistive purposes only. Thirdly, ambulatory exoskeletons, such as the ReWalk (Bionics Research Inc) and the H2 (Technaid S.L., Spain), are designed to assist leg movement, but they can only be used by patients with lower-limb weakness who still can maintain balance. These systems are of particular interest, as they can be controlled using assist-as-needed paradigms, which may be more effective than other approaches for rehabilitation and functional compensation of patients with paraplegia and also for stroke sufferers (Pons and Torricelli, 2014).

In this context, there is a growing interest toward the development of robotic devices controlled by brain–machine interfaces (BMI) to assist and rehabilitate gait function (Pfurtscheller et al., 2006; Fitzsimmons et al., 2009; Alam et al., 2014). The contingent link between neural commands and the peripheral feedback given by means of a rehabilitation device can promote neuroplasticity (Mrachacz-Kersting et al., 2012). Whereas, a BMI constitutes a natural interface that provides an easier and more intuitive control of assistive devices (Millán et al., 2010). Non-invasive technologies such, as the electroencephalogram (EEG), constitute a relatively cheap and portable option to build these BMI systems (Wolpaw et al., 2002). The use of brain-triggered rehabilitative technologies is of special relevance for incomplete SCI patients. These individuals can maintain some intact fibers below the injury level, and recent studies have shown how these spared pathways can be reinforced by the continuous association between the activation of the brain during the intention of movement and the stimulation of the paralyzed limbs (Jackson and Zimmermann, 2012).

The closed-loop control of walking exoskeletons using neural commands presents two main challenges. The first one corresponds to the development of robust and reliable BMIs to decode neural signals associated with gait movement intention. In contrast to upper-limb, which is generally the focus of BMI research for motor rehabilitation/restoration of paralyzed patients (Lebedev and Nicolelis, 2006; Millán et al., 2010), decoding of gait has not been so deeply studied. The recording of neural signals during walking might be affected by motion artifacts, which could bias the decoding and lead to misinterpretation of the neural dynamics associated with the movement (Castermans et al., 2014), although there is evidence showing that the influence of these artifacts can be reduced by using carefully designed set-ups (Nathan and Contreras-Vidal, 2016). Nonetheless, recent studies with healthy subjects have shown that EEG neural correlates can be used to decode the gait initiation before it occurs (Jiang et al., 2015; Sburlea et al., 2015) and to distinguish between different walking directions (Velu and de Sa, 2013). However, pathologies like SCI entail a brain reorganization, which may complicate the decoding of motor information (López-Larraz et al., 2015a). Hence, it is important to validate how BMI systems can be applied effectively in these patients. The EEG signals of a paralyzed patient during his/her attempt to move the legs could be decoded without any overt movement and used to trigger the movement of an exoskeleton or prosthesis that assists his/her walking. The current state of the art in non-invasive BMI technology does not allow for precise decoding of fine limb kinematics. Therefore, an accepted approach in the literature is to have a shared control paradigm in which the brain activity is used to trigger the movement of a robot/prosthesis that can autonomously perform a functional task (e.g., walk forward two steps; Millán et al., 2010; Rohm et al., 2013).

The second challenge arises from the complexity of the set-up required to control a device for gait assistance with neural signals. In the recent years, pilot studies have shown how BMIs have been used to control weight-suspended robotic and prosthetic systems (Do et al., 2013; King et al., 2015). Furthermore, robotic exoskeletons with balance control have also been controlled using brain signals (Kilicarslan et al., 2013; Kwak et al., 2015). All these studies are performed with devices that support balance, which minimizes fall risks, and three of them demonstrated successful control with SCI patients (Do et al., 2013; Kilicarslan et al., 2013; King et al., 2015). However, the control of ambulatory exoskeletons with a BMI presents additional issues compared to those systems with balance support. Even if it is used by patients with a relatively good condition (e.g., legs weakness and/or certain degree of balance control), they are required to maintain the balance by holding on to a walker or to parallel bars, and to focus on the intention of motion to command the BMI. This kind of set-up would permit the development of assist-as-needed rehabilitative interventions for such patients, which may lead to higher motor improvements (Cai et al., 2006). Hence, the validation of a BMI to control an ambulatory exoskeleton requires the design of a protocol with special considerations, such as safety, timings and control of patients' fatigue levels during the experiments.

This paper presents an integrated system for the closed-loop control of an ambulatory exoskeleton with a BMI. The exoskeleton works under an assist-as-needed control paradigm, which can be adapted to the capabilities of each patient and assist him/her only to the extent he/she needs. The EEG neural correlates of movement are used to decode the intention of gait initiation, which is used as a volitional control signal for the exoskeleton movement. The feasibility of the proposed system is validated with two sets of experiments. The first experiment shows the viability of the whole set-up with three healthy subjects. The second experiment demonstrates the viability of the system in a realistic clinical environment, involving four incomplete SCI patients. An experimental protocol is proposed to operate the BMI in an ecological set-up, with an emphasis on patients' safety. Decoding performance, exertion levels, and satisfaction and usability scores were measured as indicators of the viability of the system for clinical applications.

2. MATERIALS AND METHODS

2.1. Participants

Three able-bodied subjects and four SCI patients participated in :he study. Demographic data of both the healthy subjects (H) ınd the patients (P) can be seen in **Table 1**. The SCI patients were hospitalized at the *Hospital Nacional de Parapléjicos*, in Toledo (Spain), where all the experimentation sessions took ›lace. The inclusion criteria for the patients were: (1) SCI with ıny lesion level, ASIA C or D with gait prognosis; (2) patients n walking rehabilitation; (3) patient's balance allows standing ›etween parallel bars; (4) no orthostatic complications during ›tanding; (5) upper-limb strength to manage a walker or crutches, ınd to transfer from the wheelchair to a chair; (6) age between 8 and 60 years; and (7) height 1.50–1.95 m and weight up o 90 kg. The exclusion criteria were: (1) inability to stand in ıpright position for at least 15 min; (2) any surgery in the ›revious 3 months; (3) spasticity higher than 3 in the Modified ıshworth Scale (Bohannon and Smith, 1987) in any of the lower-ımb muscles; (4) previous/current lower-limb bone fracture; 5) ulcers or sores in areas of contact with the exoskeleton nd/or electrodes; (6) previous/current history of cardiovascular disease of any kind or exercise contraindications; (7) upper-limb pain that limits weight bearing on crutches/walker/parallel bars; (8) significant upper/lower extremity discrepancies; (9) uncontrolled autonomic dysreflexia; (10) pregnancy; and (11) cognitive impairment of any kind. The selected patients met all inclusion and no exclusion criteria. All the subjects were duly informed about the study, and all of them gave written consent before the first session. The experimental procedure was approved by the Ethics Committee of the Hospital Complex of Toledo (Spain) (C.E.I.C. 31/02-2014).

2.2. Clinical Assessment

We evaluated the clinical condition of the SCI patients before their enrollment in the study. Their injury severity, lower extremity strength, and mobility were measured using a set of clinical tests, according to the standardized ASIA clinical exams (Marino et al., 2003). The lower extremity motor score (LEMS) was used to measure muscle strength, with 5 key muscles examined in each leg: hip flexors, knee extensors, ankle dorsiflexors, long toe extensors, and ankle plantar flexors. The grading system for the muscle strength goes from 0 to 5 (0 = absence of muscle contraction, 5 = normal active movement with full range of motion against full resistance). The cumulative score for the lower extremities ranges between 0 and 50. Modified Ashworth score was used for lower-limb spasticity measurement, ranging from 0 (no spasticity) to 4 (affected part rigid in flexion or extension). Only patient P4 presented a very slight spasticity (score 1) in the right ankle, below the level established in the exclusion criteria. Walking index for spinal cord injury (WISCI II) was used to quantify the degree of assistance required by the patient during normal walking and 10 Meter Walk Test (10 MWT) to assess walking speed (Ditunno and Ditunno, 2001; van Hedel et al., 2005). WISCII II grading system ranges from 0 (patient is unable to stand and/or participate in assisted walking) to 20 (ambulates with no devices, no braces and no physical assistance). According to the recommendations of 10 MWT, walking speed was calculated discarding the 2 initial and the 2 final meters, to only consider walking at a constant speed. Distance (6 m) was divided by the time measured to obtain gait speed (m/s). The values for each patient can be found in **Table 2**. Walking tests were performed using as little assistance as possible to ensure patient safety.

2.3. Experimental protocol

The present study was divided into two stages. The first stage aimed at validating the technology under a well-controlled scenario. This was done by performing experiments with healthy subjects and evaluating if the BMI could be effectively used to close the loop and control the ambulatory exoskeleton. The second stage sought to demonstrate that the proposed system and protocol could be safely used in a clinical environment. Experiments with SCI patients were conducted, in which the key point was to measure parameters such as exertion and fatigue levels, as well as usability and satisfaction scales.

The experimental protocol consisted of familiarization sessions and BMI sessions. The experiments with the healthy subjects included the familiarization and the BMI sessions in

TABLE 1 | Demographic information of both groups: healthy subjects and SCI patients.

ID	Age (years)	Sex	Height (meters)	Weight (kilograms)	Injury level	ASIA	Time since injury (months)	Etiology
H1	31	Male	1.74	70	–	–	–	–
H2	29	Male	1.77	73	–	–	–	–
H3	29	Male	1.75	74	–	–	–	–
P1	30	Male	1.85	90	L1	C	12	Traumatic
P2	24	Male	1.92	57	L1	C	24	Traumatic
P3	21	Male	1.80	76	T11	C	5	Traumatic
P4	49	Female	1.60	57	T12	C	11	Traumatic

TABLE 2 | Clinical scores obtained by the patients before the experiments.

ID	LEMS	WISCI II (Technical aid)	10 MWT (m/s)
P1	15	9 (walker and braces)	0.144
P2	20	12 (two crutches and braces)	0.287
P3	17	9 (walker and braces)	0.162
P4	28	15 (one crutch and braces)	0.081

1 day. The experiments with the SCI patients required one familiarization session and two BMI sessions in 3 separate days. The set-up included: the EEG equipment (only for the BMI sessions) with the amplifiers in a backpack carried by the subject, the exoskeleton attached to the subject's legs, and a walking aid to help keeping balance (**Figure 1**). In addition, a trolley table was used to carry the computers that processed the EEG signals and controlled the exoskeleton. Crutches, a walker, and parallel bars were tested as walking aids. Crutches did not provide enough balance control for the patients and were discarded. The walker, which is commonly used in gait rehabilitation by these patients, worked well with the healthy subjects. However, during some preliminary tests with the patients, we realized that they had difficulties to move it while walking with the exoskeleton. Therefore, all the SCI patients performed the BMI sessions using parallel bars, whereas the healthy subjects used the walker. The exoskeleton joints remained blocked whenever it was not in movement in order to partially support patients' weight.

The familiarization sessions allowed the subjects to get used to the protocol timings and the exoskeleton movements. On these sessions, one experimenter triggered the movements of the exoskeleton manually, warning the subject before every movement. For the healthy subjects, these sessions consisted of 5–10 min walking with the exoskeleton. For the patients, the sessions took between 20 and 30 min, in which 2 clinicians monitored every movement and informed the patient about the protocol and how to interact with the exoskeleton. If required, these sessions were repeated until both the patient and the clinicians confirmed that the patient was accustomed to the system, and ready for the first BMI session.

The BMI sessions consisted of screening blocks and closed-loop feedback blocks. Given the nature of the set-up, a cue-guided BMI was proposed, in which the EEG signals were classified asynchronously. Hence, the exoskeleton moved as soon as the intention of movement was decoded, but only during specific periods of time, avoiding sudden and unexpected movements that may result in patients' falls. The participants performed 3 or 4 screening blocks of 20 trials each, which were used to calibrate the BMI decoder. During this screening phase, the participants were standing, wearing the exoskeleton, and holding the corresponding walking aid (i.e., the walker for the healthy subjects, and the parallel bars for the patients). Neither the healthy subjects nor the patients could actually move the legs during the screening blocks (as the exoskeleton joints were blocked). Therefore, in both cases, we consider the action performed as a movement attempt and not as a movement execution. The screening blocks were composed of rest and movement attempt (MA) intervals. The rest intervals had a random duration between 4 and 7 s. An audio cue indicated the start of the MA interval, which lasted 3 s. The participants were instructed to attempt to move their right leg, as if they started walking, immediately after they heard the audio cue. The rest of the time, they were asked to stay relaxed and move as little as possible. During the MA interval, participants were explicitly asked to avoid compensatory movements with the rest of the body, especially with the hip, and to attempt to move their right leg only. The closed-loop feedback blocks were composed of trials with four intervals: (*i*) "Rest," (*ii*) "Preparation," (*iii*) "Movement Attempt," and (*iv*) "Movement." The experiments with healthy subjects included 3 blocks of 20 trials each (amounting to 60 trials), in order to acquire enough movements to have a good estimation of the performance of the BMI system. In the experiments with the SCI patients, there was a variable number of trials, and they were asked to reach a distance of 10 m (i.e., the length of the parallel bars), which corresponds to around 20–25 gait cycles. During the "Rest" state (5 s), the subjects were not required to perform any task, but just to relax after the previous trial. After that, a low tone was played, which marked the beginning of the "Preparation" interval (3 s), during which they were instructed to relax and be prepared for the upcoming cue. A high tone denoted the start of the "Movement Attempt" interval (maximum 3 s), in which they were asked to attempt to move their right leg in the same way

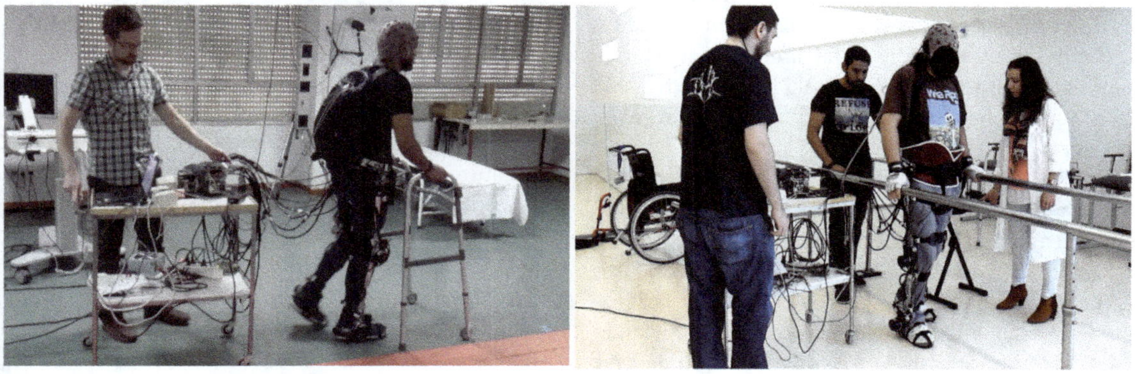

FIGURE 1 | Snapshots of experimental sessions performed by a healthy subject (left) and a SCI patient (right). The EEG cap is connected to the amplifiers that are carried in the backpack. These amplifiers are connected with long cables to a computer placed on the trolley table. The computer processes the EEG signals and sends decoder outputs to the exoskeleton controller, which sends to the joints the commands to move.

they had done in the screening blocks. If the BMI detected the intention to move at any time during these 3 s, the system started the "Movement" interval, in which the exoskeleton controller unblocked the joints and moved for one gait cycle: one step with right leg and one with left leg (6 s). Otherwise, after the 3 s, a new trial started in rest state. Supplementary Video 1 shows some trials of subject P1 triggering the exoskeleton with his motor intention.

For safety reasons, every trial required that the experimenter explicitly pressed an *activation* button during the "Rest" or "Preparation" intervals. If that button was pressed, the BMI decoder started sending its outputs to the exoskeleton controller. This would trigger the start of the gait cycle if the patient attempted to move during the "Movement Attempt" interval. If the button was not pressed, the exoskeleton did not move even if the participant attempted to move his/her leg. This mechanism was included in order to avoid starting a movement with the patient being in an unsafe position after the previous gait cycle, and to skip trials to regularly ask the patients about their fatigue levels. When required, the patients could sit for a few minutes to rest, and the trials continued when they confirmed that they were ready.

Due to the complexity of the set-up, the therapist–patient interaction was integral for the correct execution of the BMI experiments. Apart from being the control signal for the exoskeleton, the BMI was used by the therapist to guide the patient during the executions (Pichiorri et al., 2011). A therapist interface was designed to show the experimenter information of the BMI decoder output and the patient's EEG activity in real-time. The experimenter could, for instance, ask the patient to relax if the BMI was detecting movement commands during periods in which the patient should rest (e.g., due to excessive movements required to keep balance) or ask the patient to concentrate further when the BMI was not decoding any movement when they were required. In addition, an option to send manual triggers was included in the therapist interface in order to manually start exoskeleton movements, and so, reduce frustration when the BMI repeatedly failed to decode the movements.

2.4. EEG Acquisition

The EEG was recorded using a commercial g.Tec system (g.Tec GmbH, Graz, Austria), with 32 channels placed at AFz, FC3, FCz, FC4, C5, C3, C1, Cz, C2, C4, C6, CP3, CP1, CPz, CP2, CP4, FP1, FP2, F7, F3, Fz, F4, F8, T7, T8, P7, P3, Pz, P4, P8, O1, and O2 (according to the international 10/10 system). The ground and reference electrodes were placed on FPz and on the left earlobe, respectively. The EEG was digitized at a sampling frequency of 256 Hz and power-line notch-filtered to remove the 50 Hz line interference. The amplifiers connected to the EEG cap were carried in a backpack by the subject. The amplifiers were connected via long cables to a laptop placed on the trolley table.

2.5. Exoskeleton

The exoskeleton used to assist gait was a 6 degrees of freedom wearable lower-limb orthosis with anthropomorphic configuration (Bortole et al., 2015). It included three joints for each leg: hip, knee, and ankle, each of which was powered by a DC motor coupled with a harmonic drive gear. The exoskeleton was equipped with potentiometers and strain gauges to measure the joint angles and the human–robot interaction torques. Its control was conceived to work under an assist-as-needed paradigm in order to make rehabilitation more challenging for the patients. A predefined trajectory, obtained from healthy subjects, was used as the desired gait pattern. The controller updated the stiffness values in real time according to the subject's performance in order to assist him/her just to the extent he/she needed (Rajasekaran et al., 2015). The exoskeleton was connected with long cables to its controller and to the power supply, which were on the trolley table.

2.6. EEG-Based Movement Intention Decoder

After recording the screening blocks and before the closed-loop blocks, the BMI classifier was trained to distinguish between rest and movement attempt (MA) classes. The BMI decoder was based on the one proposed in López-Larraz et al. (2014). The decoding of movement attempt was dependent on the combination of two EEG movement correlates: the event-related desynchronization (ERD) of sensorimotor rhythms (Pfurtscheller and Lopes da Silva, 1999) and the movement-related cortical potentials (MRCP) (Shibasaki and Hallett, 2006). Signals from the screening datasets were trimmed down to 7-s trials (−4 to 3 s from the MA audio cue).

2.6.1. Artifact Removal

Before training, an automatized procedure based on z-scores was applied to eliminate the trials containing artifacts (López-Larraz et al., 2014). For each trial, the power in delta (1–4 Hz), theta (4–8 Hz), alpha (8–12 Hz), and beta (12–40 Hz) frequency bands, as well as the trial variance and the maximum amplitude were computed. Trials that went over a threshold set at 2.5 standard deviations of the mean in any of these parameters were discarded. Statistical methods like this are especially useful for clinical set-ups as the one presented here, since they do not require human supervision and can be used quickly to eliminate the artifacts before training the BMI (Nolan et al., 2010; Maeder et al., 2012). In principle, this method should be able to remove the most common types of artifacts that can be found in a set-up like this. For instance, analyzing the power in delta band and the signal amplitude may serve to remove low-frequency motion artifacts, whereas analyzing the power beta and signal variance could help to get rid of trials contaminated with EMG artifacts.

For the closed-loop blocks, we considered two options: (1) having an online system to detect EEG artifacts and stopping the BMI every time that it detected one; or (2) considering that the possible artifacts would not highly influence the performance of the system. Given that we trained the BMI with clean trials, the existence of artifacts during test should not deceitfully increase the performance, and at most, they would decrease it. Since we considered that this is not worse than stopping the BMI every time that an online artifact detector detects an artifact, no artifacting was performed during the closed-loop trials.

2.6.2. Feature Extraction and BMI Training

Features were computed from the clean trials using a 1-s long window with a sliding step of 250 ms. Features corresponding to the rest and MA classes were computed on the [−3, −1] s and [0, 2] s intervals, respectively (with 0 being the time when the high tone indicating the start of the MA interval was played). On these windows, the features were computed as follows:

- ERD features were calculated after applying a small Laplacian filter to the frontocentral, central, and centroparietal EEG channels. After that, a 16th order autoregressive model with a frequency resolution of 1 Hz was used to obtain the power values in the frequency range [7–25] Hz.
- MRCP features were calculated after subsampling the EEG signals to 64 Hz and applying a bandpass filter, [0.1–1] Hz, to them. Then, a common average reference (CAR) was applied to the channels FC3, FCz, FC4, C3, C1, Cz, C2, C4, CP3, CP1, CPz, CP2, and CP4, and their amplitudes were added to the feature vectors.

For each time window, 1192 features were extracted. Sparse discriminant analysis (SDA) was used to select the 30 most discriminant non-redundant features and as a linear classifier (Clemmensen et al., 2011; López-Larraz et al., 2014).

2.6.3. Closed-Loop BMI

During the closed-loop blocks, the EEG was processed continuously. A sliding window was computed every 62.5 ms and its features were extracted following the same procedure detailed in Section 2.6.2, and the classifier trained with the screening blocks generated a new BMI output. For each sliding window, the BMI classifier determined if the signal corresponded to rest or to MA classes. In order to ensure a consistent brain activation, the BMI generated a movement trigger when five consecutive windows of MA class were detected (Ramos-Murguialday et al., 2013). If the BMI was active (i.e., if the experimenter pressed the *activation* button during the "Rest" or "Preparation" intervals of a trial, see Section 2.3), the movement trigger was sent to the exoskeleton controller; otherwise, the trigger was not sent. The controller ignored those triggers that arrived during the "Rest" and "Preparation" intervals to avoid starting an unexpected movement, which could make the patients fall. Therefore, on each feedback trial, the exoskeleton moved if the experimenter activated the BMI and the BMI generated a trigger during the "Movement Attempt" interval. In addition, the exoskeleton could also be moved if the experimenter sent a manual trigger during the "Movement Attempt" interval.

2.7. Exertion and Satisfaction Assessments

In order to evaluate the feasibility of the system for clinical applications, the patients were assessed with exertion and satisfaction scales.

The exertion level was assessed three times on each BMI session: before starting (i.e., when the patient was still sitting on the wheelchair), after the screening blocks, and after the closed-loop blocks. The Borg scale was used with values ranging from 6 ("very, very light") to 20 ("very, very hard") (Borg, 1970).

After the last BMI session, the patients were asked to evaluate how satisfied they were with the system (i.e., the complete set-up, including the exoskeleton and the EEG system) by using a modified version of the QUEST (Quebec user evaluation of satisfaction with assistive technology) scale (Demers et al., 2002).

3. RESULTS

3.1. Movement Attempt EEG Correlates

The features used by the BMI to decode the attempts of movement were based on two well-studied EEG correlates: the event-related desynchronization (ERD) of sensorimotor rhythms and the movement-related cortical potentials (MRCP). **Figure** shows a summary of these correlates computed using the signals recorded in the screening blocks after removing artifactual trials (see Section 2.6.1). For the SCI patients, the screenings from both BMI sessions were combined. Following the methodology proposed in López-Larraz et al. (2014), we used optimal spatial filters (OSF) to visualize the ERD and the MRCP activities by combining the electrodes placed over the motor cortex. Activity recorded on electrodes FC3, FCz, FC4, C3, C1, Cz, C2, C4, CP3, CP1, CPz, CP2, and CP4 was combined with an optimization

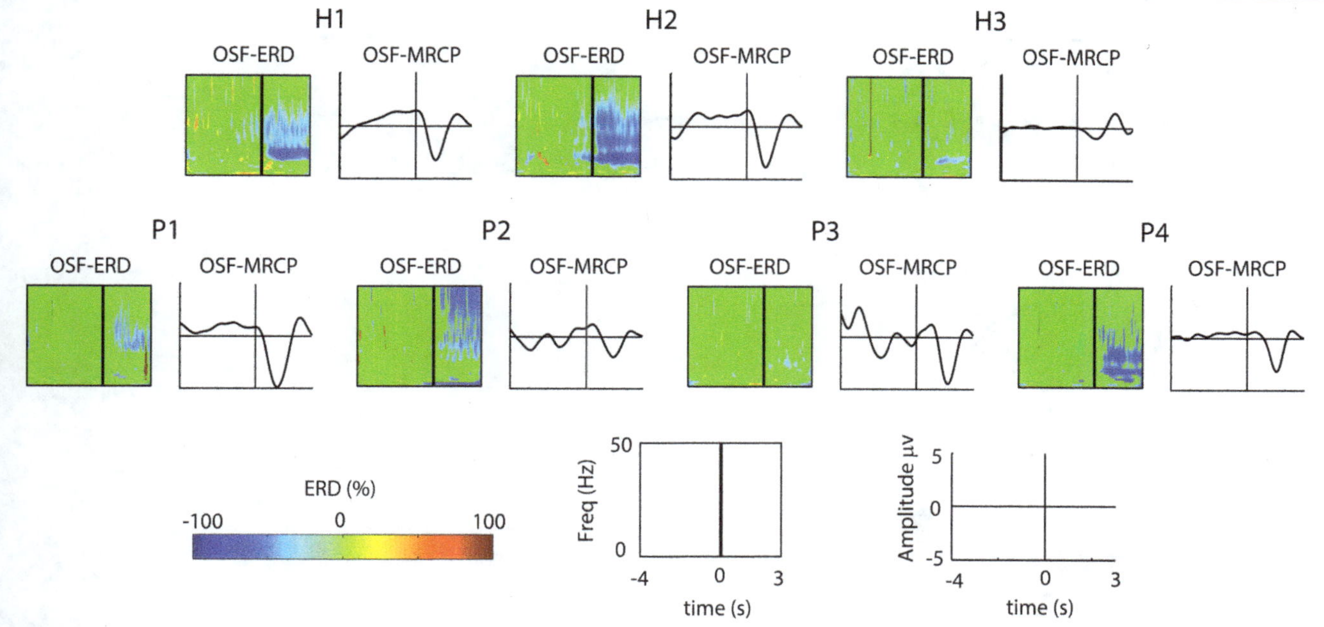

FIGURE 2 | Significant ERD and MRCP for each subject in the channels obtained by applying optimized spatial filtering. For each of the 7 subjects (the 3 healthy subjects on top and the 4 patients at the bottom), the left plot shows the ERD, and the right plot shows the MRCP. For the ERD, the *x*-axis correspond to the time interval [−4, 3] s, and the *y*-axis represent the frequency range [1–50] Hz. For the MRCPs, the *x*-axis correspond to the time interval [−4, 3] s, and the *y*-axis represent the MRCP amplitude [−5, 5] μv.

algorithm, which computed the coefficients that maximized the signal-to-noise ratio of both ERD and MRCPs (Graimann and Pfurtscheller, 2006; Niazi et al., 2011).

Two out of three healthy subjects (H1 and H2) showed strong ERD and MRCP activations, where as H3 showed weak activations of both correlates. For the SCI patients, the ERD patterns of P4 were similar to the ones of H1 and H2; P1 and P2 showed smoother ERD and only in the beta band; and P3 showed no ERD at all. Regarding the MRCPs, P1 and P4 showed similar morphology to H1 and H2, whereas P2 and P3 presented more noisy activity.

3.2. BMI Performance

On average, 14.58% of the trials were rejected before training the BMI decoder (15 ± 1.25% for the healthy subjects and 14.43 ± 2.62% for the patients). **Figure 3** shows one representative trial for one healthy subject (H1) and two patients (P2 and P3). For each subject, the following information is shown: data of 3 EEG channels (i.e., C3, Cz, and C4), the decoder output, the triggers generated (i.e., the BMI triggers and the manual triggers), the system states during the trial, the angle of both knees, and the interaction torques measured by the strain gauges of both knees. As can be seen in the left plot, a BMI trigger generated out of the "Movement Attempt" state does not start any movement of the exoskeleton. When it is generated in the appropriate state, the "Movement" period starts, first with the right leg and then followed by the left leg. In the right plot, the BMI did not detect any movement. Instead, the experimenter sent a manual trigger to start the "Movement" phase. The movement of the exoskeleton seems to cause relatively large motion artifacts in the EEG, especially in the patients (center and right plots).

Decoding results for the healthy subjects are presented in **Table 3**, and for the SCI patients in **Table 4**. Each of the healthy subjects performed 60 trials (3 blocks of 20 trials each). On average, 84.44% of the trials were correctly decoded, generating a walking movement with the exoskeleton. For the correctly decoded trials of the three subjects, the average time between the auditive cue and the beginning of the exoskeleton movement was 1.07 ± 0.63 s.

Given the complexity of the set-up and the unfamiliarity of the patients with the technology, they were asked to attend two BMI sessions. In the first session, which can be considered as a BMI-familiarization session, they were carefully informed about how the BMI system works. Then, they performed the screening blocks and a few closed-loop trials to familiarize with the whole system and protocol. On the second session, patients also performed screening blocks, and subsequently, they started with the closed-loop blocks until reaching a distance of 10 m.

Patient P1 was the only one who performed two successful BMI sessions (i.e., reaching the 10 m distance). In the first one, he achieved a high performance (84%), whereas in the second one, it dropped to 55.56%. For patients P2 and P4, the first session was prematurely interrupted, but both of them performed a successful second session, with more than 85% of decoded trials. For patient P3, performances were low in both sessions, especially in the second one, in which the experimenter had to repetitively use the manual trigger due to the lack of movement attempt commands decoded by the BMI. Notice that the decoding performances

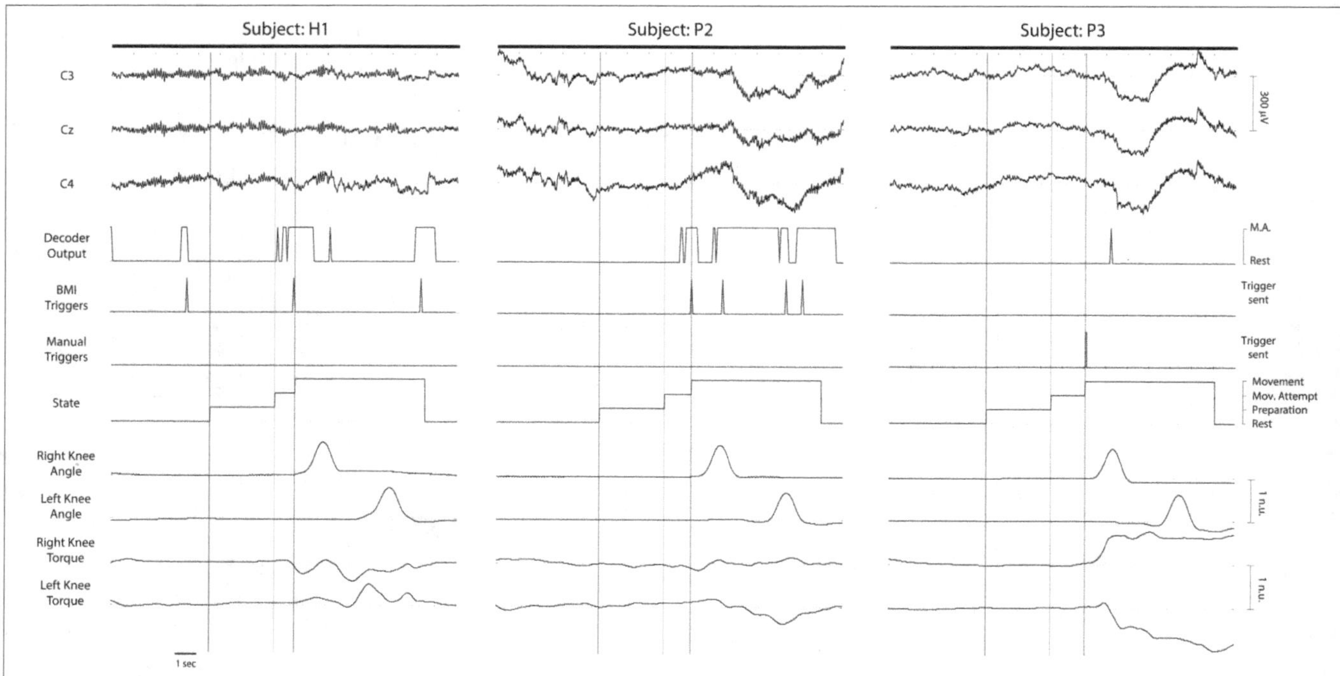

FIGURE 3 | Time series of three representative trials for healthy subject S1 (left), and patients P2 (center) and P3 (right). The three first lines correspond to three EEG channels located over the motor cortex: C3, Cz, and C4. The decoder output indicates the classifier label (Rest or MA) provided for each 1-s window in real time. The BMI triggers were generated only when five consecutive classifier outputs corresponded to MA class, after being in Rest class (they were ignored when generated out of the "Mov." Attempt period–see left plot). The manual triggers correspond to the movements generated by an explicit command sent by the experimenter (see right plot). The states of the system during a normal trial were: "Rest," "Preparation," "Movement Attempt," and "Movement." The right and left knee angles (in a normalized scale) indicate the flexion of the knee joints of the exoskeleton. The right and left knee interaction torques (in a normalized scale) measure the forces performed by the subjects in the strain gauges located on the knee joint of the robot. The vertical lines indicate the change of state of the system. The red, green and blue lines correspond to the beginning of the "Preparation," "Movement Attempt," and "Movement" phases, respectively.

presented in **Table 4** are computed as the ratio between the number of trials that the BMI correctly decoded and the total number of trials in which the experimenter did not activate the exoskeleton manually. The average decoding accuracy of the successful sessions (i.e., P1 sessions 1 and 2; P2 session 2; and P4 session 2) was 77.61 ± 14.72%, and their average time was 1.35 ± 0.71 s.

Notice that the decoding times reported in **Tables 3, 4** correspond to the average time that triggering the movement took with respect to the presentation of the audio cue that indicated the beginning of the "Movement Attempt" interval. Given that different types of delays have an influence on this time (e.g., computational, cognitive, and/or physiological), we also evaluated the average decoding time with respect to the negative peak of the MRCPs. These peaks have been observed to be aligned with the beginning of the muscular activity (Niazi et al., 2011), and hence, may constitute a better indicator of when the subjects started the attempt of movement. For the healthy subjects, the average MRCP negativity appeared 1.02 ± 0.02 s after the auditory cue (**Figure 2**, first row). Hence, the average decoding time was 50 ms after the MRCP peak. For the 3 SCI patients who performed successful BMI sessions (i.e., P1, P2, and P4), the MRCP negativity appeared on average 1.37 ± 0.20 s after the cue. Therefore, the average decoding time for the patients was 20 ms before the occurrence of their MRCP peak.

TABLE 3 | Decoding results of healthy subjects.

ID	Number of trials	Number of gait cycles	Decoding accuracy (%)	Decoding time (s) mean ± std
H1	60	53	88.33	1.26 ± 0.53
H2	60	58	96.67	0.90 ± 0.60
H3	60	41	68.33	1.09 ± 0.76

Given is the number of trials performed, the number of trials in which the BMI decoded the intention of motion (resulting in a walking movement), the decoding accuracy (i.e., the percentage of correctly decoded trials), and the time between the auditive cue and the exoskeleton movement.

Although the proposed protocol impeded that the exoskeleton could start moving during "Rest" and "Preparation" time intervals, we analyzed the offline movement triggers that were generated by the BMI in those intervals. To that end, we calculated the number of trials in which, at least, one movement trigger was generated during non-movement periods. For the healthy subjects, movement triggers were generated in 52.22 ± 16.69% of the trials during the "Preparation" interval, and in 66.67 ± 13.02% of the trials during the "Rest" interval. For the successful sessions with the patients, movement triggers were generated in 40.45 ± 16.98% of the trials during the "Preparation" interval, and in 63.42 ± 14.15% of the trials

TABLE 4 | Decoding results of SCI patients.

ID	Session number	Number of trials	Number of gait cycles	Number of manual triggers	Decoding accuracy (%)*	Decoding time (s) mean ± std
P1	1	25	21	0	84.00	1.08 ± 0.61
	2	40	20	4	55.56	1.59 ± 0.76
P2	1	2**	2	0	100.00	2.69 ± 0.01
	2	28	24	0	85.71	1.54 ± 0.84
P3	1	16	7	2	50.00	1.68 ± 0.67
	2	25	2	14	18.18	0.50 ± 0.52
P4	1	6***	5	0	83.33	1.59 ± 0.97
	2	27	23	0	85.19	1.19 ± 0.51

For each patient and session, given is the number of trials performed, the number of trials in which the BMI decoded the intention of motion (resulting in a walking movement), the number of manual triggers sent by the experimenter, the decoding accuracy (i.e., the percentage of correctly decoded trials), and the time between the auditive cue and the exoskeleton movement.

**The decoding accuracy was calculated as the number of decoded trials divided by the number of trials in which the experimenter did not send a manual trigger:*
$\%Acc = \frac{\#Gait\ cycles}{\#Trials - \#Manual\ triggers} \times 100$.

***This session was prematurely interrupted due to technical problems with the exoskeleton.*

****This session was prematurely interrupted due to temporal restrictions of the participant.*

during the "Rest" interval. We performed 3 statistical tests to compare the percentages of trials with correct triggers during the "Movement Attempt" period (true positives) and with erroneous triggers generated during "Rest" (false positives during "Rest") and "Preparation" (false positives during "Preparation") periods. For each measure, a single vector was generated by concatenating the percentages of the three healthy subjects and the four successful sessions of the patients, and paired Wilcoxon signed rank tests were used to measure significant differences. The number of true positives was significantly higher than the number of false positives generated during the "Preparation" interval ($p < 0.05$), although true positive was not significantly higher than the number of false positives during the "Rest" interval ($p = 0.08$). In addition, the number of false positives during the "Rest" interval was significantly higher than the ones generated during the "Preparation" interval ($p < 0.05$).

3.3. Features

As an automatic feature selection algorithm was used during the experiments, we performed a *post-hoc* analysis to evaluate the selected features for each participant. **Figure 4** shows the features selected by the SDA algorithm for the healthy subjects and the patients. For the patients, the reported results correspond to the second BMI session. As can be seen, more frequency (ERD) than temporal (MRCP) features were consistently selected in both groups. For the ERD features, pairs in the whole channel-frequency space were selected for all the subjects. Central and centroparietal electrodes were more consistently selected than frontocentral ones. In addition, certain subjects showed a higher density of features allocated in specific regions of the channel-frequency map. For instance, for subject H1, more features were selected in the alpha band (8–12 Hz), whereas for subject H2, there were more in beta band (15–25 Hz). MRCP features were more scarcely chosen by the algorithm, although in all of the participants, some of them were selected.

3.4. Exertion and Satisfaction Assessments

Table 5 shows the values of the Borg scale given by each patient on each session. At the beginning of the session, all the patients reported the minimum exertion level. As described above, each patient performed 3 or 4 screening blocks (each of which lasted around 3 min), resting between blocks as long as they required. After these screening blocks, all the patients reported an increase between 3 and 5 points on their exertion level. Subsequently, they started the closed-loop blocks, in which they walked a maximum of 10 m with the exoskeleton. Here, exertion levels slightly increased for 1 or 2 points in most cases. The only exceptions were P2 in session 1 (which just performed 2 gait cycles due to technical problems), who did not report any increase after screening; and P3 in session 2, who increased 5 points. None of the values of the Borg scale exceeded 17, which is considered as the limit value for maximal exertion.

The results of the satisfaction test are presented in **Table 6**. The highest score for the QUEST scale was obtained in the questions about safety and security, and easiness of use (4.25 on average), whereas the lowest was obtained by the question about comfortability (2.5 on average).

3.5. Exoskeleton Adaptive Control

An important feature of the system introduced in this paper was that, since we used an ambulatory exoskeleton, we could introduce an assist-as-needed control paradigm, which may serve to make the rehabilitation interventions more challenging (Pons and Torricelli, 2014). Although it was not one of the main goals of this study, we measured the degree of assistance that the control strategy provided to healthy subjects and patients. The gait assistance for the healthy and SCI individuals is provided based on the adaptive control model presented in Rajasekaran et al. (2015). The adaptive control applies an efficient stiffness to

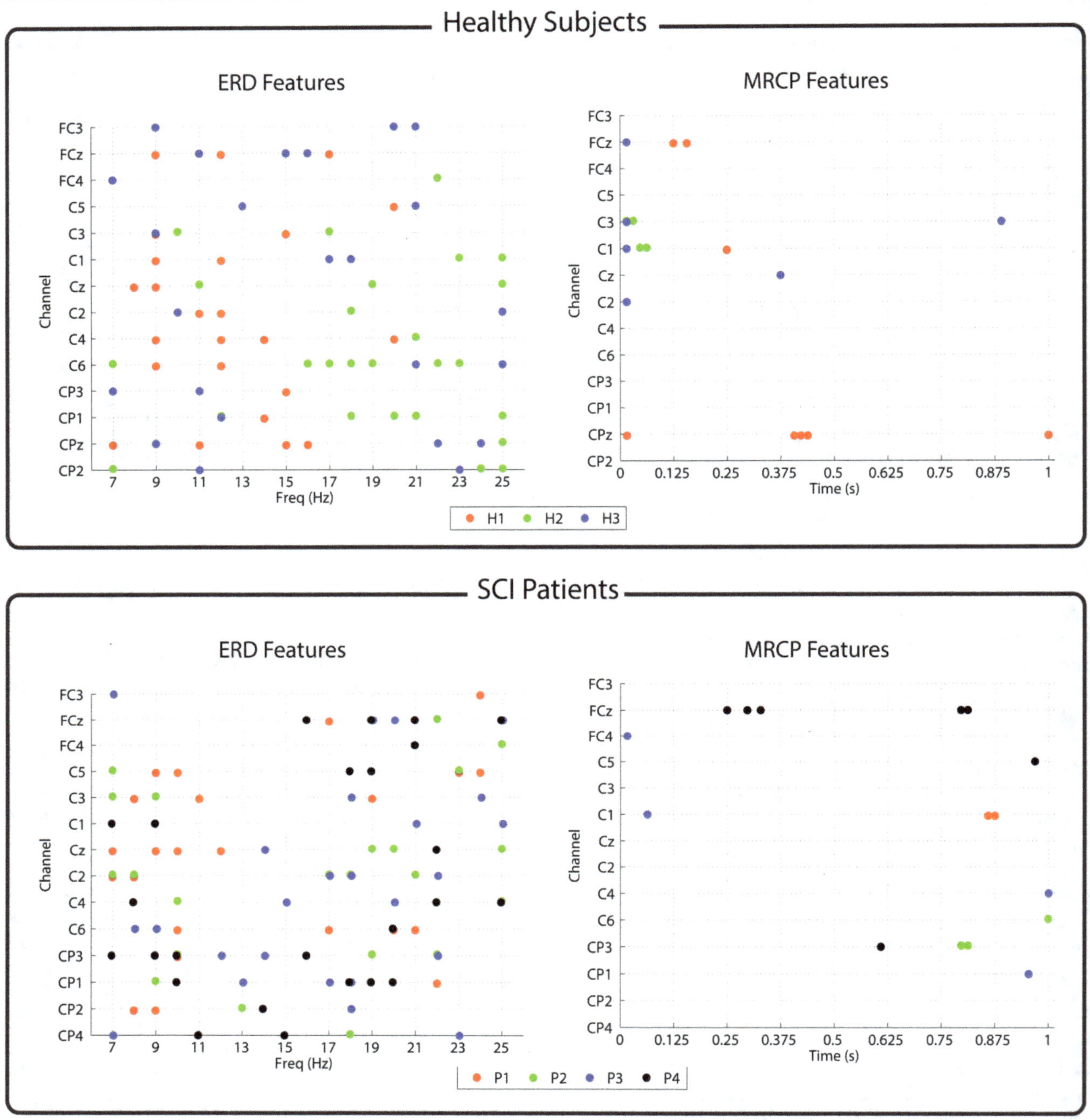

FIGURE 4 | Features selected by the SDA algorithm for each subject. Upper/lower panel corresponds to the features of the healthy subjects/patients. The left part of each panel shows the ERD features that were selected as channel-frequency pairs. The right part of each panel shows the MRCP features that were selected as channel-time pairs.

each joint, which is computed based on the interaction torques and position error of each joint. Hence, the assistance level is defined based on the variation in the stiffness parameter. For healthy subjects, the stiffness values for hip, knee, and ankle were 60 ± 4 Nm/deg, 60 ± 2 Nm/deg, and 60 ± 5 Nm/deg, respectively. For the SCI patients, the stiffness for hip, knee, and ankle were 80 ± 2 Nm/deg, 82 ± 5 Nm/deg, and 80 ± 5 Nm/deg, respectively.

4. DISCUSSION

The present study proposed a novel system BMI with a[n] ambulatory walking exoskeleton. Its feasibility has been show[n] with experiments performed by three healthy subjects and fou[r] spinal cord injury (SCI) patients. The BMI decoded the brai[n] activity related to the intention of movement and sent th[e] commands to the robotic system. The robot moved for two ste[ps] (one with the right and one with the left leg), using an assist-as-needed strategy, which assisted the patients only to the extent they needed. The degree of assistance was shown to be higher for the SCI patients, which could not perform the movement autonomously, compared to the healthy subjects, who did not have to make a high effort to follow the exoskeleton during its walking movements. This is, to the best of our knowledge, the first study in which a walking exoskeleton with no weight or balance support is controlled by incomplete SCI patients with a BMI. This may serve as a proof-of-concept for future studies in which a larger sample could allow the assessment of the rehabilitative effects of this type of BMI-controlled ambulatory exoskeletons.

In spite of the fact that EEG-based BMI technology is still far from being a practical control system for gait-assistive devices, its applicability for rehabilitation within clinical environments may be available in the next few years. In fact, its use has a great potential for rehabilitation of incomplete SCI patients. In these patients, there are still some pathways communicating the brain and the limbs, which can support some degree of functional recovery (Jackson and Zimmermann, 2012). The persistent causal relationship between the brain activation during the intention of movement and the stimulation of the limb (e.g., with an exoskeleton or electrical stimulation) has demonstrated its viability to induce Hebbian plasticity in animal studies (Jackson et al., 2006). Most BMI studies aiming to control rehabilitative devices are focused on the upper-limb, and they have demonstrated the possibility of controlling robotic systems (Gomez-Rodriguez et al., 2011; Ramos-Murguialday et al., 2012, 2013; Bhagat et al., 2016) or functional-electrical stimulation (FES) (Pfurtscheller et al., 2003; Rohm et al., 2013). For the lower-limb, there are less examples in the literature of closed-loop non-invasive brain-controlled systems. The group led by Dr. Nenadic (University of California, USA) demonstrated the BMI-based control of weight-suspended robotic (Do et al., 2013) and FES (King et al., 2015) gait-assistance systems. Furthermore, two recent studies have used brain signals to control the REX (REX Bionics Ltd), a robotic system that provides weight and balance support for patients with a high degree of gait disability (Kilicarslan et al., 2013; Kwak et al., 2015). The system proposed in this paper utilized an ambulatory exoskeleton, which does not rely on any weight support beyond the walker or the parallel bars. Hence, our approach targets patients with incomplete and lower lesions, who can walk short distances with the help of crutches or walkers, and who are the ones with best prognosis for gait rehabilitation (Nene et al., 1996; Scivoletto et al., 2014).

During the screening blocks, the exoskeleton joints were blocked, and hence, even the healthy subjects could just perform the attempt of movement, and not an overt movement. The EEG correlates of these movement attempts, namely the ERD and the MRCPs, were used as features to train the BMI decoder for the closed-loop blocks. The combination of both activation patterns has been shown to be beneficial to improve the movement intention decoding (Ibáñez et al., 2014; López-Larraz et al., 2014), as it may prime the use of features from the signals with higher degree of activation (e.g., P2 which showed a significant ERD, but an MRCP with a low amplitude, see **Figure 2**). In a *post-hoc* analysis, we observed that, in general, ERD features were

TABLE 5 | Results of the Borg scale.

ID	Session	Pre session	After screening	Post session
P1	1	6	11	12
	2	6	10	11
P2	1	6	11	11
	2	6	9	10
P3	1	6	11	13
	2	6	10	15
P4	1	6	10	11
	2	6	10	11

For each patient and session, the exertion levels were measured when the patient arrived (Pre session), after performing the screening blocks (After screening), and at the end of the session (Post session). The values of this scale range from 6 ("very, very light") to 20 ("very, very hard").

TABLE 6 | Results of each patient on the modified QUEST scale.

Question	P1	P2	P3	P4	Mean
How satisfied are you with:					
1. the **dimensions** (size, height, length width) of the device?	4	2	4	1	2.75
2. the **weight** of the device?	3	3	5	1	3
3. the **ease in adjusting** (fixing, fastening) the parts of the device?	2	4	4	2	3
4. how **safe and secure** the device is?	5	4	5	3	4.25
5. the **durability** (endurance, resistance to wear) of the device?	3	3	4	4	3.5
6. how **easy** is it to use the device?	5	3	5	4	4.25
7. how **comfortable** the device is?	3	2	4	1	2.5
. how **effective** the device is to solve the problem for which you are using it?	4	4	4	3	3.75
. What is your level of satisfaction with the device in general?	5	2	4	3	3.5
Total:	34/45	27/45	39/45	22/45	30.5/45

, Not satisfied at all; 2, Not very satisfied; 3, More or less satisfied; 4, Quite satisfied; 5, Very satisfied.

more consistently selected by the automatic feature selection algorithm than MRCP features. There is certain controversy with regard to how these correlates can be affected by motion artifacts during walking (Castermans et al., 2014; Nathan and Contreras-Vidal, 2016). In fact, we observed that slow oscillations were present in some trials during the movements of the exoskeleton, especially in the patients (see **Figure 3**, center and right plots). Anticipating this, we preferred to train the decoder using signals recorded during the attempt of movement and not during actual movement. To minimize artifacts in the training data, we used an automatic artifact rejection method that eliminated contaminated trials (e.g., by slow movement oscillations or EMG artifacts). Moreover, we carefully instructed all the participants to only perform the attempt of movement of their right leg, avoiding compensatory movements with the rest of the body. However, the attempt of movement of a paralyzed limb is a complex task, especially for the paraplegic patients, who had to concentrate on keeping balance at the same time. Therefore, in the protocol we proposed, it is not possible to guarantee that they were only attempting to move the right leg, as they may also be activating arm or trunk muscles, which normally help them to move their legs during their normal walking rehabilitation. This means that the brain activations we measured in the patients may include not only the attempt of movement of the leg but also compensations of other body parts. Comparison of the brain activation patterns between the groups of healthy subjects and patients was out of the scope of this work. Firstly, because the number of participants was small to perform an accurate neuroimaging study, and secondly, because the set-up and task performed by each group were slightly different (i.e., walker and attempt of movement of a healthy limb for the healthy subjects; parallel bars and attempt of movement of a paretic limb for the SCI patients). Nonetheless, in terms of the brain activations, we observed that the subjects who presented weaker brain activations during the attempt of movement were the ones with poorer decoding performances: H3 and P3. Three of four patients had long-term injuries, between 11 and 24 months. Curiously, these three patients were the ones with best decoding performances, showing similar values to healthy subjects, in contrast to P3, who had a 5-months injury but could not control the BMI correctly.

SCI modifies the brain activity related to movement (Müller-Putz et al., 2007; Castro et al., 2013; López-Larraz et al., 2015a). Although there is a large body of literature showing that movement intention can be decoded from EEG signals on these patients (Pfurtscheller et al., 2003; López-Larraz et al., 2012; Rohm et al., 2013; King et al., 2015), among others, this neuroplastic process may affect the reliability of rehabilitative and assistive BMI systems to be used by SCI patients. The heterogeneity of incomplete lesions will probably result in significant differences in the neural reorganization processes followed by the patients' brains (Freund et al., 2013). Hence, an interesting research pursuit for the next years will be the characterization of the brain changes following SCI, which will set the basis to personalize the systems to improve their applicability.

Regarding the decoding algorithms to detect the movement intention, extensive research is being conducted toward the optimization of signal processing and classification techniques to increase BMI performance (Bashashati et al., 2015; López-Larraz et al., 2015b). The procedure used in this work has been previously used to decode movements of the upper-limb with incomplete tetraplegic patients (López-Larraz et al., 2014), and the accuracies that we achieved were similar to other recent studies detecting gait initiation (Jiang et al., 2015; Sburlea et al., 2015). Five consecutive windows with the classifier indicating a motor attempt output were required to start the movement. Although it implied a constant delay of 250 ms with respect to the first output, this mechanism was used to ensure a consistent brain activation and not just a spurious change that may lead to false positive activations There is evidence stating that short delays are beneficial to facilitate plasticity in the brain (Mrachacz-Kersting et al., 2012), and recent studies have worked on developing methodologies to anticipate movements or to decode them with a short latency (López-Larraz et al., 2014; Xu et al., 2014; Jiang et al., 2015; Sburlea et al., 2015). However, these studies require a precise measurement of the time instant when the movement starts in order to calibrate the BMI. Due to the typology of the patients recruited for this study, we could not have a reliable signal to identify the movement onset, even measuring the muscle activity with electromyography. Therefore, we considered that the delay induced by our methodology to detect the movement intention could be acceptable to control the exoskeleton, as a similar procedure has demonstrated its efficacy for neurorehabilitation of stroke patients (Ramos-Murguialday et al., 2013). In a *post-hoc* analysis, we compared the latency of the decoder with respect to the MRCP peak negativity, and observed that the difference was minimal (+50 ms for the healthy subjects and −20 ms for the patients). MRCP negativity is, in general, aligned to the onset of muscular activity during voluntary movements (Niazi et al., 2011). Although it should not be used as a robust measurement of decoding latency, this metric allowed us to estimate how this time would be with respect to the EMG activations. In any case, we consider that more investigation is required to evaluate how different trade-offs (e.g., priming temporal precision, or guaranteeing consistent brain activation) can affect BMI performance and rehabilitative outcomes.

A cue-guided BMI protocol was proposed so that the participants always knew in which phase of the trial they were. Furthermore, the shared control strategy implemented implied that the exoskeleton movements were only enabled in specific time periods (i.e., the "Movement Attempt" intervals), ensuring that no unexpected movements could happen when the patients were not ready. The BMI analyzed the brain signals continuously, meaning that the movement triggers were generated asynchronously at any time during the trial. If these triggers were generated during the "Movement Attempt" interval, then the gait cycle gets started, and otherwise, they were ignored. The offline analysis revealed that movement triggers were generated in a high percentage of trials during the "Rest" (i.e., accommodation period, in which subjects could move and rest) and "Preparation" (i.e., relaxation period preceding the "Movement Attempt") intervals. The movement attempts were correctly decoded in 84.44 ± 14.56% and 77.61 ± 14.72% o the trials, for healthy subjects and patients, respectively. These percentages were significantly higher than the number of trials with movement triggers generated during "Preparation" interval (52.22 ± 16.69% and 40.45 ± 16.98%), but not greater than the trials with triggers generated during "Rest" interval (66.67 ± 13.02% and 63.42 ± 14.15%). Notice that in this latter period, the participants sometimes moved to accommodate their position after the previous trial. These numbers suggest that the use of shared-control strategies designed to avoid non-desired robot movements, like the one proposed in this paper, can facilitate the integration of BMI technology in clinical set-ups (Rohm et al., 2013). These take special relevance in gait rehabilitation therapies, in which keeping the balance may cause movements during rest periods that lead to more false positives.

The proposed approach aims at decoding the intention of motion to generate a functional movement (i.e., a gait cycle) with the exoskeleton. The repetitive association between the brain activation related to the motion intention and the peripheral feedback may reinforce the corticospinal circuits and promote Hebbian synaptic plasticity (Jackson and Zimmermann, 2012). An alternative and interesting approach for future would be to develop a system that continuously controls the exoskeleton movements instead of decoding the intention of movement and triggering a predefined trajectory. This should be the preferred strategy for assistive devices. Presumably, it may also improve rehabilitative effects by a more consistent association between paired firing of neurons, which may accelerate the neuroplastic changes (Jackson and Zimmermann, 2012). To date, promising results toward the continuous control of gait rehabilitations devices with EEG have been shown in preliminary studies with weight-suspended and self-supported systems (Do et al., 2013; Kilicarslan et al., 2013; King et al., 2015; Kwak et al., 2015). However, there are still several issues that need to be improved before the effective implantation of this technology in clinical practice, such as signal processing techniques or artifacts management (Castermans et al., 2014; Nathan and Contreras-Vidal, 2016). Some of these issues are of especial relevance when using ambulatory exoskeletons, which require extra considerations to improve safety, as the control strategy implemented to deal with possible false positives. Furthermore, the rehabilitative effects of each type of intervention still have to be quantified with clinical studies. For now, the development and improvement of novel interventions, like the one proposed here, aim at increasing the number of possible interventions to rehabilitate gait. Eventually, the clinicians will be in charge of evaluating the risks and benefits to recommend the most suitable interventions for each specific patient (e.g., BMI continuous control of prosthesis, or BMI-triggered predefined movements, as the one proposed in this study).

The main goals of this study were to test the BMI-exoskeleton system and to propose a methodology that may be followed in future studies combining BMI and ambulatory exoskeletons. Therefore, the design of the protocol was a key point to be able to validate the technology and the set-up with the patients. We observed that a familiarization session with the exoskeleton was necessary before the BMI session to allow the participants to get used to the dynamics of the system. While for the healthy subjects, a 5–10 min familiarization was enough, the patients required a specific session due to their poor balance and walking capabilities. Several issues have to be tailored for each patient depending on his/her capabilities, like the cadence or the distance between joints. Rehabilitative devices such as the one used in this study have to prioritize patient's safety. The recruited patients were capable of standing and ambulating without the aid of a harness, which required a complex set-up and additional safety measures to avoid falls. In this respect, the experimenter played an important role by controlling the system, which functioned as a "dead-man's" switch. This means that at the beginning of every trial, the experimenter had to make sure that the patient's legs and feet position were appropriate and ask him/her if he/she was ready for another step. This methodology tried to imitate the procedure followed by physiotherapists for patients in the early stages of gait rehabilitation with rigid leg orthoses. In addition, the experimenter had to monitor the EEG signals and the BMI output in order to verify that everything was correct and guide the patients when they lost concentration or generated artifacts by excessive movements. The use of BMI technology to provide the therapist with objective information about the patient's performance has been stated to be very important for the implantation of this type of systems in clinical environments (Mattia et al., 2013; Asín Prieto et al., 2014). We consider that the good results achieved in this study were, in part, due to the therapist–patient interaction that was augmented—thanks to the designed therapist interface.

The fatigue level of the patients was also continuously monitored, and they could ask for a pause whenever they wanted to relax for some minutes. This is, probably, the reason of the relatively low levels of exertion shown by the patients when asked at the end of the session. In terms of usability and satisfaction, the patients were not so positive as we had expected, but they provided very useful information that encourages the authors to continue working to improve the wearability and comfort of the system. Based on the high scores of the questions about safety and security, we believe that the security measures implemented in this study succeeded and they could be applied for future studies. In general, two of the patients (P1 and P3) were rather satisfied with the system, whereas the other two (P2 and P4) reported that several issues could be improved, especially those related with comfort and wearability of both the exoskeleton and the EEG system. Nonetheless, all of them appraised the potential of the combination of both technologies. Patients found the use of the conductive gel for the EEG recording as one of the main inconveniences, which is in line with other works (Rupp, 2014). We believe that the potentiality of dry electrodes will have to be explored for future prototypes to be used with patients in clinical practice. Another important limitation of the system is the difficulty to wear the exoskeleton, as at least two people had to assist the process. This is an important factor to improve for future designs of exoskeletons with clinical applicability. Ideally, the patients should be able to wear the exoskeleton by themselves. All of them reported their willingness to keep participating in rehabilitation interventions with this technology, which is a promising sign for the future of BMI-based gait rehabilitation.

It is important to mention that due to the nature of the study and the typology of patients recruited, the number of trials recorded with these patients was small. Nonetheless, the BMI performances are in line with similar works performed for the upper- and lower-limbs. The main contribution of this work is to validate the feasibility of a BMI system and protocol to control an ambulatory exoskeleton for gait rehabilitation without weight or balance support. However, this preliminary study does not allow yet to draw conclusions about the rehabilitative potential of this technology. Further experiments with a larger population of patients and with a larger number of sessions will be required to evaluate if the therapeutic potential of BMI for gait rehabilitation approaches the traditional therapies. New challenges appear when it comes to pursuing clinical trials integrating this kind of novel technologies with patients. Adapting the systems for different pathologies and personalization of the technology will be of paramount importance for the use of BMI systems in clinical practice (Rupp, 2014). In addition, standardizing metrics to evaluate system performances and clinical outcomes will facilitate the validation of BMIs for their implantation in rehabilitative centers (Venkatakrishnan et al., 2014).

AUTHOR CONTRIBUTIONS

Conceived and designed the experiments: EL, FT, VR, AD, JA, LM. Performed the experiments: EL, FT, VR, SP. Analyzed the data: EL, FT. Drafted the manuscript: EL, FT, VR. Revised the manuscript: EL, FT, VR, SP, AD, JA, JM, AG, LM.

ACKNOWLEDGMENTS

This research has been partially supported by Spanish Ministry of Science project HYPER-CSD2009-00067, and DGA-FSE, grupo T04.

REFERENCES

Alam, M., Chen, X., Zhang, Z., Li, Y., and He, J. (2014). A brain-machine-muscle interface for restoring hindlimb locomotion after complete spinal transection in rats. *PLoS ONE* 9:e103764. doi: 10.1371/journal.pone.0103764

Asín Prieto, G., Cano-de-la cuerda, R., López-Larraz, E., Metrot, J., Molinari, M., and van Dokkum, L. E. H. (2014). "Emerging perspectives in stroke rehabilitation," in *Emerging Therapies in Neurorehabilitation*, eds J. L. Pons and D. Torricelli (Berlin; Heidelberg: Springer), 3–21.

Bashashati, H., Ward, R. K., Birch, G. E., and Bashashati, A. (2015). Comparing different classifiers in sensory motor brain computer interfaces. *PLoS ONE* 10:e0129435. doi: 10.1371/journal.pone.0129435

Bhagat, N. A., Venkatakrishnan, A., Abibullaev, B., Artz, E. J., Yozbatiran, N., Blank, A. A., et al. (2016). Design and optimization of an EEG-based brain machine interface (BMI) to an upper-limb exoskeleton for stroke survivors. *Front. Neurosci.* 10:122. doi: 10.3389/fnins.2016.00122

Bohannon, R. W., and Smith, M. B. (1987). Interrater reliability of a modified Ashworth scale of muscle spasticity. *Phys. Therapy* 67, 206–207.

Borg, G. (1970). Perceived exertion as an indicator of somatic stress. *Scand. J. Rehabil. Med.* 2, 92–98.

Bortole, M., Venkatakrishnan, A., Zhu, F., Moreno, J. C., Francisco, G. E., Pons, J. L., et al. (2015). The H2 robotic exoskeleton for gait rehabilitation after stroke: early findings from a clinical study. *J. Neuroeng. Rehabil.* 12:54. doi: 10.1186/s12984-015-0048-y

Cai, L. L., Fong, A. J., Otoshi, C. K., Liang, Y., Burdick, J. W., Roy, R. R., et al. (2006). Implications of assist-as-needed robotic step training after a complete spinal cord injury on intrinsic strategies of motor learning. *J. Neurosci.* 26, 10564–10568. doi: 10.1523/JNEUROSCI.2266-06.2006

Castermans, T., Duvinage, M., Cheron, G., and Dutoit, T. (2014). About the cortical origin of the low-delta and high-gamma rhythms observed in EEG signals during treadmill walking. *Neurosci. Lett.* 561, 166–170. doi: 10.1016/j.neulet.2013.12.059

Castro, A., Díaz, F., and Sumich, A. (2013). Long-term neuroplasticity in spinal cord injury patients: a study on movement-related brain potentials. *Int. J. Psychophysiol.* 87, 205–214. doi: 10.1016/j.ijpsycho.2013.01.012

Clemmensen, L., Hastie, T., Witten, D., and Ersbøll, B. (2011). Sparse discriminant analysis. *Technometrics* 53, 406–413. doi: 10.1198/TECH.2011.08118

Demers, L., Monette, M., Lapierre, Y., Arnold, D. L., and Wolfson, C. (2002). Reliability, validity, and applicability of the Quebec User Evaluation of Satisfaction with assistive Technology (QUEST 2.0) for adults with multiple sclerosis. *Disabil. Rehabil.* 24, 21–30. doi: 10.1080/09638280110066352

Ditunno, P. L., and Ditunno, J. F. (2001). Walking index for spinal cord injury (WISCI II): scale revision. *Spinal Cord* 39, 654–656. doi: 10.1038/sj.sc.3101223

Ditunno, P. L., Patrick, M., Stineman, M., and Ditunno, J. F. (2008). Who wants to walk? Preferences for recovery after SCI: a longitudinal and cross-sectional study. *Spinal Cord* 46, 500–506. doi: 10.1038/sj.sc.3102172

Do, A. H., Wang, P. T., King, C. E., Chun, S. N., and Nenadic, Z. (2013). Brain-computer interface controlled robotic gait orthosis. *J. Neuroeng. Rehabil.* 10:111. doi: 10.1186/1743-0003-10-111

Fitzsimmons, N., Lebedev, M., Peikon, I., and Nicolelis, M. A. (2009). Extracting kinematic parameters for monkey bipedal walking from cortical neuronal ensemble activity. *Front. Integr. Neurosci.* 3:3. doi: 10.3389/neuro.07.003.2009

Freund, P., Weiskopf, N., Ashburner, J., Wolf, K., Sutter, R., Altmann, D. R., et al. (2013). MRI investigation of the sensorimotor cortex and the corticospinal tract after acute spinal cord injury: a prospective longitudinal study. *Lancet Neurol.* 12, 873–881. doi: 10.1016/S1474-4422(13)70146-7

Gomez-Rodriguez, M., Peters, J., Hill, J., Schölkopf, B., Gharabaghi, A. and Grosse-Wentrup, M. (2011). Closing the sensorimotor loop: haptic feedback facilitates decoding of motor imagery. *J. Neural Eng.* 8:036005. doi 10.1088/1741-2560/8/3/036005

Graimann, B., and Pfurtscheller, G. (2006). Quantification and visualizatior of event-related changes in oscillatory brain activity in the time-frequency domain. *Prog. Brain Res.* 159, 79–97. doi: 10.1016/S0079-6123(06)59006-5

Ibáñez, J., Serrano, J. I., del Castillo, M. D., Monge-Pereira, E., Molina Rueda, F., Alguacil-Diego, I., et al. (2014). Detection of the onset o upper-limb movements based on the combined analysis of changes in th sensorimotor rhythms and slow cortical potentials. *J. Neural Eng.* 11:056009 doi: 10.1088/1741-2560/11/5/056009

Jackson, A., Mavoori, J., and Fetz, E. E. (2006). Long-term motor corte plasticity induced by an electronic neural implant. *Nature* 444, 56–60. doi 10.1038/nature05226

Jackson, A., and Zimmermann, J. B. (2012). Neural interfaces for the brai and spinal cordrestoring motor function. *Nat. Rev. Neurol.* 8, 690–699. do 10.1038/nrneurol.2012.219

Jiang, N., Gizzi, L., Mrachacz-Kersting, N., Dremstrup, K., and Farina, D. (2015) A brain-computer interface for single-trial detection of gait initiation fror movement related cortical potentials. *Clin. Neurophysiol.* 126, 154–159. do 10.1016/j.clinph.2014.05.003

Kilicarslan, A., Prasad, S., Grossman, R. G., and Contreras-Vidal, J. L. (2013 "High accuracy decoding of user intentions using EEG to control a lower-bod exoskeleton," in *35th Annual International Conference of the IEEE Engineerir in Medicine and Biology Society (EMBC)* (Osaka), 5606–5609.

King, C. E., Wang, P. T., McCrimmon, C. M., Chou, C. C., Do, A. H., and Nenadi Z. (2015). The feasibility of a brain-computer interface functional electric stimulation system for the restoration of overground walking after paraplegi *J. Neuroeng. Rehabil.* 12:80. doi: 10.1186/s12984-015-0068-7

Kwak, N.-S., Müller, K.-R., and Lee, S.-W. (2015). A lower limb exoskeleton control system based on steady state visual evoked potentials. *J. Neural Eng.* 12:056009. doi: 10.1088/1741-2560/12/5/056009

Lebedev, M. A., and Nicolelis, M. A. L. (2006). Brain-machine interfaces: past, present and future. *Trends Neurosci.* 29, 536–546. doi: 10.1016/j.tins.2006.07.004

López-Larraz, E., Antelis, J. M., Montesano, L., Gil-Agudo, A., and Minguez, J. (2012). "Continuous decoding of motor attempt and motor imagery from EEG activity in spinal cord injury patients," in *34th Annual International Conference of the IEEE Engineering in Medicine and Biology Society (EMBC)* (San Diego, CA), 1798–1801. doi: 10.1109/EMBC.2012.6346299

López-Larraz, E., Montesano, L., Gil-Agudo, Á., and Minguez, J. (2014). Continuous decoding of movement intention of upper limb self-initiated analytic movements from pre-movement EEG correlates. *J. Neuroeng. Rehabil.* 11:153. doi: 10.1186/1743-0003-11-153

López-Larraz, E., Montesano, L., Gil-Agudo, Á., Minguez, J., and Oliviero, A. (2015a). Evolution of EEG motor rhythms after spinal cord injury: a longitudinal study. *PLoS ONE* 10:e0131759. doi: 10.1371/journal.pone.0131759

López-Larraz, E., Trincado-Alonso, F., and Montesano, L. (2015b). "Brain-machine interfaces for motor rehabilitation: is recalibration important?," in *14th International Conference on Rehabilitation Robotics (ICORR)* (Singapore), 223–228. doi: 10.1109/ICORR.2015.7281203

Maeder, C. L., Sannelli, C., Haufe, S., and Blankertz, B. (2012). Pre-stimulus sensorimotor rhythms influence brain-computer interface classification performance. *IEEE Trans. Neural Syst. Rehabil. Eng.* 20, 653–662. doi: 10.1109/TNSRE.2012.2205707

Marino, R. J., Barros, T., Biering-Sorensen, F., Burns, S. P., Donovan, W. H., Graves, D. E., et al. (2003). International standards for neurological classification of spinal cord injury. *J. Spinal Cord Med.* 26(Suppl 1), S50–S56.

Mattia, D., Pichiorri, F., Molinari, M., and Rupp, R. (2013). "Brain computer interface for hand motor function restoration and rehabilitation," in *Towards Practical Brain-Computer Interfaces*, eds B. Z. Allison, S. Dunne, R. Leeb, J. D. R. Millán, and A. Nijholt (Berlin; Heidelberg: Springer), 131–153.

Millán, J. D. R., Rupp, R., Müller-Putz, G. R., Murray-Smith, R., Giugliemma, C., Tangermann, M., et al. (2010). Combining brain-computer interfaces and assistive technologies: state-of-the-art and challenges. *Front. Neurosci.* 4:161. doi: 10.3389/fnins.2010.00161

Mrachacz-Kersting, N., Kristensen, S. R., Niazi, I. K., and Farina, D. (2012). Precise temporal association between cortical potentials evoked by motor imagination and afference induces cortical plasticity. *J. Physiol.* 590, 1669–1682. doi: 10.1113/jphysiol.2011.222851

Müller-Putz, G. R., Zimmermann, D., Graimann, B., Nestinger, K., Korisek, G., and Pfurtscheller, G. (2007). Event-related beta EEG-changes during passive and attempted foot movements in paraplegic patients. *Brain Res.* 1137, 84–91. doi: 10.1016/j.brainres.2006.12.052

Nathan, K., and Contreras-Vidal, J. L. (2016). Negligible motion artifacts in scalp electroencephalography (EEG) during treadmill walking. *Front. Hum. Neurosci.* 9:708. doi: 10.3389/fnhum.2015.00708

Nene, A. V., Hermens, H. J., and Zilvold, G. (1996). Paraplegic locomotion: a review. *Spinal Cord* 34, 507–524. doi: 10.1038/sc.1996.94

Niazi, I. K., Jiang, N., Tiberghien, O., Nielsen, J. F., Dremstrup, K., and Farina, D. (2011). Detection of movement intention from single-trial movement-related cortical potentials. *J. Neural Eng.* 8:066009. doi: 10.1088/1741-2560/8/6/066009

Nolan, H., Whelan, R., and Reilly, R. B. (2010). FASTER: fully automated statistical thresholding for EEG artifact rejection. *J. Neurosci. Methods* 192, 152–162. doi: 10.1016/j.jneumeth.2010.07.015

Pfurtscheller, G., Leeb, R., Keinrath, C., Friedman, D., Neuper, C., Guger, C., et al. (2006). Walking from thought. *Brain Res.* 1071, 145–152. doi: 10.1016/j.brainres.2005.11.083

Pfurtscheller, G., and Lopes da Silva, F. H. (1999). Event-related EEG/MEG synchronization and desynchronization: basic principles. *Clin. Neurophysiol.* 110, 1842–1857. doi: 10.1016/S1388-2457(99)00141-8

Pfurtscheller, G., Müller, G. R., Pfurtscheller, J., Gerner, H. J., and Rupp, R. (2003). 'Thought' - Control of functional electrical stimulation to restore hand grasp in a patient with tetraplegia. *Neurosci. Lett.* 351, 33–36. doi: 10.1016/S0304-3940(03)00947-9

Pichiorri, F., Cincotti, F., Fallani, F. D. V., Pisotta, I., and Morone, G. (2011). "Towards a brain computer interface-based rehabilitation : from bench to bedside," in *Proceedings of the 5th International Brain-Computer Interface Conference* (Graz), 268–271.

Pons, J. L., and Torricelli, D. (eds.). (2014). *Emerging Therapies in Neurorehabilitation, 1st Edn.* Berlin; Heidelberg: Springer-Verlag.

Rajasekaran, V., Aranda, J., and Casals, A. (2015). "Adaptive walking assistance based on human- orthosis interaction," in *IEEE/RSJ International Conference on Intelligent Robots and Systems (IROS)* (Hamburg), 6190–6195. doi: 10.1109/IROS.2015.7354260

Ramos-Murguialday, A., Broetz, D., Rea, M., Läer, L., Yilmaz, O., Brasil, F. L., et al. (2013). Brain-machine interface in chronic stroke rehabilitation: a controlled study. *Ann. Neurol.* 74, 100–108. doi: 10.1002/ana.23879

Ramos-Murguialday, A., Schürholz, M., Caggiano, V., Wildgruber, M., Caria, A., Hammer, E. M., et al. (2012). Proprioceptive feedback and brain computer interface (BCI) based neuroprostheses. *PLoS ONE* 7:e47048. doi: 10.1371/journal.pone.0047048

Rohm, M., Schneiders, M., Müller, C., Kreilinger, A., Kaiser, V., Müller-Putz, G. R., et al. (2013). Hybrid brain-computer interfaces and hybrid neuroprostheses for restoration of upper limb functions in individuals with high-level spinal cord injury. *Artif. Intell. Med.* 59, 133–142. doi: 10.1016/j.artmed.2013.07.004

Rupp, R. (2014). Challenges in clinical applications of brain computer interfaces in individuals with spinal cord injury. *Front. Neuroeng.* 7:38. doi: 10.3389/fneng.2014.00038

Sburlea, A. I., Montesano, L., and Minguez, J. (2015). Continuous detection of the self-initiated walking pre-movement state from EEG correlates without session-to-session recalibration. *J. Neural Eng.* 12:036007. doi: 10.1088/1741-2560/12/3/036007

Scivoletto, G., Tamburella, F., Laurenza, L., Torre, M., and Molinari, M. (2014). Who is going to walk? A review of the factors influencing walking recovery after spinal cord injury. *Front. Hum. Neurosci.* 8:141. doi: 10.3389/fnhum.2014.00141

Shibasaki, H., and Hallett, M. (2006). What is the Bereitschaftspotential? *Clin. Neurophysiol.* 117, 2341–2356. doi: 10.1016/j.clinph.2006.04.025

van Hedel, H. J., Wirz, M., and Dietz, V. (2005). Assessing walking ability in subjects with spinal cord injury: validity and reliability of 3 walking tests. *Arch. Phys. Med. Rehabil.* 86, 190–196. doi: 10.1016/j.apmr.2004.02.010

Velu, P. D., and de Sa, V. R. (2013). Single-trial classification of gait and point movement preparation from human EEG. *Front. Neurosci.* 7:84. doi: 10.3389/fnins.2013.00084

Venkatakrishnan, A., Francisco, G. E., and Contreras-Vidal, J. L. (2014). Applications of brain-machine interface systems in stroke recovery and rehabilitation. *Curr. Phys. Med. Rehabil. Rep.* 2, 93–105. doi: 10.1007/s40141-014-0051-4

Wirz, M., Zemon, D. H., Rupp, R., Scheel, A., Colombo, G., Dietz, V., et al. (2005). Effectiveness of automated locomotor training in patients with chronic incomplete spinal cord injury: a multicenter trial. *Arch. Phys. Med. Rehabil.* 86, 672–680. doi: 10.1016/j.apmr.2004.08.004

Wolpaw, J. R., Birbaumer, N., McFarland, D. J., Pfurtscheller, G., and Vaughan, T. M. (2002). Brain-computer interfaces for communication and control. *Clin. Neurophysiol.* 113, 767–791. doi: 10.1016/S1388-2457(02)00057-3

Wyndaele, M., and Wyndaele, J. J. (2006). Incidence, prevalence and epidemiology of spinal cord injury: what learns a worldwide literature survey? *Spinal Cord* 44, 523–529. doi: 10.1038/sj.sc.3101893

Xu, R., Jiang, N., Lin, C., Mrachacz-kersting, N., Dremstrup, K., and Farina, D. (2014). Enhanced low-latency detection of motor intention from EEG for closed-loop brain-computer interface applications. *IEEE Trans. Biomed. Eng.* 61, 288–296. doi: 10.1109/TBME.2013.2294203

2

An Improved Unscented Kalman Filter Based Decoder for Cortical Brain-Machine Interfaces

Simin Li [1,2], *Jie Li* [1,2] *and Zheng Li* [1,2]*

[1] *State Key Laboratory of Cognitive Neuroscience and Learning and IDG/McGovern Institute for Brain Research, Beijing Normal University, Beijing, China,* [2] *Center for Collaboration and Innovation in Brain and Learning Sciences, Beijing Normal University, Beijing, China*

Edited by:
Paolo Massobrio,
University of Genoa, Italy

Reviewed by:
Robert D. Flint,
Northwestern University, USA
Jacopo Tessadori,
Fondazione Istituto Italiano di Technologia, Italy

***Correspondence:**
Zheng Li
lz@bnu.edu.cn

Brain-machine interfaces (BMIs) seek to connect brains with machines or computers directly, for application in areas such as prosthesis control. For this application, the accuracy of the decoding of movement intentions is crucial. We aim to improve accuracy by designing a better encoding model of primary motor cortical activity during hand movements and combining this with decoder engineering refinements, resulting in a new unscented Kalman filter based decoder, UKF2, which improves upon our previous unscented Kalman filter decoder, UKF1. The new encoding model includes novel acceleration magnitude, position-velocity interaction, and target-cursor-distance features (the decoder does not require target position as input, it is decoded). We add a novel probabilistic velocity threshold to better determine the user's intent to move. We combine these improvements with several other refinements suggested by others in the field. Data from two Rhesus monkeys indicate that the UKF2 generates offline reconstructions of hand movements (mean CC 0.851) significantly more accurately than the UKF1 (0.833) and the popular position-velocity Kalman filter (0.812). The encoding model of the UKF2 could predict the instantaneous firing rate of neurons (mean CC 0.210), given kinematic variables and past spiking, better than the encoding models of these two decoders (UKF1: 0.138, p-v Kalman: 0.098). In closed-loop experiments where each monkey controlled a computer cursor with each decoder in turn, the UKF2 facilitated faster task completion (mean 1.56 s vs. 2.05 s) and higher Fitts's Law bit rate (mean 0.738 bit/s vs. 0.584 bit/s) than the UKF1. These results suggest that the modeling and decoder engineering refinements of the UKF2 improve decoding performance. We believe they can be used to enhance other decoders as well.

Keywords: brain-machine interface, neural decoding, encoding model, unscented Kalman filter, brain-computer interface, neuroprosthetic

INTRODUCTION

Brain-machine interfaces (BMIs) have the potential to improve the well-being of people with paralysis, locked-in syndrome, and other ailments, as well as change how humans interact with machines and each other. While there has been substantial progress (Baranauskas, 2014; Nuyujukian et al., 2015) in the accuracy or communication bandwidth of BMI, there is still room for improvement. In our previous work with the unscented Kalman filter based decoder

(Li et al., 2009), which we refer to as UKF1, we proposed a non-linear model of neural tuning which modeled the relationship between spike counts and the position and velocity of a cursor. Since that study, much progress has been made in decoder engineering and motor cortical encoding models. We have collected several novel modeling and decoder engineering refinements, as well as incorporated work from others, to form an improved unscented Kalman filter based decoder, which we call UKF2.

The refinements to the encoding model can be summarized as adding neural tuning to hand acceleration, hand position and velocity in an interactive term, and target position and modeling neuron autocorrelation and cross-neuron correlation using spiking history. We include target position as a decoded variable, i.e., the UKF2 does not require knowledge of the true target position to operate. The refinements to decoder engineering are the use of a combination of position and velocity estimates to control the cursor, probabilistically thresholding velocity to determine when the user wishes to remain still, and using estimates of future intended movement to drive the cursor. We do not modify the unscented Kalman filter algorithm itself; rather, our improvements are in the design of the filter's observation model and post-processing of filter outputs.

Using data from two Rhesus monkeys, we compare UKF2 to UKF1, as well as the popular position-velocity Kalman filter in terms of offline reconstructions of hand-controlled cursor movement, encoding model predictive power, and closed-loop neural control of cursor. We also examine the contributions of each modeling refinement. Our results show that the UKF2 reconstructs hand-controlled cursor movement more accurately than the position-velocity Kalman filter and the UKF1. Our analysis suggest that the encoding model of the UKF2 encodes neural activity better, as evidenced by better predictions of firing rate given kinematic and past spiking information. Our analysis of the modeling refinements indicates that spiking history contributed the most to encoding accuracy, but hand acceleration and target position contributed most to decoding accuracy. Finally, experiments in which monkeys used the decoders in closed-loop neural control of the cursor showed that, using the UKF2, monkeys could complete a center-out task significantly faster and with higher Fitts's Law bit rate than using the UKF1, and UKF2 performance was comparable to the FIT Kalman filter (Fan et al., 2014).

Our results indicate that the enhancements of the UKF2 improved the functionality of the decoder. Some of the enhancements, such as modeling of hand acceleration, target position, as well as the probabilistic thresholding of velocity, can be readily used by the Kalman filter and similar decoding algorithms.

MATERIALS AND METHODS

Surgical Procedures

All surgical procedures were in compliance with the U.S. National Institutes of Health Guide for the Care and Use of Laboratory Animals and were approved by the Institutional Animal Care and Use Committee of Beijing Normal University. Two adult male (6 years, 11 kg; 4 years, 8 kg) Rhesus monkeys (*Macaca mulatta*) were implanted with silicon-based electrode arrays (Utah array, Blackrock Microsystems) in the left primary motor cortex under sterile conditions. We followed standard Utah array implantation procedures. In each animal, a Utah array was implanted approximately 4 mm anterior to the central sulcus, at approximately 15 mm lateral from the midline (**Figure 1A**), targeting arm and hand areas. Photos from the implantation surgeries for monkey B and monkey M are shown in **Figures 1B,C**, respectively.

Electrode Array

We used 96-channel Utah arrays (Blackrock Microsystems) with 1.0 mm long electrode shanks (monkey B) or 1.5 mm shanks (monkey M). The arrays were arranged in a 10 × 10 grid pattern with inter-electrode separation of 400 um. The shank material was silicon with platinum coating on the electrode tip and polyimide insulation (Jones et al., 1992). Electrode diameter tapered from 80 um to a fine point (Jones et al., 1992).

Signal Acquisition and Processing

Signals were recorded from the Utah array using a Plexon Omniplex recording system in an experiment room shielded from electromagnetic interference. Signals were amplified (up to 8000x), digitized (at 16 bit, 40 kHz), and processed in the Omniplex system. A desktop personal computer (Dell Precision T3500 with an Intel Xeon W3565 3.2 GHz processor and 8 GB RAM) received the processed signals and executed the Plexon PlexControl software, as well as our experimental control and decoding software.

Spikes were detected and sorted in real time using the Omniplex hardware. The spike detection threshold and sorting parameters were set by visual inspection by the experimenter using Plexon's software. Both well-isolated single units and multiunits were used for decoding and analysis, and subsequently referred to as units without distinction.

We aggressively spike sorted, that is, we preferred to differentiate waveforms into a larger number of units when the choice was not obvious. We often sorted several multiunits per channel. Our reasoning was that if we mistakenly split the waveforms from one neuron into two units, the model fitting should not be biased (though noise due to variance would increase during decoding). If we put two neurons in the same unit, barring a specially designed decoding algorithm such as the switching Kalman filter (Wu et al., 2004), we would lose information. We illustrate the sorted spike waveforms from all channels of monkey B and monkey M in **Figures 1D,E**, respectively.

After spike sorting, spikes were counted in 50 ms duration, non-overlapping bins to estimate the instantaneous firing rate of each unit. All decoders and parameter fitting used this spike count for input.

Experiment Control and Kinematics Measurement

A custom brain-machine interface software suite (BMI3, Nicolelis Lab, Duke University) performed experiment control,

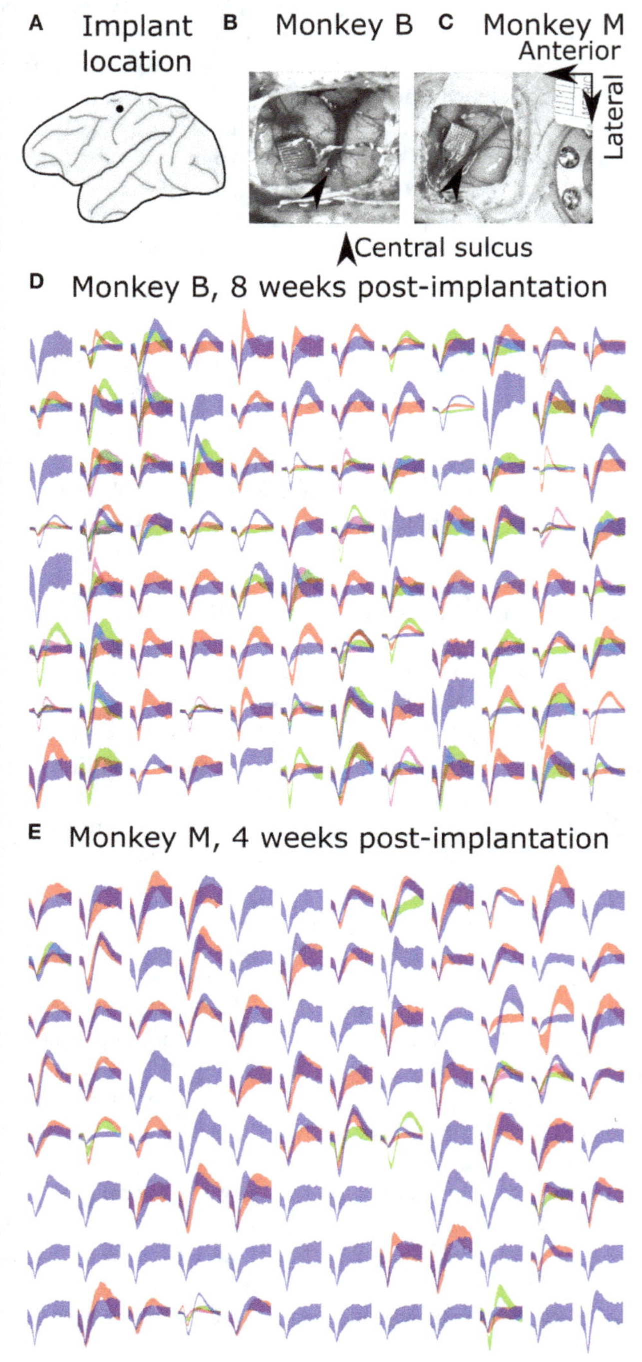

FIGURE 1 | Array implant locations and example recorded signals. (A) Implant location. **(B,C)** Photos taken during surgeries. **(D,E)** Sample waveforms. Each sub-panel shows waveforms from one channel, drawn as mean ± one standard deviation.

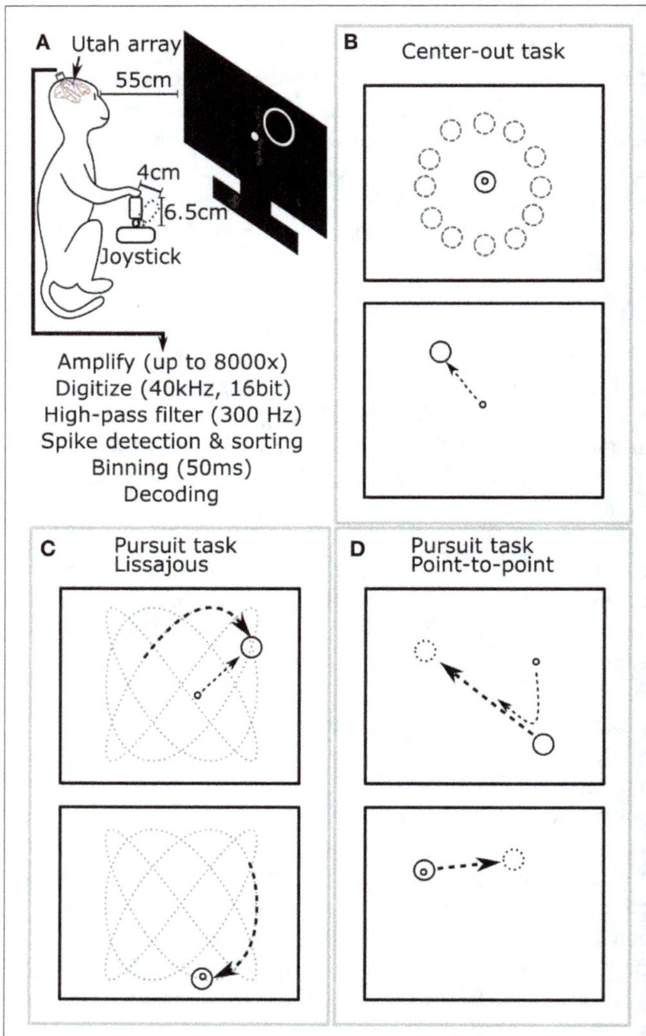

FIGURE 2 | Experimental setup and behavioral tasks. (A) The monkey sat in a primate chair 55 cm before a computer screen and grasped a 6.5 cm tall joystick with 4 cm maximum deflection in its right hand. **(B)** Center-out task. The monkey alternatively moved the cursor to center targets and peripheral targets, located at random angles and fixed distance from center. **(C)** Pursuit task with Lissajous curve: the monkey kept the cursor within a target which moved continuously following a Lissajous curve. **(D)** Pursuit task with point-to-point trajectory: the monkey kept the cursor within a target which moved continuously between randomly selected points on the screen.

model fitting, and real time decoding. This software suite communicated with the Plexon software via Plexon's C language application program interface.

An analog 3-axis potentiometer joystick (CH-400R-P3, Hangzhou Chuang Hong Electric Co.) was used to capture hand motion data. Only the x and y axes were used, and the rotation axis was ignored in these experiments. The length of the joystick including handle, was 6.5 cm, and the maximum deflection of th joystick was approximately 4 cm (**Figure 2A**). The joystick wa self-centered by a weak spring. This joystick was smaller than tha used in our previous work (Li et al., 2009); we observed that th monkey primarily moved its elbow and shoulder joints to contro the joystick.

The joystick was connected to a PCI-DAS1002 analog-to digital recording card (Measurement Computing) mounted i a separate desktop personal computer (Dell Precision T3500 Custom software read the joystick measurements and sent ther to BMI3 using a gigabit Ethernet local area network.

The position of the joystick was mapped to the position of the cursor on the screen in a one-to-one, piecewise-linear manner, with forward (anterior) joystick positions mapped to upper screen locations and backward (posterior) joystick positions mapped to lower screen locations. Joystick movements and on-screen cursor movements had a scaling ratio of approximately 1:4. Joystick measurements were recorded at 100 Hz. To match the 50 ms bin size of spike counts, the average of the five joystick position measurements within each bin was used.

Behavioral Tasks

During experiments, the monkey sat in a primate chair and a flat panel computer monitor was placed 55 cm in front of it (**Figure 2A**). Prior to experiments, all monkeys were trained on two behavioral tasks: center-out and pursuit. In the center-out task (**Figure 2B**), monkeys had to move a circular cursor (logically 0 cm diameter) into a circular target (5 cm diameter) which alternatively appeared in the screen center and the periphery. The peripheral locations were equidistant (8–10 cm) from the screen center at a random angle. Hold time was set to 500 ms. In the pursuit task, monkeys had to keep the cursor within a continuously moving target (6 cm diameter). The target moved according to a Lissajous curve (**Figure 2C**) or a smoothed point-to-point trajectory (**Figure 2D**). The center-out task was used for offline and closed-loop decoding. The pursuit task was only used for offline decoding. Details of the tasks can be found in the Supplementary Materials.

Algorithmic Overview

Our decoding method is based on the n-th order unscented Kalman filter decoder (Li et al., 2009), but with numerous enhancements, some novel and some based on prior work. The enhancements fall into two broad categories: those that modify the neural encoding model and those that modify the control mechanism during closed-loop neural control. Encoding model refinements help both offline reconstructions and closed-loop neural control, while control mechanism refinements are only applicable to closed-loop neural control.

In the neural encoding model category are four enhancements. (1) We use the Cartesian coordinates of hand acceleration and a novel acceleration magnitude. (2) We include a novel multiplicative hand position and hand velocity interaction term in the encoding model. (3) We include the target position and a novel target-cursor distance term in the encoding model. (4) We include the recent spiking history (i.e., spike count in the previous time bin) of the entire recorded population in the encoding model.

For the control mechanism, we have added three ideas: (1) we use a mixture of decoded position and decoded velocity to derive the new cursor position (Homer M. et al., 2013). (2) We use a novel probabilistic threshold for velocity, which detects when the user is trying to move in a more principled way than a simple threshold on velocity. (3) We use predicted future kinematics to drive the cursor, which is intended to improve the responsiveness of the decoder.

These refinements are specified below and discussed in the Discussion section. Table S1 in the Supplementary Materials provides an overview of which refinements are used during offline reconstructions and closed-loop decoding.

State Variables and Neural Tuning Model

The filter's state variables are the variables to be decoded, but can also include other variables which may improve the accuracy of the neural encoding model. In the standard position-velocity Kalman filter, the desired position and velocity in the x and y axis are the state variables (for a 2D task). In the UKF1, the state has multiple taps of position and velocity. That is, at time t (discrete index which counts bins), the UKF1's state variables are the position and velocity at time t, $t+1$, $t+2$, $t+3$, $t+4$, $t+5$, $t-1$, $t-2$, $t-3$, and $t-4$, for a total of 10 taps. These taps include estimates of "future" values of the kinematics as well as "past" values, relative to the current time t. By including future taps and past taps, the UKF1 is able to model neural tuning at multiple time offsets simultaneously. Since the task is two-dimensional, the number of state variables is 2 (dimensions) $\times$ 2 (position, velocity) $\times$ 10 (taps) $= 40$.

In the UKF2 decoder, hand acceleration and target position are added to the state variables. The target position is a decoded variable and not required as input to the decoder. The number of taps is reduced to five. The number of state variables is thus 2 (dimensions) $\times$ 4 (cursor position, velocity, acceleration; target position) $\times$ 5 (taps) $= 40$.

The neural encoding model or tuning model is the observation model of the (unscented) Kalman filter when it is used as a decoder. It is a generative model that predicts the binned spike count (instantaneous firing rate) given the state variables' values. The neural encoding model works in one direction, while the decoder, which wraps around it, works in the other direction by "inverting" the encoding model. To decode a variable, it must be present as a feature in the encoding model and as a state variable in the Kalman filter; however, not all encoding model features are decoded by the decoder (e.g., spiking history), and not all state variables are output by the decoder to control the cursor. The encoding model of the position-velocity Kalman filter is:

$$fr_{i,t}^{\mathrm{PVKalman}} \approx c \cdot px_t + c \cdot py_t + c \cdot vx_t + c \cdot vy_t, \tag{1}$$

where $fr_{i,t}$ is the (mean subtracted) firing rate of unit i at time t, every instance of c is a different coefficient fitted from training data, px_t and py_t are the x-axis and y-axis positions at time t, respectively, and vx_t and vy_t are the x-axis and y-axis velocities at time t, respectively.

In the UKF1, the encoding model is:

$$\begin{aligned} fr_{i,t}^{\mathrm{UKF1}} \approx\ & \text{position}\,(t+5) + \text{velocity}\,(t+5) + \text{position}\,(t+4) \\ & + \text{velocity}\,(t+4) + \cdots + \text{position}\,(t-4) \\ & + \text{velocity}\,(t-4)\,. \end{aligned} \tag{2}$$

For clarity, we have broken down the model to contributions from different kinematic features:

$$\text{position}\,(k) = c \cdot px_k + c \cdot py_k + c\sqrt{px_k^2 + py_k^2}, \tag{3}$$

$$\text{velocity}\,(k) = c \cdot vx_k + c \cdot vy_k + c\sqrt{vx_k^2 + vy_k^2}. \tag{4}$$

Again, to reduce notational clutter, every instance of c is a different coefficient (total 60).

Combining the model of UKF1 and the above outlined encoding model enhancements, and reducing the number of taps to five, we obtain the encoding model of the UKF2:

$$\begin{aligned} fr_{i,t}^{\text{UKF2}} \approx\ & \text{position}\,(t+2) + \text{velocity}\,(t+2) + \text{acceleration}\,(t+2) \\ & + \text{interaction}\,(t+2) + \text{target}\,(t+2) + \ldots \\ & + \text{position}\,(t-2) + \text{velocity}\,(t-2) + \text{acceleration}\,(t-2) \\ & + \text{interaction}\,(t-2) + \text{target}\,(t-2) + \text{spiking}\,(t-1), \end{aligned} \tag{5}$$

$$\text{acceleration}\,(k) = c \cdot ax_k + c \cdot ay_k + c\sqrt{ax_k^2 + ay_k^2}, \tag{6}$$

$$\text{interaction}\,(k) = c \cdot (px_k \cdot vx_k) + c \cdot (py_k \cdot vy_k), \tag{7}$$

$$\begin{aligned} \text{target}\,(k) =\ & c \cdot tx_k + c \cdot ty_k \\ & + c\sqrt{(tx_k - px_k)^2 + (ty_k - py_k)^2}, \end{aligned} \tag{8}$$

$$\text{spiking}\,(k) = c \cdot fr_{1,k}^{\text{actual}} + c \cdot fr_{2,k}^{\text{actual}} + \ldots + c \cdot fr_{n,k}^{\text{actual}}, \tag{9}$$

where ax_t and ay_t are the x-axis and y-axis hand accelerations at time t, respectively, tx_t and ty_t are the x-axis and y-axis target positions at time t, respectively, n is the number of units, and as before every instance of c is a different coefficient (total $70 + n$). Note that our use of target position in the encoding model includes a target-to-cursor distance term. The five taps of kinematic features are followed by spiking history terms for the entire population of n units [in spiking($t - 1$)]. This spiking history is the spike count in the previous bin for the entire population.

Mixing Position and Velocity Outputs

Now we describe the first of the control mechanism refinements. These refinements operate on the output of the unscented Kalman filter. The outputs, or "decoded" variables, are the means of the state variables of the unscented Kalman filter after it has performed its filtering operations. These decoded variables are processed further by the methods described below to get the final on-screen cursor position.

Instead of using only the decoded position to control the cursor as in UKF1, for the UKF2, both the decoded velocity and the decoded position are used to update the cursor during closed-loop operation. The two inputs are mixed together using a mixing coefficient (Homer M. et al., 2013):

$$\bar{x}_t = \bar{x}_{t-1} + c_m \cdot \mathrm{dt} \cdot \bar{v}_t + (1 - c_m)\,\mathrm{dt}\frac{\|\bar{v}_t\|}{\|\bar{e}_t\|}\bar{e}_t, \tag{10}$$

$$\bar{e}_t = \bar{p}_t - \bar{x}_{t-1}, \tag{11}$$

where $\bar{x}_t$ is the vector of on-screen cursor position at time t, c_m is the mixing coefficient (0.5), dt is the delta time between time steps (50 ms), $\bar{v}_t$ is the decoded velocity vector at time t [i.e., $\bar{v}_t = (vx_{t+2}, vy_{t+2})$, the +2 is due to use of future predictions, described below], $\bar{e}_t$ is an intermediate variable representing the difference between the decoded position and previous on-screen cursor location, and $\bar{p}_t$ is the decoded position vector at time t [i.e., $\bar{p}_t = (px_{t+2}, py_{t+2})$]. One way to interpret these equations is that the decoded velocity magnitude acts as a gate or limit for the amount that the decoded position can affect the cursor. We did not use this feature in offline reconstructions and analysis. Note this control mechanism refinement is orthogonal to the position-velocity interaction refinement in the encoding model.

Movement Thresholding

We add a probability-based mechanism to help the user stop the cursor during closed-loop control (only) which applies a threshold on the decoded velocity. Since the Kalman filter provides a covariance estimate for the velocity state variable, we can perform a check using the decoded mean and covariance values that allows us to place a threshold in terms of false positive rate. Since the distribution of the state variables is assumed to be multivariate normal, the x-axis and y-axis velocity values together form a vector that has a two-dimensional multivariate normal distribution. Given the mean vector ($\bar{v}$) and covariance matrix (C_v) of this distribution, we can compute the statistic:

$$X = \bar{v}^{\mathrm{T}} C_v^{-1} \bar{v}, \quad X \sim \mathcal{X}^2(2) \tag{12}$$

X has a chi-squared distribution with 2 degrees of freedom. We can consult the cumulative distribution function of the chi-squared distribution to test if the velocity is significantly different from zero with a given α-value.

During decoding, the decoded velocity outputted by the UKF2 is tested using this method. If the null hypothesis is rejected, i.e., the user is deemed to want to move the cursor, unscented Kalman filtering proceeds as normal and the decoded position and velocity are mixed as described in the previous section. Otherwise, the cursor is not moved (skipping mixing of position and velocity) and in the next iteration, instead of adding the velocity to the position in the execution of the transition model, we do not modify the position. Note that this procedure does not set the velocity variable in the state to zero. If we were to do that, accelerating from zero velocity might be difficult: if the velocity increases from zero to a small value, but does not pass the threshold, it is then set to zero again. By not editing the velocity in the state, we allow it to build up over time to exceed the probabilistic threshold. In our experience, a p-value of around 0.3 worked well, and we used values in the range 0.1–0.5 in closed-loop experiments, varying with session. We did not use this enhancement in offline reconstructions and analysis.

Use of Future Predictions

During closed-loop neural control, we used filter predictions of future intentions to drive the cursor for the UKF2. The UKF1 included multiple taps in its state. This allowed the filter's observation model to capture tuning relationships between kinematic variables and neural firing rates at multiple time offsets simultaneously. A concrete example is that the x-axis velocity at time bins $t - 4$, $t - 3$... $t + 5$ are all included in the function that models the spike count at time bin t. However, for the UKF1 the position in the filter state corresponding to time t is used to control the cursor when the filter is processing neural activity at time t, i.e., there is no temporal offset.

We keep five taps of kinematic variables in the state of the UKF2, $t-2$, $t-1$, t, $t+1$, $t+2$, where t is the time of the bin of neural activity the filter is currently processing. We use the estimated kinematics at the $t+2$ tap to control the cursor during closed-loop neural control of the cursor. With our bin size of 50 ms, this amounts to a temporal offset of 100 ms. This offset is in the causal direction, i.e., compatible with the notion that neural activity encodes for movement occurring 100 ms later. For offline reconstructions and analysis, the UKF2 used the zero offset temporal tap (t), otherwise we would introduce error due to temporal misalignment.

Decoder Comparison

We compared the improved unscented Kalman filter based decoder (UKF2) with the previously published unscented Kalman filter based decoder (UKF1). The settings for UKF1 differ from Li et al. (2009) in several ways. First, the bin size was 50 ms instead of 100 ms, so as to be easily comparable to UKF2 using the same training data. Second, in offline reconstructions the UKF1 transition model used one time tap of kinematics to estimate the future-most tap of kinematics, whereas, in our previous work, the UKF1 estimate was based on all (10) taps in the state. This change improved filter stability: when all 10 taps are used, forming a 10th order autoregressive model, the fitted transition model was more likely to cause filter instability. In closed-loop experiments, the transition model was pre-designed around physical laws of motion, as described in the Model Fitting section. This contrasts to our previous work, where the transition model was always fit to data. We made this change so that all three decoders would use transition models based on physical laws of motion, since transition model design is not the focus of this study.

We also compare with a Kalman filter which includes position and velocity in its state space (position-velocity Kalman filter). During closed-loop decoding, this Kalman filter used two refinements developed by other researchers: modeling position as a feedback signal (Gilja et al., 2012) and using intention estimates to fit observation model parameters (Gilja et al., 2012; Fan et al., 2014), which makes it equivalent to the FIT Kalman filter (Fan et al., 2014). We do not use the re-training paradigm of the ReFIT Kalman filter (Gilja et al., 2012), because we needed to keep the training data for all of the tested decoders the same to achieve a fair comparison. Moreover, adding a re-training phase to the experiment protocol would allow more time to practice using the Kalman filter decoder, and inject additional variation in animal behavior. Since Fan et al. (2014) reported that intention estimation applied to initial training data had comparable benefits as retraining with intention estimation, we opted to use intention estimation on initial training data in our experimental protocol. See the Supplementary Materials for the implementation of the two refinements.

A brief description of the Kalman and unscented Kalman filters and a table summarizing the compared decoders can be found in the Supplementary Materials.

Model Fitting

We fitted the encoding models of all decoders using the same training portion of each session. This data consisted of population binned spike counts and simultaneously recorded cursor positions (equivalent to transformed hand positions), velocities, accelerations, and target positions, if applicable. The encoding models included terms which were non-linear in the state variables, but the coefficients for them can be fitted in a linear regression since the non-linear terms can be pre-calculated as features. We used Tikhonov regularized linear regression (ridge regression) to fit the coefficients of the models, with automatic finding of the best ridge parameter. The parameter fitting procedure is very similar to the one in Li et al. (2009), except for the details of the ridge parameter selection scheme (see Supplementary Materials). We used this parameter fitting procedure to fit the coefficients of the encoding models for all analysis.

In offline reconstructions, the transition model of all three decoders were fitted to training data in the same way as Li et al. (2009), except that we used the newer scheme described in the Supplementary Materials for choosing the ridge regression parameter. Note that this means the target position is decoded, but otherwise does not directly affect the other variables.

In closed-loop neural control, the transition models of all three decoders were set to be similar to the equations describing physical laws. For the Kalman filter:

$$\overline{p}_{t+1} = \overline{p}_t + \overline{v}_t \cdot \mathrm{dt}, \quad (13)$$

$$\overline{v}_{t+1} = c_{\mathrm{v}} \cdot \overline{v}_t + \overline{\epsilon}_{\mathrm{v}}, \quad (14)$$

where $\overline{p}_t$ and $\overline{v}_t$ are the position and velocity vectors at time t, respectively, c_{v} is the coefficient representing friction (0.85), dt is delta time between filter iterations, i.e., the bin width (50 ms), and $\overline{\epsilon}_{\mathrm{v}}$ is the random noise on the velocity (details below for fitting procedure). The position lacks a noise term since we used the position-as-feedback scheme. The friction term gives the cursor a virtual mass, which makes it easier to control.

The transition model for the UKF1 is slightly different since it has multiple taps in the state space. We set the leading tap similar to above:

$$\overline{p}_{t+6} = \overline{p}_{t+5} + \overline{v}_{t+5} \cdot \mathrm{dt} + \overline{\epsilon}_{\mathrm{p}}, \quad (15)$$

$$\overline{v}_{t+6} = c_{\mathrm{v}} \cdot \overline{v}_{t+5} + \overline{\epsilon}_{\mathrm{v}}. \quad (16)$$

Note that position also has a random noise term. For the other taps, values are propagated through time without change.

The UKF2 model includes acceleration, thus we change our equation for velocity and include an equation for acceleration. Acceleration is constant except for a decay coefficient and random noise. Furthermore, target position is included as a constant value modified by random noise. Target position attracts the cursor by affecting acceleration during closed loop control. The UKF2 transition model for the leading tap is:

$$\overline{p}_{t+3} = \overline{p}_{t+2} + \overline{v}_{t+2} \cdot \mathrm{dt} + \overline{\epsilon}_{\mathrm{p}}, \quad (17)$$

$$\overline{v}_{t+3} = c_v \cdot \overline{v}_{t+2} + \overline{a}_{t+2} \cdot \mathrm{dt} + \overline{\epsilon}_v, \tag{18}$$

$$\overline{a}_{t+3} = c_a \cdot \overline{a}_{t+2} + c_g(\overline{g}_{t+2} - \overline{p}_{t+2})/\mathrm{dt}^2 + \overline{\epsilon}_a, \tag{19}$$

$$\overline{g}_{t+3} = \overline{g}_{t+2} + \overline{\epsilon}_g, \tag{20}$$

where $\overline{a}_t$ and $\overline{g}_t$ are the vectors of acceleration and target position at time t, respectively, c_a is the coefficient representing acceleration decay (0.75), and c_g is the gain on the attraction effect of the target position (0.01). We add acceleration decay to prevent an error in acceleration decoding from affecting decoded output for an unlimited duration. For the other taps, values are propagated through time without change. The values of the constants were picked to be similar to typical values seen when fitting transition models to training data in our preliminary analysis. We did this so that the values would be similar to fitted values, but do not change per closed-loop recording session.

The transition model noise covariance matrices, which describe the joint distribution of the noise terms ($\overline{\epsilon}_p$, $\overline{\epsilon}_v$, $\overline{\epsilon}_a$, and $\overline{\epsilon}_g$) were fitted under the above specified models. That is, the above physics-based models were used to predict the variables (using one time step as the input and having the next time step be the desired output), and the sample covariance matrix of the prediction residuals was used as the transition model noise covariance matrix. Note that, for the FIT Kalman filter, we set the positional noise's variance and covariance entries to zero to achieve the position-as-feedback enhancement of Gilja et al. (2012).

Experiment Procedure

We first compared the performance of decoders in making offline reconstructions. For this, we used portions of sessions where the monkey controlled the cursor with its hand. We reconstructed the cursor movements with each decoder and measured the accuracy of the reconstructions vs. the actual cursor movements. The data was divided into training and testing portions. We ignored the first 30 s of data to avoid transient problems, used the subsequent 10 min for the training portion, and set aside the remainder as the testing portion. If the session had less than 12.5 min of hand control data, we used 5 min of data for training (the shortest session had 8 min).

We measured accuracy of reconstructions by computing the correlation coefficient (CC) and signal to noise ratio (SNR, see below for equation). CC or SNR for each Cartesian axis' position and velocity were computed separately and combined by averaging. For SNR, the arithmetic mean in decibels was calculated. We did not use mixing of position and velocity (Homer M. et al., 2013) or the position-as-feedback scheme (Gilja et al., 2012) in reconstructions, as those are designed for closed-loop control.

We compared the encoding accuracy of the UKF2 encoding model with the encoding model of the UKF1 and the position-velocity linear model of the Kalman filter decoder. To do this, we again used portions of sessions where the monkey controlled the cursor with its hand. Since the number of parameters differs substantially between models, a comparison of model fit may be biased toward the more complex model. Therefore, we compared the ability of the models to predict binned spike counts on testing data that was not used to fit model parameters. Model predictions on separate testing data are unbiased toward more complex models, since prediction accuracy reflects generalization accuracy.

We split the data into training and testing portions using a two-fold cross-validation procedure. We used the training portions to fit the parameters of the encoding models. Then we tested the encoding models by providing kinematics data (and past spike counts, if applicable) and then predicting spike counts. We compared the predicted spike counts with the actual spike counts in the testing portion and calculated accuracy using the correlation coefficient or the signal-to-noise ratio (SNR). We repeated this procedure, switching training and testing data, and averaged results between the two repetitions. For model predictions, we only used one tap of kinematics for all models, since our previous work has already shown the advantage of using multiple taps (Li et al., 2009) and that is not the focus of this study.

Finally, we compared the ability of monkeys to use the decoders, in turn, to control a cursor in closed-loop neural control. All the decoders' parameters were fitted on the same initial training data (10 min.), collected at the beginning of each session when the monkey used its hand to control the cursor. The order of use of the decoders was shuffled across sessions to average out order effects. In each session (day), each decoder was used for 10 min, with the first 5 min for familiarization and the last 5 min used for accuracy calculation. During neural control of cursor, the monkey continued to manipulate the joystick, even though it was disconnected (i.e., brain control with hand movements).

When analyzing the closed-loop performance data, we calculated fraction of targets acquired, movement time, and Fitts's Law bit rate (Gilja et al., 2012). Shorter movement durations meant the monkey could move and hold the cursor in the target faster, which reflects better controllability. Since we kept target sizes and reach distances constant, the Fitts's Law bit rate was monotonic with the movement time. For fraction of targets acquired, we included acquisition of the center target as well as peripheral targets. We only considered movements from the center to the periphery for movement time and Fitts's Law bit rate. Since the monkey sometimes paused during performance of the task due to lack of motivation or distraction, failure in the task may occur due to inactivity. We observed that, when the monkey was actively participating, the percentage of successful trials was high (>90%). Thus, to eliminate failures due to inactivity from the time and rate calculations, which are confounds not related to decoder performance, we only analyzed the movement time and Fitts's Law bit rate of successful center to peripheral trials which followed successful acquisition of the center target.

The SNR, in decibels, was calculated by:

$$SNR_{dB} = 10 \cdot log_{10}\left(\frac{Var_s}{MSE}\right), \tag{21}$$

where Var_s is the variance of the desired signal, e.g., recorded position during reconstructions or measured spike counts during encoding model analysis, and MSE is the mean squared error between the desired signal and decoded value, e.g., reconstructed kinematics or predicted spike counts. The SNR can be seen as a normalized, inverted, and log-transformed mean squared error. Unlike the CC, SNR does not saturate. It also detects scale and offset errors which CC cannot. We believe it is better than the mean squared error because it is normalized and thus more comparable across experimental setups, does not saturate, and naturally increases with quality.

For statistical analysis, we used two-factor analysis of variance (decoder × session, or model × unit) with single replication, and we focus on the decoder and model differences. *Post-hoc* multiple comparison testing was conducted with two-tailed paired *t*-tests with *p*-values corrected by the Holm-Bonferroni method. All testing used a significance level of $\alpha = 0.05$.

RESULTS

Offline Reconstructions

We compared the ability of the decoders to reconstruct hand-controlled cursor trajectories. We analyzed 16 sessions from monkey B, recorded 24–97 days post-implant, and 16 sessions from monkey M, recorded 17–162 days post-implant. Hand-controlled portions of these sessions ranged from 8 to 73 min in length, with mean 27.2 min. For each session, reconstructions were performed by using up to 10 min to fit parameters of models and then reconstructing the remainder of the hand-controlled portion of the session (see Experiment Procedure). The results are summarized in **Table 1** and graphed in **Figure 3**.

We calculated the SNR of the trajectory reconstructions for each decoder (**Figure 3A**). ANOVA found a main effect of decoder [monkey B: $F_{(2, 15)} = 27.03$, $p = 1.94 \times 10^{-7}$, monkey M: $F_{(2, 15)} = 42$, $p = 2.01 \times 10^{-9}$] and *post-hoc* testing showed that all three decoders were significantly different from each other (monkey B: all corrected $p < 0.0024$, monkey M: all corrected $p < 0.00007$). We also quantified accuracy in terms of correlation coefficient (CC) (**Figure 3B**). ANOVA found a main effect of decoder [monkey B: $F_{(2, 15)} = 15.59$, $p = 2.28 \times 10^{-5}$, monkey M: $F_{(2, 15)} = 53.86$, $p = 1.18 \times 10^{-10}$] and *post-hoc* testing showed that all three decoders were significantly different from each other (monkey B: all corrected $p < 0.015$, monkey M: all corrected $p < 0.00002$). The UKF2 reconstructed most accurately among the three decoders.

We pooled data from both monkeys and analyzed the contributions of each of the different encoding model enhancements used in the UKF2 decoder, in terms of CC (**Figure 3C**, white bars). To do this, we added to the UKF1 model each of the model enhancements in turn: acceleration (+A), position-velocity interactions (+PVI), target position (+T), which includes the target-to-cursor distance term, and spiking history of the population (+SH). For the pooled data, ANOVA found a main effect of decoder [$F_{(6, 31)} = 29.32$, $p < 10^{-10}$] and *post-hoc* comparisons showed that UKF2 was significantly more accurate than KF (corrected $p < 10^{-6}$) and UKF1 (corrected $p = 6 \times 10^{-6}$) and UKF1 was significantly more accurate than KF (corrected $p = 0.000014$). In terms of feature contributions, UKF1+A was significantly more accurate than UKF1 alone (corrected $p = 0.00006$). UKF1+PVI was significantly less accurate than UKF1 alone (corrected $p = 0.0035$). UKF1+T was significantly more accurate than UKF1 alone (corrected $p = 0.00092$). UKF1+SH was not significantly different from UKF1 (corrected $p = 0.39$). UKF2 was significantly more accurate than UKF1 augmented with PVI (corrected $p = 3 \times 10^{-6}$) and SH (corrected $p = 0.000014$). Significance testing results when using SNR values were similar [main effect of decoder, $F_{(6, 31)} = 33.49$, $p < 10^{-10}$], except that UKF2 was also significantly better than UKF1+A (corrected $p = 0.0019$) and UKF1+T (corrected $p = 0.00081$). Comparing the contribution of individual features in terms of CC, UKF1+A was better than UKF1+PVI (corrected $p = 0.000013$) and UKF1+SH (corrected $p = 0.0011$), and UKF1+T was better than UKF1+PVI (corrected $p = 0.00023$) and UKF1+SH (corrected $p = 0.0017$). These comparisons indicate acceleration and target tuning contributed the most to reconstruction accuracy.

It was concerning that the UKF1+PVI reconstructed less accurately than UKF1 alone. When we examined behavioral tasks separately, we found that for the pursuit task (both variants combined), UKF1+PVI (0.831 ± 0.026, mean CC±SEM) was nominally higher than UKF1 alone (0.829 ± 0.025), though the difference was not significant (two-tailed paired *t*-test, uncorrected, $n = 6$, $p = 0.103$). We think this is due to the more

TABLE 1 | Offline reconstruction accuracy.

Mean ± SEM	CC, monkey B	CC, monkey M	CC, pooled	CC, pooled, merged units	SNR (dB), monkey B	SNR (dB), monkey M	SNR (dB), pooled	SNR (dB), pooled, merged units
UKF2	0.873 ± 0.013	0.829 ± 0.013	0.851 ± 0.010	0.836 ± 0.011	6.484 ± 0.409	5.113 ± 0.349	5.799 ± 0.292	5.295 ± 0.266
Kalman	0.850 ± 0.011	0.775 ± 0.009	0.812 ± 0.010	0.786 ± 0.010	5.423 ± 0.320	3.917 ± 0.233	4.670 ± 0.237	4.008 ± 0.200
UKF1	0.859 ± 0.011	0.806 ± 0.012	0.833 ± 0.009	0.806 ± 0.010	5.824 ± 0.349	4.568 ± 0.292	5.196 ± 0.251	4.488 ± 0.226
UKF1+A	0.868 ± 0.010	0.828 ± 0.016	0.848 ± 0.010	0.828 ± 0.010	6.019 ± 0.370	5.009 ± 0.389	5.514 ± 0.279	4.854 ± 0.249
UKF1+PVI	0.852 ± 0.012	0.799 ± 0.012	0.826 ± 0.010	0.798 ± 0.011	5.663 ± 0.352	4.437 ± 0.295	5.050 ± 0.251	4.349 ± 0.230
UKF1+T	0.871 ± 0.010	0.819 ± 0.015	0.845 ± 0.010	0.824 ± 0.011	6.193 ± 0.361	4.839 ± 0.364	5.516 ± 0.280	4.847 ± 0.253
UKF1+SH	0.865 ± 0.013	0.794 ± 0.010	0.830 ± 0.010	0.808 ± 0.010	6.160 ± 0.379	4.422 ± 0.231	5.291 ± 0.268	4.712 ± 0.228

A, acceleration; PVI, position-velocity interaction; T, target; SH, spiking history of population; Pooled, combining data from two monkeys; Merged units, undoing spike sorting by merging units in each channel.

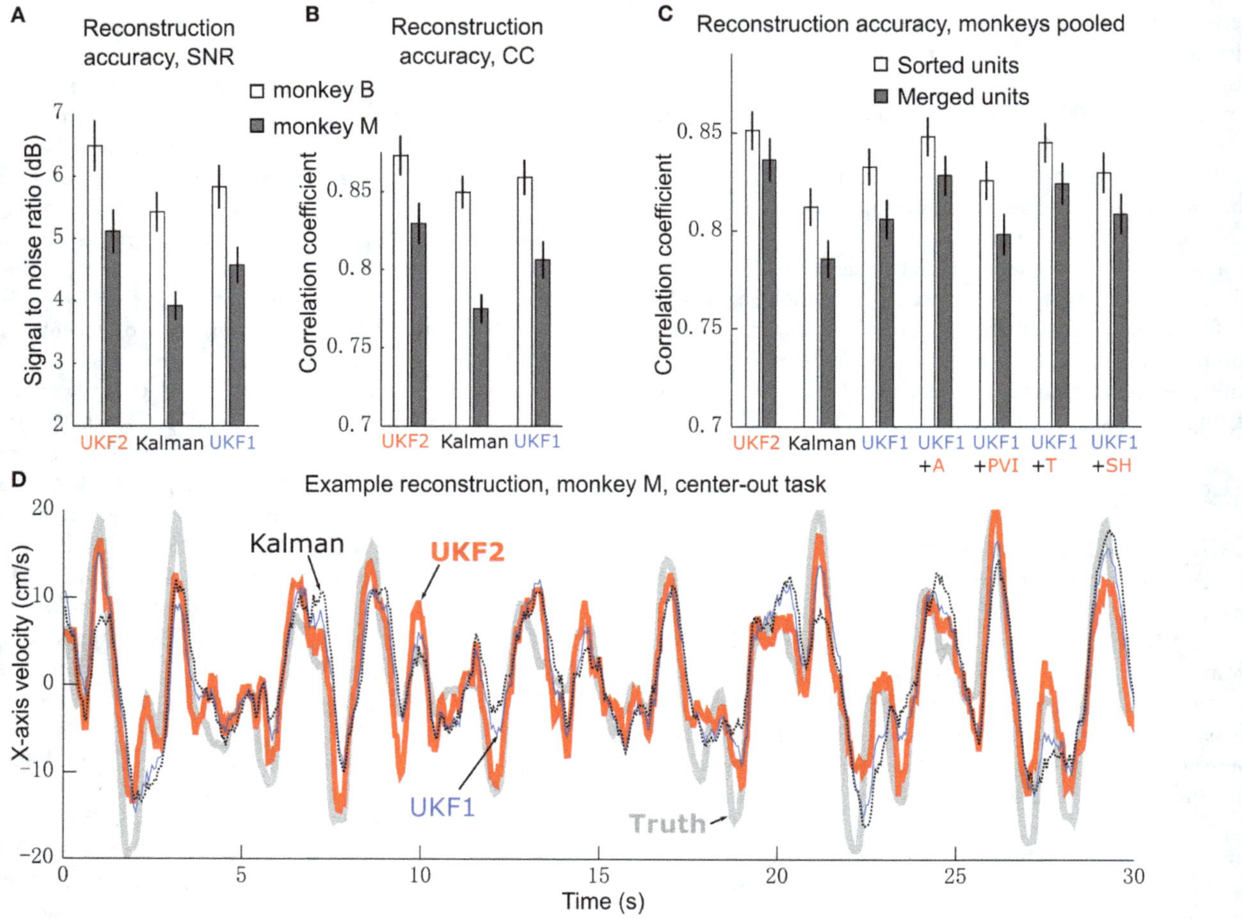

FIGURE 3 | Offline reconstruction accuracy. (A) Mean ± SEM of signal-to-noise ratios. **(B)** Mean±SEM of correlation coefficients. **(C)** Reconstruction accuracy when pooling data from two monkeys. White bars show accuracy when using spike sorting. Gray bars show accuracy when using unsorted spikes derived by merging all sorted units on each channel. Right side bars show UKF1 augmented with each of: +A, acceleration; +PVI, position-velocity interaction; +T, target; +SH, spiking history of population. **(D)** Example reconstruction of x-axis velocity from one session of monkey M.

thorough sampling of the space of possible position/velocity combinations seen in the pursuit task data.

Accuracy for monkey M was generally poorer, and upon examining fitted model parameters, we suspected that the spiking history features were not fitted as well for monkey M. Thus, we examined the contribution of spiking history per monkey. For monkey B, in terms of CC, UKF1+SH was significantly more accurate than UKF1 alone (two-tailed paired t-test, uncorrected, $n = 16$, $p = 0.04995$), but for monkey M, UKF1+SH was significantly less accurate than UKF1 alone (two-tailed paired t-test, uncorrected, $n = 16$, $p = 0.0001$). The significance testing results were the same for SNR.

As described in the methods, we spike sorted aggressively, which resulted in a large number of multiunits. We wondered if our aggressive spike sorting affected the observed trends. Thus, we tried performing reconstructions using unsorted spiking data. We merged all units on each channel, undoing the process of spike sorting. Note that this is different from using all threshold crossings, since waveforms which crossed the threshold but did not match any unit's template are excluded. The reconstruction results from merged units are shown by the gray bars in **Figure 3C**. The mean accuracy when using merged units was significantly and substantially worse than the mean accuracy when using sorted units under every decoder variant (two-tailed paired t-tests, all corrected $p <$ 0.000035). ANOVA (merged decoders x session) found a main effect of decoder [$F_{(6, 31)} = 34{,}31$, $p < 10^{-10}$]. The trends in accuracy among UKF2, KF, UKF1 and when enhancements are individually added to UKF1 for merged units were similar to the trends from sorted units (except that UKF2 was significantly better than UKF1+T, corrected $p = 0.0028$), confirming that our aggressive spike sorting did not influence the trends we observed.

We illustrate sample reconstructions of the UKF2, position velocity Kalman filter, and UKF1 in **Figure 3D**. In this panel we show the 30 s of reconstructed x-axis velocity vs. time from one center-out session of monkey M. We can see that the UKF2 reconstruction follows the cursor velocity better at several peaks and valleys, though there are also instances where UKF2's reconstruction is farthest from the true value.

Encoding Model Predictions

We next compared the encoding model of the UKF2 with that of UKF1 and the position-velocity Kalman filter. The purpose of this is to better understand what motor cortical neurons encode and to explain the improvements in decoding accuracy—it would be unsatisfying if the source of decoding improvements were unknown—and not as evidence for better decoding accuracy. We analyzed the same 16 sessions from monkey B and 16 sessions from monkey M, which together had a total of 8582 single units and multiunits. These units represent a far smaller number of distinct neurons, since electrodes usually record the same neurons between sessions. Due to this, we also conducted analysis on a single session from each monkey, so as to obtain unique units for significance testing. The results are summarized in **Table 2** and graphed in **Figure 4**.

We first plotted the distribution of encoding model prediction accuracy (in CC), among all units in all sessions, as a histogram in **Figure 4A**. In this figure, the dashed vertical lines represent the mean correlation values for each model. We see that the UKF2 model predicted spike counts more accurately for many unit instances (which include repeated observations of the same units over different sessions), with substantially higher mean prediction accuracy (UKF2: 0.210, p-v Kalman: 0.098, UKF1: 0.138). These values are substantially lower than decoding accuracy values, which is not surprising given our limited understanding of what individual neurons are doing and the intrinsic noise in spiking. The fact that we can achieve higher decoding accuracies despite this is because the decoding algorithm is aggregating information from hundreds of units.

We wanted to know how each new enhancement of the UKF2 model contributed to the improvement in encoding accuracy. In addition to the four improvements, we also tested intention estimation (Gilja et al., 2012; Fan et al., 2014), applying it to both training and testing data, to see if this improves encoding accuracy for the Kalman filter's position-velocity linear model. We plot the resulting mean correlation coefficient and SNR in **Figure 4B**. We see that adding spiking history to the UKF1 model resulted in the largest increase in accuracy. Adding the other features resulted in smaller increases in accuracy. Intention estimation did not improve the mean encoding accuracy of the position-velocity linear model.

We wanted to know if these improvements were significant. However, the prediction accuracy of different units is not independent in this analysis since units from different sessions may be the same neuron. Thus, we chose one session from each monkey to perform significance testing. We chose a relatively long center-out session for each monkey with a large number of units sorted. We show the mean prediction accuracy for one session from each monkey in **Figure 4C**. As measured by correlation, ANOVA found a main effect on decoding method [monkey B: $F_{(10,\,410)} = 716.58, p < 10^{-10}$, monkey M: $F_{(10,\,218)} = 96.68, p < 10^{-10}$]. *Post-hoc* comparisons showed that the mean prediction accuracy of the UKF2 model was significantly higher than that of the position-velocity Kalman and UKF1 models for both monkeys (all corrected $p < 10^{-6}$). The differences in mean prediction accuracies were all significant (all corrected $p < 10^{-6}$) between UKF1 and UKF1 augmented with each enhancement, as well as between UKF2 and UKF1 augmented with each enhancement. The UKF1 model also had significantly higher (corrected $p < 10^{-6}$) mean prediction accuracy than the position-velocity linear model of the Kalman filter decoder. Comparing the contribution of different enhancements when added to UKF1, all pair-wise tests were significant (all corrected $p < 10^{-6}$), except UKF1+A vs. UKF1+PVI for monkey M

TABLE 2 | Encoding model prediction accuracy.

Mean ± SEM	CC, pooled	CC, monkey B, one session	CC, monkey M, one session	CC, monkey B, one session, top 10 percentile units	CC, monkey M, one session, top 10 percentile units	SNR(dB), pooled	SNR(dB), monkey B, one session	SNR(dB), monkey M, one session
UKF2	0.210 ± 0.002	0.239 ± 0.006	0.137 ± 0.006	0.294 ± 0.024	0.245 ± 0.039	0.216 ± 0.005	0.285 ± 0.019	0.075 ± 0.017
Kalman	0.098 ± 0.001	0.101 ± 0.003	0.091 ± 0.005	0.137 ± 0.013	0.189 ± 0.031	0.020 ± 0.002	0.050 ± 0.004	0.033 ± 0.010
Kalman intention estimation	0.087 ± 0.001	0.099 ± 0.003	0.084 ± 0.005	0.133 ± 0.013	0.169 ± 0.028	0.008 ± 0.002	0.047 ± 0.004	0.023 ± 0.008
UKF1	0.138 ± 0.001	0.148 ± 0.004	0.099 ± 0.005	0.163 ± 0.014	0.196 ± 0.032	0.070 ± 0.003	0.109 ± 0.007	0.041 ± 0.010
UKF1+A	0.145 ± 0.001	0.163 ± 0.004	0.103 ± 0.005	0.184 ± 0.015	0.198 ± 0.032	0.082 ± 0.003	0.133 ± 0.007	0.043 ± 0.010
UKF1+PVI	0.145 ± 0.001	0.157 ± 0.004	0.102 ± 0.005	0.181 ± 0.016	0.201 ± 0.033	0.081 ± 0.003	0.125 ± 0.007	0.044 ± 0.011
UKF1+T	0.156 ± 0.001	0.179 ± 0.004	0.107 ± 0.005	0.189 ± 0.015	0.199 ± 0.032	0.101 ± 0.003	0.160 ± 0.008	0.046 ± 0.010
UKF1+SH	0.206 ± 0.001	0.234 ± 0.006	0.134 ± 0.006	0.286 ± 0.023	0.241 ± 0.039	0.208 ± 0.005	0.272 ± 0.018	0.071 ± 0.016
Self history	–	0.130 ± 0.005	0.063 ± 0.005	0.224 ± 0.022	0.160 ± 0.037	–	0.104 ± 0.010	0.024 ± 0.011
Others history	–	0.218 ± 0.006	0.114 ± 0.005	0.232 ± 0.021	0.177 ± 0.030	–	0.225 ± 0.016	0.034 ± 0.011
Population history	–	0.229 ± 0.006	0.121 ± 0.006	0.277 ± 0.023	0.214 ± 0.037	–	0.259 ± 0.018	0.054 ± 0.015

Kalman, linear encoding model of the position-velocity Kalman filter decoder; Kalman intention estimation, training and testing hand velocity data were modified using the intention estimation scheme; A, acceleration; PVI, position-velocity interaction; T, target; SH, spiking history of population; Self history, using past spiking of neuron to predict its future spiking; Others history, using past spiking of other neurons in population to predict future spiking; Population history, using past spiking of all neurons in population to predict future spiking. For details, see text. Pooled: combining data from two monkeys. Top 10 percentile units: using only units with mean spike height (peak to trough) in the top 10 percentile of all units in the session.

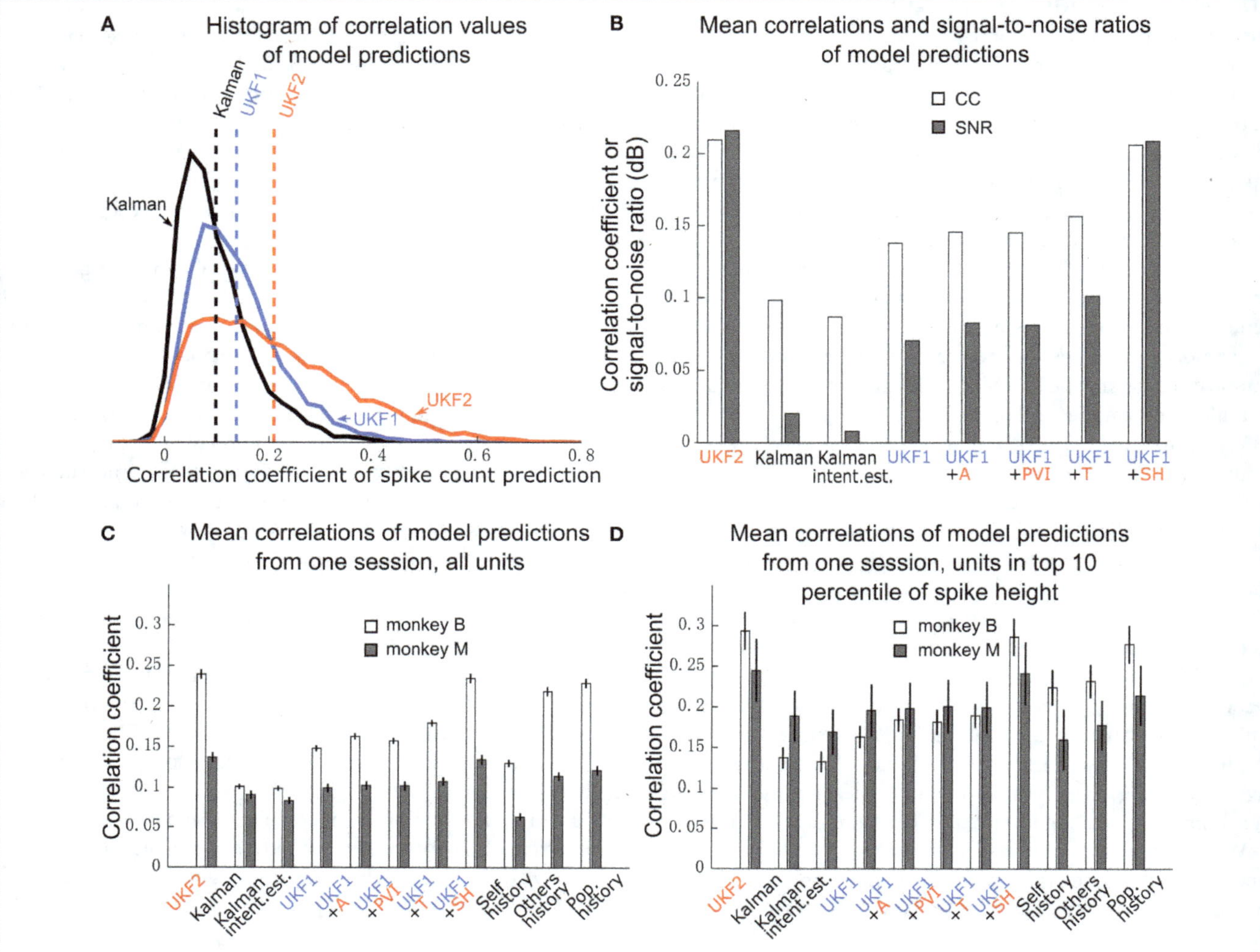

FIGURE 4 | Encoding model prediction accuracy. (A) Histogram of spike count prediction accuracies measured by correlation coefficient. Dashed vertical lines indicate means for each encoding model. **(B)** Mean CC and SNR of each encoding model, including UKF1 augmented with each of: +A, acceleration; +PVI, position-velocity interaction; +T, target; +SH, spiking history of population. SEM was not calculated since data likely includes repeated observations of neurons. **(C)** Mean±SEM of CC from one session of each monkey when using all sorted units. **(D)** Mean ± SEM of CC from one session of each monkey when using units with mean spike height (peak to trough) in the top 10 percentile of all units in the session.

(corrected $p = 0.25$). For both monkeys, the linear position-velocity model with intention estimation had lower mean correlation than without intention estimation (corrected $p \leq 1.7 \times 10^{-5}$).

We wondered whether the trends in encoding model prediction accuracies would be the same when we only consider units which are more likely to be single units. Thus, we looked at units whose spike height (peak to trough) was in the top 10 percentile of units in their respective sessions. These are the units most likely to be well-isolated single units, and the encoding model prediction accuracies for them were higher under all models. We plot the mean prediction accuracy for top 10 percentile spike height units in **Figure 4D**. ANOVA found a main effect on decoding method [monkey B: $F_{(10, 40)} = 53.96$, $p < 10^{-10}$, monkey M: $F_{(10, 20)} = 4.96$, $p < 10^{-10}$]. Some *post-hoc* comparisons between features were no longer significant, particularly for monkey M, since the amount of data was less (monkey B: $n = 41$, monkey M: $n = 21$), but the trends remaine the same.

We were curious how much spiking history alone coul predict firing rates. Thus, we compared three simple encodin models that did not use any kinematics or target position, onl firing rate history. The *self history* model uses one bin of firin rate history of neuron i to predict neuron i's instantaneous firin rate:

$$fr_{i,t}^{\text{self history}} \approx c \cdot fr_{i,t-1}^{\text{actual}}, \quad (22$$

where c is a fitted coefficient. The *others history* model uses on bin of the firing rate history of the entire population, except th neuron we are trying to model:

$$fr_{i,t}^{\text{others history}} \approx c \cdot fr_{1,t-1}^{\text{actual}} + \cdots + c \cdot fr_{i-1,t-1}^{\text{actual}} + c \cdot fr_{i+1,t-}^{\text{actual}} + \cdots + c \cdot fr_{n,t-1}^{\text{actual}}, \quad (23$$

where *cs* are n-1 different fitted coefficients, and n is the size of the population. The *population history* model uses one bin of the entire population, including the neuron we are trying to model:

$$fr_{i,\,t}^{\text{population history}} \approx c{\cdot}fr_{1,\,t-1}^{\text{actual}} + \cdots + c{\cdot}fr_{i,\,t-1}^{\text{actual}} + \cdots + c{\cdot}fr_{n,\,t-1}^{\text{actual}}, \tag{24}$$

where *cs* are n different fitted coefficients. The mean model prediction correlations are shown in **Figures 4C,D** in the right-most bars.

When considering all units (**Figure 4C**), self history had the lowest accuracy. Others history was substantially higher, and population history was only a small amount higher than others history. Pair-wise differences between the three models were all significant (all corrected $p \leq 2.0 \times 10^{-6}$). Notably, for monkey B, all three models were significantly more accurate than the position-velocity model with and without intention estimation (all corrected $p < 10^{-6}$), and the others history and population history models were significantly more accurate than the UKF1 model (all corrected $p < 10^{-6}$). For monkey M, the others history and population history models were significantly more accurate than the position-velocity model with and without intention estimation (all corrected $p < 10^{-6}$) and UKF1 ($p < 0.00076$). The UKF2 and UKF1+SH models were significantly more accurate than all three history models for both monkeys (all corrected $p < 10^{-6}$), which is expected since they include the history models.

When considering top 10 percentile spike height units (**Figure 4D**), the trends are similar, but fewer comparisons were significant due to less data. Population history was significantly more accurate than the self history model for both monkeys (all corrected $p \leq 0.0033$). For monkey B, all three history models were significantly more accurate than the position-velocity model with and without intention estimation and the UKF1 model (all corrected $p \leq 0.0013$). For monkey M, differences between the three history models vs. the position-velocity model (with and without intention estimation) and vs. the UKF1 model were not significant. The UKF2 and UKF1+SH models were significantly more accurate than all three history models for both monkeys (all corrected $p \leq 0.00086$), as expected.

To illustrate tuning to position-velocity interactions, we depict an example single unit from monkey B with relatively strong position-velocity interaction in **Figure 5**. **Figure 5B** shows representative spike shapes from this single-unit. **Figure 5A** consists of nine panels, where each panel shows tuning in a different portion of the work space. For example, the lower right panel shows velocity tuning when the cursor is near the lower right (hand is near the right and posterior) portion of the work space. Within each panel, the axes represent cursor velocity, with the center of the panel representing zero velocity. Firing rate is indicated by the shading. For example, the shading in the lower right of a panel is the firing rate of the single unit when the hand is moving toward the right and posterior. The visualization was created by performing Gaussian kernel smoothing on a 7 by 7 grid (per panel). All kinematic variables were normalized to be unit-variance and the smoothing kernel width was 3.

We can see differences in the velocity tuning at different positions in the work space. For example, the firing rate was higher for lower-right velocities in the lower-right position (4.26 Hz at the red dot) than in the upper-left position (2.55 Hz at the red dot).This suggests a multiplicative interaction between position and velocity. This figure illustrates why, for 349 out of 411 (monkey B) and 153 out of 219 (monkey M) units, UKF1+PVI predicted spiking rates better than UKF1, and why PVI is a tuning phenomenon which next-generation neural encoding models should probably take into account.

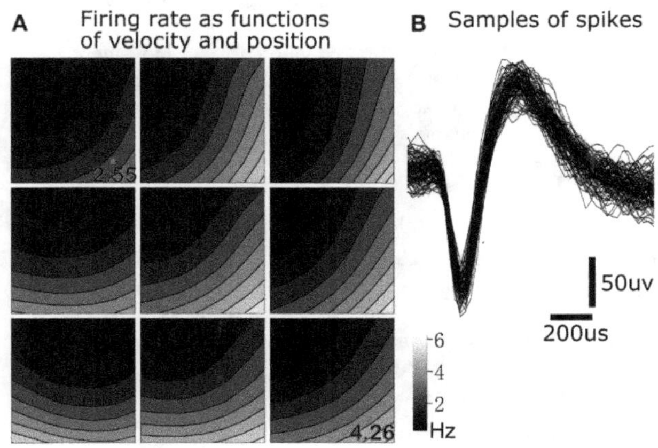

FIGURE 5 | Position-velocity interaction in the encoding of a motor cortical single unit. (A) Illustration of position-velocity interaction tuning. Shading indicates firing rate. Each sub-panel depicts velocity tuning when the cursor was in a portion of the position work space, with the sub-panel's position corresponding to the cursor position. Location within each sub-panel corresponds to the 2D cursor velocity, with zero velocity in the center. See text for details. **(B)** Example spike waveforms from this single unit.

Closed-Loop Neural Control Experiments

We compared the ability of monkeys to complete a center-out task using the decoders in closed-loop neural control. We recorded 7 sessions with monkey B, 153–184 days post-implant, and 30 sessions with monkey M, 15–70 days post-implant. Each session was recorded on a separate day and contains one 10-min block of each condition (UKF2, KF, UKF1), and the last 5 min of each 10-min block were analyzed for performance. We recorded fewer sessions with monkey B because the difference between decoders was larger, and monkey B was tasked with other experiments. The results of closed-loop comparisons are summarized in **Table 3** and graphed in **Figure 6**.

We calculated the mean (across sessions) of the fraction of targets acquired (**Figure 6A**), time to move to a peripheral target (**Figure 6B**), and Fitts's Law bit rate (**Figure 6C**) for each decoder, as well as hand control of the cursor via joystick.

The fractions of targets acquired were not significantly different between conditions for monkey B [ANOVA $F_{(3,\,6)} = 1.13$, $p = 0.36$]. For monkey M, ANOVA found a main effect on mode of control [$F_{(3,\,29)} = 5.4474$, $p = 0.0018$], and *post-hoc* tests showed that fractions of targets acquired for the decoders were not significantly different, but all decoders had significantly lower fractions than hand control (all corrected $p < 0.034$). The high variance in fraction of targets acquired by monkey B (session MS = 0.02718, compared to control condition MS = 0.02309, while other closed-loop control

TABLE 3 | Comparison of decoders during closed-loop neural control of cursor.

Mean ± SEM	Fraction of targets acquired, monkey B	Fraction of targets acquired, monkey M	Movement time (s), monkey B	Movement time (s), monkey M	Movement time (s), pooled	Fitts's Law bit rate (bits/s), monkey B	Fitts's Law bit rate (bits/s), monkey M	Fitts's Law bit rate (bits/s), pooled
UKF2	0.961 ± 0.016	0.906 ± 0.025	1.201 ± 0.150	1.640 ± 0.065	1.557 ± 0.065	0.980 ± 0.122	0.682 ± 0.026	0.738 ± 0.036
FIT Kalman filter	0.980 ± 0.014	0.847 ± 0.037	1.766 ± 0.217	1.722 ± 0.092	1.730 ± 0.083	0.666 ± 0.084	0.668 ± 0.032	0.668 ± 0.030
UKF1	0.850 ± 0.091	0.909 ± 0.026	2.456 ± 0.489	1.959 ± 0.103	2.053 ± 0.124	0.545 ± 0.100	0.593 ± 0.032	0.584 ± 0.031
Hand control	0.934 ± 0.062	0.987 ± 0.008	0.689 ± 0.065	1.182 ± 0.050	1.089 ± 0.053	2.248 ± 0.186	1.178 ± 0.050	1.381 ± 0.087

Pooled, combining data from two monkeys.

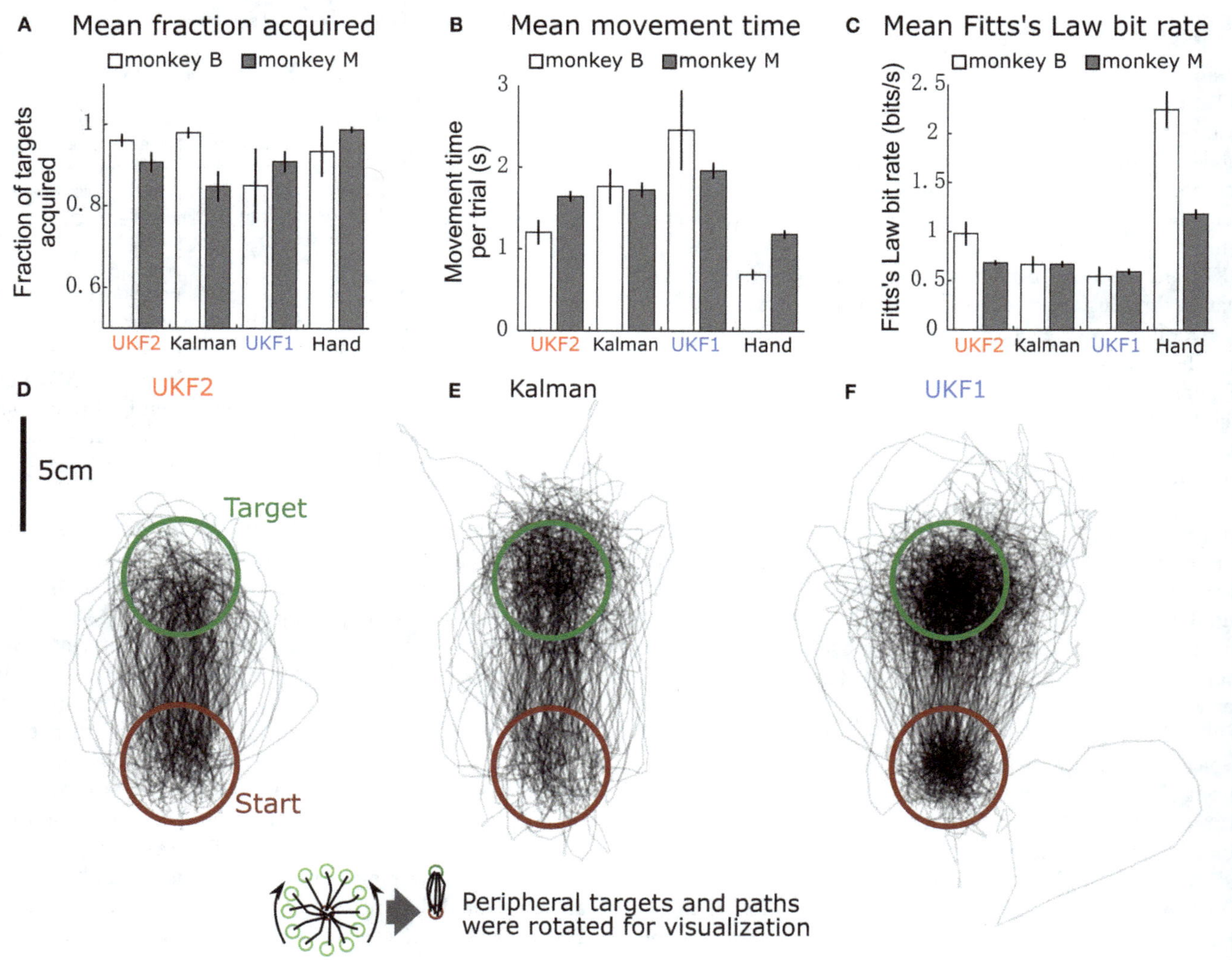

FIGURE 6 | Comparison of decoders during closed-loop neural control of cursor. (A) Mean ± SEM of fraction of targets acquired. "Hand" indicates performance when monkey controlled the cursor using its hand via the joystick. **(B)** Mean ± SEM of movement time per peripheral target. **(C)** Mean ± SEM of Fitts's Law bit rate. **(D)** Example movement trajectories generated under UKF2 control. Peripheral targets and paths have been rotated so that all peripheral targets align. **(E)** Trajectories under Kalman control. **(F)** Trajectories under UKF1 control.

metrics had control condition MS which were 4–20 times larger than session MS) was due to poor parameter fits in some experimental sessions leading to relatively poorer control, which led to monkey non-participation during the evaluation period, as the monkey had grown used to very good neura control.

In terms of time to move to a peripheral target, for monkey B ANOVA found a main effect on mode of control [$F_{(3, 6)} = 9.9, p =$

0.0004]. *Post-hoc* tests showed that UKF2 times were significantly shorter than UKF1 times (corrected $p = 0.049$), other decoder comparisons were not significant. Hand control had significantly shorter times than every decoder (all corrected $p < 0.040$). For monkey M, ANOVA found a main effect on mode of control [$F_{(3,\,29)} = 36.8127, p = 1.87 \times 10^{-15}$], and *post-hoc* tests showed that UKF2 and FIT Kalman filter times were significantly shorter than UKF1 times (corrected $p = 0.0012$, $p = 0.020$, respectively), the UKF2 and FIT Kalman comparison was not significant. Hand control had significantly shorter times than every decoder (all corrected $p < 2 \times 10^{-6}$).

In terms of Fitts's Law bit rates, for monkey B, ANOVA found a main effect on mode of control [$F_{(3,\,6)} = 90.09, p < 10^{-10}$]. *Post-hoc* tests showed that UKF2 bit rates were significantly higher than UKF1 bit rates (corrected $p = 0.00061$), and other decoder comparisons were not significant. Hand control had significantly higher bit rate than every decoder (all corrected $p < 0.00057$). For monkey M, ANOVA found a main effect on mode of control [$F_{(3,\,29)} = 155.2043$, $p = 8.2 \times 10^{-35}$]. *Post-hoc* tests showed that UKF2 and FIT Kalman filter bit rates were significantly higher than UKF1 bit rates (corrected $p = 0.0030$, $p = 0.012$, respectively). UKF2 bit rates and FIT Kalman bit rates were not significantly different, and hand control had significantly higher bit rate than every decoder (all corrected $p < 10^{-6}$).

When we pooled the data between the two monkeys, the mean movement times were significantly different among the three decoders and hand control [ANOVA $F_{(3,\,36)} = 34.94$, $p = 7.3 \times 10^{-16}$, *post-hoc* UKF2 < FIT Kalman, corrected $p = 0.045$; UKF2 < UKF1, corrected $p = 0.00024$; FIT Kalman < UKF1, corrected $p = 0.013$]. Mean Fitts's law bit rates were also significantly different among the three decoders and hand control [ANOVA $F_{(3,\,36)} = 80.19$, $p = 2.3 \times 10^{-27}$, *post-hoc* UKF2 > FIT Kalman corrected $p = 0.046$; UKF2 > UKF1 corrected $p = 0.00006$; FIT Kalman > UKF1 corrected $p = 0.0039$]. The hand movement times (all corrected $p < 10^{-6}$), and bit rates (all corrected $p < 10^{-6}$) were significantly better than that for every decoder. For fraction of targets acquired, there was a main effect on mode of control [ANOVA $F_{(3,\,36)} = 3.81$, $p = 0.012$], but *post-hoc* testing did not find significant differences among the decoders. The hand control fraction correct was better than that for the FIT Kalman (corrected $p = 0.036$) and UKF1 (corrected $p = 0.040$).

Figures 6D–F show all center to peripheral movement trajectories generated during UKF2 control, FIT Kalman filter control, and UKF1 control, respectively, for one session from monkey B. For clarity of visualization, the trajectories have been rotated so that the peripheral target locations are aligned at the top. Thus, all trajectories start from the lower, red circle and end in the upper, green circle. We can see that the trajectories generated during UKF2 control start movement in the wrong direction and overshoot the target the least among the three decoders. From the movement time and bit rate comparisons and the trajectory illustrations, we can see that UKF2 allows the monkey to perform center-out movements more quickly and accurately than the UKF1 and comparably to the FIT Kalman filter.

One may ask why the plot of trajectories for UKF1 (**Figure 6F**) looks darker within the targets. This is because the decoded cursor positions are more "jumpy" during the hold period. This is due to the use of position as the signal to control the cursor, and noisy neural activity causes the estimated position to jump. We conjecture that the position-velocity mixing scheme (Homer M. et al., 2013) and our probabilistic velocity thresholding refinement solve this problem for the UKF2.

DISCUSSION

The UKF2 reconstructed kinematics offline more accurately than the position-velocity Kalman filter and UKF1. Examining why the UKF2 performed better, analysis of the encoding model found that the UKF2's encoding model made more accurate predictions of neural activity. In closed-loop neural control experiments, the UKF2 allowed better task performance than the UKF1, but comparisons with the FIT Kalman filter were not significant on a per-monkey basis, though they were significant when data from two monkeys were combined.

The differences between monkeys were quite large. Monkey B was more proficient at the center-out task under hand control, with lower movement times and higher bit rate. Offline reconstructions were generally more accurate with monkey B. The differences between decoders in closed-loop control were larger for monkey B. A particularly pronounced area of disparity was encoding model predictions. Monkey B and monkey M had similar encoding model prediction accuracy for the Kalman filter, but quite different accuracy for the UKF1 and UKF2. For monkey B, adding spiking history to UKF1 resulted in the largest improvement, with target tuning also large. For monkey M, improvements from these two features were substantially smaller. The trends suggest that spiking history is less beneficial for modeling the activity of monkey M's units, and even harmful for decoding accuracy, which hints at some qualitative differences in the populations recorded from these two monkeys. Overall, the differences between monkeys may be due to: electrode length (B: 1.0 mm, M: 1.5 mm), age (B: 6, M: 4), amount of practice with the center-out task (B: 4 months, M: 2 months), and spike sorting performed by different experimenters.

During the design of the UKF2 algorithm, we used pursuit task data from another monkey, which we cannot publish here. We froze the design of our algorithm, as much as possible, before starting closed-loop experiments and data collection for reconstructions. Thus, we included refinements such as PVI and SH which were not universally beneficial.

Our results with CC and SNR are, in some cases, quite different in absolute terms. This is understandable since they are very different measures, with SNR including a logarithm to avoid saturation.

All decoders we tested, including the FIT Kalman filter, had significantly worse performance, in terms of movement time and Fitts's Law bit rate, than hand control via the joystick. These differences were large, for example, hand control had 1.9 times the bit rate of UKF2 and 2.1 times the bit rate of the FIT Kalman filter. This indicates there is still much room for improvement in decoding and signal acquisition methodology.

In terms of the contributions of the different refinements, our closed-loop results are limited in granularity; future work may investigate the individual contributions in closed-loop, which would greatly assist practitioners in optimizing their decoder design.

Acceleration

Acceleration of the hand has been decoded in past studies (Ashe and Georgopoulos, 1994; Gao et al., 2003), and force has long been known to contribute to encoding (Evarts, 1968 and many others). In our previous work, we considered using acceleration as a feature in the encoding model, but did not detect a substantial benefit. After UKF1's publication, we continued to look for ways to improve the neural encoding model using new kinematic features. Our recent analysis included temporal smoothing (sliding window moving average) of kinematics before parameter fitting for the encoding model (see Supplementary Materials). Doing this, the quickly-changing acceleration signal is smoothed out, and neural encoding strength for acceleration is increased, resulting in worthwhile decoding accuracy increases. Similar to position and velocity, upon visualization of acceleration tuning, we found spatial patterns consistent with the existence of a relationship between the acceleration magnitude (in any direction) and the firing rate of many neurons. Thus, we have also included the magnitude of the acceleration vector as a novel feature of the UKF2 encoding model. Even though we do not use the acceleration in the filter state to directly control the cursor, the acceleration interacts with the other variables in the state space via the state transition model (movement model).

Position-Velocity Interaction

In our quest for a better encoding model, we visualized neural tuning patterns in various ways (for example, **Figure 5A**). We found that the encoding of velocity changes with the position of the hand in a systematic way. Thus, we surmised that there is an interaction between position and velocity tuning. Differences in preferred directions at different limb postures have previously been found (Caminiti et al., 1990; Sergio and Kalaska, 2003), and gain-field encoding has been suggested for limb position and velocity (Hwang et al., 2003). To capture this interaction, we added a multiplicative feature to our encoding model which is a simple multiplication of the position and velocity for each dimension separately. This encoding model refinement was used both in offline and closed-loop decoding. We found that by adding this novel encoding feature, significantly more accurate predictions of firing rate could be achieved (**Figure 4C**).

However, in terms of offline reconstructions, using position-velocity interaction was actually detrimental when considering both center-out and pursuit tasks, and slightly helpful (though not significant, since $n = 6$) when considering the pursuit task only. In the center-out task, position (with respect to center of workspace) and velocity are either very correlated (outward movement), very anti-correlated (inward movement), or independent (hold), with few instances of other relationships. This is not true for the pursuit task, which samples the possible space of position and velocity values much more thoroughly. We believe this difference accounts for the results we found. For neural control of a prosthetic, where movements throughout the space of possible position and velocity values need to be supported, the position-velocity interaction term will likely help.

Target

Inspired by studies which included the target of reaches in the trajectory decoding process (Shanechi et al., 2012; Shanechi M. et al., 2013; Shanechi M. M. et al., 2013; Shanechi and Carmena, 2013), we investigated adding information about the target into the encoding model. In preliminary analysis we found that some neurons show significant encoding of target position, which has been found in the past (Fu et al., 1995). Though using the neurons we recorded to decode target position alone provides very noisy results, the rough information that can be decoded is still valuable. We set the target position to weakly attract the cursor during closed-loop control. This, in effect, gives a small assistance to the cursor decoding by using the rough estimate of the target location. This is somewhat similar to the mechanism that Shanechi and Carmena (2013) used, where the target position is used in an optimal feedback controller, which can be understood as biasing decoded movement toward the target.

In addition to target position in Cartesian coordinates, our preliminary analysis showed that there was significant encoding of the distance between target position and cursor position, which is similar to the reach distance found by Fu et al. (1995). Thus, we included this novel feature in our encoding model as well.

Spiking History

In multiple previous studies (Paninski et al., 2004b; Truccolo et al., 2005; Lawhern et al., 2010; Saleh et al., 2010, 2012; Truccolo et al., 2010; Park et al., 2014; Xu et al., 2014) the past spiking of a neuron as well as the past spiking of other neurons in the population have been used to better model the probability of spiking in a point process framework, sometimes leading to very accurate models (Truccolo et al., 2010). The past neural activity of all neurons in the population may capture correlations in firing due to functional connectivity or common inputs. Another advantage of this modeling approach is the ability to indirectly capture tuning to latent neural states. One disadvantage of this approach is the large number of additional parameters that must be fitted, with the accompanying increase in over-fitting risk.

We wanted to include spiking history in our encoding model to capture these benefits. However, instead of using complex temporal features as in the point process studies, we use a comparatively simple idea: we include only the spike counts in the previous bin for the entire population. In preliminary analysis we investigated using more than one previous bin and found the benefit to be small in comparison to the additional cost in number of parameters that needed to be fit.

During closed-loop decoding, the spike count of the previous time bin is available, and is directly provided to the neural encoding model as point values without uncertainty. In other words, unlike the filter state variables in the encoding model, the previous spike counts are not decoded; their benefit comes from improving the fit of the encoding model. This is similar to the role of the position state variables in the ReFIT Kalman filter

By including spiking history, we aim to remove more systematic variation (e.g., from autocorrelation) from the encoding model's residual, making the remaining residual closer to white noise, which better fits the theoretical assumptions of the Kalman filter framework. However, it is still beneficial to include improved kinematic features in the encoding model: these provide the "conduits" through which information flows from neural activity to kinematic variables during the operation of the unscented Kalman filter.

Our results show that adding spiking history improved encoding model predictions substantially. However, offline reconstruction accuracy only improved when adding spiking history for monkey B, with possible reasons discussed above.

Mixing Position and Velocity Outputs

In our previous work with the unscented Kalman filter, we used the decoder's position output to directly drive the cursor. As the position is decoded from noisy firing rates, we observed that the decoded position jumped around in a small area at high frequency. One benefit of the position-as-feedback enhancement of the ReFIT Kalman filter is that by controlling position only through decoded velocity, this "jumpy" cursor phenomenon is avoided.

We believe that while some neurons in the motor cortex do encode for the current position of the limb in a feedback or mental representation sense, there also exist neurons which encode for the desired position in the immediate future (as opposed a distant future time, i.e., the ultimate target of a reach). If we do not make use of encoded desired position, we may be losing information potentially helpful for controlling a neuroprosthetic, particularly because UKF2's encoding model includes position-velocity interaction terms.

Thus, we chose to retain position as a directly decoded variable in the state space. However, in an effort to avoid the "jumpy" cursor of the UKF1, we adopted the method for mixing position and velocity proposed by Homer M. et al. (2013). In this scheme, if the decoded velocity is zero, the position decode cannot change the cursor. This mechanism assists the user in stopping the cursor, as well as reduces the jumpiness of the cursor. By partially controlling the cursor using the position output, we also stabilize the cursor, preventing velocity decode errors from accumulating, which was a problem we discovered in preliminary experiments when combining the position-velocity interaction enhancement and the position-as-feedback refinement of the ReFIT Kalman filter.

Movement Thresholding

The ability to stop and hold the cursor (or prosthetic limb) is important for various tasks. Several studies have examined how to stop the cursor more accurately. Golub et al. (2014) used a refinement of the transition model which allows the user to perform a "hockey stop," that is, the user changes the movement direction quickly to slow the cursor to a stop. Another approach (Velliste et al., 2014) decoded a speed term, separately from the Cartesian velocity coordinates. This speed term is used to scale the position and velocity uncertainties in the transition model, effectively acting as a gate for movements. In the mixture method of Homer M. et al. (2013), decoded velocity also acted like a gate for the influence of decoded position on the cursor. Another related decoding engineering feature is the detection of idle states—when the user is not actively using the neuroprosthetic. Aggarwal et al. (2013) and Velliste et al. (2014) detected states using a linear discriminant analysis classifier, separate from the movement decoder. When an idle or hold state was detected, the decoder output is ignored and movement was set to zero. Recently, Sachs et al. (2016) detected posture vs. movement states using linear discriminant analysis and used Wiener filters with different coefficients during each.

To improve the user's ability to stop the cursor within the target during closed-loop control, we added our own mechanism to detect movement intention, a probabilistic threshold for movement which is computed using the uncertainty output of the unscented Kalman filter. Using a probabilistic threshold means we can set the threshold in terms of a false positive rate. This probabilistic threshold is similar to a significance test; the null hypothesis is that the user wants to remain still. We check if there is enough evidence to reject the null hypothesis under the specified false positive rate. This framework, while more complex than a simple threshold on the decoded velocity, allows one threshold to work under different amounts of uncertainty in the decoded output, e.g., for both fast and imprecise (more uncertain) movements and slower and more precise (more certain) movements.

In this study, we set the desired false positive rate by hand. Larger false positive rates mean the cursor is rarely stopped through this mechanism, and holding inside a target may be more difficult if control is poor. Smaller false positive rates may make the cursor too difficult to move. Future decoders with multiple modes of operation may find it advantageous to use a lower false positive rate for certain modes where unwanted movements are dangerous or highly undesirable, e.g., when the user is asleep. While the position and velocity mixing method (Homer M. et al., 2013) also helps stop the cursor, it is dependent on accurate decoding of velocity. Our probabilistic threshold complements this method by verifying that the velocity is not non-zero due to mere noise.

Use of Future Predictions

Motor cortex neurons encode for movements that occur up to a few hundreds of milliseconds later (Ashe and Georgopoulos, 1994; Schwartz et al., 2004; Paninski et al., 2004a; Wu et al., 2006; Wang et al., 2007; Wang and Principe, 2010), making decoding of intentions at $t + 100$ ms to $t + 300$ ms possible given neural activity at time t. These "future predictions" are merely a reflection of the built-in delays in the natural motor system. Most previous work used the decoded kinematics for time t as the output at time t, in effect mimicking the delay of the natural motor system. In the UKF1, even though future intended movements are decoded, we did not choose to use future predictions to control the cursor.

Cunningham et al. (2011) found that reducing the bin width during closed-loop neural control with feedback improves performance, and Willett et al. (2013) found that using predictions of future intentions can compensate for delays in the

BMI system. Inspired by these studies, we wondered whether using future predictions could improve neural control. Our temporal offset was 100 ms in size, i.e., we use the decoded kinematics for $t + 100$ at time t, which is reasonable considering the 75–100 ms average offset found in prior work (Ashe and Georgopoulos, 1994; Paninski et al., 2004a; Schwartz et al., 2004).

One may ask why include the other taps in the filter state, if they are not used to control the cursor. The answer is that they help model the firing rate of neurons, which may encode for movements in a temporally persistent manner or specifically encode for movements in the past. Similar to adding spiking history to the encoding model or the position-as-feedback enhancement, the other taps do not directly affect the decoder output, but may improve decoder accuracy by explicitly modeling what would otherwise be thrown in to the catch-all error term.

Related Work

Reviews of research in decoding for BMIs can be found elsewhere (Homer M. L. et al., 2013; Andersen et al., 2014; Baranauskas, 2014; Bensmaia and Miller, 2014; Kao et al., 2014; Li, 2014). Here we discuss the decoders compared in the present study.

The improved unscented Kalman filter decoder proposed in this study is a development of our previous unscented Kalman filter decoder (Li et al., 2009). That filter, which we refer to here as UKF1, used an encoding model with non-linear dependence on kinematic variables which modeled tuning to the speed or velocity magnitude of movements. The UKF1 modeled tuning at multiple temporal offsets, using an n-th order hidden Markov model framework where n taps of kinematics ($n = 10$ was tested) are held in the state space. Encoding studies by Paninski et al. (2004a,b), Hatsopoulos et al. (2007), Hatsopoulos and Amit (2012) and Saleh et al. (2010) found tuning to position and velocity trajectories, called movement fragments or pathlets. The n-th order framework makes the encoding model of the UKF1 flexible enough to capture such tuning. Even though including taps of position also indirectly includes velocity, explicitly including taps of velocity reduces the amount of non-linearity needed in the neural encoding model, which helps improve the approximation accuracy of the UKF. On the basis of UKF1, we expand the neural encoding model and add decoder engineering improvements developed by ourselves and other groups to make the UKF2.

The ReFIT Kalman filter (Gilja et al., 2012) has demonstrated high communications bit rate by using two advances in decoder engineering. In closed-loop experiments, we compared the UKF2 with the FIT Kalman filter (Fan et al., 2014), which is similar to the ReFIT Kalman filter in using position-as-feedback and intention estimation, but does not have the online re-training component. The bin size in this study, 50 ms, was the same as the Gilja et al. study. Our Fitts's Law bit rate values for the FIT Kalman filter are lower than those reported by Gilja et al. for the ReFIT Kalman filter, likely due to a combination of factors. First, online re-training separates the FIT and ReFIT Kalman filters. In terms of experimental setup, Gilja et al. used video tracking of natural reaching movements, whereas we used a joystick during hand control of the cursor. The use of an unnatural joystick made our task more difficult: the mean movement time during hand control in our task was approximately double those reported by Gilja et al. we used a joystick due to the limitations of our experimental platform and to compare with our previous work (Li et al., 2009). While using the same Fitts's law bit rate measure, our task used circular targets, which have a smaller acceptance area for the same width compared to the square targets of Gilja et al. We used circular targets because they are more natural in terms of determining whether the cursor is within the target by using a distance criterion. We also spike sorted and did not include unsorted or "hash" threshold crossings, whereas Gilja et al. used threshold crossing counts.

Latent Neural State

Models proposed by many previous studies have modeled latent neural states explicitly (Brockwell et al., 2007; Kulkarni and Paninski, 2007; Wu et al., 2009; Lawhern et al., 2010; Macke et al., 2011; Petreska et al., 2011; Aghagolzadeh and Truccolo, 2014, 2016; Deng et al., 2015; Kao et al., 2015; Lakshmanan et al., 2015). In Aghagolzadeh and Truccolo (2014) and Kao et al. (2015), the latent neural state comprises the entirety of the Kalman filter state, and kinematics are decoded from this latent neural state after it is decoded from the spike counts. When modeling latent states like this, some form of unsupervised learning is required to fit the observation model of the filter. The typical approach is Expectation-Maximization applied to linear dynamical systems (Shumway and Stoffer, 1982).

An alternative approach is to implicitly model latent states by adding spiking history to the observation model. By adding spiking history, one may (partially) capture latent shared variables if they have temporal autocorrelation. In other words, if a unobserved common input of many neurons is changing slowly, by using the past neural activity, which partially encodes this hidden input, to predict the current neural activity, one is including this hidden common input in the encoding model by proxy.

Two engineering advantages of explicitly modeling the latent variable using additional state variables are: (1) lower dimensionality; (2) ability to impose prior assumptions on the model structure, such as in the transition model or observation model (Aghagolzadeh and Truccolo, 2016). Additionally, investigating these latent states may yield neuroscientific insights. However, it is not obvious this approach is always better from a decoding point of view, since the unsupervised learning of latent variables cannot be checked against a gold standard and, in practice, it is vulnerable to local optima. Some of the autocorrelation or cross-correlation captured by spiking history may not be due to low-dimensional latent variables, but are due to biophysics and actual neuronal connectivity. The effect of these phenomena may not be easily captured by low dimensional latent states.

CONCLUSION

We have shown in offline analysis and closed-loop experiments with two Rhesus monkeys that our encoding model features and decoder engineering refinements improve encoding and decoding accuracy. Some of the enhancements used in this work, particularly the probabilistic velocity thresholding and the inclusion of hand acceleration and target position (without the non-linear terms) are compatible with the standard Kalman filter, are fairly easy to implement, and are likely to bring the largest benefits. We hope that these enhancements will be utilized by others, just as we have improved our decoder using innovations published by others.

AUTHOR CONTRIBUTIONS

SL and ZL designed the algorithm. SL and JL collected the data. SL, JL, and ZL analyzed the results. ZL drafted the manuscript. SL, JL, and ZL revised the manuscript.

ACKNOWLEDGMENTS

This work was supported by the National Natural Science Foundation of China (61431002), National Key Basic Research Program of China (2014CB846101), National Natural Science Foundation of China (61401028), and Fundamental Research Funds for the Central Universities. We thank Wu Li, Dajun Xing, Feng Wang, Xibin Xu, Shujie Wang, Xing Ma, Lüyan Zhong, Yin Yan, Minggui Chen, Rujia Chen, Zhihan Li, Yang Li, Tian Wang, Chen Yang, Guanzhong Yang, Yi Yang, Xiuli Chen, and Chenguang Zhang for technical assistance and assistance during animal surgeries. We also thank Joseph O'Doherty, Wu Li, and the reviewers for helpful comments on the manuscript. We thank Miguel Nicolelis for permission to use the BMI3 software suite.

REFERENCES

Aggarwal, V., Mollazadeh, M., Davidson, A. G., Schieber, M. H., and Thakor, N. V. (2013). State-based decoding of hand and finger kinematics using neuronal ensemble and LFP activity during dexterous reach-to-grasp movements. *J. Neurophysiol.* 109, 3067–3081. doi: 10.1152/jn.01038.2011

Aghagolzadeh, M., and Truccolo, W. (2014). "Latent state-space models for neural decoding," in *Engineering in Medicine and Biology Society (EMBC), 2014, 36th Annual International Conference of the IEEE* (Chicago, IL), 3033–3036.

Aghagolzadeh, M., and Truccolo, W. (2016). Inference and decoding of motor cortex low-dimensional dynamics via latent state-space models. *IEEE Trans. Neural Syst. Rehabil. Eng.* 24, 272–282. doi: 10.1109/TNSRE.2015.2470527

Andersen, R. A., Kellis, S., Klaes, C., and Aflalo, T. (2014). Toward more versatile and intuitive cortical brain-machine interfaces. *Curr. Biol.* 24, R885–R897. doi: 10.1016/j.cub.2014.07.068

Ashe, J., and Georgopoulos, A. P. (1994). Movement parameters and neural activity in motor cortex and area 5. *Cereb. Cortex* 4, 590–600. doi: 10.1093/cercor/4.6.590

Baranauskas, G. (2014). What limits the performance of current invasive brain machine interfaces? *Fron. Syst. Neurosc.* 8:68. doi: 10.3389/fnsys.2014.00068

Bensmaia, S. J., and Miller, L. E. (2014). Restoring sensorimotor function through intracortical interfaces: progress and looming challenges. *Nat. Rev. Neurosci.* 15, 313–325. doi: 10.1038/nrn3724

Brockwell, A. E., Kass, R. E., and Schwartz, A. B. (2007). Statistical signal processing and the motor cortex. *Proc. IEEE* 95, 881–898. doi: 10.1109/JPROC.2007.894703

Caminiti, R., Johnson, P. B., Burnod, Y., Galli, C., and Ferraina, S. (1990). Shift of preferred directions of premotor cortical cells with arm movements performed across the workspace. *Exp. Brain Res.* 83, 228–232. doi: 10.1007/bf00232214

Cunningham, J. P., Nuyujukian, P., Gilja, V., Chestek, C. A., Ryu, S. I., and Shenoy, K. V. (2011). A closed-loop human simulator for investigating the role of feedback control in brain-machine interfaces. *J. Neurophysiol.* 105, 1932–1949. doi: 10.1152/jn.00503.2010

Deng, X., Faghih, R., Barbieri, R., Paulk, A., Asaad, W., Brown, E., et al. (2015). "Estimating a dynamic state to relate neural spiking activity to behavioral signals during cognitive tasks," in *Engineering in Medicine and Biology Society (EMBC), 2015, 37th Annual International Conference of the IEEE* (Milan), 7808–7813.

Evarts, E. V. (1968). Relation of pyramidal tract activity to force exerted during voluntary movement. *J. Neurophysiol.* 31, 14–27.

Fan, J. M., Nuyujukian, P., Kao, J. C., Chestek, C. A., Ryu, S. I., and Shenoy, K. V. (2014). Intention estimation in brain-machine interfaces. *J. Neural Eng.* 11:016004. doi: 10.1088/1741-2560/11/1/016004

Fu, Q. G., Flament, D., Coltz, J. D., and Ebner, T. J. (1995). Temporal encoding of movement kinematics in the discharge of primate primary motor and premotor neurons. *J. Neurophysiol.* 73, 836–854.

Gao, Y., Black, M., Bienenstock, E., Wu, W., and Donoghue, J. P. (2003). "A quantitative comparison of linear and non-linear models of motor cortical activity for the encoding and decoding of arm motions," in *First International IEEE EMBS Conference on Neural Engineering* (Capri), 189–192.

Gilja, V., Nuyujukian, P., Chestek, C. A., Cunningham, J. P., Yu, B. M., Fan, J. M., et al. (2012). A high-performance neural prosthesis enabled by control algorithm design. *Nat. Neurosci.* 15, 1752–1757. doi: 10.1038/nn.3265

Golub, M. D., Yu, B. M., Schwartz, A. B., and Chase, S. M. (2014). Motor cortical control of movement speed with implications for brain-machine interface control. *J. Neurophysiol.* 112, 411–429. doi: 10.1152/jn.00391.2013

Hatsopoulos, N. G., and Amit, Y. (2012). Synthesizing complex movement fragment representations from motor cortical ensembles. *J. Physiol. Paris* 106, 112–119. doi: 10.1016/j.jphysparis.2011.09.003

Hatsopoulos, N. G., Xu, Q., and Amit, Y. (2007). Encoding of movement fragments in the motor cortex. *J. Neurosci.* 27, 5105–5114. doi: 10.1523/JNEUROSCI.3570-06.2007

Homer, M., Harrison, M., Black, M., Perge, J., Cash, S., Friehs, G., et al. (2013). "Mixing decoded cursor velocity and position from an offline Kalman filter improves cursor control in people with tetraplegia," in *2013 6th International IEEE/EMBS Conference on Neural Engineering (NER)* (San Diego, CA), 715–718.

Homer, M. L., Nurmikko, A. V., Donoghue, J. P., and Hochberg, L. R. (2013). Sensors and decoding for intracortical brain computer interfaces. *Annu. Rev. Biomed. Eng.* 15, 383–405. doi: 10.1146/annurev-bioeng-071910-124640

Hwang, E. J., Donchin, O., Smith, M. A., and Shadmehr, R. (2003). A gain-field encoding of limb position and velocity in the internal model of arm dynamics. *PLoS Biol.* 1:e25. doi: 10.1371/journal.pbio.0000025

Jones, K. E., Campbell, P. K., and Normann, R. A. (1992). A glass/silicon composite intracortical electrode array. *Ann. Biomed. Eng.* 20, 423–37. doi: 10.1007/BF02368134

Kao, J. C., Nuyujukian, P., Ryu, S. I., Churchland, M. M., Cunningham, J. P., and Shenoy, K. V. (2015). Single-trial dynamics of motor cortex and their applications to brain-machine interfaces. *Nat. Commun.* 6, 7759. doi: 10.1038/ncomms8759

Kao, J., Stavisky, S., Sussillo, D., Nuyujukian, P., and Shenoy, K. (2014). Information systems opportunities in brain-machine interface decoders. *Proc. IEEE* 102, 666–682. doi: 10.1109/JPROC.2014.2307357

Lakshmanan, K. C., Sadtler, P. T., Tyler-Kabara, E. C., Batista, A. P., and Yu, B. M. (2015). Extracting low-dimensional latent structure from time series in the presence of delays. *Neural Comput.* 27, 1825–1856. doi: 10.1162/NECO_a_00759

Kulkarni, J. E., and Paninski, L. (2007). Common-input models for multiple neural spike-train data. *Netw. Comput. Neural Syst.* 18, 375–407. doi: 10.1080/09548980701625173

Lawhern, V., Wu, W., Hatsopoulos, N., and Paninski, L. (2010). Population decoding of motor cortical activity using a generalized linear model with hidden states. *J. Neurosci. Methods* 189, 267–280. doi: 10.1016/j.jneumeth.2010.03.024

Li, Z. (2014). Decoding methods for neural prostheses: where have we reached? *Front. Syst. Neurosci.* 8:129. doi: 10.3389/fnsys.2014.00129

Li, Z., O'Doherty, J. E., Hanson, T. L., Lebedev, M. A., Henriquez, C. S., and Nicolelis, M. A. L. (2009). Unscented Kalman filter for brain-machine interfaces. *PLoS ONE* 4:e6243. doi: 10.1371/journal.pone.0006243

Macke, J. H., Buesing, L., Cunningham, J. P., Yu, B. M., Shenoy, K. V., and Sahani, M. (2011). "Empirical models of spiking in neural populations," in *Advances in Neural Information Processing Systems 24,* eds J. Shawe-Taylor, R. Zemel, P. Bartlett, F. Pereira, and K. Weinberger (Granada: Curran Associates, Inc.), 1350–1358.

Nuyujukian, P., Fan, J. M., Kao, J. C., Ryu, S. I., and Shenoy, K. V. (2015). A high-performance keyboard neural prosthesis enabled by task optimization. *IEEE Trans. Biomed. Eng.* 62, 21–29. doi: 10.1109/TBME.2014.2354697

Paninski, L., Fellows, M. R., Hatsopoulos, N. G., and Donoghue, J. P. (2004a). Spatiotemporal tuning of motor cortical neurons for hand position and velocity. *J. Neurophysiol.* 91, 515–532. doi: 10.1152/jn.00587.2002

Paninski, L., Shoham, S., Fellows, M. R., Hatsopoulos, N. G., and Donoghue, J. P. (2004b). Superlinear population encoding of dynamic hand trajectory in primary motor cortex. *J. Neurosci.* 24, 8551–8561. doi: 10.1523/JNEUROSCI.0919-04.2004

Park, I. M., Meister, M. L. R., Huk, A. C., and Pillow, J. W. (2014). Encoding and decoding in parietal cortex during sensorimotor decision-making. *Nat. Neurosci.* 17, 1395–403. doi: 10.1038/nn.3800

Petreska, B., Yu, B. M., Cunningham, J. P., Santhanam, G., Ryu, S. I., Shenoy, K. V., et al. (2011). "Dynamical segmentation of single trials from population neural data," in *Advances in Neural Information Processing Systems 24,* eds J. Shawe-Taylor, R. Zemel, P. Bartlett, F. Pereira, and K. Weinberger (Granada: Curran Associates, Inc.), 756–764.

Sachs, N. A., Ruiz-Torres, R., Perreault, E. J., and Miller, L. E. (2016). Brain-state classification and a dual-state decoder dramatically improve the control of cursor movement through a brain-machine interface. *J. Neural Eng.* 13:016009. doi: 10.1088/1741-2560/13/1/016009

Saleh, M., Takahashi, K., Amit, Y., and Hatsopoulos, N. G. (2010). Encoding of coordinated grasp trajectories in primary motor cortex. *J. Neurosci.* 30, 17079–17090. doi: 10.1523/JNEUROSCI.2558-10.2010

Saleh, M., Takahashi, K., and Hatsopoulos, N. G. (2012). Encoding of coordinated reach and grasp trajectories in primary motor cortex. *J. Neurosci.* 32, 1220–1232. doi: 10.1523/JNEUROSCI.2438-11.2012

Schwartz, A. B., Moran, D. W., and Reina, G. A. (2004). Differential representation of perception and action in the frontal cortex. *Science* 303, 380–383. doi: 10.1126/science.1087788

Sergio, L. E., and Kalaska, J. F. (2003). Systematic changes in motor cortex cell activity with arm posture during directional isometric force generation. *J. Neurophysiol.* 89, 212–228. doi: 10.1152/jn.00016.2002

Shanechi, M., and Carmena, J. (2013). "Optimal feedback-controlled point process decoder for adaptation and assisted training in brain-machine interfaces," in *2013, 6th International IEEE/EMBS Conference on, Neural Engineering (NER)* (San Diego, CA), 653–656.

Shanechi, M. M., Hu, R. C., Powers, M., Wornell, G. W., Brown, E. N., and Williams, Z. M. (2012). Neural population partitioning and a concurrent brain-machine interface for sequential motor function. *Nat. Neurosci.* 15, 1715–1722. doi: 10.1038/nn.3250

Shanechi, M. M., Wornell, G. W., Williams, Z. M., and Brown, E. N. (2013). Feedback-controlled parallel point process filter for estimation of goal-directed movements from neural signals. *Neural Syst. Rehabil. Eng. IEEE Trans.* 21, 129–140. doi: 10.1109/TNSRE.2012.2221743

Shanechi, M. M., Williams, Z. M., Wornell, G. W., Hu, R. C., Powers, M., and Brown, E. N. (2013). A real-time brain-machine interface combining motor target and trajectory intent using an optimal feedback control design. *PLoS ONE* 8:e59049. doi: 10.1371/journal.pone.0059049

Shumway, R. H., and Stoffer, D. S. (1982). An approach to time series smoothing and forecasting using the EM algorithm. *J. Time Series Anal.* 3, 253–264. doi: 10.1111/j.1467-9892.1982.tb00349.x

Truccolo, W., Eden, U. T., Fellows, M. R., Donoghue, J. P., and Brown, E. N. (2005). A point process framework for relating neural spiking activity to spiking history, neural ensemble, and extrinsic covariate effects. *J. Neurophysiol.* 93, 1074–1089. doi: 10.1152/jn.00697.2004

Truccolo, W., Hochberg, L. R., and Donoghue, J. P. (2010). Collective dynamics in human and monkey sensorimotor cortex: predicting single neuron spikes. *Nat. Neurosci.* 13, 105–111. doi: 10.1038/nn.2455

Velliste, M., Kennedy, S. D., Schwartz, A. B., Whitford, A. S., Sohn, J.-W., and McMorland, A. J. (2014). Motor cortical correlates of arm resting in the context of a reaching task and implications for prosthetic control. *J. Neurosci.* 34, 6011–6022. doi: 10.1523/JNEUROSCI.3520-13.2014

Wang, Y., and Principe, J. C. (2010). Instantaneous estimation of motor cortical neural encoding for online brain-machine interfaces. *J. Neural Eng.* 7:056010. doi: 10.1088/1741-2560/7/5/056010

Wang, Y., Sanchez, J. C., and Principe, J. C. (2007). "Information theoretical estimators of tuning depth and time delay for motor cortex neurons," in *Third International IEEE EMBS Conference on Neural Engineering* (Kohala), 502–505.

Willett, F. R., Suminski, A. J., Fagg, A. H., and Hatsopoulos, N. G. (2013). Improving brain-machine interface performance by decoding intended future movements. *J. Neural Eng.* 10:026011. doi: 10.1088/1741-2560/10/2/026011

Wu, W., Black, M. J., Mumford, D., Gao, Y., Bienenstock, E., and Donoghue, J. P. (2004). Modeling and decoding motor cortical activity using a switching Kalman filter. *IEEE Trans. Biomed. Eng.* 51, 933–942. doi: 10.1109/TBME.2004.826666

Wu, W., Gao, Y., Bienenstock, E., Donoghue, J. P., and Black, M. (2006). Bayesian population decoding of motor cortical activity using a Kalman filter. *Neural Comput.* 18, 80–118. doi: 10.1162/089976606774841585

Wu, W., Kulkarni, J. E., Hatsopoulos, N. G., and Paninski, L. (2009). Neural decoding of hand motion using a linear state-space model with hidden states. *IEEE Trans. Neural Syst. Rehabil. Eng.* 17, 370–378. doi: 10.1109/TNSRE.2009.2023307

Xu, K., Wang, Y., Wang, F., Liao, Y., Zhang, Q., Li, H., et al. (2014). Neural decoding using a parallel sequential Monte Carlo method on point processes with ensemble effect. *BioMed. Res. Int.* 2014:685492. doi: 10.1155/2014/685492

3

A Sliced Inverse Regression (SIR) Decoding the Forelimb Movement from Neuronal Spikes in the Rat Motor Cortex

Shih-Hung Yang [1†], You-Yin Chen [2†], Sheng-Huang Lin [3,4], Lun-De Liao [5,6], Henry Horng-Shing Lu [7], Ching-Fu Wang [2], Po-Chuan Chen [2], Yu-Chun Lo [8], Thanh Dat Phan [1], Hsiang-Ya Chao [9], Hui-Ching Lin [10], Hsin-Yi Lai [11] and Wei-Chen Huang [12]*

[1] Department of Mechanical and Computer Aided Engineering, Feng Chia University, Taichung, Taiwan, [2] Department of Biomedical Engineering, National Yang Ming University, Taipei, Taiwan, [3] Institute of Biomedical Engineering, College of Medicine, National Taiwan University, Taipei, Taiwan, [4] Department of Neurology, Tzu Chi General Hospital, Tzu Chi University, Hualien, Taiwan, [5] Institute of Biomedical Engineering and Nanomedicine, National Health Research Institutes, Zhunan Township, Taiwan, [6] Singapore Institute for Neurotechnology, National University of Singapore, Singapore, Singapore, [7] Institute of Statistics, National Chiao Tung University, Hsinchu, Taiwan, [8] The Ph.D. Program for Neural Regenerative Medicine, College of Medical Science and Technology, Taipei Medical University, Taipei, Taiwan, [9] Department of Electrical Engineering, National Taiwan University, Taipei, Taiwan, [10] Department and Institute of Physiology, School of Medicine, National Yang Ming University, Taipei, Taiwan, [11] Interdisciplinary Institute of Neuroscience and Technology, Qiushi Academy for Advanced Studies, Zhejiang University, Hangzhou, China, [12] Department of Materials Science and Engineering, Carnegie Mellon University, Pittsburgh, PA, USA

Edited by:
Timothée Levi,
University of Bordeaux 1, France

Reviewed by:
Alireza Mousavi,
Brunel University London, UK
Inaki Iturrate,
École Polytechnique Fédérale de Lausanne, Switzerland

***Correspondence:**
Hsin-Yi Lai
laihy@zju.edu.cn

† These authors have contributed equally to this work.

Several neural decoding algorithms have successfully converted brain signals into commands to control a computer cursor and prosthetic devices. A majority of decoding methods, such as population vector algorithms (PVA), optimal linear estimators (OLE), and neural networks (NN), are effective in predicting movement kinematics, including movement direction, speed and trajectory but usually require a large number of neurons to achieve desirable performance. This study proposed a novel decoding algorithm even with signals obtained from a smaller numbers of neurons. We adopted sliced inverse regression (SIR) to predict forelimb movement from single-unit activities recorded in the rat primary motor (M1) cortex in a water-reward lever-pressing task. SIR performed weighted principal component analysis (PCA) to achieve effective dimension reduction for nonlinear regression. To demonstrate the decoding performance, SIR was compared to PVA, OLE, and NN. Furthermore, PCA and sequential feature selection (SFS) which are popular feature selection techniques were implemented for comparison of feature selection effectiveness. Among SIR, PVA, OLE, PCA, SFS, and NN decoding methods, the trajectories predicted by SIR (with a root mean square error, RMSE, of 8.47 ± 1.32 mm) was closer to the actual trajectories compared with those predicted by PVA (30.41 ± 11.73 mm), OLE (20.17 ± 6.43 mm), PCA (19.13 ± 0.75 mm), SFS (22.75 ± 2.01 mm), and NN (16.75 ± 2.02 mm). The superiority of SIR was most obvious when the sample size of neurons was small. We concluded that SIR sorted the input data to obtain the effective transform matrices for movement prediction, making it a robust decoding method for conditions with sparse neuronal information.

Keywords: sliced inverse regression (SIR), neural decoding, forelimb movement prediction, neural networks (NN), principle component analysis (PCA)

INTRODUCTION

In order to improve daily life activities for paralyzed patients, the establishment of a non-muscular communication interface between brain neurons and machines has rapidly developed over the last two decades (Schwartz, 1993, 1994; Donoghue, 2002; Schwartz et al., 2006; Velliste et al., 2008). With assistance from stable generated brain-derived control signals incorporated with prosthetic devices and motor functions, paralyzed patients now possibly regain their ability to move a computer cursor (Kennedy et al., 2000; Hochberg et al., 2006; Gilja et al., 2015), control an anthropomorphic prosthetic arm (Wodlinger et al., 2015), and drive a prosthetic device (Hochberg et al., 2012; Collinger et al., 2013) through a brain-machine interface (BMI). One important challenge to BMI is how to design an appropriate neural decoder (Pohlmeyer et al., 2014). To address the challenge, previous studies have carefully utilized training paradigms that have been designed for a BMI decoder and controller. For brain-derived control signals, neural decoding is an indispensable technique that translates neuronal activities to physical states, such as the position of a foraging rat (Brown et al., 1998), arm movement (Ashe and Georgopoulos, 1994), movement speed (Moran and Schwartz, 1999), hand position (Paninski et al., 2004), and joint angular velocity (Reina et al., 2001).

A population vector algorithm (PVA), one method for decoding motor cortical activity, assumed that a neuron's firing rate is related to the velocity vector of movement. PVA categorizes each neuron's contribution into directional and distance information of the movement by a directional tuning function under uniform variance conditions (Georgopoulos et al., 1988). A previous study showed that PVA decoding could expose the visuomotor coordinate transformations between visual and motor information by processing masses of neuronal activities recorded from relative brain regions (Takeda and Funahashi, 2004; Watanabe et al., 2009). PVA presented superior performance in predicting hand path throughout reaching tasks (Schwartz, 1994). However, a uniformity constraint is usually not the case for real experiments, and the equality of the tuning function is variable because of the small amount of unit recordings in realistic applications (Schwartz et al., 2001). To compensate for the non-uniform preferred directions in the population of recorded neurons, an optimal linear estimator (OLE) was proposed to define the preferred direction of each neuron using the center of mass of the tuning function (Salinas and Abbott, 1994). Requiring large numbers of neurons with a temporal solution of 10–100 ms, PVA and OLE studies successfully predicted the kinematic parameters of a primate arm movement (Schwartz et al., 2001; Takeda and Funahashi, 2004; Watanabe et al., 2009).

A Bayesian decoder, a probabilistic decoding technique, could achieve accurate offline trajectory reconstructions by combing simple trajectory models (Yu et al., 2007). However, off-line reconstruction may not be suitable for online prosthesis control because the essential features of a real prosthesis are not acquired, and the system dynamics may vary because the user is in a closed loop. Furthermore, offline and online approaches resulted in different parameter choices for decoding algorithms (Cunningham et al., 2011). Therefore, the neural decoders and the motor prosthesis must be tested online even though online control experiments are more expensive both in terms of physical resources and time (Gilja et al., 2011). A recursive Bayesian decoder, i.e., a Kalman filter, was developed to decode the neural data recorded in the monkey motor and premotor cortex in response to goal-directed reaching movements (Shenoy and Carmena, 2014). It yielded high decoding performance and accurate trajectory prediction when the probability modeling assumptions were satisfied. For online purposes, a modified Kalman filter that transforms the acquired neural signals into a controller input was further designed for online cursor-control tasks and resulted in high performance in rhesus monkeys (Gilja et al., 2012). To adapt decoders to the dynamics of a prosthetic device and its environment, a likelihood gradient ascent and a self-recalibrating classifier were proposed to update decoder parameters during closed-loop BMI operation and normal use (Dangi et al., 2013; Bishop et al., 2014). Additionally, neural networks developed from probabilistic aspects were designed in an online setting (Sussillo et al., 2012) and in a real-time setting (Dethier et al., 2013).

A selection of cortical neurons, instead of all available neurons, used in the encoding process could improve the control performance of the neuroprosthetic system, such as robotic arms (Wahnoun et al., 2006). However, neural coding mechanisms evolve with time, individual experience, and the learning process (Nicolelis, 2001), i.e., the contribution from individual neurons may vary considerably from day to day (Carmena et al., 2003). It has been observed that neuronal activity for monkey was not as stable from day to day (Sadtler et al., 2014). The decoding algorithms which require previous day's observation of neural activity, such as PVA and OLE, may be affected by neuron's stability. For this reason, the selection of cortical neurons becomes an essential issue for the decoding processes, especially after continuous practice and learning. Furthermore, long-term inflammatory responses lead to a gradual decrease of recording quality and the eventual breakdown of the electrode's recording ability (Polikov et al., 2005; Schwartz et al., 2006). Losing neural signals over time will result in chronic coding failure. Thus, a decoder that has the capability to process recorded signals from a small number of neurons will become more important.

Sliced inverse regression (SIR) is a data-analytic tool that can effectively perform nonlinear regression based on a small number of inputs (Li, 1991). It divides the range of output variable into several intervals and partitions the input data into several slices according to the corresponding output value. Each slice consists of data with a similar contribution to output estimation. SIR then applies a weighted principal component analysis (PCA) to theses slice means of data to find effective dimension reduction directions for general and flexible setups. Each slice gains weight according to its contribution to output estimation. With a simple inverse regression model, SIR requires a low computational cost and retains reliably stable subspaces to extract primary information from noisy data with effective dimension reduction directions. Because of the good performance in dimension reduction and data de-noising, SIR has been widely applied to data-intensive marketing environments (Naik et al., 2000), dat classification (Dai et al., 2006; Wu, 2008), and medical images (Wu and Lu, 2007; Lu, 2008; Tu et al., 2015).

It has been known that the number of recorded neurons in rodents is less than primates in BMI applications. Owing to the abilities of processing small number of input variables and slicing data for inverse regression model, SIR was considered as a neural decoding algorithm to provide realistic behavior interpretation for brain-derived control tasks in this study. A surrogate driving task with lever-pressing was designed for evaluating the efficacy of the proposed decoding algorithm in predicting motor functions of rats. The signals of lever-pressing and the spike trains related to the intended forelimb movement trajectories were simultaneously acquired during the task. This study adopts SIR to predict intended forelimb movement trajectories according to the recorded neurons from primary motor (M1) cortex. We presented experimental validation of the proposed decoding system using the recorded neurons to predict forelimb movement. We demonstrated that the proposed SIR decoding algorithm can not only extract primary features from the small number of neurons but perform more accurate prediction of intended forelimb movement trajectories than PVA and OLE which usually require hundreds of neurons in primates.

MATERIALS AND METHODS

Animal Preparation

Four male Wistar rats weighing 250–300 g (BioLASCO Taiwan Co., Ltd., Taiwan) were used in this study. All rats were individually housed in a 12 h light-dark cycle (light from 7.00 to 19.00 h) at room temperature (22 ± 1°C) with access to food and water *ad libitum* in the experimental animal center of National Yang Ming University. All experiments were conducted according to standards established in the Guide for the Care and Use of Laboratory Animals, which has been approved by the Institutional Animal Care and Use Committee at the National Yang Ming University.

Animal Training and Behavioral Tasks

The rats were trained to use their right forelimb to press a lever to obtain the water reward for a week before electrode implantation, as shown in **Figure 1**. The rat was placed in the lab-designed Plexiglas testing box with a 15-cm tall lever above the floor on the left side (**Figure 1A**) and a water-feeder with a flow rate of 1 ml/time on the right side as shown in **Figure 1B** (Lin et al., 2016). **Figure 1C** shows the experimental setup where a rat was pressing lever for the water reward. Before achieving the successful lever-pressing training, all rats underwent water deprivation for 8 h per day. In this study, we have defined the criterion for the successful training was to consecutively repeat the lever-pressing and water-drinking for five times during daily 5-h sessions (9:00–14:00), for days at the most. Once the rats learned the association, they always kept the skilled concept (Lin et al., 2016).

Surgery and Electrophysiological Mapping

Animals were anesthetized with pentobarbital (50 mg/Kg, i.p.) and were placed on a stereotaxic apparatus (Model 900, Kopf Instruments, Tujunga, CA, USA). A 16-channel stainless microwire electrode array (diameter of 0.002 ft., California Fine Wire Co., Ltd, Grover Beach, CA, USA) was inserted vertically and was implanted into layer V of the M1 cortex (2–4 mm anterior and 2–4 mm left-lateral to bregma; 1.7 mm ventral to the cortical surface) by referring to a previous work . Here, a standard intracortical microstimulation (ICMS) technique was conducted to deduce maps of rat forelimb movement representations in the M1 cortex, which could help assess the functional integrity of M1 cortex and activate pyramidal cell fibers. ICMS delivered a 40 ms stimulus train with 0.2 ms square-wave monophasic cathodal pulses at 350 Hz to the electrodes (impedance: 200–400 kΩ at 1 kHz) by an isolated pulse stimulator at a rate of 1/s (Model 2100, A-M Systems Inc., Sequim, WA, USA). Because the intensity of the stimulating current depends on the distance between the neuron and the stimulating electrode, the threshold current intensity can be estimated by a strength-distance relationship as follows:

$$I = kr^2 + I_m \tag{1}$$

where $k = 1292\mu A/mm^2$ for direct activation, r is the distance, and $I_m = 1\mu A$. An implantation location of the electrode site was defined as valid when the rat forelimb was activated by ICMS with a current intensity less than $60\mu A$. Then, a stainless steel screw was secured to the skull over the cerebellum as a reference electrode. Finally, the microwire electrode array was secured in the skull using dental acrylic (Type 1 Class 1, Hygenic Corp., Akron, OH, USA) and was covered with a small amount of 2% agar. For a better recovery, all rats were given an analgesia (Buprenorphine/Buprenex, 0.05 mg/kg s.c.; Reckitt Benckiset Healthcare Ltd, Hull, UK) every 8–12 h for 3 days and antibiotic treatment (Ampicillin, 100 mg/kg s.c. twice daily; Bristol Myers Squibb, New York, NY, USA) for 7 days after surgery. Following a 1-week post-surgery recovery period, all implanted rats received the behavioral task to use their forelimb to press a lever for water reward. The forelimb movements in the rat were captured by a charge coupled device (CCD) camera (DFK 21F04, Imaging Source, Bremen, Germany) and the neuronal signals were recorded by a Multi-channel Acquisition Processor (MAP, Plexon Inc., Dallas, TX, USA) through a 16-channel stainless microwire electrode array implanted in the rat M1 cortex. The detailed data recordings for forelimb movement and neuronal signals are described in the Supplementary Note 1.

Trajectory Prediction Model

This study assumed that lever-pressing forelimb movement, which was considered to be a stereotyped movement, was performed at a nearly constant distance from the CCD in each trial, i.e., the distance did not vary dramatically. The recorded trajectory might consist of major forelimb movement and minor whole body movement which led to the coupling mechanism of two-dimensional forelimb movement (see Supplementary Note 1). The coupling mechanism resulted in a nonlinear relationship between neural activity and forelimb movement, and thus caused general linear regression to fail at forelimb movement prediction. SIR performs as a nonlinear regression since it can recover the most severe nonlinearity of the data by estimating effective dimensional reduction (*e.d.r.*) space (Li, 1991). Therefore, SIR

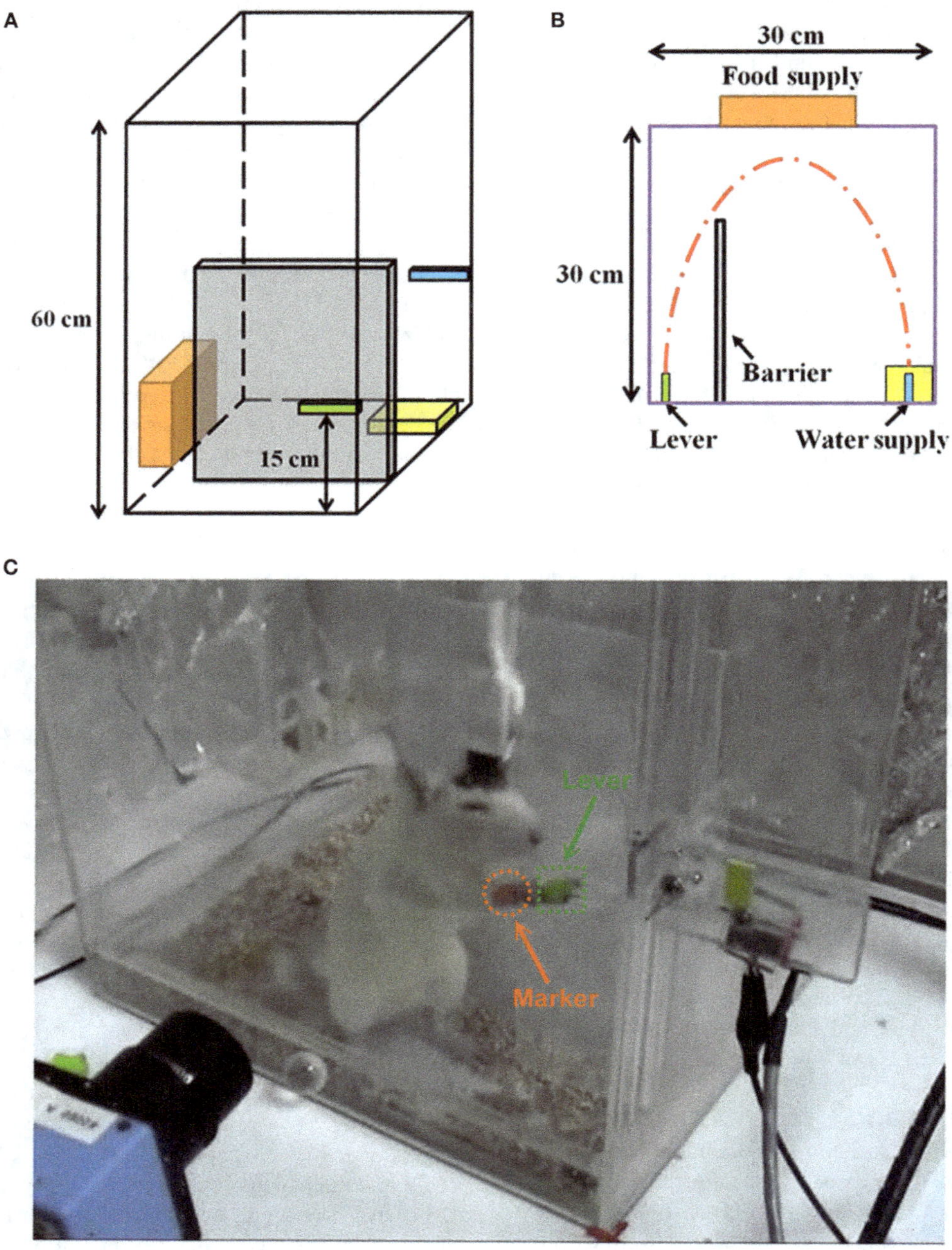

FIGURE 1 | Experimental setup and protocol. A perspective drawing **(A)** and vertical view **(B)** of the Plexiglas testing box. A lever is on the left side of the barrier and a water supply is on the right side. **(C)** A rat is using his right forelimb to press the lever to obtain a water reward. Simultaneously, his forelimb movement trajectory is videotaped by a camcorder approximately 25 cm away from the box, and the neuronal activities are recorded by the implanted electrode.

was adopted to predict the forelimb movement according to the neural activity in this study.

The two-dimensional trajectory movement vectors v_x and v_y in Cartesian coordinates are transformed into polar coordinates as follows:

$$v_r = \sqrt{v_x^2 + v_y^2} \tag{2}$$

$$v_\theta = \tan^{-1}\frac{v_y}{v_x} \tag{3}$$

where v_r and v_θ are the magnitude and direction, respectively.

The movement response g is assumed to be given by deterministic function f with additive noise ε, so that

$$g = f(\beta_1 z, ..., \beta_K z, \varepsilon) \quad (4$$

where g is v_r or v_θ, and z is firing rate data in $\mathbf{R}^p$. Here, β' are unknown linearly independent projection row vectors, an K is the sufficient number of β's. The p-dimensional variabl z is projected onto the K-dimensional space by functiona relationship f, where $p \geq K$. The combinations of β's are called the *e.d.r.* direction and the linear space produced by the β's are called *e.d.r.* space. The present study assumes the movement response g was predictable from K projected variables. To train the functional relationship f, a set of training data consisting of N training samples was prepared. According to the model assumptions, the centered inverse regression curve $E(z|g) - E(z)$ is included in the linear subspace, which is spanned by $\beta_k \Sigma_{zz}$ $(k = 1, \ldots, K)$, where Σ_{zz} represents the covariance matrix of z. SIR sorts and divides the whole data z into H intervals (slices) according to the g value. Each slice has almost equally number of observations. SIR then performs an eigenvalue decomposition of the weighted covariance matrix $\Sigma_{E(z|g)}$ with respect to Σ_{zz}. The weighted covariance matrix $\Sigma_{E(z|g)}$ is constructed as:

$$\Sigma_{E(z|g)} = \frac{\sum_{h=1}^{H} m_h(\bar{z}_h - \bar{z})(\bar{z}_h - \bar{z})'}{(N-1)} \tag{5}$$

where m_h denotes the size of each slice, $\bar{z}$ is the sample mean of z, and $\bar{z}_h$ is the sample mean of the hth slice. The *e.d.r.* directions could be estimated by solving the generalized eigen-problem:

$$\Sigma_{E(z|g)}\beta_j = \lambda_j \Sigma_{zz}\beta_j \tag{6}$$

where $j = 1, \ldots, p$ and $\lambda_1 \geq \lambda_2 \geq \cdots \geq \lambda_p$. Then, z was further projected onto the *e.d.r.* space by the first K *e.d.r.* directions as follows:

$$w = [\beta_1 z, ..., \beta_K z] \tag{7}$$

Then, a linear combination of w was performed to predict the forelimb movement. Although a linear combination approach was adopted, SIR was considered as a nonlinear regression since there is no linearity constraint on the prediction rules. Note that the user-specified parameters of SIR are only the number of slices H and the number of components K. It has been known that SIR can provide root n consistent estimates regardless of the choice of H. A previous study has demonstrated that the performance of SIR is less sensitive to the selection of H when H was set 5, 10, and 20 (Li, 1991). Furthermore, it has been found that the first component ($K = 1$) is close to the *e.d.r.* space. Therefore, H and K were set to 10 and one, respectively, in this study.

Time-Lags and Temporal Orders

In fact, the physical relationship between the neuronal signal and the forelimb movement may imply time-lags in the neuronal signal. Previous work indicates that a model that assumes that all cells exhibit the same time-lags is computationally simple (Wu et al., 2004). Then, the optimal time-lags could be found with an empirical setting for further improvement of the decoding task. A number of time-lags (0–5 time bins, at levels corresponding from 33 to 165 ms) were evaluated for trajectory prediction by SIR.

In addition to the time-lags, the temporal order of the input is another interesting factor for the decoding issue. The information at the nth time bin may have a relationship with that at the $(n-1)^{\text{th}}$ time bin. Hence, both current and previous neuronal activities are important and are considered as the inputs for prediction. Therefore, a tapped delay line model of neuronal activities is adopted in this study where a third-order model would consider the nth, $(n-1)^{\text{th}}$, and $(n-2)^{\text{th}}$ time bins as the input.

Performance Evaluation and Statistical Analysis

This study computed the root mean square error (RMSE) between true and predicted forelimb movements from movement start to endpoint in order to examine the performance of proposed decoding algorithm (Srinivasan and da Silva, 2011). The experimental trails were randomly split 70/30% into training and testing sets for each rat. Therefore, the performance of the proposed decoding algorithm on the testing set could be evaluated on each rat individually. A 10-fold cross validation was applied to avoid capitalization on chance (Efron and Tibshirani, 1994).

For statistical analysis, the predicted performance (RMSE) from 4 testing sets (145 trails; rat 74: 24 trials, rat 102: 18 trails, rat 106: 78 trails and rat 129: 25 trails) were represented as the mean ± standard error of mean (SEM). Two-way ANOVA was calculated using effects of time-lag (bin number 0, 1, 2, 3, 4, and 5) and temporal order (1-oder, 2-order, and 3-oder of time bins) as the independent variables in order to determine if there were any differences in the decoding ability based on which parameters was employed. *Post-hoc* comparisons were conducted using a Tukey HSD *post-hoc* test and the significance level was corrected to $*P < 0.002$ using a Bonferroni correction for the comparison of six time-lags and three temporal order. MATLAB (MathWorks, Natick, MA, USA) was used for all statistical analyses.

RESULTS

To evaluate the decoding performance of the proposed algorithm for trajectory prediction, the majority of decoding methods, PVA, OLE, and NN, were implemented for comparison. Furthermore, two popular feature selection techniques, PCA (Wold et al., 1987) and sequential feature selection (SFS) (Aha and Bankert, 1996), were implemented for comparison of feature selection effectiveness. Although PCA was developed as dimension reduction of feature space, it could be considered as a way to select features from principle components. Then a linear regression approach was adopted to perform regression whose inputs were the features provided by PCA and outputs were forelimb movements. The number of principal components was selected according to the variance of the reconstruction error (Valle et al., 1999). The same regression procedure was applied to SFS. A set of time-lags (0–5 time-lags) was carried out to observe the effect of different delays between the neuronal activity and the forelimb movement in each method. Furthermore, a set of experiments was conducted to evaluate the effect of various temporal orders (1–3 temporal orders) used in each decoding method. The experimental data were recorded from four rats where the number of trials and number of neurons per trial for each rat are shown in **Table 1**. The average number of successful trials was 45.9 ± 4.3, and the average number of recorded neurons was 21.2 ± 2.6 units. The period of each trial was 0.4–0.7 s before lever-pressing and 0.2–0.4 s after the lever-pressing.

Neuronal Signal Pattern during Behavior Task

The task timeline in **Figure 2** presents the sequential images of the lever-pressing (**Figure 2A**) and the corresponding spike trains (**Figure 2B**). The spike trains were acquired from five neurons related to right forelimb movement and were represented as the neuronal activity histogram with 33 ms time bins. The neuronal activities distinctly increased approximately 0.4 s before lever-pressing (**Figure 2B**), corresponding to the second image at 01:56.332 s (**Figure 2A**). The maximum value in the histogram appears approximately 0.1 s before the lever-pressing. The neuronal activity has a substantial reduction after the rat completes the lever-pressing and then it re-strengthens gradually because of the redundant movement off of the lever.

Effects of Different Time-Lags and Temporal Orders

Results of a particular test trial (Rat 106, 29 units, and 52th trial) were shown in **Figure 3** where the trajectories were reconstructed by six decoding methods with delay activity of four time-lags. The actual trajectory (blue solid line) was compared with the decoded trajectories by SIR (black dashed line), OLE (red dashed line), PVA (green dashed line), PCA (magenta dashed line), SFS (cyan dashed line), and NN (yellow dashed line) in **Figure 3**. Furthermore, the results of one and three temporal orders were conducted to demonstrate the advantage of SIR with the requisite amount of input data as shown in **Figures 3A,B**, respectively. In the one temporal order experiment, the trajectories reconstructed by PVA and OLE obviously deviated from the actual trajectory more than that reconstructed by SIR. PCA and SFS, which perform feature selection, could achieve accurate prediction in the previous time steps but did not predict the latter time steps well. Similarly, a NN, which has learning ability for nonlinear regression, could predict the trajectory well in the first few time steps, but it did not have robust prediction performance because of the random initialization of weights that leads to prediction error. As the temporal order increased to three, all methods had more accurate prediction compared to those of one temporal order. Overall, SIR shows the best performance among the other methods, especially when the decoding methods used less neuronal activity information.

TABLE 1 | Experimental data characteristics.

Subject	Number of trials	Number of neurons per trial
Rat 74	80	18 ± 3.1
Rat 102	60	11.1 ± 1.5
Rat 106	263	32.9 ± 5.2
Rat 129	83	24.9 ± 5.4

Figure 4 presents the effects of various time-lags and temporal orders in each method. **Figure 4A** shows the results of SIR where the smallest RMSE (8.47 ± 1.32 mm) was obtained by using four time-lags (132 ms) and one temporal order. It can be seen that SIR with four time-lags could achieve a significantly smaller RMSE than those with various time-lags [$F_{(5, 54)} = 4.22$, $^*P < 0.002$ with Two-way ANOVA with Bonferroni correction, $N = 145$]. Furthermore, the RMSE of SIR had no conspicuous variations among the three different temporal orders. As shown in **Figure 4B**, OLE achieved the smallest RMSE (17.22 ± 3.80 mm) by using four time-lags and three temporal orders. However, there was no significant enhancement of the prediction performance using OLE decoding with different time-lags and temporal orders. **Figure 4C** shows the results of PVA where the RMSE decreased as the number of temporal orders increases. PVA resulted in an average RMSE of 21.76 ± 8.11 mm when using one time-lag and three temporal orders. **Figures 4D,E** showed the results of PCA and SFS, respectively, where the features were selected via these two algorithms. PCA achieved a decreasing RMSE as the number of time-lags increased and obtained the smallest RMSE (19.13 ± 0.75 mm) when using four time-lags and three temporal orders. The results of SFS did not present a decreasing RMSE as the number of time-lags increased. SFS achieved the smallest RMSE (22.75 ± 2.01 mm) when using five time-lags and three temporal orders. **Figure 4F** shows the results of NN where the smallest RMSEs (16.75 ± 2.02 mm) were achieved by using three time-lags and two temporal orders. The RMSEs of NN did not present a regular trend as the number of time-lags increased. The forelimb movement predictions using OLE, PVA, PCA, SFS, and NN were not affected by either time-lag or temporal order. No significant interaction of time-lag and temporal order was found in the decoding methods of OLE, PVA, PCA, SFS, and NN in comparison to SIR. These results indicated that SIR outperformed other methods for trajectory prediction.

DISCUSSION

The main finding of this study is that a rat's forelimb movement could be successfully predicted and reconstructed using relatively few motor cortical neurons. In comparison with competing neural decoding algorithms including PVA, OLE, PCA, SFS, and NN, SIR presented an extremely superior RMSE in distance deviation between the reconstructed and real forelimb movement trajectories.

Previous studies indicated that neuronal activity discharged before the onset of the desired movement, such as the motor preparation period, and encoded behaviors (Chapin et al., 1999; Churchland et al., 2006). The kinematic parameters therefore were decoded and reconstructed with high accuracy using the neuronal activity before the onset of the movement. Hence in this study, SIR and the competing algorithms decoded the neuronal activities during the motor preparation period for reconstruction of introduced upcoming lever-pressing. The results showed that SIR, OLE, and PCA achieved optimal efficiency when using the neuronal activities that led to the onset of forelimb movement for 132 ms. PVA, SFS and NN each

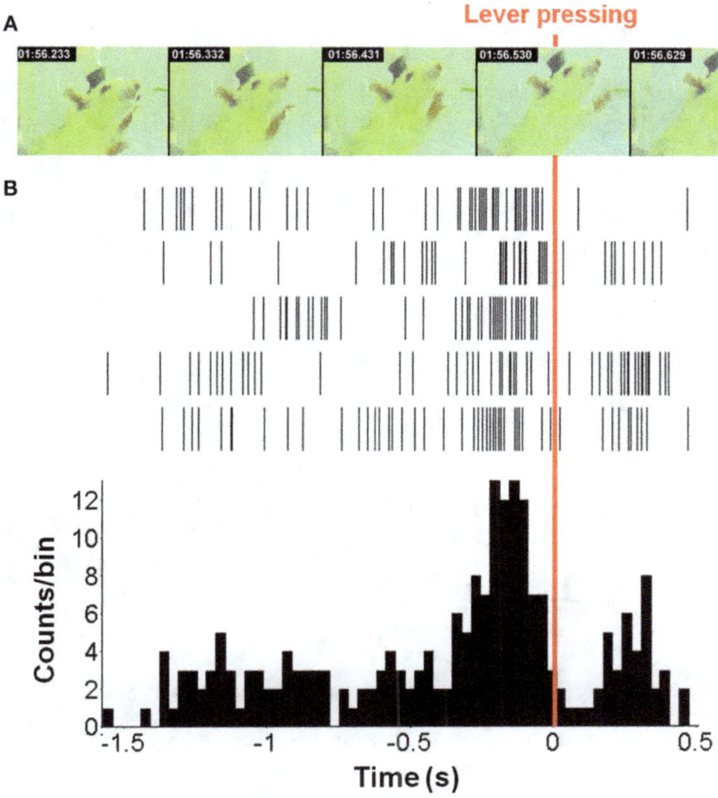

FIGURE 2 | One example of forelimb movement over time. (A) The movement video of forelimb movement. **(B)** The neuronal activities were recorded from five neurons during one movement displayed as spike trains and the neuronal activity histogram (a bin size of 33 ms). The red line indicated the moment when the rat presses down the lever with the right-forelimb. Moreover, our results showed that neuronal firing rates highly correlated with forelimb movement; >71% (41/57) neurons exhibited specific firing changes during movement used to discriminate directional pairs.

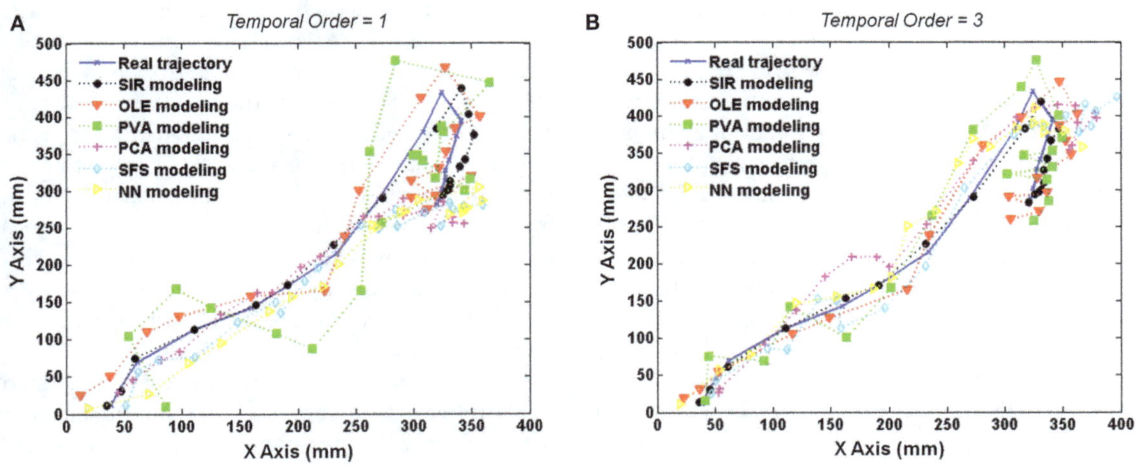

FIGURE 3 | Reconstructed trajectories of the test trial with the use of delayed activity with four time-lags (132 ms). The actual trajectory (blue solid line) and the trajectories predicted by SIR (black dashed line), OLE (red dashed line), PVA (green dashed line), PCA (magenta dashed line), SFS (cyan dashed line), and NN (yellow dashed line) are shown for an example trial using **(A)** one- and **(B)** three- temporal orders. The trajectory reconstructed by SIR is more accurate than the other methods.

chieved optimal efficiency by using the neuronal activities that ed to the onset of forelimb movement for 33, 165, and 99 ms, espectively. In **Figure 2B**, the peak of the spike train occurred at four time-lags, prior to the onset of lever-pressing. The neuronal firing rate then declined for 0.2 s as a result of the completion of motor command transmission. Because the rat performed an

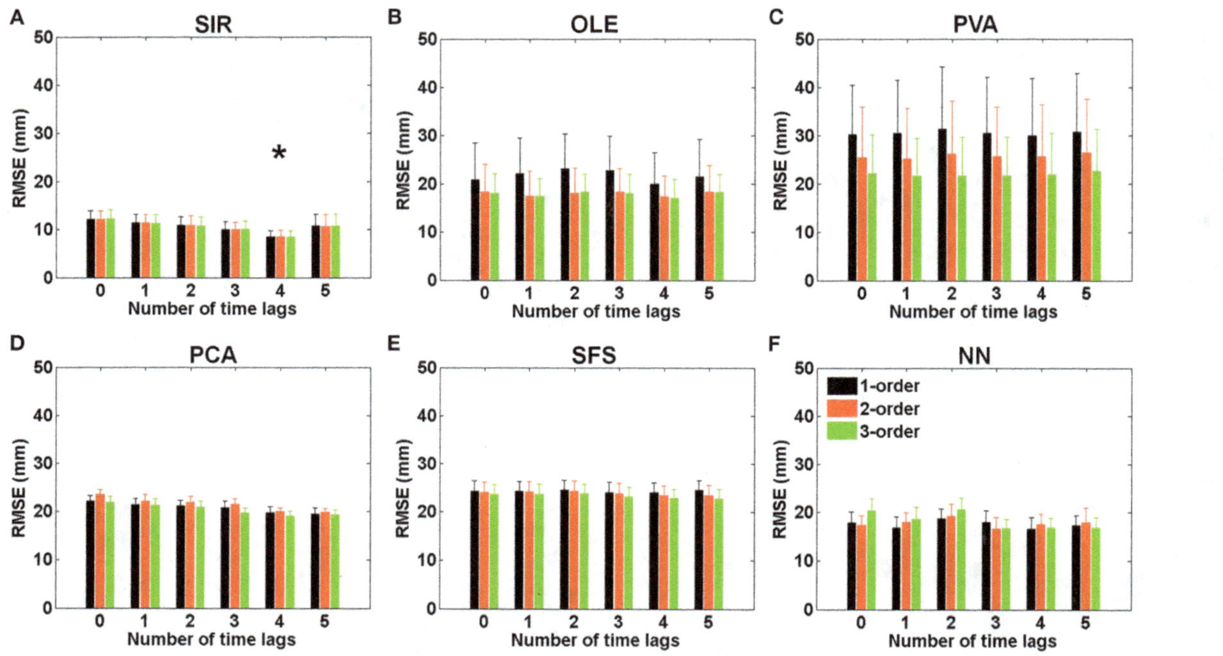

FIGURE 4 | RMSEs of (A) SIR, **(B)** OLE, **(C)** PVA, **(D)** PCA, **(E)** SFS, and **(F)** NN decoding methods plotted with various time-lags (33 ms/lag) and temporal orders. The error bars denote standard error of the mean (Mean ± SEM). The results showed that SIR is superior to the other methods for trajectory reconstruction. SIR is unaffected by temporal orders, and the best performance was achieved with four time-lags (132 ms). The symbol * indicates significant different means with $P < 0.002$ and analyzed by Bonferroni correction for multiple comparisons, $N = 145$. Mean ± SEM%.

unexpected forelimb swing, the neuronal firing rate increased again approximately 0.2 s after to the onset of lever-pressing.

The performance of cortical neural decoding hinged on the exploited information in chronically-recorded neuronal activities. Previous studies using PVA (Schwartz, 1994) and OLE (Salinas and Abbott, 1994) show that cortical neurons with known motor associations were chronically sampled and as many as possible were recorded. Because of the lack of a precise technique to target the modulated neurons that largely contributed to goal-directed behavior, PVA and OLE summed the weighted vectors across all neurons, performing a neuronal vote, to predict the kinematic parameters (Salinas and Abbott, 1994; Schwartz, 1994). A large number of electrodes and sample neurons (usually up to hundreds) was required for reconstruction of kinematic parameters with a high degree of accuracy (Chapin et al., 1999; Wessberg et al., 2000; Serruya et al., 2002; Taylor et al., 2002). However, the neuronal activity was not as stable from day to day (Sadtler et al., 2014). PVA and OLE may be affected by neuron's stability since they extract movement information from the selected cortical population.

In this study, we recorded only tens of neurons from rat M1 where the amount of recorded neurons was insufficient for PVA and OLE, which usually require hundreds of neurons to provide a robust neural decoding process (Takeda and Funahashi, 2004; Wahnoun et al., 2006). Compared to PVA and OLE, SIR can effectively achieve nonlinear regression from a small number of inputs (Li, 1991). SIR adopted a sliced regression framework with a sorting procedure to divide the neuronal dataset into several slices according to the sorted output variable value. Each slice contained neurons with a similar contribution to the introduced lever-pressing and was then modified by a weight. Slices containing neurons with tiny or even a null contribution to the lever-pressing may gain zero weight and can be removed from the decoding model. Multiplied by a proper weight according to the weighted PCA, a slice containing a few neurons with a high contribution presented a comparable influence on the prediction and reconstruction of the introduced lever-pressing to the neuronal vote from hundreds of neurons. Hence, SIR is able to perform forelimb prediction through a small number of neurons. On the other hand, dimensionality reduction technique factor analysis is usually adopted to describe population activity using low-dimensional set of factors and highlight feature of interest in data from a large number of recorded neurons (Sadtler et al., 2014). Although SIR could perform dimensionality reduction through weighted PCA, it preserved all recorded neurons and assigned weights to the slices according to their contribution. It learned forelimb movement prediction from whole neuronal activities regardless of neuron's stability across days. Thus, SIR was robust to uncertain variation of movements and neuronal activities across days due to the success of inverse regression and effective dimension reduction. Furthermore, using this SIR, the size of the neural decoding model topology was significantly reduced, burdened with data storage and reduced computational loading, indicating that efficiency in neural decoding in comparison to PVA and OLE was attainable. Compared to PCA and SFS, which perform feature selection and dimensional reduction, PCA could further project the data onto another space, which could lead to better reconstruction than SFS. However, SIR outperformed PCA and SFS because SIR clusters data into each slice accordin to the output values. NN performed better prediction than PCA and SFS because of its nonlinearity and learning ability. Nevertheless, NN did not result in a robust reconstruction because of the mechanism of random initialization and the existence of many local optima. These comparisons indicate that the neural decoding based on SIR with one temporal order presents a smaller RMSE in reconstructing limb movement than those based on PVA or OLE with three temporal orders and those based on feature selection and learning ability. It indicates that SIR can be a more suitable solution than the commonly used linear progression methods using the neuronal ensemble inputs to predict and reconstruct the introduced limb movement.

CONCLUSIONS

Neural decoding models that require hundreds of input variables, such as PVA and OLE, not only require considerable computation but also have detrimental effects in the decoding process because of errors in assigning neuronal spikes or non-stationary noise, especially for non-adaptive models. Reducing the neurons that may cause model over-fitting emerges as a significant neural decoding issue. However, with the help of the proposed approached based on SIR, researchers can predict and reconstruct the limb movement of interest with high accuracy using only tens of neurons in a single setting. Furthermore, SIR outperformed other feature selection methods, such as PCA and SFS because of its clustering ability. SIR further achieved more robust performance than NN because there is no random initialization and local optimization problems in SIR. By indexing the contribution of multiple cortical areas with different sizes, it has become feasible to ascertain the importance of selected areas for the motor commands. This will provide valuable insights for follow-up studies in the future.

ETHICS STATEMENT

The animal use protocol listed below has been reviewed and approved by the Institutional Animal Care and Use Committee (IACUC) at the National Yang Ming University. Protocol Title: Peripheral Nerve Prostheses: A Paradigm Shift in Restoring Dexterous Limb Function. IACUC Approval No: 1050622. Period of Protocol: Valid From: 08/01/2016. To: 07/31/2020. There is no endangered animal species involved in this study.

AUTHOR CONTRIBUTIONS

SY, HYL, and YC designed the project, organized the entire research. SL, LL conceived the experiments. CW, PC, TP, HCL, and WH conducted the experiments. HC, HHSL, and YL analyzed the results. SY, HYL, and YC wrote the manuscript. All authors discussed the results and reviewed on the manuscript.

ACKNOWLEDGMENTS

This research is financially supported by the Ministry of Science and Technology of the Republic of China, Taiwan under Contract numbers of MOST 105-2221-E-010-014-MY2, 103-2320-B-010-014-MY2, 103-2321-B-010-016, 102-2221-E-010-011-MY3, 103-2515-S-035-002 and National Health Research Institutes grant of BN-105-PP-15 and the Zhenjiang University, China under the Fund number of 181110- 193544B01/007.

REFERENCES

Aha, D. W., and Bankert, R. L. (1996). "A comparative evaluation of sequential feature selection algorithms," in *Learning from Data*, eds D. Fisher and H. J. Lenz (New York, NY: Springer-Verlag), 199–206.

Ashe, J., and Georgopoulos, A. P. (1994). Movement parameters and neural activity in motor cortex and area 5. *Cereb. Cortex* 4, 590–600. doi: 10.1093/cercor/4.6.590

Bishop, W., Chestek, C. C., Gilja, V., Nuyujukian, P., Foster, J. D., Ryu, S. I., et al. (2014). Self-recalibrating classifiers for intracortical brain–computer interfaces. *J. Neural Eng.* 11:026001. doi: 10.1088/1741-2560/11/2/026001

Brown, E. N., Frank, L. M., Tang, D., Quirk, M. C., and Wilson, M. A. (1998). A statistical paradigm for neural spike train decoding applied to position prediction from ensemble firing patterns of rat hippocampal place cells. *J. Neurosci.* 18, 7411–7425.

Carmena, J. M., Lebedev, M. A., Crist, R. E., O'Doherty, J. E., Santucci, D. M., Dimitrov, D. F., et al. (2003). Learning to control a brain-machine interface for reaching and grasping by primates. *PLoS Biol.* 1:e42. doi: 10.1371/journal.pbio.0000042

Chapin, J. K., Moxon, K. A., Markowitz, R. S., and Nicolelis, M. A. (1999). Real-time control of a robot arm using simultaneously recorded neurons in the motor cortex. *Nat. Neurosci.* 2, 664–670. doi: 10.1038/10223

Churchland, M. M., Santhanam, G., and Shenoy, K. V. (2006). Preparatory activity in premotor and motor cortex reflects the speed of the upcoming reach. *J. Neurophysiol.* 96, 3130–3146. doi: 10.1152/jn.00307.2006

Collinger, J. L., Wodlinger, B., Downey, J. E., Wang, W., Tyler-Kabara, E. C., Weber, D. J., et al. (2013). High-performance neuroprosthetic control by an individual with tetraplegia. *Lancet* 381, 557–564. doi: 10.1016/S0140-6736(12)61816-9

Cunningham, J. P., Nuyujukian, P., Gilja, V., Chestek, C. A., Ryu, S. I., and Shenoy, K. V. (2011). A closed-loop human simulator for investigating the role of feedback control in brain-machine interfaces. *J. Neurophysiol.* 105, 1932–1949. doi: 10.1152/jn.00503.2010

Dai, J. J., Lieu, L., and Rocke, D. (2006). Dimension reduction for classification with gene expression microarray data. *Stat. Appl. Genet. Mol. Biol.* 5, 6. doi: 10.2202/1544-6115.1147

Dangi, S., Gowda, S., and Carmena, J. M. (2013). Likelihood gradient ascent (LGA): a closed-loop decoder adaptation algorithm for brain-machine interfaces. *Conf. Proc. IEEE Eng. Med. Biol. Soc.* 2013, 2768–2771. doi: 10.1109/embc.2013.6610114

Dethier, J., Nuyujukian, P., Ryu, S. I., Shenoy, K. V., and Boahen, K. (2013). Design and validation of a real-time spiking-neural-network decoder for brain–machine interfaces. *J. Neural Eng.* 10:036008. doi: 10.1088/1741-2560/10/3/036008

Donoghue, J. P. (2002). Connecting cortex to machines: recent advances in brain interfaces. *Nat. Neurosci.* 5, 1085–1088. doi: 10.1038/nn947

Efron, B., and Tibshirani, R. J. (1994). *An Introduction to the Bootstrap*. New York, NY: CRC press.

Georgopoulos, A. P., Kettner, R. E., and Schwartz, A. B. (1988). Primate motor cortex and free arm movements to visual targets in three-dimensional space. II.

Coding of the direction of movement by a neuronal population. *J. Neurosci.* 8, 2928–2937.

Gilja, V., Chestek, C., Diester, I., Henderson, J. M., Deisseroth, K., and Shenoy, K. V. (2011). Challenges and opportunities for next-generation intracortically based neural prostheses. *IEEE Trans. Biomed. Eng.* 58, 1891–1899. doi: 10.1109/TBME.2011.2107553

Gilja, V., Nuyujukian, P., Chestek, C. A., Cunningham, J. P., Byron, M., Yu, B. M., et al. (2012). A high-performance neural prosthesis enabled by control algorithm design. *Nat. Neurosci.* 15, 1752–1757. doi: 10.1038/nn.3265

Gilja, V., Pandarinath, C., Blabe, C. H., Nuyujukian, P., Simeral, J. D., Sarma, A. A., et al. (2015). Clinical translation of a high-performance neural prosthesis. *Nat. Med.* 21, 1142–1145. doi: 10.1038/nm.3953

Hochberg, L. R., Bacher, D., Jarosiewicz, B., Masse, N. Y., Simeral, J. D., Vogel, J., et al. (2012). Reach and grasp by people with tetraplegia using a neurally controlled robotic arm. *Nature* 485, 372–375. doi: 10.1038/nature11076

Hochberg, L. R., Serruya, M. D., Friehs, G. M., Mukand, J. A., Saleh, M., Caplan, A. H., et al. (2006). Neuronal ensemble control of prosthetic devices by a human with tetraplegia. *Nature* 442, 164–171. doi: 10.1038/nature04970

Kennedy, P. R., Bakay, R. A. E., Moore, M. M., Adams, K., and Goldwaithe, J. (2000). Direct control of a computer from the human central nervous system. *IEEE Trans. Rehabil. Eng.* 8, 198–202. doi: 10.1109/86.847815

Li, K. C. (1991). Sliced inverse regression for dimension reduction. *J. Am. Stat. Assoc.* 86, 316–327. doi: 10.1080/01621459.1991.10475035

Lin, H. C., Pan, H. C., Lin, S. H., Lo, Y. C., Shen, E. T.-H., Liao, L.-D., et al. (2016). Central thalamic deep-brain stimulation alters striatal-thalamic connectivity in cognitive neural behavior. *Front. Neural Circuits.* 9:87. doi: 10.3389/fncir.2015.00087

Lu, H. H. S. (2008). "Reconstruction, visualization and analysis of medical images," in *Handbook of Computational Statistics: Vol. 3, Data Visualization,* eds C. H. W. Chen, W. Hardle, and A. Unwin (Berlin; Heidelberg: Springer-Verlag), 813–830.

Moran, D. W., and Schwartz, A. B. (1999). Motor cortical representation of speed and direction during reaching. *J. Neurophysiol.* 82, 2676–2692.

Naik, P. A., Hagerty, M. R., and Tsai, C. L. (2000). A new dimension reduction approach for data-rich marketing environments: sliced inverse regression. *J. Marketing. Res.* 37, 88–101. doi: 10.1509/jmkr.37.1.88.18715

Nicolelis, M. A. L. (2001). Actions from thoughts. *Nature* 409, 403–408. doi: 10.1038/35053191

Paninski, L., Fellows, M. R., Hatsopoulos, N. G., and Donoghue, J. P. (2004). Spatiotemporal tuning of motor cortical neurons for hand position and velocity. *J. Neurophysiol.* 91, 515–532. doi: 10.1152/jn.00587.2002

Pohlmeyer, E. A., Mahmoudi, B., Geng, S., Prins, N. W., and Sanchez, J. C. (2014). Using reinforcement learning to provide stable brain-machine interface control despite neural input reorganization. *PLoS ONE* 9:e87253. doi: 10.1371/journal.pone.0087253

Polikov, V. S., Tresco, P. A., and Reichert, W. M. (2005). Response of brain tissue to chronically implanted neural electrodes. *J. Neurosci. Methods* 148, 1–18. doi: 10.1016/j.jneumeth.2005.08.015

Reina, G. A., Moran, D. W., and Schwartz, A. B. (2001). On the relationship between joint angular velocity and motor cortical discharge during reaching. *J. Neurophysiol.* 85, 2576–2589.

Sadtler, P. T., Quick, K. M., Golub, M. D., Chase, S. M., Ryu, S. I., Tyler-Kabara, E. C., et al. (2014). Neural constraints on learning. *Nature* 512, 423–426. doi: 10.1038/nature13665

Salinas, E., and Abbott, L. F. (1994). Vector reconstruction from firing rates. *J. Comput. Neurosci.* 1, 89–107. doi: 10.1007/BF00962720

Schwartz, A. B. (1993). Motor cortical activity during drawing movements: population representation during sinusoid tracing. *J. Neurophysiol.* 70, 28–36.

Schwartz, A. B. (1994). Direct cortical representation of drawing. *Science* 265, 540–542. doi: 10.1126/science.8036499

Schwartz, A. B., Cui, X. T., Weber, D. J., and Moran, D. W. (2006). Brain-controlled interfaces: movement restoration with neural prosthetics. *Neuron* 52, 205–220. doi: 10.1016/j.neuron.2006.09.019

Schwartz, A. B., Taylor, D. M., and Tillery, S. I. (2001). Extraction algorithms for cortical control of arm prosthetics. *Curr. Opin. Neurobiol.* 11, 701–708. doi: 10.1016/S0959-4388(01)00272-0

Serruya, M. D., Hatsopoulos, N. G., Paninski, L., Fellows, M. R., and Donoghue, J. P. (2002). Brain-machine interface: instant neural control of a movement signal. *Nature* 416, 141–142. doi: 10.1038/416141a

Shenoy, K. V., and Carmena, J. M. (2014). Combining decoder design and neural adaptation in brain-machine interfaces. *Neuron* 84, 665–680. doi: 10.1016/j.neuron.2014.08.038

Srinivasan, L., and da Silva, M. (2011). Breaking the fixed-arrival-time restriction in reaching movements of neural prosthetic devices. *IEEE Trans. Biomed. Eng.* 58, 1555–1564. doi: 10.1109/TBME.2010.2101599

Sussillo, D., Nuyujukian, P., Fan, J. M., Kao, J. C., Stavisky, S. D., Ryu, S., et al. (2012). A recurrent neural network for closed-loop intracortical brain–machine interface decoders. *J. Neural Eng.* 9:026027. doi: 10.1088/1741-2560/9/2/026027

Takeda, K., and Funahashi, S. (2004). Population vector analysis of primate prefrontal activity during spatial working memory. *Cereb. Cortex* 14, 1328–1339. doi: 10.1093/cercor/bhh093

Taylor, D. M., Tillery, S. I., and Schwartz, A. B. (2002). Direct cortical control of 3D neuroprosthetic devices. *Science* 296, 1829–1832. doi: 10.1126/science.1070291

Tu, Y., Tan, A., Fu, Z., Hung, Y. S., Hu, L., and Zhang, Z. (2015). Supervised nonlinear dimension reduction of functional magnetic resonance imaging data using Sliced Inverse Regression. *Conf. Proc. IEEE Eng. Med. Biol. Soc.* 2015, 2641–2644. doi: 10.1109/EMBC.2015.7318934

Valle, S., Li, W., and Qin, S. J. (1999). Selection of the number of principal components: the variance of the reconstruction error criterion with a comparison to other methods. *Ind. Eng. Chem. Res.* 38, 4389–4401. doi: 10.1021/ie990110i

Velliste, M., Perel, S., Spalding, M. C., Whitford, A. S., and Schwartz, A. B. (2008). Cortical control of a prosthetic arm for self-feeding. *Nature* 453, 1098–1101. doi: 10.1038/nature06996

Wahnoun, R., He, J., and Helms-Tillery, S. I. (2006). Selection and parameterization of cortical neurons for neuroprosthetic control. *J. Neural Eng.* 3, 162–171. doi: 10.1088/1741-2560/3/2/010

Watanabe, Y., Takeda, K., and Funahashi, S. (2009). Population vector analysis of primate mediodorsal thalamic activity during oculomotor delayed-response performance. *Cereb. Cortex* 19, 1313–1321. doi: 10.1093/cercor/bhn170

Wessberg, J., Stambaugh, C. R., Kralik, J. D., Beck, P. D., Laubach, M., Chapin, J. K., et al. (2000). Real-time prediction of hand trajectory by ensembles of cortical neurons in primates. *Nature* 408, 361–365. doi: 10.1038/35042582

Wodlinger, B., Downey, J., Tyler-Kabara, E., Schwartz, A., Boninger, M., and Collinger, J. (2015). Ten-dimensional anthropomorphic arm control in a human brain—machine interface: difficulties, solutions, and limitations. *J. Neural Eng.* 12:016011. doi: 10.1088/1741-2560/12/1/016011

Wold, S., Esbensen, K., and Geladi, P. (1987). Principal component analysis. *Chemometr. Intell. Lab. Syst.* 2, 37–52. doi: 10.1016/0169-7439(87)80084-9

Wu, H. M. (2008). Kernel sliced inverse regression with applications to classification. *J. Comput. Graph. Stat.* 17, 590–610. doi: 10.1198/106186008X345161

Wu, H. M., and Lu, H. H. S. (2007). Iterative sliced inverse regression for segmentation of ultrasound and MR images. *Pattern Recognit.* 40, 3492–3502 doi: 10.1016/j.patcog.2007.04.019

Wu, W., Black, M. J., Mumford, D., Gao, Y., Bienenstock, E., and Donoghue J. P. (2004). Modeling and decoding motor cortical activity using a switching Kalman filter. *IEEE Trans. Biomed. Eng.* 51, 933–942 doi: 10.1109/TBME.2004.826666

Yu, B. M., Kemere, C., Santhanam, G., Afshar, A., Ryu, S. I., Meng, T. H., et al (2007). Mixture of trajectory models for neural decoding of goal-directed movements. *J. Neurophysiol.* 97, 3763–3780. doi: 10.1152/jn.00482.2006

4

An FPGA Platform for Real-Time Simulation of Spiking Neuronal Networks

Danilo Pani [1], Paolo Meloni [1], Giuseppe Tuveri [1], Francesca Palumbo [2], Paolo Massobrio [3] and Luigi Raffo [1]*

[1] EOLab - Microelectronics and Bioengineering Lab, Department of Electrical and Electronic Engineering, University of Cagliari, Cagliari, Italy, [2] Information Engineering Unit, PolComIng Department, University of Sassari, Sassari, Italy, [3] Neuroengineering and Bio-nano Technology Lab, Dibris, University of Genova, Genova, Italy

Edited by:
Eberhard E. Fetz, University of Washington, USA

Reviewed by:
Stavros Zanos, University of Washington Tacoma, USA
Francesco Leporati, University of Pavia, Italy

***Correspondence:**
Danilo Pani
pani@diee.unica.it

In the last years, the idea to dynamically interface biological neurons with artificial ones has become more and more urgent. The reason is essentially due to the design of innovative neuroprostheses where biological cell assemblies of the brain can be substituted by artificial ones. For closed-loop experiments with biological neuronal networks interfaced with *in silico* modeled networks, several technological challenges need to be faced, from the low-level interfacing between the living tissue and the computational model to the implementation of the latter in a suitable form for real-time processing. Field programmable gate arrays (FPGAs) can improve flexibility when simple neuronal models are required, obtaining good accuracy, real-time performance, and the possibility to create a hybrid system without any custom hardware, just programming the hardware to achieve the required functionality. In this paper, this possibility is explored presenting a modular and efficient FPGA design of an *in silico* spiking neural network exploiting the Izhikevich model. The proposed system, prototypically implemented on a Xilinx Virtex 6 device, is able to simulate a fully connected network counting up to 1,440 neurons, in real-time, at a sampling rate of 10 kHz, which is reasonable for small to medium scale extra-cellular closed-loop experiments.

Keywords: FPGA, fixed-point, neural simulator, closed-loop hardware accelerator, real-time

1. INTRODUCTION

In the past decades, spiking neuronal networks (SNN) progressively acquired relevance due to possibility to exploit them in several application scenarios. Typical artificial intelligence applications take advantage of the learning capabilities of SNN for classifiers and autonomous controls. Nevertheless, SNN represent a powerful instrument in neuroscience, allowing to simulate living neuronal assemblies trying to gather from the characteristics of a fitted artificial neuronal network clues on the properties of the living tissue (Bonifazi et al., 2013). From this perspective, it is interesting not only the accurate evaluation of the single neuron behavior but, primarily, the study of the emergent properties of the neuronal assembly dynamics (van Pelt et al., 2004). This can be studied through intracellular recordings (single cell models, by voltage clamp techniques) or extracellular recordings (*in vitro* cultures of neurons or cortical implants, by Micro-Electrode Arrays MEAs). In this case, the adoption of SNN software simulators (Brette et al., 2007) is widely accepted and the use of such tools is cumbersome only when it is required to simulate very large networks, because of the explosion of the computational cost and, in turn, of the processing time.

This limitation fostered the research toward the development of hardware accelerators able to carry out such simulations in a shorter time (Cheung et al., 2016), possibly comparable to the time scales of a real evolving neuronal network, in order to enable complex simulations otherwise impossible. With the advancements of the technology, it is possible to look at such hardware simulators as enabling tools for new neuroscience experiments. For instance, closed-loop electrophysiological systems are characterized by the tight interaction between the living neuronal tissue and a controlling electronic unit able to interact with it through sensing and stimulation (Le Masson et al., 2002). Compared to open-loop experiments, closed-loop ones enable the study of both the input and output side of the neuronal assembly at the same time (Rolston et al., 2010). The largest part of systems for closed-loop experiments aim to study this aspect by means of an integration between a sensing interface, simple and abstracted computational models and a stimulation interface. Examples of interfacing with muscles for real-time control have been already presented in the literature (Zbrzeski et al., 2016). One aspect, paving the way to the development of neuroprostheses, would be the direct interface of a population of living neurons to an artificial SNN in order to evaluate the capability of the living system to interact with the simulated one (Bonifazi et al., 2013). This poses severe constraints on the hardware implementation of the SNN, particularly for everything concerning the timing, which is no more a matter of performance improvement over a simple PC implementation, but an aspect connected to the feasibility of the neuroprosthetic approach. Examples of the integration of living neurons into artificial SNN can be already found in the literature (Nawrot et al., 2003).

The goal of this paper is to describe and validate a scalable and modular hardware architecture to simulate the dynamics generated by biologically-plausible synthetic neuronal assemblies in real-time. This architecture was completely manually coded and optimized in Verilog Hardware Description Language (HDL) for a single Field Programmable Gate Array (FPGA) chip, thus it can be easily adopted in any lab for small-to-medium SNN sizes. This, along with a fixed-point implementation of the Izhikevich (IZ) neuronal model (Izhikevich, 2003), confers to the architecture a considerable real-time performance up to 0.1 ms, joined to a programmable delay that can be reduced down to such bound. The architecture is parametric in the number of neurons that can be simulated, with limitations imposed by the hardware only in terms of the possibility of fitting the SNN in a commercial FPGA. The long-term goal of the so developed architecture is to bi-directionally interface the SNN with a biological one. Three different experimental scenarios can be envisioned:

- Use the real-time SNN on FPGA as a stimulator. The signals generated by the SNN can be used to trigger the spontaneous dynamics of the biological networks. Different stimulation protocols can be imagined, for example using the onset of the network bursts, or the frequency of the bursts. The possibility to generate a "natural" stimulation can be used to shift the dynamical states of the biological network;
- Connect in a bi-directional way the real-time SNN on FPGA and a biological neuronal assembly. Although closed-loop stimulation experiments have been already performed (Wagenaar et al., 2005; Wallach et al., 2011), such works have the intrinsically drawback to use "artificial stimulation," i.e., stereotyped stimuli delivered by a controlled stimulator. By means of the proposed architecture, it becomes feasible to deliver stimuli modulated by the intrinsic dynamics.
- In the long term, the real-time SNN could be used as a tool to replace a damaged biological network. In fact, in the last years, researchers started to develop a new family of prostheses applied to the central nervous system (neuroprostheses). As an example, Berger et al. developed a hippocampal prosthesis improving memory function in behaving rats (Berger et al., 2011, 2012).

2. MATERIALS AND METHODS

SNNs are more realistic than the conventional neural networks for neuroscientific simulations, taking into consideration not only the neuronal and the synaptic state, but also the concept of time into their operating model. Artificial neurons' firing activity is determined by the evolution of their membrane potential, which follows the model equations. Not only different models produce different firing behaviors, but within the same model it is often possible to tune the parameters so that the artificial neuron is able to reproduce different firing patterns proper of specific cells.

The architecture is currently based on the implementation of the IZ neuronal model (Izhikevich, 2003), which is characterized by an excellent trade-off between computational complexity and biological accuracy, being able to reproduce several spiking patterns by simply tuning its parameters. The proposed version of the architecture implements the model in fixed-point arithmetic, in order to primarily reduce the memory requirements (known to be a limiting factor for hardware SNN) and the latency of the mathematical computations. The architecture is conceived to be a customizable framework, where the neuronal model can be easily replaced while preserving the global structure, and the same holds for the synapses. The main features pursued in the design phase were the low latency, with a real-time timing constraint of 0.1 ms and a programmable delay between firing activity and its reflection on the network activity. In turn, this means that the output sample rate is 10 ksample/s, which is adequate for closed-loop experimental systems.

2.1. Izhikevich Spiking Model

The simple model of spiking neurons proposed by Izhikevich (2003) is composed of a two-dimensional system of ordinary differential equations.

$$\frac{dv}{dt} = 0.04v^2 + 5v + 140 - u - I \quad (1$$

$$\frac{du}{dt} = a(bv - u) \quad (2$$

v is the *membrane potential* of the neuron and it is modeled according to Equation (1), whereas Equation (2) provides the dynamic of u that is the *membrane recovery variable.* The term I, in Equation (1), is meant to take into account the contribution of the connected nodes to the considered neuron, by means of the sum of the synaptic currents or injected dc-currents. When a spike is fired, meaning v has reached its threshold, the following resetting condition is applied:

$$v \geq v_{th} \Rightarrow \begin{cases} v = c; \\ u = u + d \end{cases} \tag{3}$$

Both the membrane potential and the membrane recovery value are normally measured in mV. The IZ spiking model is capable to reproduce several different firing patterns, 20 in the original article (e.g., chattering, fast spiking, low-threshold spiking, etc.) but others are being studied, representing the known types of neo-cortical and thalamic neurons, by tuning the a, b, c, and d dimensionless parameters:

- a represents the time scale of the recovery variable u. Smaller values result in slower recovery;
- b represents the sensitivity of the recovery variable u to possible sub-threshold fluctuations of the membrane potential v. Larger values indicate v and u are strongly coupled, resulting in possible sub-threshold oscillations and low-threshold spiking dynamics;
- c is the after-spike reset value of v;
- d determines the after-spike reset value of u.

2.2. Hardware Spiking Neural Network

In this work, a SNN hardware emulation platform, based on the IZ spiking neuron model, was developed and tested. **Figure 1** depicts an overview of the system. The entire neural network is subdivided in *units*, which are the building blocks of the SNN. Each unit produces, according to the IZ spiking neuron model, a sub-set of spikes whose occurrence is stored in the binary *spike register*, which keeps trace of the whole network spiking activity. It is composed of one bit per neuron under emulation. The bit corresponding to a neuron is set high when the neuron has fired a spike. The chosen simulation paradigm is synchronous (or clock-driven), meaning that all neurons are updated at every simulation step, regardless of the spiking activity (Brette et al., 2007). From a macroscopic point of view, each simulation cycle is composed as follows:

1. The *units* process their subset of neurons. They receive the content of the *spike register*, accounting for the whole SNN firing activity (the architectures assumes a fully-connected structure) and, according to the IZ model, they determine which neurons within their subset should fire;
2. The firing activities estimated by the *units* are grouped together by a dedicated *concatenation logic* and sent back to the *spike register*;
3. The *spike register* is updated and represents the updated status of the overall SNN.

Additional details, regarding what happens within the *units* in each simulation step, are provided hereafter in Section 2.2.2. It is worth to notice now that the architecture gives the possibility to set at design time a delay for the spike propagation, exploiting a register chain strategy. The firing activity is propagated back to the units with a delay of several (up to ten) emulation cycles, to mimic a physiological delay of up to 1 ms between firing and its reflection on the network status.

Figure 1 depicts an exemplary instance of the proposed platform, parameterized in order to emulate a network of 256 neurons only for the sake of clarity. The platform instance integrates four *units*, emulating 64 IZ neurons each. According to the signal activity of all the 256 neurons, each unit generates up to 64 spikes per simulation cycle. The four different 64-bit signals, representing each *unit*'s neuronal activity, are concatenated to create a single 256-bit signal and fed back to the *spike register*.

2.2.1. Units: Architectural Overview

The *units* are responsible for the implementation of Equations (1) and (2) and for estimating the firing activity of the subset of neurons assigned to each of them. Equations (1) and (2) represent two derivatives and they have been implemented in hardware exploiting the finite-difference method, which is a numerical method for solving differential equations by approximating them with finite differences, as specified hereafter:

$$\frac{v(k+1) - v(k)}{h} = 0.04v(k)^2 + 5v(k) + 140 - u(k) - I \tag{4}$$

$$\frac{u(k+1) - u(k)}{h} = a(bv(k) - u(k)) \tag{5}$$

The smaller is h (i.e., the time interval between k and $k+1$) the better Equations (4) and (5), respectively, approximate Equations (1) and (2). In the current implementation, h is fixed to 0.1 ms, which turned out to be an excellent compromise between the approximation quality and the overall processing time required to update the status of the entire SNN. Furthermore, such a delta-cycle is compatible with hybrid closed-loop experiments.

Each *unit*, as depicted on the right hand side of **Figure 1**, is composed of a *Neuron Section* and of a *Synapses Section*, which are, respectively, responsible for computing the overall neuronal activity of the considered *unit* and for determining, for each neuron, the synaptic current (I) that has to be subtracted in Equation (4).

Figure 2 presents an overview of the *Neuron Section* of each single *unit* block. Equations (4) and (5) are physically computed by the *Izhikevich* block, which receives $v(k)$ and $u(k)$ values from the *u-v RAM* block, a, b, c, and d parameters from the *parameter RAM* block, and finally I from the *Synapses Section*. The interactions with the *u-v RAM* and *parameter RAM* blocks, and the synchronization with the *Synapses Section* are controlled by a dedicated Finite State Machine (FSM), the *neuron FSM*. The *neuron FSM* also masters the execution of the different phases of the *Izhikevich* block itself. In terms of library IP module, the latter includes only a multicycle multiplier, which is re-used for all the

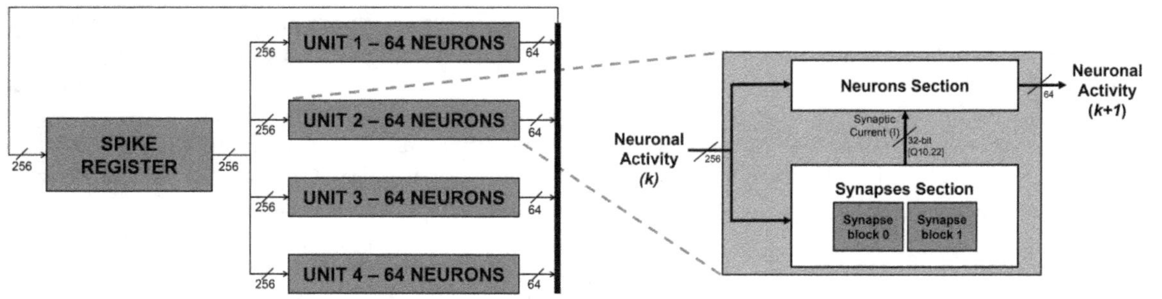

FIGURE 1 | SNN block diagram (on the left) and *unit* block high-level architecture (on the right). The numbers reported in the scheme are referred to an exemplary embodiment with a fully connected network of 256 neurons.

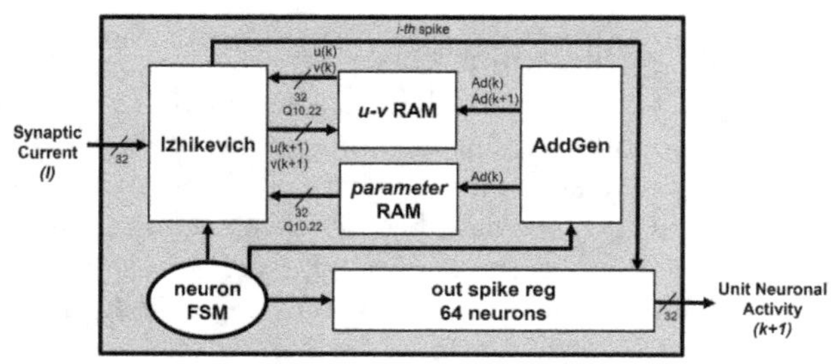

FIGURE 2 | *Unit*—Overview of the *Neuron Section*.

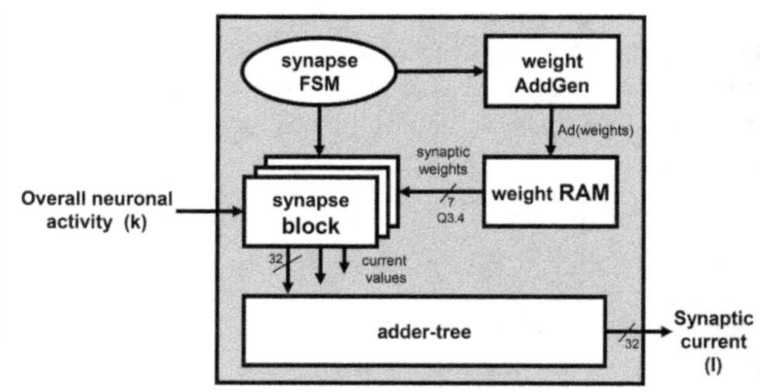

FIGURE 3 | *Unit*—Overview of the *Synapses Section*.

multiplications in Equations (4) and (5); all the other modules are HDL-coded. In this way, it is possible to save as much hardware resources as possible (by re-using the same processing element rather than instantiating several of them in parallel) and to maintain the operating frequency high (by pipelining the operations and, in turn, breaking down the critical path). The *Izhikevich* block processes one neuron at a time; its output is written on the *out_spike_reg* module, which contains the spikes of all the neurons within the given *unit*. The output of the *Neuron Section* is the updated *unit*'s contribution to the firing activity of the SNN, to be sent to the *concatenation logic*.

The *Synapses Section* is depicted in the block diagram in **Figure 3**. The figure shows how the synaptic current is computed on the basis of the overall firing activity (i.e., the content of the *spike register*). It computes the weighted sum of the contribution of the pre-synaptic neurons, connected to the processed one by means of the synapses. Only the synaptic weights associated to those neurons that fired (having a 1 in the corresponding bit of the *spike register*) are eventually accumulated. The *synaptic weights* are provided by the *weight RAM* block. The contribution of each connected neuron is computed by a set of *synapses* blocks, placed in parallel to speed-up the computation since all the incoming neuronal activity has to be scanned to determine the *synaptic weights* associated to the pre-synaptic neurons that fired and, accordingly, retrieve and accumulate them. As an example, the Synapse section of the platform instance in **Figure 1** integrates 2 *synapse* blocks per unit, which means that each synapse block calculates the contribution given by 128 neurons. The outputs of the of *synapses* blocks are summed-up by an *adder-tree* module to produce *I*. The interactions with the *weight RAM* block and the synchronization with the *Neuron Section* block is controlled by a dedicated FSM, the *synapses-FSM*.

2.2.2. Units: Execution Flow

The execution flow of a *unit* within each simulation cycle can be described as follows:

1. According to the currently processed neuron index, the *neuron_FSM* drives the *AddGen* block, which generates the address $Ad(k)$, used to correctly fetch the current $v(k)$ and $u(k)$ values from the *u-v RAM* block, and to retrieve the IZ parameters from the *parameter RAM* blocks;
2. The *Izhikevich* block executes all the multiplications in Equations (4) and (5), the *Synapses Section* determines *I*. The *neuron_FSM* and the *synapses_FSM* exchange control signals to synchronize these two operations, in order to make sure that the proper value *I* is added in Equation (4);
3. As already said, *I* is a weighted sum, depending on the firing neurons. The *synapses_FSM* drives the *weight AddGen* to correctly access the *weight RAM* that stores the *synaptic weights* of the excitatory and inhibitory neurons. *Ad(weights)* represents the addresses of the memory locations storing the weights associated to the excitatory and inhibitory neuron connected to the currently processed one;

4. As soon as Equations (4) and (5) are completely computed, the *neuron_FSM* enables the possibility of writing back the updated $v(k+1)$ and $u(k+1)$ values on the *u-v RAM* block. The *neuron_FSM* drives the *AddGen* to access the correct location of address $Ad(k+1)$;
5. The final processing stage of each single neuron requires to evaluate whether the spike has to be fired or not. The result is written in the correct position (determined by the currently processed neuron index) of the *out_spike_reg* module.

All these steps are iterated for all the neurons within the *unit* to evaluate and update the status of the SNN. The *neuron_FSM* is responsible of verifying whether all the neurons have been processed or not and to notify that the content of the *out_spike_reg* module is the complete updated *unit* contribution to the neuronal activity that can be sent to the *concatenation logic*. Depending on the initialization data stored within *u-v RAM*, *parameter RAM* and *weight RAM* blocks, the platform is thus capable to fully emulate an arbitrary IZ-based SNN.

A fixed-point arithmetic was adopted in order to pursue a fast execution and a compact hardware implementation. A Q3.4 format for the weights (meaning that a Q format is adopted, with the decimal point virtually placed in order to leave 4 bits for the fractional portion over a 7-bit word) was chosen. Such a solution limits the dynamic ranges of the weights with minor effects, since the low values are usually swamped by the thalamic noise term (Thomas and Luk, 2009). A more conservative approach based on the worst-case design, which is unrealistic in this kind of applications, would limit the SNN weights in the $[-1,1)$ range. Multiple iterations with NEST have been performed in order to define a format for the weights able to reduce the memory requirements while preserving an acceptable accuracy. In order to avoid intermediate overflows, the synapse accumulators use 8 bits for the input and 32 bits for the outputs, and they are connected to a 32-bit in 32-bit out adder tree. Both of them are implemented using DSP48 macros for Xilinx FPGAs. In order to be able to represent the IZ parameters with enough flexibility to accommodate typical models and novel ones, a Q10.22 was selected for them. The internal computations rely on pre-computed constants, full-precision adders and multi-cycle multipliers with 32-bit in and 32-bit out.

The communication between the emulation platform and the external environment is required, at start-up, to allow the pre-loading of neuron parameters and synaptic weights for the target experiment inside the system memory blocks. Moreover, emulation results must be sent to the external environment, respecting real-time constraints, during the whole emulation time. Communication interface can be implemented in different ways, exploiting the connectivity in modern FPGA boards and the support offered by design tools and programming environment. Two different communication methods were tested. Firstly, the exploitation of a host general-purpose processor, implemented as a Microblaze soft-core on the FPGA, was evaluated. The processor reads system memories as part of its memory map and communicates with the external environment using an Ethernet connection or a serial UART connection. This solution is easy to implement and provides comfortable coupling of the processor with the emulator, but presents the disadvantage to occupy resources on the reconfigurable device, which may be exploited to emulate more neurons. A second solution is available using FPGA families that embed hard-wired processing cores, such as the Xilinx Zynq family, which includes chips integrating programmable logic and an ARM dual-core processor. In this case, an interface between the emulator, implemented on the programmable logic, and the ARM sub-system, serving as a host processor and providing adequate connectivity with the external environment, was developed. A master IP that loads ad stores data on the DDR memory connected to the ARM when needed, exploiting a set of 4 AXI-based interfaces natively available in the system, was mapped on the FPGA. Each of the AXI interfaces provides a bandwidth of 64 bits/cycle and can be clocked at more than 100 MHz, thus is sufficient to sustain output of emulation results in real time.

However, it must be noticed that the best interface implementation depends on the target FPGA device and on the target use-case of the emulation infrastructure.

2.3. Platform Validation Approach

2.3.1. Architectural Performance Evaluation Metrics

The main performance evaluation metrics for the FPGA-based hardware implementation are timing and resource utilization. In the proposed parametric architecture, both depend on the chosen configuration of the architectural parameters, i.e., the number of units, the number of synapse modules inside each unit and the precision of the weights. The main limiting factors for the proposed implementation are the DSP modules and the RAM modules. In particular:

- DSP48E1 modules are computing modules used to implement *add* and *multiply* operations,
- RAMB36E1 modules are RAM memory macros that are used to implement memories in the architecture. Each macro has a capacity of 32 kbits.

Obviously, the amount of DSP48E1 and RAMB36E1 needed to implement a given configuration is dependent on the architectural parameters. Performance will be evaluated considering the maximum number of neurons that can be emulated in real-time by the platform. This metric is impacted by several factors:

- real-time constraint,
- architectural parameters,
- implementation level variables (such as working clock frequency and FPGA resource utilization).

In order to provide an overview of the involved dependencies, a model, described in Section 3.1.1, was developed to enable a prospective user to estimate the achievable performance level for different architectural configurations implemented on different FPGA devices.

2.3.2. Accuracy Evaluation Tests

To evaluate the accuracy of the simulations performed using the hardware SNN, a sister-pool of simulations with NEST (Gewaltig and Diesmann, 2007) was performed. In this way, it was possible to compare the so generated dynamics of the *in silico* (implemented in NEST) and hardware SNN, by means of well-known statistics commonly used to analyze the electrophysiological activity of large-scale neuronal networks coupled to Micro-Electrode Arrays (MEAs). For this purpose, an heterogeneous 1,024-neuron SNN with 768 excitatory neurons and 256 inhibitory ones was simulated. Compared to the maximum number of synthesizable neurons, which is 1,440, this number represents the highest power of two and was chosen in order to simplify the scripting operations required, for the time being, to load the parameters and analyze the results. The DC input currents are 4 pA and 2 pA for excitatory and inhibitory neurons respectively; neurons are randomly connected, according to the generation model in Izhikevich (2003); inhibitory neurons have stronger synaptic connections. In order to achieve heterogeneity (i.e., to model all exctitatory and inhibitory neurons), excitatory cells are generated by assigning $(a_i, b_i) = (0.02, 0.2)$ and $(c_i, d_i) = (-65, 8) + (15, -6)r_i^2$, where r_i is a random variable uniformly distributed on the interval [0,1] and i is the neuron index; similarly, each inhibitory cell has $(a_1, b_i) = (0.02, 0.25) + (0.08, -0.05)r_i^2$ and $(c_i, d_i) = (-65, 2)$.

To characterize the spiking activity, the mean firing rate (MFR) of the network and the inter spike interval distribution (ISI) of the excitatory and inhibitory neurons were evaluated. The bursting activity was characterized by means of the mean bursting rate (MBR), burst duration (BD), and inter-burst interval (IBI). Bursts have been detected by using the algorithm devised in Chiappalone et al. (2005). Detected bursts are sequences of spikes having an ISI smaller than a reference value (set at 100 ms in our simulations), and containing at least a minimum number of consecutive spikes (set at 4 spikes in our simulations). Briefly, MFR and MBR are the number of detected spikes per second and bursts per minute falling in a temporal window equal to the duration of the simulation. The ISI and IBI distributions are the probability density functions of time intervals between consecutive spikes and bursts, respectively (Dayan and Abbott, 2001). Finally, BD is the duration of the detected bursts.

In addition to the aforementioned statistics, the spike jitter between *in silico* and hardware simulations was also computed. Practically speaking, by considering as reference the spike timing of the NEST simulations, the temporal distance of the correspondent spikes generated by the hardware SNN was computed.

The evolution of the membrane potential of a single neuron in the two simulations were also compared. Five experiments were performed, in order to analyze the dynamics of the u and v potentials of a modeled neuron respectively belonging to three classes of excitatory neurons (*regular spiking*, *intrinsically bursting* and *chattering*), and two classes of inhibitory neurons (*fast spiking* and *low-threshold spiking*). The a, b, c and d parameters belonging to each of the emulated cortical cells are reported in **Table 1**; the DC input current, for all considered experiments, is 4 pA. The behavior of the emulated potentials with the potential evolution obtained by means of a NEST simulation were also compared.

TABLE 1 | Parameters of emulated cortical cells.

	a	*b*	*c*	*d*
RS	0.02	0.2	−65	8
IB	0.02	0.2	−55	4
CH	0.02	0.2	−50	2
FS	0.1	0.2	−65	2
LTS			−65	2

3. RESULTS

In this section, the results have been organized in order to discuss at first those related to the architectural performance evaluation and then those related to the accuracy evaluation.

3.1. Architectural Performance Evaluation Results

As previously mentioned, the assessment of the quality of the proposed architecture has to consider two main factors: resource utilization and emulation performance. In the following, a description of the timing and utilization figures that can be obtained changing the architectural parameters is presented. At first, the timing characteristics of the architectures modules and their dependence on the selected architectural parameters have to be studied, within the real-time constraints imposed by the emulation. Then, the optimal parameter values have to be selected, in the range actually allowed by the target FPGA device. All the presented results were verified after synthesis and implementation.

3.1.1. Timing Characteristics of the Architecture Modules

The real-time constraint to be considered defines how often the SNN output has to be evaluated. Such a metric, in emulation/simulation, is usually referred to as *delta cycle*. A delta cycle of 0.1 ms was chosen, aiming to be aligned with an acceptable sampling frequency in the scope of acquisition of signals from neuronal cultures with MEAs. The same time step was also used for the differential equations discretization hereafter called T_{sample}.

As mentioned, hardware structures are reused to emulate more neurons, in the considered interval. Emulation of one neuron occupies the set of hardware resources in a unit for a determined number of cycles, that will be indicated in the following as T_{emu}. In order to relate T_{emu} with the real time constraint, actual clock period, which will be indicated as T_{clock} in the following, used as synchronization reference within the architecture, shall be considered. In synchronous digital systems, the minimum clock period that can be chosen by the designer is related to the propagation delay of gates implementing combinational paths through the design. In the design of the proposed architecture, a pipeline strategy that allows the minimum clock period to be independent from the architectural configuration was adopted. After the implementation on the FPGA device, the optimal value of T_{clock}

can be evaluated to be 10 ns, corresponding to a maximum working frequency of 100 MHz. It was proven that this frequency can be substained for all the configurations that may fit in mid-to-high end FPGA devices, confirming the scalability of the proposed architecture.

Thus, the number of cycles available for emulation in a sampling interval is $T_{sample}/T_{clock} = 10,000$ cycles. Then, each unit can emulate N_{neu} neurons in one sampling interval, where

$$N_{neu} = 10,000/T_{emu} \tag{6}$$

T_{emu} is a function of the number of synapse modules N_{syn} and units N_{units} in the system. The number of cycles needed to emulate one neuron is the sum of two contributions:

$$T_{emu} = log_2(N_{syn}) + \frac{N_{neu} * N_{units}}{2 * N_{syn}} \tag{7}$$

Equation (7) was constructed on the basis of the architectural details of the hardware modules and its validity was verified in HDL-level simulation and after actual implementation. The first contribution is an offset related to the pipeline stages in the adder tree connecting the output of the synapse modules. The second contribution is the actual time needed to perform all the accumulation routine that calculates the synaptic current. In the second term the numerator represents the total number of neurons constituting the emulated network, the denominator takes into account that the workload related with the accumulation is divided between the synapse modules in the unit, each one performing two *add* operations per cycle.

Combining Equations (6) and (7), N_{neu} can be calculated solving a quadratic equation, on the basis of the architectural parameters N_{syn} and units N_{units}. Eventually, the total number of neurons that can be emulated is $N_{units} \times N_{neu}$.

Figure 4 shows how such numbers changes varying N_{units} for two different N_{syn} values. The selection of the values for such parameters is obviously bounded by the amount of resources available on the target FPGA device, as it will be described in more detail in the next section.

Even though the proposed architecture was not conceived as an hardware accelerator but, rather, a real-time simulation platform enabling closed-loop neurophysiological experiments, a rough performance comparison against NEST can be presented. When running on a PC platform (Ubuntu 14.04 LTS, kernel 3.13.0-96-generic, CPU Intel(R) Core(TM) i7-2600 CPU @ 3.40 GHz, 16 GB RAM), the emulation of the SNN with 1,440 neurons requires 6.3 s per second of simulation, which is far from the real-time achieved with the proposed architecture. Nevertheless, caution should be used when considering such numbers for a fair comparison. In fact, on one hand, the architecture is clocked in order to provide the real-time performance at 10 kHz, so the actual processing time is masked by the (higher) wall time, which is 0.1 ms. The same does not hold for a PC-based emulation, not constrained by such a wall time. On the other hand, different programming styles, programming language and

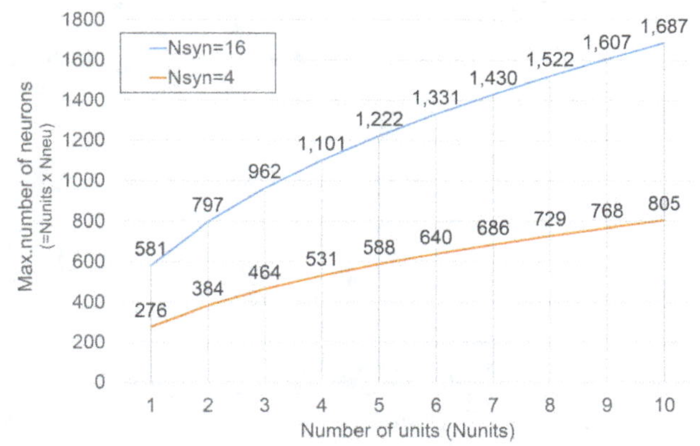

FIGURE 4 | Dependence of the maximum number of neurons under emulation on N_{units}. Results corresponding to two different numbers of synapse modules (N_{syn}) are presented.

processor architectures can lead to very different results, so the performance of PC-based solutions could seem unfairly poor.

3.1.2. Hardware Resources Utilization

In order to select the correct architectural parameters, it is mandatory to understand their impact on the utilization of hardware resources in the target device.

When the architectural configuration is known, it is very easy to estimate the number of required DSP48E1 macros. Each unit uses 3 macros for each synapse module and 3 macros to implement the hardware emulating the neuronal dynamic. The amount of RAM macros depends on the total number of neurons to be emulated. The architecture should embed enough storage to contain all the weights determining the contribution of each pre-synaptic neuron to the post-synaptic ones. Such neurons are prospectively disjointed, thus the utilization of resources roughly has a quadratic dependence on the size of the emulated network. Some memory resources are also needed to store neurons' parameters and evolving values of u and v.

Considering the number of resources in commercial FPGA devices, for typical network configurations, the limiting factor is very often the availability of Block RAM (BRAM). This can sometimes limit the maximum number of neurons under emulation with respect to the possibilities offered by a given parameterization of the unit hardware modules.

In order to provide an estimation of the architecture configurations that may be implemented on mid-range commercial devices, the hardware-related features of a configuration featuring 8 units, each one embedding 16 synapse modules, realized on a XC6VLX240T Xilinx device, are presented. **Table 2** represents the device utilization summary.

This configuration occupies 94% of the BRAM resources and 53% of the DSP48 macros, and it is capable of emulating 1,440 neurons in real time.

Although power consumption analysis has been considered as a secondary development objective in this work, it is worth to provide some hints about the power-related features of the proposed architecture. Obviously, the actual power dissipation

TABLE 2 | Summary of the resource utilization.

	Used	Available	Utilization
Registers	48,502	301,440	16%
LUTs	55,884	150,720	37%
RAMB36E1	392	416	94%
DSP48E1	408	768	53%

Target FPGA platform is a XC6VLX240T Xilinx device. The implemented architecture features 8 units with 16 synapses, capable of emulating 1,440 neurons.

depends on the specific FPGA platform selected as target. However, for every FPGA device considered in the developed experiments, a significant part of the power consumption is related to the usually called quiescent power, that is the power dissipation of the idle FPGA, before its actual programming. Moreover, recent all-programmable FPGA-based SoCs as Xilinx Zynq devices, present an additional contribution to the power consumption due to the host processing system implemented on the chip. Finally, in general FPGA chips are mounted on a development board including several peripherals, that add a further contribution unrelated with the emulation. Thus, the power consumption of the overall emulation platform is weakly dependent on the number of emulated neurons. As an example, in the presented experiments, a Xilinx ZC706 evaluation board featuring a XC7Z045 FPGA chip dissipates 6.8 W in the idle state and 8.5 W when executing emulation with a 100 MHz clock on the FPGA.

3.2. Accuracy Evaluation Results

3.2.1. Single Neuron Membrane Potential Evolution

From the single neuron simulation, it is possible to find a good adherence between the membrane potential evolution as obtained with the proposed architecture and with NEST. This is clearly visible in **Figures 5**, **6** respectively for low-threshold spiking and fast spiking neurons.

3.2.2. Fully-Connected Network of N Neurons

By using the NEST simulations as reference, the electrophysiological patterns of activity generated by the hardware implementation of the network model were compared. The raster plot of **Figure 7A** shows the spike timing of the 1024 neurons of the network. The first neurons (id: from 1 to 768) are excitatory whereas the others inhibitory (id: from 769 to 1024). Blue circles and red crosses are representative for the two simulation approaches (i.e., software, blue circles, and hardware red crosses, respectively). The zoom of **Figure 7A** shows a good overlap of the spike timing. In order to quantify such a jitter, the histogram (bin width equal to 0.3 ms) of the occurrences relative to the excitatory (**Figure 7B**) and inhibitory neurons (**Figure 7C**) was plotted. Both the neuronal populations display significant jitters less than 2.0 ms in 95% of the occurrences, indicating good performances of the hardware implementation of the network model.

In terms of number of spikes, both the software and hardware models present the same number of spikes, as the plot of the MFR displays (**Figure 8**). MFR values are 1.05 $\pm$ 0.48 spikes/s

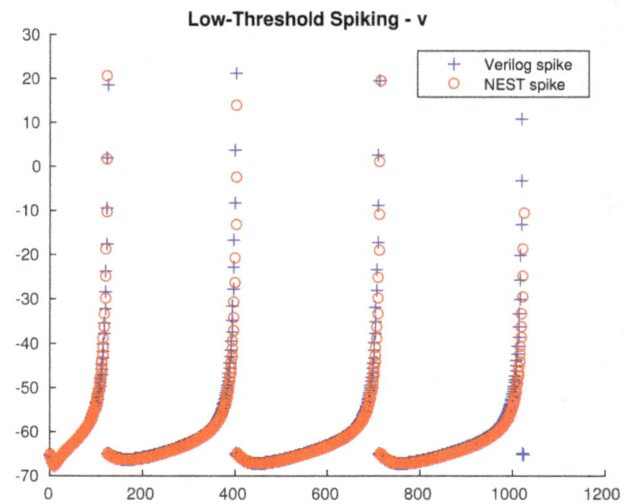

FIGURE 5 | Low-threshold spiking neuron membrane potential evolution: comparison between the proposed architecture and NEST.

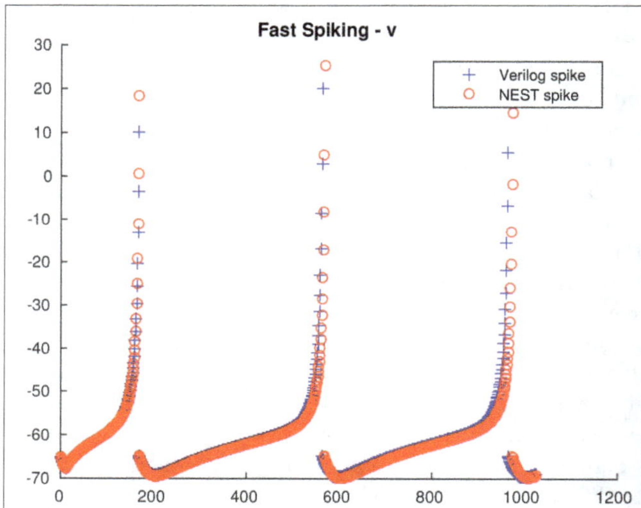

FIGURE 6 | Fast spiking neuron membrane potential evolution: comparison between the proposed architecture and NEST.

in the NEST implementation of the model and 1.05 $\pm$ 0.49 spikes/s in the hardware one. Finally, the ISI distributions (**Figure 8B**, relative to the software, and **Figure 8C**, relative to the hardware model) by splitting the contribution of the excitatory (red line) and inhibitory (black line) populations, were evaluated. This analysis shows a good agreement of the two model implementations too. Qualitatively, the shape of the ISI distributions is similar, as well as the temporal position of the peaks of the curves (hardware: 2.54 ms vs. software: 2.50 ms).

The validation of the hardware network model was carried out by comparing the bursting dynamics (**Figure 9**). **Figures 9A–C** compare the values of MBR, BD, and IBI of the software and hardware network models, respectively. Although slight differences can be appreciated, such differences are no

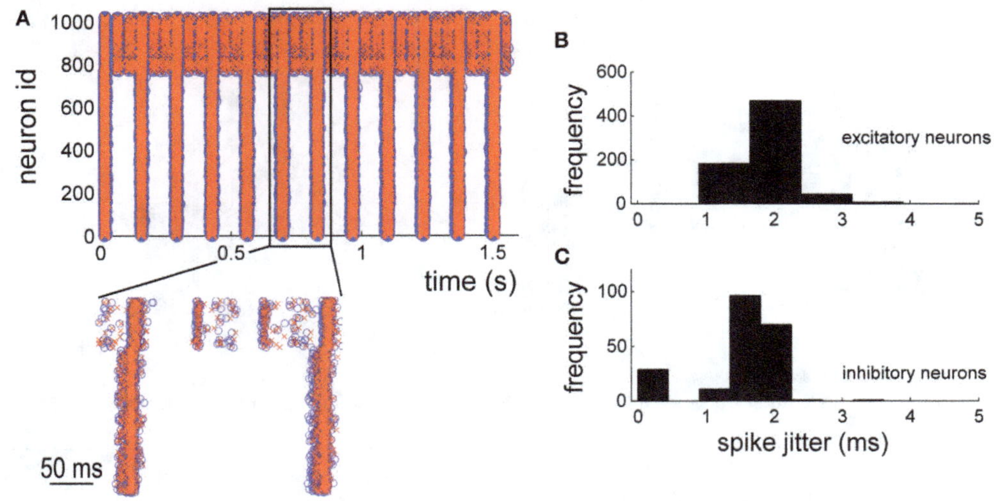

FIGURE 7 | Network dynamics characterization: comparison between *in silico* and hardware simulations. (A) 2 s of electrophysiological activity. Blue circles and red crosses are representative for software and hardware approaches, respectively. **(B,C)** histograms of the spike jitter between software and hardware simulations evaluated for excitatory **(B)** and inhibitory **(C)** neurons of the network.

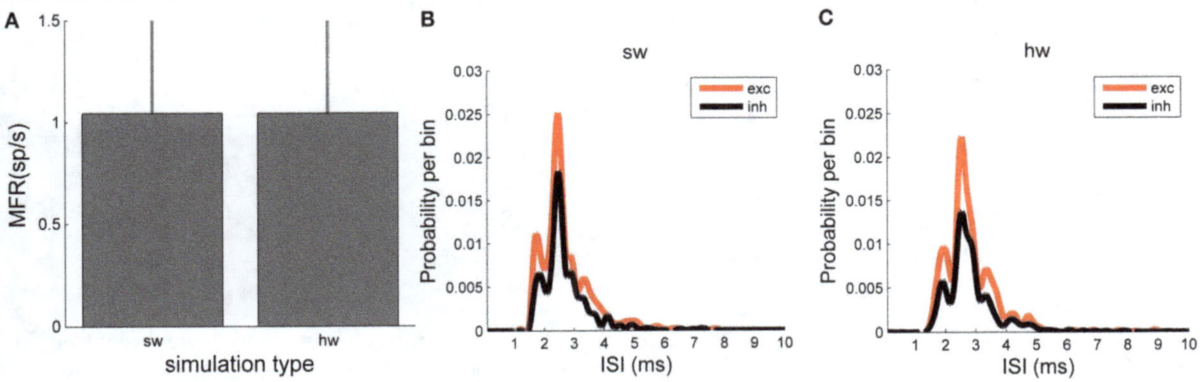

FIGURE 8 | Network dynamics characterization: comparison between *in silico* and hardware simulations. (A) MFR (evaluated over the whole neurons of the network). No statistical difference can be evaluated between the two simulation approaches. **(B,C)** ISI distributions of the excitatory (red) and inhibitory (black) neuronal populations evaluated in the *in silico* **(B)** and in hardware **(C)** simulations: the same trend can be appreciated.

tatistically significant (p >0.05, Mann-Whitney, non-parametric est). The Mann-Whitney U-test was chosen since the analysed lata do not follow a normal distribution, as revealed by neans of the Kolmogorov-Smirnov normality test applied to hem. The chosen p-value is assumed to be adequate for the onsidered problem. Similar considerations can be done for the BI distributions (**Figures 9B,C**).

4. DISCUSSION

everal SNN hardware accelerators have been proposed so far n the scientific literature (Maguire et al., 2007). They usually ry to overcome the performance limitations of purely software imulators (Brette et al., 2007) such as NEURON (Carnevale nd Hines, 2006), NEST (Gewaltig and Diesmann, 2007), BRIAN Goodman and Brette, 2009), etc., widely accepted as research ools in the community of computational neuroscience. However, unless an explicitly parallel processing is pursued on large multiprocessors high performance computing platforms, such simulators suffer the intrinsic scalability limits of the underlying object of the simulation, becoming soon too slow for large-scale networks of biologically plausible neuronal models (Rast et al., 2010). In this section, a discussion about some relevant architectures for SNN simulations in hardware is presented, along with a comparison with the proposed approach. Among the different architectures cited hereafter, those aimed to simulate a large number of neurons have been grouped in **Table 3**, reporting the main relevant data gathered from the cited sources. Without being exhaustive, this table enables a quick overview of the present state of the art.

Despite the purely software solutions present the aforementioned limitations, it is obvious that they usually pursue simplicity (in the creation and simulation of the model), precision (typically double) and flexibility (the

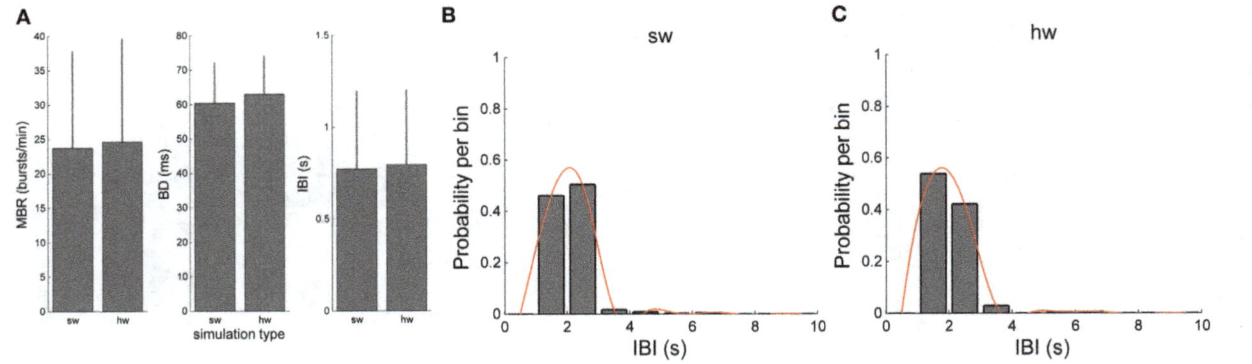

FIGURE 9 | Comparison of the bursting features of the simulated network by using the software and hardware approaches: (A) MBR, BD, IBI **(B,C)** IBI distributions.

TABLE 3 | Summary of some relevant state-of-the-art architectures for SNN hardware simulation.

Work	Target	♯Neurons/core	♯Cores	Model	♯Synapses/neuron	Time res
Schoenauer et al., 1998	ASIC	$\approx 30{,}000$	4	LIF	> 30	$< 1\,ms$
Wolff et al., 1999	Multi-processor (DSP)	$\approx 1{,}900$	64	Eckhorn	> 30	$> 1\,ms$
Glackin et al., 2005	FPGA	$\approx 1{,}000$	4	I&F	$\approx 500\,k$	–
Upegui et al., 2005	FPGA	30	1	custom	30	$\approx 1\,ms$
Pearson et al., 2007	FPGA	112	10	LIF	$\approx 912/112$	$0.5\,ms$
Cassidy et al., 2007	FPGA	51	1	LIF	128	320 ns
Jin et al., 2008	Multi-processor (ARM)	1,000	1	IZ	100	$1\,ms$
Thomas and Luk, 2009	FPGA	1,024	1	IZ	1,024	$10\,\mu s$
Ambroise et al., 2013	FPGA	117	1	IZ	117	$1\,ms$
Cheung et al., 2016	FPGA	$> 98{,}000$	6	IZ	$1{,}000 - 10{,}000$	$1\,ms$

For some architectures flexible enough to implement several neuronal models, only one published result is reported.

possibility to change topology, parameters, synaptic model, neuron model, etc.). For this reason, when moving toward the hardware simulation systems, it is obvious the success of architectures exploiting efficient signal processing cores, such as ParSPIKE (Wolff et al., 1999), which is based on the Analog Devices ADSP21060 Digital Signal Processor. In fact, Digital Signal Processors revealed better performance than high-end mainstream processors in several biomedical and signal processing applications, with a power consumption that could be even two orders of magnitude lower (Pani et al., 2013, 2014) and they are currently being used for studies in neuroprosthetics (Pani et al., 2011, 2016).

A very successful implementation of a hardware architecture for SNN based on general purpose (embedded) processors is SpiNNaker (Furber et al., 2014). It is a multilevel tiled architecture, i.e., an architecture composed, at different levels, of a regular mesh of computing elements called tiles, mixing the flexibility of a software implementation of the neuronal model with the performance of a custom architecture (at macroscale). The smallest tile is a node, i.e., a custom chip consisting of multiple (up to 18 in the latest versions) ARM968 processors clocked at 200 MHz, without embedded floating-point units and exploiting a network-on-chip infrastructure for the communications. These nodes are assembled in boards comprising 48 of them, and exploiting highly customized self-timed connections. These boards communicate each other through custom serial links implemented on FPGA. This architecture is being used in the human brain project (www.humanbrainproject.eu). Despite the impressive work behind this platform, it is neither suited for a neuroengineering lab with limited budget nor for closed-loop applications. Furthermore compared to our design, each core is able to model up to a few hundred neurons (LIF or IZ) with about one thousand inpu synapses each. The time resolution scales down to 1 ms only which is inadequate for interfacing with the living tissue. Recen completely asynchronous extensions of the software framework on the SpiNNaker platform allowed performing simulation with networks implementing sub-millisecond tasks, such a sound localization, (Lagorce et al., 2015). However, some specifi conditions apply, as the use of even-driven LIF neurons, th adoption of a dendritic delay core for every particular delay valu (leveraging the large number of cores available), etc.

The same holds for the NeuroFlow architecture, which fo sure represents the state of the art in the field of FPG architectures for SNN (Cheung et al., 2016). Compared to i the proposed architecture targets a real-time performance c

0.1 ms, which can be ever reduced by changing the size of the network or speculating on the connectivity (assumed to be full in our tests). In particular, the time step of 0.1 ms is one order of magnitude less then that of the NeuroFlow architecture. Furthermore, the impressive numbers of simulated neurons provided by NeuroFlow (up to 600,000 units) can be reached with 6 FPGAs, with a toroidal network configuration, limiting the number of synapses to 1,000–10,000, when the connection probability follows a Gaussian probability of the synaptic distance with standard deviation ranging from 32 to 512. This unfortunately makes a point comparison hard and potentially unfair. Overall, NeuroFlow targets larger networks than the proposed architecture, with a different aim which is closer to that of SpiNNaker. This is reflected by the choice of a large off-chip Dynamic Random Access Memory (DRAM) compared to the BRAM used in our and other designs, and by the higher flexibility in the simulation setup.

On the other end of the flexibility axis, it is possible to find neural architectures based on application-specific integrated circuits (ASIC). They usually range from the analog neuromorphic chips (Hofstoetter et al., 2005), which exploit the possibility to make the transistors work on the current flow as the ion channels do on the ions flow, to the custom VLSI digital neurocomputers (Van Sickle and Abdel-Aty-Zohdy, 2009). Typically, the former are more complex to design but achieve better performance than the latter, both in terms of silicon area and power consumption (Joubert et al., 2012). In order to take the best in terms of performance while preserving the flexibility of software solutions, programmable hardware progressively gained interest in the computational neuroscience community. If field programmable analog arrays are still not completely convincing in terms of performance, even though some reconfigurable analog VLSI neuromorphic chips exist (Yu et al., 2010), on the digital side there is a growing interest toward the use of FPGA for these purposes (Maguire et al., 2007). FPGAs, providing the user the possibility to reconfigure the device by full or partial reload of the configuration bitstream, present the advantages of a custom architectures (as for the ASIC) and a flexibility approaching that of software implementations. Furthermore, the presence of IP cores enables the creation of multiprocessors systems on chip even on FPGA (Glackin et al., 2005).

In the largest part of cases, the effort toward the development of very fast architectures had a negative impact on the biological plausibility of the adopted neuronal model. In fact, the neuronal models that have been presented in the scientific literature so far are characterized by different biological plausibility and computational complexity (Paugam-Moisy and Bohte, 2012). Despite even the most complex Hodgkin-Huxley model was implemented in hardware (Graas et al., 2004), not all of them are suited for medium to large scale SNNs on digital hardware, because they should be computationally simple and at the same time capable of representing the wide variety of firing patterns exhibited by the different biological neurons. For this reason, some of the architectures use simplified custom neuronal models (Upegui et al., 2003, 2005), much more use integrate-and-fire (I&F) (Glackin et al., 2005) or leaky-integrate-and-fire (LIF) (Cassidy et al., 2007; Pearson et al., 2007). A recent interesting investigation on the limits of computer based approaches, FPGAs and Graphics Processing Units (GPUs) on highly complex biologically-plausible models of neurons belonging to the cerebellar cortex was reported in Florimbi et al. (2016). This work, in the main framework of the Human Brain Project, remarks how such complex neuronal models require huge hardware resources so that single-chip FPGAs cannot be an effective platform for cell networks, even though ASICs could, whereas GPUs can provide speedups that are still far from the real-time bound.

The proposed architecture exploits the very efficient IZ model (Izhikevich, 2003). Other works at the state of the art implemented the same neuronal model. Usually, for computational complexity reasons, the fixed-point processing is preferred. Despite this approach obviously limits the precision of the operations, compared to a floating-point solution, it has been shown to be adequate for several practical applications. First thing to notice is that several papers in the past described the implementation of the IZ model on FPGA without embedding it into a SNN. For instance, in Cassidy and Andreou (2008) a hardware implementation on the neuronal model alone is described (the model equations were changed in order to exploit power-of-two arithmetic, leading to less precision). The absence of the synapses is a remarkable limitation because of the quadratic dependence from the number of neurons of the synaptic weights, which is the main issue for scalability.

Other works, such as Rice et al. (2009), even though introducing the synapses, present topologies such that synapses connectivity is a minor issue. In that case, for instance, the number of neurons in very high (about 96 × 96, as much as the pixels of the input images) but the synapses are not as much as the square of such a value but rather only 48 times it. In that case, a Q4.12 format was used for the parameters, with the weights represented in Q4.12 format. The format depends on a trial and error procedure. SpiNNaker, for instance, uses different scaling factors for different parameters and values, showing that the best results can be achieved with a Q8.8 format for u, v, c, and d, whereas the Q0.16 format was chosen for parameter a and ab (since b alone is not used in that implementation), limiting such parameters to be <1 (Jin et al., 2008). With such an approach, the architecture is able to simulate up to 1000 IZ neurons on a single fascicle in a network with a low connectivity level (10%). Nevertheless, such a low connectivity is unrealistic: in Thomas and Luk (2009) a connectivity with 1,000 synapses per neuron, claimed to be a common-sense choice, is simulated. In this case, the fixed point representation used for the weight and the arithmetic of the adder tree is used, due to the limits imposed by the memory limits of the chosen platform, and weights are limited to 9 bits. Our architecture, with its 7 bits for the weights with a Q3.4 format, follows a similar approach, considering that on a physical platform it is acceptable to fix limits to the range of such parameters (Thomas and Luk, 2009). Spikes accumulation is performed at 32 bits to preserve as much as possible the precision. In Ambroise et al. (2013), the authors present a similar approach, that is capable of emulating up to 167 neurons (it is worth to notice that these results have been achieved on a smaller device: no data is provided on large FPGAs). Compared to the proposed one, such a work uses a higher number of resources due to higher data precision and to a fairly more complex processing of the synaptic current. It also considers a reduced sampling frequency (1 kHz) with respect to our work. In Glackin et al. (2005), the I&F model is implemented in fixed point with a Q8.10 precision for the membrane voltage and 12-bit precision for the synaptic conductance (no further details on the data size), using powers of 2 for the scaling parameters in the model, to avoid multipliers and dividers, with some precision loss.

In the proposed work, precision of the computation is demonstrated by the achieved results. The architecture is capable to obtain the same firing patterns of NEST, with a real-time performance that reaches 0.1 ms. The slight differences cannot be considered a limiting factor for the exploitation of the architecture in real-time closed-loop experiments, since the global firing patterns are respected. Even though the proposed architecture is not highly optimized, because of the need to ensure flexibility at this development stage, it is possible to pursue energy/performance efficiency by means of fine application-driven customization of the hardware architecture, that requires adequate support by advanced design tools (Jozwiak et al., 2012, 2013). The proposed approach can evolve in such a direction for closed-loop implantable implementations.

In perspective, the possibility to have a valid and efficient hardware tool to simulate and generate in real-time realistic spiking dynamics could pave the way to the design of new devices to interface synthetic neuronal assemblies to biological excitable tissues. Indeed, the so developed architecture could be used to generate realistic signals (in terms of time and spatial constants) to stimulate biological networks (open-loop application) as well as to realize closed-loop systems in which, in a bi-directional way, biological and hardware networks are mutually stimulated. In such scenarios, similar to state-of-the-art closed-loop experiments (Wagenaar et al., 2005; Wallach et al., 2011), the availability of an embedded system implementing in hardware (e.g., FPGA) a biologically plausible SNN would be the only enabling technology. In fact, purely software simulations could not be used to interface *in silico* neuronal models with living beings.

In the meanwhile, the real-time performance of an FPGA platform as the one proposed in this work, overcoming the limitations of the software simulators, can be exploited to study the fundamentals of the interaction between living neuronal assemblies and synthetic ones, in closed-loop, opening to hitherto unexplored neurophysiological experiments.

AUTHOR CONTRIBUTIONS

All the authors substantially contributed to the manuscript. In particular, PMa, DP, and LR conceived the study, PMa and DP defined the methods and analyzed the performance results, PMe and FP defined the architectural features and coding approach, GT performed the hardware parameterization, debug and co-simulations HDL-NEST. All the authors drafted and revised the manuscript and agree with the current version.

ACKNOWLEDGMENTS

The authors wish to thank Mr. R. Montano for his precious work in coding a preliminary version of the architecture.

REFERENCES

Ambroise, M., Levi, T., Bornat, Y., and Saighi, S. (2013). "Biorealistic spiking neural network on FPGA," in *Information Sciences and Systems (CISS), 2013 47th Annual Conference on* (Baltimore, MD), 1–6.

Berger, T. W., Hampson, R. E., Song, D., Goonawardena, A., Marmarelis, V. Z., and Deadwyler, S. A. (2011). A cortical neural prosthesis for restoring and enhancing memory. *J. Neural Eng.* 8:046017. doi: 10.1088/1741-2560/8/4/046017

Berger, T. W., Song, D., Chan, R. H. M., Marmarelis, V. Z., LaCoss, J., Wills, J., et al. (2012). A hippocampal cognitive prosthesis: multi-input, multi-output nonlinear modeling and VLSI implementation. *IEEE Trans. Neural Syst. Rehabil. Eng.* 20, 198–211. doi: 10.1109/TNSRE.2012.2189133

Bonifazi, P., Difato, F., Massobrio, P., Breschi, G. L., Pasquale, V., Levi, T., et al. (2013). *In vitro* large-scale experimental and theoretical studies for the realization of bi-directional brain-prostheses. *Front. Neural Circ.* 7:40. doi: 10.3389/fncir.2013.00040

Brette, R., Rudolph, M., Carnevale, T., Hines, M., Beeman, D., Bower, J. M., et al. (2007). Simulation of networks of spiking neurons: a review of tools and strategies. *J. Comput. Neurosci.* 23, 349–398. doi: 10.1007/s10827-007-0038-6

Carnevale, N., and Hines, M. (2006). *The NEURON Book.* Cambridge: Cambridge University Press.

Cassidy, A., and Andreou, A. G. (2008). "Dynamical digital silicon neurons," in *2008 IEEE Biomedical Circuits and Systems Conference* (Baltimore, MD), 289–292.

Cassidy, A., Denham, S., Kanold, P., and Andreou, A. (2007). "FPGA based silicon spiking neural array," in *2007 IEEE Biomedical Circuits and Systems Conference* (Montreal, QC), 75–78.

Cheung, K., Schultz, S. R., and Luk, W. (2016). NeuroFlow: a general purpose spiking neural network simulation platform using customizable processors. *Front. Neurosci.* 9:516. doi: 10.3389/fnins.2015.00516

Chiappalone, M., Novellino, A., Vajda, I., Vato, A., Martinoia, S., and Pelt, J. V. (2005). Burst detection algorithms for the analysis of spatio-temporal patterns in cortical networks of neurons. *Neurocomputing* 65–66, 653–662. doi: 10.1016/j.neucom.2004.10.094

Dayan, P., and Abbott, L. (2001). *Theoretical Neuroscience.* Cambridge: MIT Press.

Florimbi, G., Torti, E., Masoli, S., D'Angelo, E., Danese, G., and Leporati, F. (2016). The human brain project: parallel technologies for biologically accurate simulation of granule cells. *Microprocess. Microsyst.* 47(Pt B), 303–313. doi: 10.1016/j.micpro.2016.05.015

Furber, S. B., Galluppi, F., Temple, S., and Plana, L. A. (2014). The SpiNNaker project. *Proc. IEEE* 102, 652–665. doi: 10.1109/JPROC.2014.2304638

Gewaltig, M.-O., and Diesmann, M. (2007). NEST (neural simulation tool). *Scholarpedia* 2:1430. doi: 10.4249/scholarpedia.1430

Glackin, B., McGinnity, T. M., Maguire, L. P., Wu, Q. X., and Belatreche, A. (2005). *A Novel Approach for the Implementation of Large Scale Spiking Neural Networks on FPGA Hardware.* Berlin; Heidelberg: Springer.

Goodman, D. F. M., and Brette, R. (2009). The brian simulator. *Front. Neurosci.* 3:26. doi: 10.3389/neuro.01.026.2009

Graas, E. L., Brown, E. A., and Lee, R. H. (2004). An FPGA-based approach to high-speed simulation of conductance-based neuron models. *Neuroinformatics* 2, 417–436. doi: 10.1385/NI:2:4:417

Hofstoetter, C., Gil, M., Eng, K., Indiveri, G., Mintz, M., Kramer, J., et al. (2005). "The cerebellum chip: an analog VLSI implementation of a cerebellar model of classical conditioning," in *Advances in Neural Information Processing Systems 17*, eds L. K. Saul, Y. Weiss, and L. Bottou (Vancouver, BC: MIT Press), 577–584.

Izhikevich, E. M. (2003). Simple model of spiking neurons. *IEEE Trans. Neural Netw.* 14, 1569–1572. doi: 10.1109/TNN.2003.820440

Jin, X., Furber, S. B., and Woods, J. V. (2008). "Efficient modelling of spiking neural networks on a scalable chip multiprocessor," in *2008 IEEE International Joint Conference on Neural Networks (IEEE World Congress on Computational Intelligence)* (Hong Kong), 2812–2819.

Joubert, A., Belhadj, B., Temam, O., and Heliot, R. (2012). "Hardware spiking neurons design: analog or digital?" in *The 2012 International Joint Conference on Neural Networks (IJCNN)* (Brisbane, QLD), 1–5.

Jozwiak, L., Lindwer, M., Corvino, R., Meloni, P., Micconi, L., Madsen, J., et al. (2012). "ASAM: automatic architecture synthesis and application mapping," in *Proceedings - 15th Euromicro Conference on Digital System Design, DSD 2012* (Çeşme), 216–225.

Jozwiak, L., Lindwer, M., Corvino, R., Meloni, P., Micconi, L., Madsen, J., et al. (2013). ASAM: automatic architecture synthesis and application mapping. *Microprocess. Microsyst.* 37(8 Pt C), 1002–1019. doi: 10.1016/j.micpro.2013.08.006

Lagorce, X., Stromatias, E., Galluppi, F., Plana, L. A., Liu, S.-C., Furber, S. B., et al. (2015). Breaking the millisecond barrier on SpiNNaker: implementing asynchronous event-based plastic models with microsecond resolution. *Front. Neurosci.* 9:206. doi: 10.3389/fnins.2015.00206

Le Masson, G., Renaud-Le Masson, S., Debay, D., and Bal, T. (2002). Feedback inhibition controls spike transfer in hybrid thalamic circuits. *Nature* 417, 854–858. doi: 10.1038/nature00825

Maguire, L., McGinnity, T., Glackin, B., Ghani, A., Belatreche, A., and Harkin, J. (2007). Challenges for large-scale implementations of spiking neural networks on FPGAs. *Neurocomputing* 71, 13–29. doi: 10.1016/j.neucom.2006.11.029

Nawrot, A. P., Pistohl, T., Schrader, S., Hehl, U., Rodriguez, V., and Aertsen, A. (2003). "Embedding living neurons into simulated neural networks," in *Neural Engineering, 2003. Conference Proceedings. First International IEEE EMBS Conference on* (Capri Island), 229–232.

Pani, D., Barabino, G., Citi, L., Meloni, P., Raspopovic, S., Micera, S., et al. (2016). Real-time neural signals decoding onto off-the-shelf DSP processors for neuroprosthetic applications. *IEEE Trans. Neural Syst. Rehabil. Eng.* 24, 993–1002. doi: 10.1109/TNSRE.2016.2527696

Pani, D., Barabino, G., and Raffo, L. (2013). NInFEA: an embedded framework for the real-time evaluation of fetal ECG extraction algorithms. *Biomed. Eng.* 58, 13–26. doi: 10.1515/bmt-2012-0018

Pani, D., Pani, A., and Raffo, L. (2014). Real-time blind audio source separation: performance assessment on an advanced digital signal processor. *J. Supercomput.* 70, 1555–1576. doi: 10.1007/s11227-014-1252-4

Pani, D., Usai, F., Citi, L., and Raffo, L. (2011). "Real-time processing of tfLIFE neural signals on embedded DSP platforms: a case study," in *Proceedings of 5th International IEEE EMBS Conference on Neural Engineering* (Cancun), 44–47.

Paugam-Moisy, H., and Bohte, S. (2012). "Computing with spiking neuron networks," in *Handbook of Natural Computing*, eds G. Rozenberg, T. Bäck, and J. N. Kok (Berlin; Heidelberg: Springer), 335–376.

Pearson, M. J., Pipe, A. G., Mitchinson, B., Gurney, K., Melhuish, C., Gilhespy, I., et al. (2007). Implementing spiking neural networks for real-time signal-processing and control applications: a model-validated FPGA approach. *IEEE Trans. Neural Netw.* 18, 1472–1487. doi: 10.1109/TNN.2007.891203

Rast, A. D., Jin, X., Galluppi, F., Plana, L. A., Patterson, C., and Furbe, S. (2010). "Scalable event-driven native parallel processing: the spinnaker neuromimetic system," in *Proceedings of the 7th ACM International Conference on Computing Frontiers* (Bertinoro: ACM), 21–30.

Rice, K. L., Bhuiyan, M. A., Taha, T. M., Vutsinas, C. N., and Smith, M. C. (2009). "FPGA implementation of izhikevich spiking neural networks for character recognition," in *2009 International Conference on Reconfigurable Computing and FPGAs* (Quintana Roo), 451–456.

Rolston, J. D., Gross, R. E., and Potter, S. M. (2010). Closed-loop, open-source electrophysiology. *Front. Neurosci.* 4:31. doi: 10.3389/fnins.2010.00031

Schoenauer, T., Mehrtash, N., Jahnke, A., and Klar, H. (1998). "MASPINN: novel concepts for a neuro-accelerator for spiking neural networks," in *Proc. SPIE 3728, Ninth Workshop on Virtual Intelligence/Dynamic Neural Networks*, eds T. Lindblad, M. L. Padgett, and J. M. Kinser (Stockholm), 87–97.

Thomas, D., and Luk, W. (2009). "FPGA accelerated simulation of biologically plausible spiking neural networks," in *Field Programmable Custom Computing Machines, 2009. FCCM '09. 17th IEEE Symposium on* (Napa, CA), 45–52.

Upegui, A., Peña-Reyes, C. A., and Sanchez, E. (2003). *A Functional Spiking Neuron Hardware Oriented Model.* Berlin; Heidelberg: Springer.

Upegui, A., Peña-Reyes, C. A., and Sanchez, E. (2005). An FPGA platform for on-line topology exploration of spiking neural networks. *Microprocess. Microsyst.* 29, 211–223. doi: 10.1016/j.micpro.2004.08.012

van Pelt, J., Wolters, P. S., Corner, M. A., Rutten, W. L. C., and Ramakers, G. J. A. (2004). Long-term characterization of firing dynamics of spontaneous bursts in cultured neural networks. *IEEE Trans. Biomed. Eng.* 51, 2051–2062. doi: 10.1109/TBME.2004.827936

Van Sickle, K., and Abdel-Aty-Zohdy, H. (2009). "A reconfigurable spiking neural network digital ASIC simulation and implementation," in *Proceedings of the IEEE 2009 National Aerospace Electronics Conference (NAECON)* (Dayton, OH), 275–280.

Wagenaar, D. A., Madhavan, R., Pine, J., and Potter, S. M. (2005). Controlling bursting in cortical cultures with closed-loop multi-electrode stimulation. *J. Neurosci.* 25, 680–688. doi: 10.1523/JNEUROSCI.4209-04.2005

Wallach, A., Eytan, D., Gal, A., Zrenner, C., and Marom, S. (2011). Neuronal response clamp. *Front. Neuroeng.* 4:3. doi: 10.3389/fneng.2011.00003

Wolff, C., Hartmann, G., and Ruckert, U. (1999). "ParSPIKE a parallel DSP-accelerator for dynamic simulation of large spiking neural networks," in *Proceedings of the 7th International Conference on Microelectronics for Neural, Fuzzy and Bio-Inspired Systems* (Granada: IEEE Computer Society), 324–332.

Yu, T., Sejnowski, T. J., and Cauwenberghs, G. (2010). "Biophysical neural spiking and bursting dynamics in reconfigurable analog VLSI," in *2010 Biomedical Circuits and Systems Conference (BioCAS)* (Paphos), 186–189.

Zbrzeski, A., Bornat, Y., Hillen, B., Siu, R., Abbas, J., Jung, R., et al. (2016). Bio-inspired controller on an FPGA applied to closed-loop diaphragmatic stimulation. *Front. Neurosci.* 10:275. doi: 10.3389/fnins.2016.00275

5

Detecting a Cortical Fingerprint of Parkinson's Disease for Closed-Loop Neuromodulation

*Kevin Kern [1], Georgios Naros [1], Christoph Braun [2,3], Daniel Weiss [4] and Alireza Gharabaghi [1]**

[1] Division of Functional and Restorative Neurosurgery and Centre for Integrative Neuroscience, Eberhard Karls University Tuebingen, Tuebingen, Germany, [2] Magnetoencephalography Center, Eberhard Karls University Tuebingen, Tuebingen, Germany, [3] Center for Mind/Brain Sciences (CIMeC), University of Trento, Italy, [4] Department for Neurodegenerative Diseases and Hertie Institute for Clinical Brain Research and German Centre of Neurodegenerative Diseases (DZNE), Eberhard Karls University Tuebingen, Tuebingen, Germany

Edited by:
Michela Chiappalone,
Istituto Italiano di Tecnologia, Italy

Reviewed by:
Nader Pouratian,
University of California, Los Angeles, USA
Daniela S. Andres,
University Zurich and Federal Institute of Technology (ETH Zurich), Switzerland

***Correspondence:**
Alireza Gharabaghi
alireza.gharabaghi@uni-tuebingen.de

Recent evidence suggests that deep brain stimulation (DBS) of the subthalamic nucleus (STN) in Parkinson's disease (PD) mediates its clinical effects by modulating cortical oscillatory activity, presumably via a direct cortico-subthalamic connection. This observation might pave the way for novel closed-loop approaches comprising a cortical sensor. Enhanced beta oscillations (13-35 Hz) have been linked to the pathophysiology of PD and may serve as such a candidate marker to localize a cortical area reliably modulated by DBS. However, beta-oscillations are widely distributed over the cortical surface, necessitating an additional signal source for spotting the cortical area linked to the pathologically synchronized cortico-subcortical motor network. In this context, both cortico-subthalamic coherence and cortico-muscular coherence (CMC) have been studied in PD patients. Whereas, the former requires invasive recordings, the latter allows for non-invasive detection, but displays a rather distributed cortical synchronization pattern in motor tasks. This distributed cortical representation may conflict with the goal of detecting a cortical localization with robust biomarker properties which is detectable on a single subject basis. We propose that this limitation could be overcome when recording CMC at rest. We hypothesized that—unlike healthy subjects—PD would show CMC at rest owing to the enhanced beta oscillations observed in PD. By performing source space analysis of beta CMC recorded during resting-state magnetoencephalography we provide preliminary evidence in one patient for a cortical *hot spot* that is modulated most strongly by subthalamic DBS. Such a spot would provide a prominent target region either for direct neuromodulation or for placing a potential sensor in closed-loop DBS approaches, a proposal that requires investigation in a larger cohort of PD patients.

Keywords: deep brain stimulation, Parkinson's disease, beta cortico-muscular coherence, source space, neurophysiological biomarker, cortical targeting, closed-loop stimulation

INTRODUCTION

Cortico-subcortical networks of Parkinson's disease (PD) patients are characterized by pathological circuit dynamics such as dysfunctional synchronization in the beta-frequency (12–35 Hz) band (Little and Brown, 2014). Dopaminergic medication and electrical stimulation may rebalance and clinically improve these altered interactions both locally and on a network level

(Kühn et al., 2008; Litvak et al., 2011; Eusebio et al., 2012; Hirschmann et al., 2013b; Weiss et al., 2015). Even in PD patients with early motor complications, deep brain stimulation (DBS) of the subthalamic nucleus (STN) provides better relief (alleviating motor symptoms and improving life quality) than medication (Schuepbach et al., 2013).

Two lines of evidence nominate the cortex as a target for modulating the dysfunctional network dynamics in PD: In patients, cortical beta activity precedes pathological subcortical synchronization (Marreiros et al., 2013). Furthermore, findings in both animal models of DBS (Gradinaru et al., 2009; Li et al., 2012) and patients (de Hemptinne et al., 2015) suggest that anti-dromically activated responses in the motor cortex are involved in the beneficial effects of STN DBS. Although previous studies of electrical cortical stimulation (CS) in PD revealed lower efficacy compared to DBS (Cilia et al., 2007; Moro et al., 2011; Bentivoglio et al., 2012), recent technological developments of implantable devices for simultaneously sensing and stimulating (Afshar et al., 2012) have refueled the interest in CS by applying closed-loop devices (Rosin et al., 2011; Beuter et al., 2014). Simultaneous magnetoencephalography (MEG) and local field potential (LFP) recordings in the STN of PD patients (using implanted DBS electrodes with externalized leads) detected long-range functional connectivity between STN and the ipsilateral sensorimotor and premotor cortex in the beta frequency range, suggesting the involvement of the hyperdirect pathway (Hirschmann et al., 2011; Litvak et al., 2011). More recently, electroencephalography (EEG) has also been applied to capture cortical beta-gamma phase-amplitude coupling (PAC) as a functional marker in PD while demonstrating its modulation by levodopa (Swann et al., 2015). However, the elevation of the EEG PAC signal in PD patients compared to healthy controls was not demonstrable on a single subject basis, but only at the group level (Swann et al., 2015). We therefore still lack a non-invasive technique that could be applied before surgery on a single subject basis to functionally localize a cortical target area informative on pathological beta oscillatory characteristics for either direct CS or as a sensor for closed-loop DBS.

There is converging evidence, that enhanced cortical beta activity is a prominent feature in the pathophysiology of PD (Kühn et al., 2008; Eusebio et al., 2011; Airaksinen et al., 2012; Little and Brown, 2012). Moreover, the hyperdirect pathway, connecting the STN and the motor cortical area is believed to mediate a DBS-related decrease of this exaggerated beta activity in parallel to alleviation of bradykinesia-rigidity symptoms (Kühn et al., 2006; Whitmer et al., 2012). Therefore, the most intuitive candidate marker is expected within the beta frequency range in order to detect a reliable cortical biomarker for PD. Oscillatory activity in the beta range, however, is widely distributed over the cortical surface. Additional measures are warranted to spot the cortical area reliably modulated by DBS. Cortico-muscular coherence (CMC) might provide such an additional measure. During motor tasks, CMC generally displays a spatially distributed cortical representation (Crone et al., 1998a,b; Grosse-Wentrup et al., 2011; Hipp et al., 2011), thereby conflicting with the goal of detecting a cortical hot spot. There is also a large inter-subject variability of CMC in PD patients during a motor task (Kühn, 2004; Kühn et al., 2008; Tropini et al., 2011; Weiss et al., 2012; Selzler et al., 2013) most probably explaining the variable findings in previous motor task related CMC studies in PD (Airaksinen et al., 2015).

We propose that this limitation could be overcome when performing the CMC measurement at rest. We suggest that—unlike in healthy subjects—(I) CMC would be detectable in the PD condition even in the absence of movement due to the disease-specific enhanced beta oscillations. Furthermore, we hypothesize that (II) the cortical CMC spot would topographically converge with the cortical spot modulated most strongly by subthalamic DBS. To provide proof-of-concept evidence, we implemented a MEG set-up for resting-state CMC and DBS to perform source space analysis of related cortical activity.

EXPERIMENTAL SET-UP

Recording

The measurements were performed inside a magnetically shielded room (Vakuumschmelze, Hanau, Germany) with a whole-head 275-channel MEG (CTF, VSM Medtech, Port Coquitlam, Canada) at a sampling rate of 1172 Hz. Recordings included bipolar electromyography (EMG) from the right flexor carpi radialis muscle (grounded to elbow), bipolar electrooculography (EOG) and electrocardiography (ECG). The patient was seated comfortably and asked to remain motionless. Her gaze was focused on a fixation cross at eye level. The pre-programmed stimulation was switched off 30 min beforehand to obtain reliable wash-out of subthalamic DBS effects (Cooper et al., 2013; Weiss et al., 2013). We recorded 6 min (360 s) of resting-state MEG without stimulation (rest). This baseline measurement was followed by recordings during 10 stimulation trials, each lasting 2 min; 1 min stimulation-on followed by 1 min stimulation-off. For data analysis, we selected the first 40 s of the stimulation-off period of each trial. This resulted in an overall time-period of ~360 s after artifact rejection. Time periods immediately following DBS were compared with the 360 s of baseline measurement at rest before the stimulation trials. This approach was chosen because: (i) methods for suppressing the stimulation artifact in MEG recordings during simultaneous monopolar DBS might not be sufficiently effective for interpreting stimulation results (Devos, 2004; Silberstein et al., 2005; Airaksinen et al., 2012). By analyzing the period immediately after stimulation, stimulation artifacts are avoided. (ii) Even short term stimulation has neuronal effects that last for several seconds or minutes after stimulation (Kühn et al., 2008; Bronte-Stewart et al., 2009; Whitmer et al., 2012). The time period immediately following stimulation might therefore provide information on stimulation-induced physiological effects. (iii) By comparing this data to the resting measurements before stimulation trials, any carry-over effects in the data used as baseline can be excluded. Source space analysis was performed using a T2-weighted individual MRI.

Pre-processing

Notwithstanding stimulation, the DBS hardware itself induced relevant MEG artifacts. These were removed using temporal signal space separation (tSSS; Taulu and Simola, 2006; Taulu and Hari, 2009), which was applied with a subspace correlation limit of 0.9 (Medvedovsky et al., 2009; Airaksinen et al., 2011). The Dynamic Imaging of Coherent Sources (DICS) beamformer has been shown to reliably suppress metal artifacts of implanted DBS electrode leads in the stimulation-off mode as well as with externalized extension cables, i.e., an impulse generator (IPG) outside the body (Litvak et al., 2010). However, it has not yet been shown that this approach also removes the artifacts induced by an implanted IPG during breathing or even during stimulation.

By contrast, tSSS has been shown to overcome these additional artifacts when applied in an Electa Neuromag. Together with the developers of tSSS, we have therefore implemented tSSS in our CTF MEG system. The data presented here was preceded by phantom and *in vivo* studies to optimize the device settings so as to reliably suppress artifacts. When signal quality did not allow a reliable rejection of artifacts, the algorithm refused the artifact rejection *per se*. In these pre-studies, we reliably localized movement-related activity and event-related potentials to their anticipated cortical localization during stimulation (unpublished data).

The patient's magnetic resonance images (MRI) were interpolated to a resolution of 256 × 256 × 256 voxels. Fiducial (nasion, left, and right preauricular) and anatomical landmarks (anterior and posterior commissure, mid-sagittal plane) were used to align the MRI to standard space of the Montreal Neurological Institute (MNI). Finally, the source space was defined by a single shell segmented model and lead fields with a resolution of 8 mm.

We applied a first order zero-phase lag finite impulse response bandpass filter (1–40 Hz) to the MEG time series, and highpass filters of 0.5 Hz to the ECG, 0.05 Hz to the EOG, and 2 Hz to the EMG, respectively, to preserve relevant spectral components in the signals. Thereafter, we applied an independent component analysis (ICA) and correlation analysis to identify and remove eye movement, blink, and cardiac-related artifacts. We decorrelated each trial of the MEG sensor time series into 40 independent components via fast independent component analysis. Both independent components, which maximally correlated with the ECG and EOG, were labeled artifacts and skipped during back-projection of the independent components to sensor level. An additional visual inspection, where we focused on the eye movement, blink, and cardiac-related artifacts in the time series of the components, verified the respective artifacts. The magnetic fields of the single sensors were recomputed using an interpolation toward average head position throughout the recordings. All trials and conditions were divided into 5-s epochs. Finally, z-value-transformed epoch-wise artifact rejection was performed using a cutoff-value of 20.

Data Analysis

We applied a previously described approach (Litvak et al., 2011) to identify the frequency band with maximal cortico-muscular coherence (CMC) and to calculate source space CMC. We rectified the EMG channel (Myers et al., 2003; Yao et al., 2007) and calculated cross-spectra with all MEG sensor time series from 2 to 40 Hz by tapering the 5-s epochs using slepian functions (Mitra and Pesaran, 1999) and 2 Hz spectral smoothing resulting in a frequency resolution of $\delta f = 0.2$ Hz (see **Figure 1A**). Source space CMC was then calculated by using these cross-spectra and Dynamic Imaging of Coherent Sources (DICS) beamforming (Gross et al., 2001). Pre-processing with tSSS has previously been shown not to restrict the usage of a subsequent beamformer analysis (Hillebrand et al., 2013). Common spatial DICS filter of both conditions, i.e., rest and stimulation, were calculated beforehand and used for source space CMC calculation. Calculating a common spatial filter for beamforming is usually applied when comparing different conditions after beamforming to avoid biased results due to different spatial filters of the conditions.

For the statistical comparison of the rest and stimulation condition for both CMC and power, a non-parametric cluster-based permutation approach was used to correct for multiple comparisons (Maris and Oostenveld, 2007; Oostenveld et al., 2011). We computed voxel-wise t-values between the rest and stimulation condition and clustered voxels exceeding $p < 0.001$ (uncorrected). The sum of the t-value within the clustered voxel area defined the cluster-level statistics. By randomly permuting the data between rest and stimulation condition for 1000 times, we obtained a reference null distribution of the maximum cluster-level statistics. In order to correct for multiple comparisons, the maximum cluster-level statistics that differed from the reference null distribution with $p < 0.05$ (corrected) were considered significant. All data analysis was performed offline with custom written scripts and FieldTrip toolbox (Oostenveld et al., 2011) in MATLAB® (R2011a, The MathWorks® Inc.,).

EMPIRICAL DATA

An idiopathic akinetic-rigid PD patient (female; age: 69 years; disease duration: 12 years; UPDRS III (motor part) stimulation on/off: 15/20) participated after giving written informed consent. We examined the patient 5 months after DBS surgery with bilateral electrode implantation in the STN (Medtronic 3389 leads and Activa PC® stimulator, Minneapolis, USA). The physiological effects of unilateral DBS (left hemisphere) were studied using the same stimulation parameters as applied clinically (monopolar, contact 2-G+, 1.5 V, 60 µs, 125 Hz) while the patient was in medication-on (levodopa equivalent dose = 581 mg; Deuschl et al., 2006). The study was conducted with the patients' informed consent and in accordance with the guidelines approved by the local ethics committee of the University Hospital Tuebingen.

Spectral analysis of CMC at baseline, i.e., in rest and stimulation-off, revealed that the strongest connectivity occurred in the beta-band (**Figure 1A**). Scanning all sensors showed predominant involvement of the hemisphere contralateral to the EMG recording (**Figure 1B**) with a topography suggestive of one major source in MEG sensor space (**Figure 1C**). Source space CMC analysis showed the maximum of the beta-CMC within the motor cortex of the hemisphere contralateral to the muscle (**Figure 2A**) as opposed to a distributed pattern of cortical activation in the beta-band (**Figure 2B**).

During STN-DBS, the same beta-CMC (**Figure 3A**) and beta power (**Figure 3B**) source-cluster revealed the strongest stimulation-induced changes, i.e., decreases of CMC and cortical power in the beta-band.

DISCUSSION

We performed source space analysis of beta CMC recorded during resting-state MEG and DBS and provide proof-of-concept evidence for a cortical *hot spot* that is most strongly modulated by subthalamic DBS. Since this study is carried out in only one subject, this proposal requires investigation in a larger cohort of PD patients to probe the robustness of this approach, e.g., for different disease states.

The present work suggests that a circumscribed cortical area involved in the pathologically synchronized cortico-subcortical-muscular motor network can be detected non-invasively in PD on single subject level, which constitutes a mandatory prerequisite for future closed-loop neurostimulation strategies on the basis of a cortical sensor. Due to its high spatial resolution of ~2 mm (Pizzella and Romani, 1990), MEG is as an excellent tool for non-invasive mapping prior to neurosurgical procedures. Up to date, MEG examinations have been successfully used for presurgical evaluation of epilepsy patients (Knowlton and Shih, 2004) and patients with tumors in eloquent areas (Rezai et al., 1996; Orrison, 1999). Integration of the MEG information in the stereotactic planning software has been used for electrode placement (Agirre-Arrizubieta et al., 2014) and to aid safe resection of tumors (Kelly, 1996; Rezai et al., 1996; Orrison, 1999). The knowledge acquired with the presented approach may thus be integrated in stereotactic planning for the placement of cortical implants for direct neuromodulation or for placing a potential sensor in closed-loop DBS approaches. We did not intend to describe a specific extent or location of such a cortical area, since these parameters may vary between patients. However, in accordance with previous literature on the hyperdirect cortico-subthalamic pathway recorded with cortico-subthalamic coherence (Hirschmann et al., 2011), the data presented here suggests that this cortical area covers a part of the medial motor and premotor cortex.

The involvement of the cortical areas associated with motor processing in Parkinson tremor is well-documented (Timmermann et al., 2003; Hirschmann et al., 2013a). However, source space topographic information about CMC in akinetic-rigid PD and in the absence of movement is rather sparse. As a conceptual novelty of this work, we captured the cortical spot of pathological resting-state CMC in the beta band. An implantable cortical sensor for closed-loop applications needs to be spatially restricted from a neurosurgical point of view. Therefore, the cortical target point would be defined as the area which addresses both networks, i.e., the rigidity/bradykinesia and the tremor network. The cortical area involved most strongly in the rigidity/bradykinesia network observed here seems to be more restricted than the tremor network reported by Timmermann and colleagues. Since still being part of the latter such an area would qualify as the common hotspot.

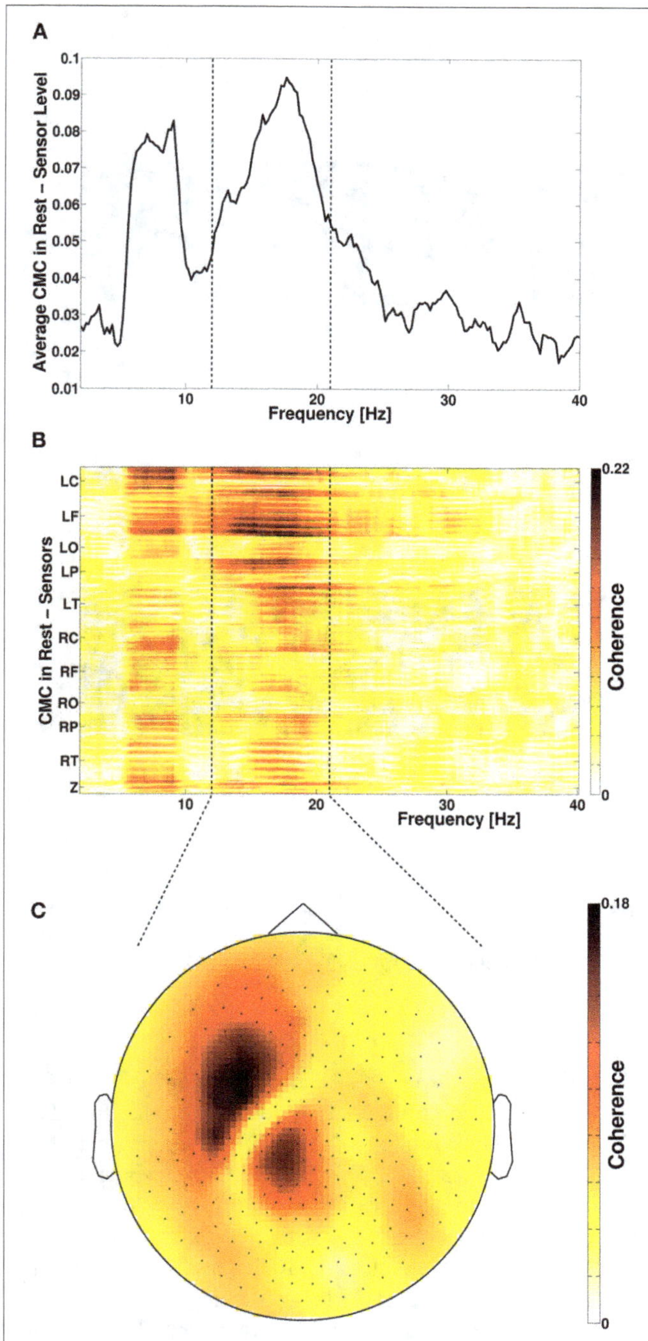

FIGURE 1 | (A) Frequency spectrum of resting-state cortico-muscular coherence (CMC) of all sensors. Dotted vertical lines indicate the beta-frequency range which was analyzed. **(B)** Spatial distribution of CMC. **(C)** Topoplot of beta-band CMC in MEG sensor space. L, left; R, right; C, central; F, frontal; O, occipital; P, parietal; T, temporal; Z, midline.

Our concept suggests capturing a cross spectrum for every patient to detect the individual peak frequency band of CMC (see **Figure 1A**). As expected, the presented case also showed the peak CMC in the beta-band followed by the alpha-band. This observation is in accordance with a large body of literature reporting relating enhanced beta oscillations both in the STN

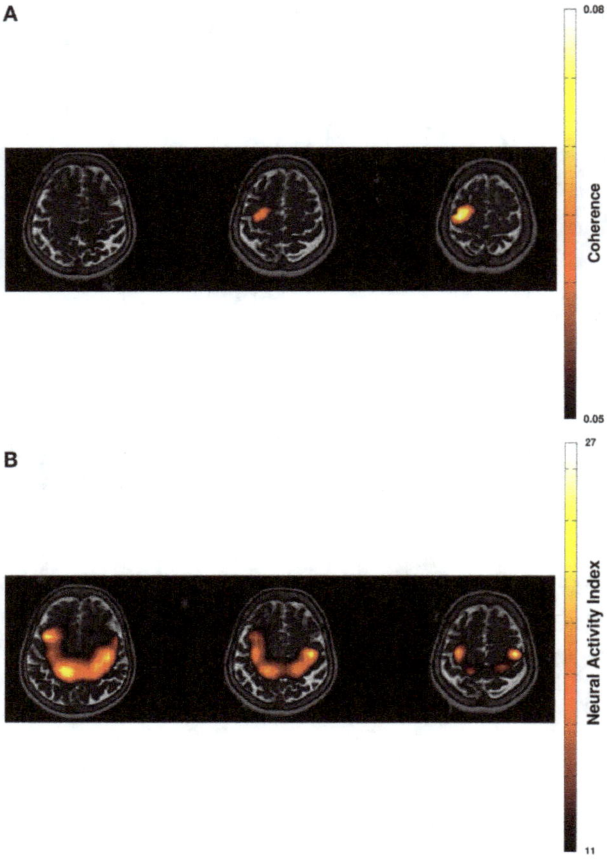

FIGURE 2 | Projection of beta-band cortico-muscular coherence (A) and of cortical beta power (B) in resting-state on transversal slices of individual T2-weighted MRI with 60% thresholding.

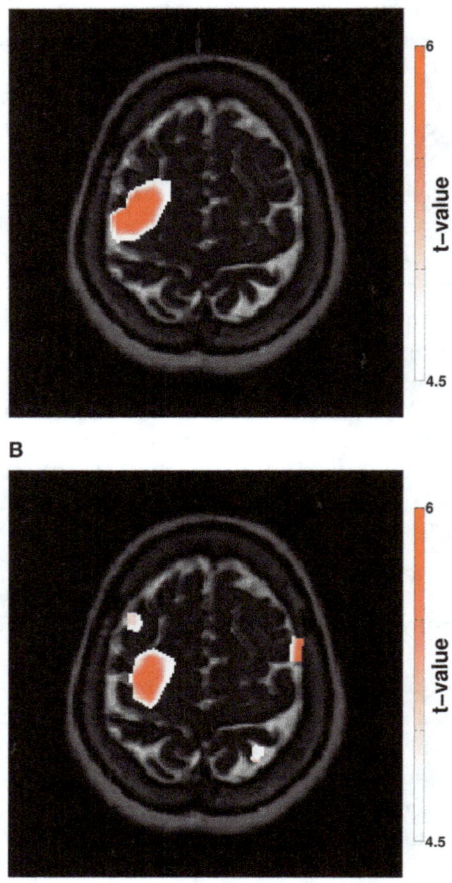

FIGURE 3 | (A) Stimulation modulated beta-CMC showing the difference between the rest and the stimulation condition. **(B)** Stimulation modulated cortical beta power showing the difference between the rest and the stimulation condition. The color bar indicates the *t*-values according to a non-parametric cluster-based permutation approach ($p < 0.05$, corrected).

and on the cortical level to the pathophysiology of PD (Kühn et al., 2008; Eusebio et al., 2011; Airaksinen et al., 2012; Little and Brown, 2012; Whitmer et al., 2012). Moreover, beta-band oscillations have repeatedly been shown to mediate cortico-muscular communication (Salenius et al., 2002; Baker, 2007; Engel and Fries, 2010; Weiss et al., 2012; Airaksinen et al., 2015). In contrast to beta-CMC, alpha-CMC is not consistently found (Kilner et al., 2000; Budini et al., 2014) and may be confounded by coherence occuring at double tremor frequency (Timmermann et al., 2003). Therefore, it is not surprising that we did not find any significant source cluster for alpha-CMC in the resting state and in the absence of tremor.

STN stimulation is known to modulate spontaneous activity and somatosensory evoked responses over the sensorimotor cortex (Mäkelä et al., 2007; Airaksinen et al., 2011). Furthermore, excessive beta oscillatory activity is suppressed by STN-DBS in PD along with symptom alleviation (Kühn et al., 2008; Whitmer et al., 2012; Little and Brown, 2014). This correlation of therapeutic beta activity modulation and motor symptom alleviation is not surprising, given that oscillatory beta activity relates to motor processing, sensorimotor control, and cortico-peripheral interactions (Brovelli et al., 2004; Schoffelen et al., 2005; Baker, 2007; Chakarov et al., 2009; Engel and Fries 2010). Cortical beta band activity may parallel the maintenance of the sensorimotor state (status quo; Engel and Fries, 2010) Therefore, decreased motor cortical beta power, as found in this study, may represent a release of cognitive resources, which restores the ability of motor self-control mediated by cortico basal ganglia-thalamo-cortical loops (Kringelbach et al., 2010 McIntyre and Hahn, 2010; Little and Brown, 2012). As already described previously (Whitmer et al., 2012; Weiss et al., 2015) STN stimulation suppresses cortical beta band activity in motor related areas. Thus, the findings reported here are in line with these previous results.

Cortico-peripheral interactions as measured by CMC in the beta frequency band may be increased by levodopa administration (Salenius et al., 2002). The effect of STN stimulation was more variable showing a slight beta band CMC increase on fine-motor integration (Weiss et al., 2012) and variable outcomes during joint movement (Airaksinen et al. 2015). This case study suggests that, in the resting state, this long-distance corticomuscular synchronization is decreased b

STN-DBS. This tallies with the anticipated dysbalanced drive from cortex to muscle in PD (Salenius et al., 2002; Hirschmann et al., 2013b). The concept of maintaining the status quo via sensorimotor activity in beta band may therefore be extended to beta band CMC as well (Baker, 2007; Engel and Fries, 2010). Decreasing beta CMC in the resting state through STN-DBS may thus represent a reduction of an abnormal persistence of the status quo, i.e., of the pathological oscillatory drive to the muscle in PD (Brown et al., 2001; Marsden et al., 2001). It should be noted, however, that CMC in itself may have a functional role in the motor system apart from the cortical oscillatory activity (Baker and Baker, 2003), thus deserving a consideration independent from cortical beta band power modulation.

However, previous work performing resting-state MEG recordings in PD patients with DBS has neither captured CMC nor has it analyzed source level oscillatory activity (Cao et al., 2015). Only movement-related beta-CMC is currently being investigated as a physiological marker in PD patients undergoing DBS surgery (Hirschmann et al., 2011; Airaksinen et al., 2015). Although, these studies focused on the impact of levodopa medication and DBS on CMC as physiological predictors of clinical outcome, an application of this technique for delineating a cortical *hot spot* for surface stimulation remains elusive. Airaksinen and co-workers suggested that the cortical representation of beta-CMC and the cortical area modulated by DBS might even differ (Airaksinen et al., 2015). Based on our findings, we suggest that the cortical representation of beta-CMC during resting state might be more restricted.

We therefore suggest that resting-state CMC may eliminate the large inter-individual variability inherent to movements in PD patients in general (Kühn, 2004; Kühn et al., 2008; Tropini et al., 2011; Selzler et al., 2013) and of the related CMC in particular as observed by Airaksinen et al. (2015). Moreover, we demonstrate that source reconstruction—and co-location—of both CMC (**Figure 3A**) and oscillatory power (**Figure 3B**) during DBS reveals the cortical convergence of pathological synchronization within a cortical hot spot.

Using simultaneous MEG and LFP recordings, motor cortical areas directly connecting STN and cortex, i.e., mediated via the hyperdirect pathway, were identified in source space thereby disentangling different sub-frequency bands within the beta-band and attributing the upper beta-band to cortico-subcortical interactions (Hirschmann et al., 2011). In the present study, we did not capture cortico-subcortical coherence, which would have necessitated externalized leads. Future studies will therefore need to explore frequency-specific interactions between local beta activity and rather long-range interaction with the sensorimotor loop, i.e., for STN/cortex, muscles/cortex, and STN/muscles. Corroborating results for a direct connection between STN and cortex were however obtained by quantitative modeling of axonal fiber activation (Hartmann et al., 2015) or a combination of diffusion tensor imaging (DTI) and electrocorticographic (ECoG) electrodes (Whitmer et al., 2012).

More recently, ECoG (de Hemptinne et al., 2015) and EEG (Swann et al., 2015) have also been applied to capture cortical beta-gamma phase-amplitude coupling (PAC) as a functional marker, while demonstrating its modulation by DBS (de Hemptinne et al., 2015) and levodopa (Swann et al., 2015); PAC might provide an even more robust biomarker than beta oscillations in PD patients (de Hemptinne et al., 2015; Swann et al., 2015). Capturing PAC in MEG source space, however, poses methodological challenges. We are therefore currently applying EEG to compare different physiological markers in PD patients, e.g., for determining topographic and functional differences between PAC and beta oscillations. Future physiological studies will moreover need to compare the interactions in medication on/off and to capture clinical lateralization scores as well. Medication may modulate the very same networks that are modulated by DBS, and the observed DBS effects might even be more pronounced in the medication off state.

This proof-of-concept is however the first to show that beta-CMC delineates the very same cortical area as modulated by STN-DBS, and is meant to inspire and encourage other groups to challenge this testable hypothesis by examining their patients with resting-state CMC as well. These future larger scale studies will then have to address further questions, such as (1) can resting-state CMC be detected in all PD patients, (2) is resting-state CMC correlated with the severity of the disease, (3) does the cortical hot spot vary between patients, and (4) do peak frequencies vary between patients?

CONCLUSION

We argue that the particular pathophysiology, i.e., the increased synchronization in the oscillatory beta-frequency band, in advanced Parkinson's disease (PD) would facilitate the non-invasive detection of a cortical *hot spot* since cortico-muscular communication is also mediated in the very same frequency band.

We demonstrated that both clusters projected to the same anatomically plausible area in the primary motor/ premotor area and that these overlapping source clusters revealed the strongest stimulation induced changes for CMC (**Figure 3A**) and cortical power (**Figure 3B**). The decreases of CMC and cortical power were both in the same beta-band. Only a circumscribed area of the whole extended region with increased cortical beta activity (**Figure 2B**) was significantly reduced by DBS (**Figure 3B**). All these complementary and consistent findings cannot be explained by random collocation and are therefore not compromised by the sample size of one. However, the inherent intersubject variability in signals will necessitate the study of further patients to draw definite conclusions.

The novelty of this concept is grounded in the new combination of methods rather than in a new methodology, i.e., by combining resting-state (instead of the usual movement related) cortico-muscular coherence (CMC) with source space analysis of magnetencephalography recordings. Future studies will need to reveal which cortical recording technique, MEG or EEG, is better suited to detect the cortical *hot spot* before surgery.

The underlying hypotheses are (a) that resting-state CMC would be detectable in PD (other than in healthy subjects), (b) that resting-state CMC would avoid the known variability of movement related CMC in PD, and (c) that pathologically synchronized loops would converge on the cortical level. Such a topographic convergence within a cortical-subcortical-muscular network would provide a prominent target region either for direct neuromodulation or for placing a potential *sensor* in closed-loop DBS approaches since DBS was recently shown to mediate its therapeutic effects also via remote cortical modulation.

AUTHOR CONTRIBUTIONS

KK designed and performed research, analyzed data, and wrote the paper. GN designed and performed research. CB designed research and edited the paper. DW designed research and edited the paper. AG designed research, analyzed data, and wrote the paper.

ACKNOWLEDGMENTS

KK was supported by the Graduate Training Centre of Neuroscience, International Max Planck Research School for Cognitive and Systems Neuroscience, Tuebingen, Germany, GN was supported by a grant from the German Research Council [DFG EC 307], and AG was supported by grants from the German Research Council [DFG EC 307], and from the Federal Ministry for Education and Research [BFNT 01GQ0761, BMBF 16SV3783, BMBF 0316064B, BMBF 16SV5824].

REFERENCES

Afshar, P., Khambhati, A., Stanslaski, S., Carlson, D., Jensen, R., Linde, D., et al. (2012). A translational platform for prototyping closed-loop neuromodulation systems. *Front. Neural Circuits* 6:117. doi: 10.3389/fncir.2012.00117

Agirre-Arrizubieta, Z., Thai, N. J., Valentín, A., Furlong, P. L., Seri, S., Selway, R. P., et al. (2014). The value of Magnetoencephalography to guide electrode implantation in epilepsy. *Brain Topogr.* 27, 97–207. doi: 10.1007/s10548-013-0330-x

Airaksinen, K., Butorina, A., Pekkonen, E., Nurminen, J., Taulu, S., Ahonen, A., et al. (2012). Somatomotor mu rhythm amplitude correlates with rigidity during deep brain stimulation in Parkinsonian patients. *Clin. Neurophysiol. Off. J. Int. Fed. Clin. Neurophysiol.* 123, 2010–2017. doi: 10.1016/j.clinph.2012.03.004

Airaksinen, K., Mäkelä, J. P., Nurminen, J., Luoma, J., Taulu, S., Ahonen, A., et al. (2015). Cortico-muscular coherence in advanced Parkinson's disease with deep brain stimulation. *Clin. Neurophysiol.* 126, 748–755. doi: 10.1016/j.clinph.2014.07.025

Airaksinen, K., Mäkelä, J. P., Taulu, S., Ahonen, A., Nurminen, J., Schnitzler, A., et al. (2011). Effects of DBS on auditory and somatosensory processing in Parkinson's disease. *Hum. Brain Mapp.* 32, 1091–1099. doi: 10.1002/hbm.21096

Baker, M. R., and Baker, S. N. (2003). The effect of diazepam on motor cortical oscillations and corticomuscular coherence studied in man. *J. Physiol. (Lond).* 546, 931–942. doi: 10.1113/jphysiol.2002.029553

Baker, S. N. (2007). Oscillatory interactions between sensorimotor cortex and the periphery. *Curr. Opin. Neurobiol.* 17, 649–655. doi: 10.1016/j.conb.2008.01.007

Bentivoglio, A. R., Fasano, A., Piano, C., Soleti, F., Daniele, A., Zinno, M., et al. (2012). Unilateral extradural motor cortex stimulation is safe and improves Parkinson disease at 1 year. *Neurosurgery* 71, 815–825. doi: 10.1227/NEU.0b013e318266e6a5

Beuter, A., Lefaucheur, J.-P., and Modolo, J. (2014). Closed-loop cortical neuromodulation in Parkinson's disease: an alternative to deep brain stimulation? *Clin. Neurophysiol. Off. J. Int. Fed. Clin. Neurophysiol.* 125, 874–885. doi: 10.1016/j.clinph.2014.01.006

Bronte-Stewart, H., Barberini, C., Koop, M. M., Hill, B. C., Henderson, J. M., and Wingeier, B. (2009). The STN beta-band profile in Parkinson's disease is stationary and shows prolonged attenuation after deep brain stimulation. *Exp. Neurol.* 215, 20–28. doi: 10.1016/j.expneurol.2008.09.008

Brovelli, A., Ding, M., Ledberg, A., Chen, Y., Nakamura, R., and Bressler, S. L. (2004). Beta oscillations in a large-scale sensorimotor cortical network: directional influences revealed by Granger causality. *Proc. Natl. Acad. Sci. U.S.A.* 101, 9849–9854. doi: 10.1073/pnas.0308538101

Brown, P., Marsden, J., Defebvre, L., Cassim, F., Mazzone, P., Oliviero, A., et al. (2001). Intermuscular coherence in Parkinson's disease: relationship to bradykinesia. *Neuroreport* 12, 2577–2581. doi: 10.1097/00001756-200108080-00057

Budini, F., McManus, L. M., Berchicci, M., Menotti, F., Macaluso, A., Di Russo, F., et al. (2014). Alpha band cortico-muscular coherence occurs in healthy individuals during mechanically-induced tremor. *PLoS ONE* 9:e115012. doi: 10.1371/journal.pone.0115012

Cao, C., Li, D., Jiang, T., Ince, N. F., Zhan, S., Zhang, J., et al. (2015). Resting state cortical oscillations of patients with Parkinson disease and with and without subthalamic deep brain stimulation: a magnetoencephalography study. *J. Clin. Neurophysiol.* 32, 109–118. doi: 10.1097/WNP.0000000000000137

Chakarov, V., Naranjo, J. R., Schulte-Mönting, J., Omlor, W., Huethe, F., and Kristeva, R. (2009). Beta-range EEG-EMG coherence with isometric compensation for increasing modulated low-level forces. *J. Neurophysiol.* 102, 1115–1120. doi: 10.1152/jn.91095.2008

Cilia, R., Landi, A., Vergani, F., Sganzerla, E., Pezzoli, G., and Antonini, A. (2007). Extradural motor cortex stimulation in Parkinson's disease. *Mov. Disord.* 22, 111–114. doi: 10.1002/mds.21207

Cooper, S. E., McIntyre, C. C., Fernandez, H. H., and Vitek, J. L. (2013). Association of deep brain stimulation washout effects with Parkinson disease duration. *JAMA Neurol.* 70, 95–99. doi: 10.1001/jamaneurol.2013.581

Crone, N. E., Miglioretti, D. L., Gordon, B., and Lesser, R. P. (1998a). Functional mapping of human sensorimotor cortex with electrocorticographic spectral analysis. II. Event-related synchronization in the gamma band. *Brain J. Neurol.* 121(Pt 12), 2301–2315.

Crone, N. E., Miglioretti, D. L., Gordon, B., Sieracki, J. M., Wilson, M. T., Uematsu, S., et al. (1998b). Functional mapping of human sensorimotor cortex with electrocorticographic spectral analysis. I. Alpha and beta event-related desynchronization. *Brain J. Neurol.* 121(Pt 12), 2271–2299.

de Hemptinne, C., Swann, N. C., Ostrem, J. L., Ryapolova-Webb, E. S., San Luciano, M., Galifianakis, N. B., et al. (2015). Therapeutic deep brain stimulation reduces cortical phase-amplitude coupling in Parkinson's disease. *Nat. Neurosci.* 18, 779–786. doi: 10.1038/nn.3997

Deuschl, G., Schade-Brittinger, C., Krack, P., Volkmann, J., Schäfer, H., Bötzel, K., et al. (2006). A randomized trial of deep-brain stimulation for Parkinson's disease. *N. Engl. J. Med.* 355, 896–908. doi: 10.1056/NEJMoa060281

Devos, D. (2004). Subthalamic nucleus stimulation modulates motor cortex oscillatory activity in Parkinson's disease. *Brain* 127, 408–419. doi: 10.1093/brain/awh053

Engel, A. K., and Fries, P. (2010). Beta-band oscillations–signalling the status quo? *Curr. Opin. Neurobiol.* 20, 156–165. doi: 10.1016/j.conb.2010.02.015

Eusebio, A., Cagnan, H., and Brown, P. (2012). Does suppression of oscillatory synchronisation mediate some of the therapeutic effects of DBS in patients with Parkinson's disease? *Front. Integr. Neurosci.* 6:47. doi: 10.3389/fnint.2012.0004

Eusebio, A., Thevathasan, W., Doyle Gaynor, L., Pogosyan, A., Bye, E., Foltynie, T., et al. (2011). Deep brain stimulation can suppress pathological synchronisation in parkinsonian patients. *J. Neurol. Neurosurg. Psychiatr.* 82, 569–573. doi: 10.1136/jnnp.2010.217489

Gradinaru, V., Mogri, M., Thompson, K. R., Henderson, J. M., and Deisseroth, K. (2009). Optical deconstruction of parkinsonian neural circuitry. *Science* 324, 354–359. doi: 10.1126/science.1167093

Gross, J., Kujala, J., Hamalainen, M., Timmermann, L., Schnitzler, A., and Salmelin, R. (2001). Dynamic imaging of coherent sources: studying neura interactions in the human brain. *Proc. Natl. Acad. Sci. U.S.A.* 98, 694–699. doi: 10.1073/pnas.98.2.694

Grosse-Wentrup, M., Schölkopf, B., and Hill, J. (2011). Causal influence of gamma oscillations on the sensorimotor rhythm. *Neuroimage* 56, 837–842. doi: 10.1016/j.neuroimage.2010.04.265

Hartmann, C. J., Chaturvedi, A., and Lujan, J. L. (2015). Quantitative analysis of axonal fiber activation evoked by deep brain stimulation via activation density heat maps. *Front. Neurosci.* 9:28. doi: 10.3389/fnins.2015.00028

Hillebrand, A., Fazio, P., de Munck, J. C., and van Dijk, B. W. (2013). Feasibility of clinical Magnetoencephalography (MEG) functional mapping in the presence of dental artefacts. *Clin. Neurophysiol.* 124, 107–113. doi: 10.1016/j.clinph.2012.06.013

Hipp, J. F., Engel, A. K., and Siegel, M. (2011). Oscillatory synchronization in large-scale cortical networks predicts perception. *Neuron* 69, 387–396. doi: 10.1016/j.neuron.2010.12.027

Hirschmann, J., Hartmann, C. J., Butz, M., Hoogenboom, N., Ozkurt, T. E., Elben, S., et al. (2013a). A direct relationship between oscillatory subthalamic nucleus-cortex coupling and rest tremor in Parkinson's disease. *Brain J. Neurol.* 136, 3659–3670. doi: 10.1093/brain/awt271

Hirschmann, J., Özkurt, T. E., Butz, M., Homburger, M., Elben, S., Hartmann, C. J., et al. (2011). Distinct oscillatory STN-cortical loops revealed by simultaneous MEG and local field potential recordings in patients with Parkinson's disease. *Neuroimage* 55, 1159–1168. doi: 10.1016/j.neuroimage.2010.11.063

Hirschmann, J., Özkurt, T. E., Butz, M., Homburger, M., Elben, S., Hartmann, C. J., et al. (2013b). Differential modulation of STN-cortical and cortico-muscular coherence by movement and levodopa in Parkinson's disease. *Neuroimage* 68, 203–213. doi: 10.1016/j.neuroimage.2012.11.036

Kelly, P. J. (1996). The interactive use of magnetoencephalography in stereo- tactic image-guided neurosurgery. *Neurosurgery* 39, 92–102. doi: 10.1097/00006123-199607000-00018

Kilner, J. M., Baker, S. N., Salenius, S., Hari, R., and Lemon, R. N. (2000). Human cortical muscle coherence is directly related to specific motor parameters. *J. Neurosci. Off. J. Soc. Neurosci.* 20, 8838–8845.

Knowlton, R. C., and Shih, J. (2004). Magnetoencephalography in epilepsy. *Epilepsia* 45(Suppl. 4), 61–71. doi: 10.1111/j.0013-9580.2004.04012.x

Kringelbach, M. L., Green, A. L., Owen, S. L. F., Schweder, P. M., and Aziz, T. Z. (2010). Sing the mind electric - principles of deep brain stimulation. *Eur. J. Neurosci.* 32, 1070–1079. doi: 10.1111/j.1460-9568.2010.07419.x

Kühn, A. A. (2004). Event-related beta desynchronization in human subthalamic nucleus correlates with motor performance. *Brain* 127, 735–746. doi: 10.1093/brain/awh106

Kühn, A. A., Kempf, F., Brücke, C., Gaynor Doyle, L., Martinez-Torres, I., Pogosyan, A., et al. (2008). High-frequency stimulation of the subthalamic nucleus suppresses oscillatory beta activity in patients with Parkinson's disease in parallel with improvement in motor performance. *J. Neurosci. Off. J. Soc. Neurosci.* 28, 6165–6173. doi: 10.1523/JNEUROSCI.0282-08.2008

Kühn, A. A., Kupsch, A., Schneider, G. H., and Brown, P. (2006). Reduction in subthalamic 8–35 Hz oscillatory activity correlates with clinical improvement in Parkinson's disease. *Eur. J. Neurosci.* 23, 1956–1960. doi: 10.1111/j.1460-9568.2006.04717.x

Li, Q., Ke, Y., Chan, D. C. W., Qian, Z.-M., Yung, K. K. L., Ko, H., et al. (2012). Therapeutic deep brain stimulation in Parkinsonian rats directly influences motor cortex. *Neuron* 76, 1030–1041. doi: 10.1016/j.neuron.2012.09.032

Little, S., and Brown, P. (2012). What brain signals are suitable for feedback control of deep brain stimulation in Parkinson's disease? *Ann. N.Y. Acad. Sci.* 1265, 9–24. doi: 10.1111/j.1749-6632.2012.06650.x

Little, S., and Brown, P. (2014). The functional role of beta oscillations in Parkinson's disease. *Parkinsonism Relat. Disord.* 20(Suppl.) 1, S44–S48. doi: 10.1016/S1353-8020(13)70013-0

Litvak, V., Eusebio, A., Jha, A., Oostenveld, R., Barnes, G. R., Penny, W. D., et al. (2010). Optimized beamforming for simultaneous MEG and intracranial local field potential recordings in deep brain stimulation patients. *Neuroimage* 50, 1578–1588. doi: 10.1016/j.neuroimage.2009.12.115

Litvak, V., Jha, A., Eusebio, A., Oostenveld, R., Foltynie, T., Limousin, P., et al. (2011). Resting oscillatory cortico-subthalamic connectivity in patients with Parkinson's disease. *Brain J. Neurol.* 134, 359–374. doi: 10.1093/brain/awq332

Mäkelä, J., Taulu, S., Pohjola, J., Ahonen, A., and Pekkonen, E. (2007). Effects of subthalamic nucleus stimulation on spontaneous sensorimotor MEG activity in a Parkinsonian patient. *Int. Congr. Ser.* 1300, 345–348. doi: 10.1016/j.ics.2007.02.003

Maris, E., and Oostenveld, R. (2007). Nonparametric statistical testing of EEG- and MEG-data. *J. Neurosci. Methods* 164, 177–190. doi: 10.1016/j.jneumeth.2007.03.024

Marreiros, A. C., Cagnan, H., Moran, R. J., Friston, K. J., and Brown, P. (2013). Basal ganglia-cortical interactions in Parkinsonian patients. *Neuroimage* 66, 301–310. doi: 10.1016/j.neuroimage.2012.10.088

Marsden, J., Limousin-Dowsey, P., Fraix, V., Pollak, P., Odin, P., and Brown, P. (2001). Intermuscular coherence in Parkinson's disease: effects of subthalamic nucleus stimulation. *Neuroreport* 12, 1113–1117. doi: 10.1097/00001756-200105080-00013

McIntyre, C. C., and Hahn, P. J. (2010). Network perspectives on the mechanisms of deep brain stimulation. *Neurobiol. Dis.* 38, 329–337. doi: 10.1016/j.nbd.2009.09.022

Medvedovsky, M., Taulu, S., Bikmullina, R., Ahonen, A., and Paetau, R. (2009). Fine tuning the correlation limit of spatio-temporal signal space separation for magnetoencephalography. *J. Neurosci. Methods* 177, 203–211. doi: 10.1016/j.jneumeth.2008.09.035

Mitra, P. P., and Pesaran, B. (1999). Analysis of Dynamic Brain Imaging Data. *Biophys. J.* 76, 691–708. doi: 10.1016/S0006-3495(99)77236-X

Moro, E., Schwalb, J. M., Piboolnurak, P., Poon, Y. Y. W., Hamani, C., Hung, S. W., et al. (2011). Unilateral subdural motor cortex stimulation improves essential tremor but not Parkinson's disease. *Brain*, 134, 2096–2105. doi: 10.1093/brain/awr072

Myers, L. J., Lowery, M., O'Malley, M., Vaughan, C. L., Heneghan, C., St Clair Gibson, A., et al. (2003). Rectification and non-linear pre-processing of EMG signals for cortico-muscular analysis. *J. Neurosci. Methods* 124, 157–165. doi: 10.1016/S0165-0270(03)00004-9

Oostenveld, R., Fries, P., Maris, E., and Schoffelen, J.-M. (2011). FieldTrip: open source software for advanced analysis of MEG, EEG, and invasive electrophysiological data. *Comput. Intell. Neurosci.* 2011, 1–9. doi: 10.1155/2011/156869

Orrison, W. W. Jr. (1999). Magnetic source imaging in stereotactic and functional neurosurgery. *Stereotact. Funct. Neurosurg.* 72, 89–94. doi: 10.1159/000029705

Pizzella, V., and Romani, G. (1990). "Principles of magnetoencephalography," in *Magnetoencephalography*, ed S. Sato (New York, NY: Raven Press), 1–9.

Rezai, A. R., Hund, M., Kronberg, E., Zonenshayn, M., Cappell, J., Ribary, U., et al. (1996). The interactive use of magnetoencephalography in stereotactic image-guided neurosurgery. *Neurosurgery* 39, 92–102. doi: 10.1097/00006123-199607000-00018

Rosin, B., Slovik, M., Mitelman, R., Rivlin-Etzion, M., Haber, S. N., Israel, Z., et al. (2011). Closed-loop deep brain stimulation is superior in ameliorating parkinsonism. *Neuron* 72, 370–384. doi: 10.1016/j.neuron.2011.08.023

Salenius, S., Avikainen, S., Kaakkola, S., Hari, R., and Brown, P. (2002). Defective cortical drive to muscle in Parkinson's disease and its improvement with levodopa. *Brain, J. Neurol.* 125, 491–500. doi: 10.1093/brain/awf042

Schoffelen, J.-M., Oostenveld, R., and Fries, P. (2005). Neuronal coherence as a mechanism of effective corticospinal interaction. *Science* 308, 111–113. doi: 10.1126/science.1107027

Schuepbach, W. M. M., Rau, J., Knudsen, K., Volkmann, J., Krack, P., Timmermann, L., et al. (2013). Neurostimulation for Parkinson's disease with early motor complications. *N. Engl. J. Med.* 368, 610–622. doi: 10.1056/NEJMoa1205158

Selzler, K., Burack, M., Bender, R., and Mapstone, M. (2013). Neurophysiological correlates of motor and working memory performance following subthalamic nucleus stimulation. *J. Cogn. Neurosci.* 25, 37–48. doi: 10.1162/jocn_a_00306

Silberstein, P., Pogosyan, A., Kühn, A. A., Hotton, G., Tisch, S., Kupsch, A., et al. (2005). Cortico-cortical coupling in Parkinson's disease and its modulation by therapy. *Brain J. Neurol.* 128, 1277–1291. doi: 10.1093/brain/awh480

Swann, N. C., de Hemptinne, C., Aron, A. R., Ostrem, J. L., Knight, R. T., and Starr, P. A. (2015). Elevated synchrony in Parkinson disease detected with electroencephalography. *Ann. Neurol.* 78, 742–750. doi: 10.1002/ana.24507

Taulu, S., and Hari, R. (2009). Removal of magnetoencephalographic artifacts with temporal signal-space separation: demonstration with single-trial auditory-evoked responses. *Hum. Brain Mapp.* 30, 1524–1534. doi: 10.1002/hbm.20627

Taulu, S., and Simola, J. (2006). Spatiotemporal signal space separation method for rejecting nearby interference in MEG measurements. *Phys. Med. Biol.* 51, 1759–1768. doi: 10.1088/0031-9155/51/7/008

Timmermann, L., Gross, J., Dirks, M., Volkmann, J., Freund, H.-J., and Schnitzler, A. (2003). The cerebral oscillatory network of parkinsonian resting tremor. *Brain* 126, 199–212. doi: 10.1093/brain/awg022

Tropini, G., Chiang, J., Wang, Z. J., Ty, E., and McKeown, M. J. (2011). Altered directional connectivity in Parkinson's disease during performance of a visually guided task. *Neuroimage* 56, 2144–2156. doi: 10.1016/j.neuroimage.2011.03.018

Weiss, D., Breit, S., Hoppe, J., Hauser, A.-K., Freudenstein, D., Krüger, R., et al. (2012). Subthalamic nucleus stimulation restores the efferent cortical drive to muscle in parallel to functional motor improvement. *Eur. J. Neurosci.* 35, 896–908. doi: 10.1111/j.1460-9568.2012.08014.x

Weiss, D., Klotz, R., Govindan, R. B., Scholten, M., Naros, G., Ramos-Murguialday, A., et al. (2015). Subthalamic stimulation modulates cortical motor network activity and synchronization in Parkinson's disease. *Brain* 138(Pt 3), 679–693. doi: 10.1093/brain/awu380

Weiss, D., Walach, M., Meisner, C., Fritz, M., Scholten, M., Breit, S., et al. (2013). Nigral stimulation for resistant axial motor impairment in Parkinson's disease? A randomized controlled trial. *Brain J. Neurol.* 136, 2098–2108. doi: 10.1093/brain/awt122

Whitmer, D., de Solages, C., Hill, B., Yu, H., Henderson, J. M., and Bronte-Stewart, H. (2012). High frequency deep brain stimulation attenuates subthalamic and cortical rhythms in Parkinson's disease. *Front. Hum. Neurosci.* 6:155. doi: 10.3389/fnhum.2012.00155

Yao, B., Salenius, S., Yue, G. H., Brown, R. W., and Liu, J. Z. (2007). Effects of surface EMG rectification on power and coherence analyses: an EEG and MEG study. *J. Neurosci. Methods* 159, 215–223. doi: 10.1016/j.jneumeth.2006.07.008

6

Prediction of STN-DBS Electrode Implantation Track in Parkinson's Disease by Using Local Field Potentials

*Ilknur Telkes [1], Joohi Jimenez-Shahed [2], Ashwin Viswanathan [3], Aviva Abosch [4] and Nuri F. Ince [1]**

[1] Clinical Neural Engineering Lab., Biomedical Engineering Department, University of Houston, Houston, TX, USA, [2] Department of Neurology, Baylor College of Medicine, Houston, TX, USA, [3] Department of Neurosurgery, Baylor College of Medicine, Houston, TX, USA, [4] Department of Neurosurgery, University of Colorado, Aurora, CO, USA

Edited by:
Paolo Bonifazi,
Tel Aviv University, Israel

Reviewed by:
Alessandro Stefani,
University of Rome, Italy
J. Luis Lujan,
Mayo Clinic, USA

***Correspondence:**
Nuri F. Ince
nfince@uh.edu

Optimal electrophysiological placement of the DBS electrode may lead to better long term clinical outcomes. Inter-subject anatomical variability and limitations in stereotaxic neuroimaging increase the complexity of physiological mapping performed in the operating room. Microelectrode single unit neuronal recording remains the most common intraoperative mapping technique, but requires significant expertise and is fraught by potential technical difficulties including robust measurement of the signal. In contrast, local field potentials (LFPs), owing to their oscillatory and robust nature and being more correlated with the disease symptoms, can overcome these technical issues. Therefore, we hypothesized that multiple spectral features extracted from microelectrode-recorded LFPs could be used to automate the identification of the optimal track and the STN localization. In this regard, we recorded LFPs from microelectrodes in three tracks from 22 patients during DBS electrode implantation surgery at different depths and aimed to predict the track selected by the neurosurgeon based on the interpretation of single unit recordings. A least mean square (LMS) algorithm was used to de-correlate LFPs in each track, in order to remove common activity between channels and increase their spatial specificity. Subband power in the beta band (11–32 Hz) and high frequency range (200–450 Hz) were extracted from the de-correlated LFP data and used as features. A linear discriminant analysis (LDA) method was applied both for the localization of the dorsal border of STN and the prediction of the optimal track. By fusing the information from these low and high frequency bands, the dorsal border of STN was localized with a root mean square (RMS) error of 1.22 mm. The prediction accuracy for the optimal track was 80%. Individual beta band (11–32 Hz) and the range of high frequency oscillations (200–450 Hz) provided prediction accuracies of 72 and 68% respectively. The best prediction result obtained with monopolar LFP data was 68%. These results establish the initial evidence that LFPs can be strategically fused with computational intelligence in the operating room for STN localization and the selection of the track for chronic DBS electrode implantation.

Keywords: local field potentials, subthalamic nucleus, microelectrode recordings, least mean square algorithm, LDA classification

INTRODUCTION

Deep brain stimulation (DBS) of the subthalamic nucleus (STN) is an effective therapy for the treatment of the motor symptoms of Parkinson's disease (PD) (Herzog et al., 2004; Hariz, 2012). DBS surgery involves localization of the motor territory of the STN, for permanent implantation of a DBS electrode at this site. Although the exact mechanism of DBS remains to be elucidated, STN stimulation is well-tolerated and improves all of the cardinal symptoms of PD (Levy et al., 2002). However, STN stimulation can result in side effects arising from the spread of stimulation to structures surrounding the STN (Richardson et al., 2009). Moreover, sub-optimal positioning of DBS electrodes accounts for up to 40% of cases of inadequate efficacy of stimulation postoperatively (Okun et al., 2005). Thus, developing quantitative electrophysiological methods to define the optimal site of stimulation may help optimize DBS outcomes.

The task of the neurosurgeon is to place the DBS electrode within the motor territory of the STN, and well within the STN borders such that current does not spread to the surrounding structures, thereby resulting in stimulation-limiting side effects (Richardson et al., 2009). Although the surgical procedure varies somewhat between medical centers, targeting of the STN during DBS surgery generally includes preoperative stereotactic imaging (MRI), used in conjunction with stereotactic atlases. This step is followed by intraoperative electrophysiological techniques consisting of the conversion of neural activity, in the form of single-unit neuronal activity (SUA) recorded at the microelectrode tip, into audio and visual signals. This procedure is experience-based and depends critically on the neurosurgeon's and neurophysiologist's ability to recognize entry into the STN, based on a variety of cues.

In order to obtain a three-dimensional map of the STN and surrounding structures, multiple microelectrode recording tracks (typically up to five) (Benabid et al., 2009) are carried out, either sequentially or simultaneously. Determination of the optimal track for DBS implantation is a key component to successful therapeutic outcome. Optimal track selection is primarily based on microelectrode recording of single unit activity (MER/SUA), which is used to identify cells with firing characteristics consistent with STN neurons and response characteristics confirming the motor sub-territory of the STN (Falkenberg et al., 2006). Despite the common usage of MER/SUA during stereotactic surgery for PD, limitations of this technique include difficulties interpreting complex signal patterns to localize the anatomical borders of the STN, highly overlapping spiking characteristics of single neurons around the target structure, recording SUA from a very small region, sensitivity of SUA to noise, susceptibility of SUA to small amounts of blood or edema within the microelectrode track, and the binary nature of SUA (unlike local field potentials; LFP), all of which may affect the accuracy of STN localization in PD (Chen et al., 2006; Gross et al., 2006; Novak et al., 2011). The caliber of single-unit recordings can be easily diminished due to drift of the recorded unit away from the electrode tip, as a consequence of transmitted pulsations of the brain and other environmental conditions (Sanghera and Grossman, 2004).

Interpretation of SUA recordings with computational intelligence was proposed as a new approach to help clinical decision making in the operating room (Wong et al., 2009). However, such approaches are still susceptible to the challenges of isolating single neurons in the operating room. LFPs represent the aggregate activity of neuronal populations, and are particularly sensitive to synchronous and oscillatory firing patterns (Priori et al., 2004; Gross et al., 2006). Recent studies indicate that LFPs in PD correlate with both motor and non-motor symptoms of the disease, and their signals are more robust than SUA (Priori et al., 2013; Thompson et al., 2014). Importantly, LFPs are an objective and quantitative metric while MER/SUA is more qualitative and subject to inter-practitioner variability. Although, the functional role of LFPs during DBS surgery is not fully established, we propose that they can be used to contribute to target localization in PD. In the present study, for the purpose of assisting with clinical decision making, we aimed to develop an automated approach by processing LFPs from multiple tracks to localize the dorsal border of STN and predict the macroelectrode implantation track identified by the neurosurgeon based on SUA interpretation. In the next sections first we describe our data collection methods and then detail our signal processing and classification techniques. We study the role of LFP sub-bands in prediction of the location of the dorsal border of STN. Moreover, we explore different decision criteria fused with LFP sub-band features toward prediction of optimal track selected by the neurosurgeons. We show experimental results obtained from 22 patients and discuss our results and demonstrate that LFPs can be used effectively in the operating room for clinical decision making.

METHODS

Patients and Surgical Procedure

This is a multicenter study in which patients were recruited in either University of Minnesota Medical Center or Baylor St. Luke's Medical Center. The experimental protocol was approved by the Institutional Review Boards of the University of Minnesota and Baylor College of Medicine. All patients provided written informed consent to participate in the study. Intraoperative LFPs were recorded from 22 patients (14 men, 8 women), who were diagnosed with idiopathic PD, and exhibited typical motor symptoms which were tremor, rigidity, and bradykinesia. Disease duration ranged between 1 and 20 years, with a mean of 10.55 years (standard deviation of 4.7 years) (**Table 1**). All patients discontinued short-acting Parkinson's medications at 12 h prior to surgery, and long-acting medications at least 24 h prior to surgery. As per standard clinical protocol, target coordinates and trajectory to the STN, were identified by preoperative stereotactic MRI, which was fused to a stereotactic computed tomography (CT), on a neuro-navigational platform (StealthStation, Medtronic Corp, MN). Then, again based on standard clinical protocol, three simultaneous tracks were performed in each subject (**Figure 1A**). The superior and inferior borders of STN, along with the optimal depth for positioning the DBS electrode, were determined by the clinical team via electrophysiological mapping using MER/SUA, and the DBS

TABLE 1 | Clinical characteristics of the PD patients included in this study.

Number of patients	22
Gender (women/men)	8/14
Age (mean ± std in years)	57 ± 11
Disease duration (mean ± std in years)	10.5 ± 4.7
PHENOTYPES:	
Typical	12
Tremor dominant	5
Bradykinetic/Rigid	5
OFF/ON UPDRS[†] scores (mean)[‡]	45.60%
Number of microelectrodes recording (total)	75 in total

[†] *UPDRS = Unified Parkinson's Disease Rating Scale.*
[‡] *Pre-Operative Medication OFF-to-ON UPDRS Scores: Total Improvement.*

electrode was implanted by the neurosurgeon based on these spatial data, followed by macro stimulation to confirm electrode location based on benefit and side effect profile—i.e., location within motor territory of STN, but not so close to border with adjacent internal capsule or medial lemniscus, that low-threshold stimulation- induced side effects were detected—followed by confirmatory intra-operative imaging modalities. Surgeries were performed in awake patients, under the benefits of local anesthesia. In 3 of 22 patients, microelectrode mapping of right and left STN occurred on different surgical dates, as the surgical procedures were staged for clinical reasons. Therefore, these recordings were counted as separate, enabling 25 individual STN microelectrode recordings for LFP-based optimal track prediction.

Intra-Operative Recordings and Track Selection

Following standard stereotactic techniques, and insertion of three brain cannulas and microelectrodes (Abosch et al., 2002), MER/SUA recording was carried out using a Microguide system (AlphaOmega Inc., USA) at 12 kHz. Simultaneous LFPs were recorded with an XLTEK-EMU128FS system (Natus, San Carlos, California) at 2 kHz with 16 bit A/D resolution or gHIAmp (gTec Inc., Graz, Austria), 38.4 kHz with 24 bit A/D resolution. The LFP recordings were obtained from a 1 mm wide stainless steel contact which is 3 mm (NeuroProbe, AlphaOmega Inc., USA) or 1 mm (MicroTargeting™, FHC Inc., USA) above the SUA recording tip and referenced to the cannula (**Figure 1B**). All microelectrodes were advanced toward the estimated target using a NeuroDrive (AlphaOmega Inc., USA) with micrometer resolution. In order to synchronize the SUA and LFP recordings, the digital depth information of the NeuroDrive is transmitted from the MicroGuide system to LFP recording system using a TCP/IP connection. Initial recordings began 20 mm above the intended final location of the electrode tip ("target") as determined by direct targeting methods and proceeded until the electrode reached 3 mm below the MER-determined target, within the substantia nigra. Electrodes were lowered in 1 mm steps until 10 mm above "target," and then in 0.5 mm steps. Duration of recordings at each depth was 15–30 s.

At each depth, the subjects sequentially rested and after a certain depth (<10 mm) executed limb movements for 10–15 s period. The neurosurgeon used standard clinical techniques for localizing the STN, via real-time auditory and visual analysis of the recorded SUA. The dorsal, ventral, and posterior borders of the STN were identified by noting increased background noise and cell firing rate, and the STN neurons were examined for movement-responsive receptive fields. In particular, the superior border of STN was determined when the background activity increased and border cells were first observed among one of the tracks in MER-SUA. This position was used as the target value in STN border identification. Among three tracks, the track with the longest span of bursting cell firing and movement responsive fields was selected for the chronic DBS electrode implantation. This track was labeled as the "optimal track" and used as the target variable in LFP based track number prediction. The neurosurgeons were blinded to the LFP recordings in the operating room and the identification of STN dorsal border and the selection of optimal track for chronic DBS electrode implantation was not influenced by the LFP recordings. The STN border and the track selected by the neurosurgeon are predicted with the LFP data using the signal processing methods detailed below.

Signal Processing

All data were analyzed offline. Before any processing, all recorded signals were visualized with a custom in-house developed software and annotated to distinguish artifact and/or epochs of resting, active, and passive movements. Based on these annotations, resting state data were extracted into MATLAB (Mathworks, Natick, Massachusetts) and the data recorded by XLTEK system and gHIAmp system were downsampled to 1 and 1.2 kHz, respectively, for analysis.

A schematic diagram of our signal processing pipeline is given in **Figure 2**. As an initial step the raw signals were visualized and it was observed that tracks were difficult to distinguish, due to a high amount of common activity masking spatially localized activity and/or artifacts resulting from abrupt movements of the patient and other environmental factors. In order to eliminate the common activity among tracks, but still preserve the track-specific neural activity, the LFP data on each track were de-correlated using a least mean square (LMS) algorithm with a steepest descent update. The general formula for the de-correlation method is as follows:

$$\text{Initialization: } w(0) = 0.5,\ n = 0, 1, 2, \ldots$$

$$y(n) = w^T(n)x(n) \quad (1)$$

$$e(n) = d(n) - y(n) \quad (2)$$

$$\hat{e}(n) = \begin{cases} sign\,(e(n)) * 20 & \text{if } |e(n)| > 20 \\ e(n) & \text{otherwise} \end{cases} \quad (3)$$

$$w(n+1) = w(n) + \mu\hat{e}(n)\,x(n) \quad (4)$$

where $y(n)$ is the filter output, $\hat{e}(n)$ is the residual which is the de-correlated signal, $d(n)$ is the desired signal, μ is the step size, and $w(n)$ is time varying filter coefficient (Hayes, 1996). In the current method, each channel, $d(n)$, was predicted by using a

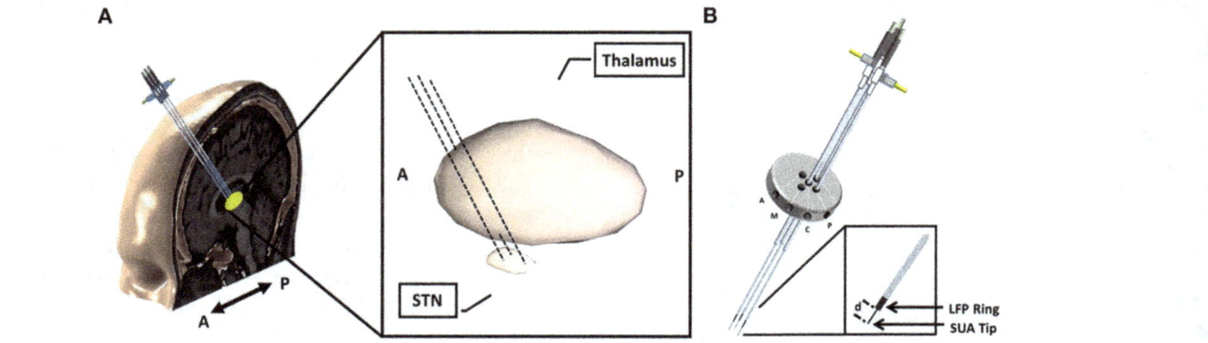

FIGURE 1 | Implantation of microelectrodes into STN using 3 simultaneous tracks. (A) Schematic of 3-track- microelectrode implantation into STN. The schematic in the middle shows the 3D-structure of STN and thalamus. The anatomical structures are viewed from sagittal plane. **(B)** Schematic of 5-port Bengun routinely used in STN localization in PD and penetration of multiple microelectrodes through the Bengun. Among these three tracks, optimal track is used as the DBS electrode implantation track. The LFP recording surfaces of both AO recording microelectrode (NeuroProbe, AlphaOmega Inc., USA) and FHC microelectrode (MicroTargetingTM, FHC, Inc., USA) are identical with a 1 mm stainless steel semi-macro contact situated 3 and 1 mm proximal to the micro-recording tip (electrode offset "d"), respectively. A, anterior; M, medial; C, center; P, posterior. The fifth trajectory, not visualized in the figure, is lateral.

linear weighted combination of other two channels, $x(n)$. LFP activity from three tracks were recorded continuously during the entire surgery while the microelectrodes were traveling to the estimated target. Consequently, the signal characteristic varied over depths. Since in each depth the signal was recorded for 15–30 s, temporal variability exists in the signal. Therefore, the filter coefficients, $w^T(n)$, were updated on a sample by sample basis recursively to make the system to adapt to depth and time varying signal properties. At each iteration, the error, $e(n)$, was calculated and this residual was used as the de-correlated LFP data in future steps for feature extraction and visualization. At 20 mm above the estimated target, all three tracks showed very similar signal characteristics indicating that they were in the white matter. Therefore, the initial filter coefficients were selected as the average of two channels with equal weights with the initialization of the filter coefficients $w(n) = 0.5$. By using this adaptive approach, we aimed to eliminate the common activity across tracks and suppress localized artifacts caused by patient movements and environmental factors. In order to prevent the system from being affected by high amplitude artifacts and to preserve the robustness, the error was saturated by using a 20 µV threshold (Equation 3). This threshold was determined experimentally and we observed that the system recovered from localized artifacts pretty fast even if the artifact amplitude was too large.

Due to differences in spatial correlation of low and high frequency bands, the monopolar data were, first, decomposed into two frequency bands which were 8–200 and 200–450 Hz by using a 2nd order Butterworth IIR filter (**Figure 2**). The LMS algorithm was individually applied to these subbands with step size of $\mu = 0.0002$. Each track was de-correlated by using LFPs on the other two tracks. The algorithm was applied to each depth by transferring filter coefficients to the next depth. In this way, filter coefficients were not required to start from 0.5 at each new depth so that the algorithm would adapt faster and can use both temporal and spatial information of the past. Decomposed and de-correlated data were re-merged and spectral analysis was performed. In this regard, a modified Welch periodogram method with a robust statistics was used (Telkes et al., 2014). Specifically, a fast Fourier transform (FFT) was computed with a 1024 samples long Hanning window and the window was shifted with 50% overlap. Since some artifacts destroy or dominate the power spectrum estimate obtained with mean operator, the median of the spectra of all sliding windows was calculated to eliminate localized artifacts in the spectrum. The method was repeated for each depth and all spectra were combined to visualize depth-varying power spectrum of LFPs on multi tracks. Generated depth-frequency maps (DFMs) were resampled with a 0.25 mm depth resolution and linearly interpolated to obtain equidistance depth values. The maps were smoothed using a Gaussian kernel filter to suppress noise and to reveal beta and high frequency band oscillations (HFOs). Then, DFMs were normalized with the average baseline of three tracks and transformed into log scale using the Equations (5) and (6). The tracks were not normalized by their own baseline but by the mean of all three tracks in order to compare the signal power between them. The baseline used for normalization was selected as the highest depths which assumed to be in the white matter. Therefore, the baseline was determined as top 5 depths (20–15 mm above the estimated target) in 22 recordings. However in rest of the three recordings, since the analysis started from lower than 20 mm (such that 18 mm) due to artifacts, the baseline segment was kept shorter and selected as top 3 depths. The purpose of using higher depths was to avoid from including any thalamic activity in normalization segment. The baseline normalization formula is noted below:

$$\bar{b}_{avg} = \frac{\left(\bar{b}_1 + \bar{b}_2 + \bar{b}_3\right)}{3} \quad (5)$$

$$\bar{n}_{dfm} = 20 \times \log_{10} \left(\frac{\bar{r}_{dfm}}{\bar{b}_{avg} + \Phi(f)} \right) \quad (6)$$

where $\bar{b}_1$, $\bar{b}_2$, $\bar{b}_3$ are the baseline spectrum of each 3 track, $\bar{b}_{avg}$ is the average baseline power, $\bar{r}_{dfm}$ indicates the DFM, $\Phi(f$

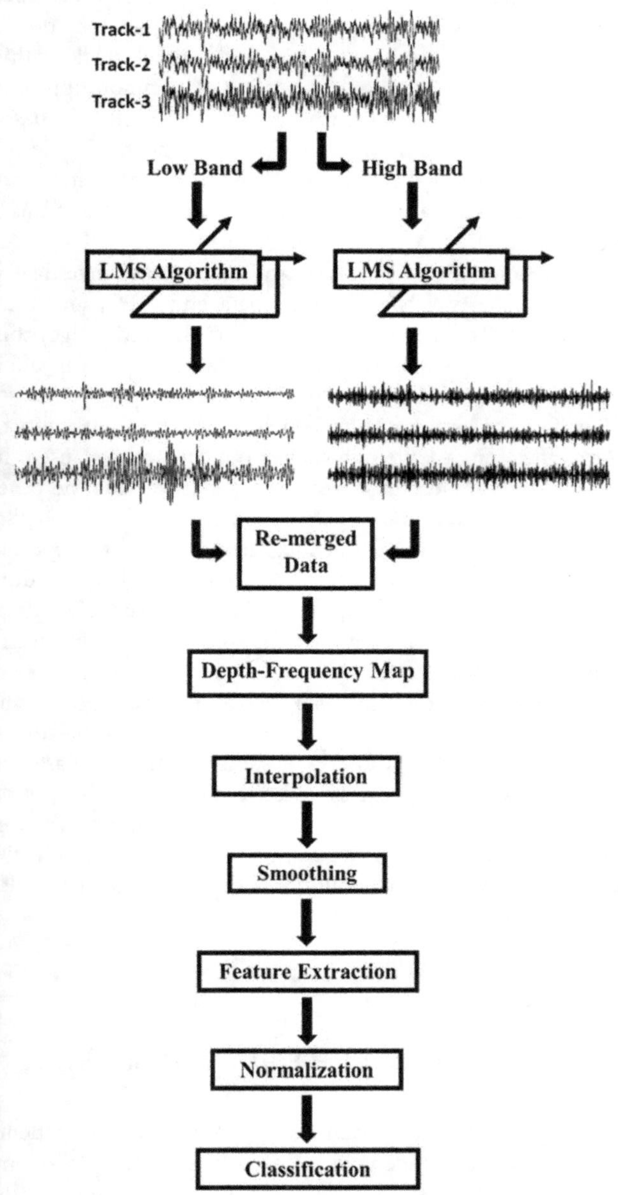

FIGURE 2 | Schematic of the work flow. LFPs recorded by 3 tracks of microelectrodes were decomposed into low (8–200 Hz) and high (200–450 Hz) frequency bands. Each track was de-correlated using LMS algorithm at each frequency band. De-correlated signals were combined and the frequency domain features were extracted for classification.

s a small regularization parameter which is applied for each requency f and $\overline{n}_{dfm}$ is the normalized DFM.

In order to observe the depth-varying frequency content of .FPs, DFMs of the patients were visualized. We noted that vhen the electrodes reached the STN border identified by the ıeurosurgeon, generally there was also an excessive activity in he beta and HFO range. In order to identify the most beneficial rack along with the dorsal border of the STN, the sub-band ›wer was extracted from all tracks and normalized by using subject-specific average baseline. Based on the distribution of neural activity on the tracks, the sub-band frequencies were designated 11–32 Hz for beta band and 200–450 Hz for HFOs. The distribution of power in the STN among all tracks and the distribution of power only on the selected track inside and outside of STN (above the dorsal border of STN) were investigated by box and whisker plots. Student's t-test with two-sample was used to check if the distributions were significantly different or not.

Classification

After sub-band power features were normalized between zero and one with a Max-Min normalization method for inter-subject comparison, a linear discriminant analysis (LDA) was used for classification. The principle of LDA is to maximize the separation of classes while keeping the within class densities small by using linear combination of features, $\vec{v} \cdot \vec{z}$ (Alpaydin, 2010). The linear discriminant function:

$$g_i(z|v_i, v_{i0}) = v_i^T z + v_{i0} = \sum_{j=1}^{d} v_{ij} z_j + v_{i0} \quad (7)$$

where $g_i(z)$ is the discriminant function for the input features z_j with sum of the weights v_j and threshold values v_{i0}.

Localization of the Dorsal Border of STN

In the present study, the dorsal border of STN identified by clinical team is predicted from the depth varying LFP data by using the decision distance of a linear classifier as shown in **Figure 3A**. First an LDA classifier was trained by contrasting the LFP sub-band features coming from inside and outside of STN (above the dorsal border of STN). This classifier was evaluated at each depth and the returned decision distance was used as a measure of confidence. The depth with the highest confidence for IN-STN decisions was marked. Then we traced the decision distances above this depth and found the location where the LDA classifier voted for OUT-STN. This point where the classifier made IN vs. OUT decision transition was finally chosen as the predicted dorsal border of STN. The difference between prediction and the STN border identified by MER-SUA was calculated in each patient and the root mean square (RMS) of the prediction errors was used to quantify the performance of the classifier. Further, statistical analysis by using Student's t-test and F-test was conducted in order to compare the mean and the variance of predictions obtained by different subband features, respectively.

Prediction of the Optimal Track

The optimal track selection among three tracks is done by the neurosurgeons through interpreting the excessive single cell firings within the STN. Consequently, for the prediction of the optimal track using LFP data, an LDA classifier was trained by contrasting the LFP subband features of selected track vs. unselected tracks below the dorsal border of STN. This classifier was evaluated at all depths as in the STN border prediction and the returned decision distance was used as a measure of confidence. The distance returned by the linear classifier

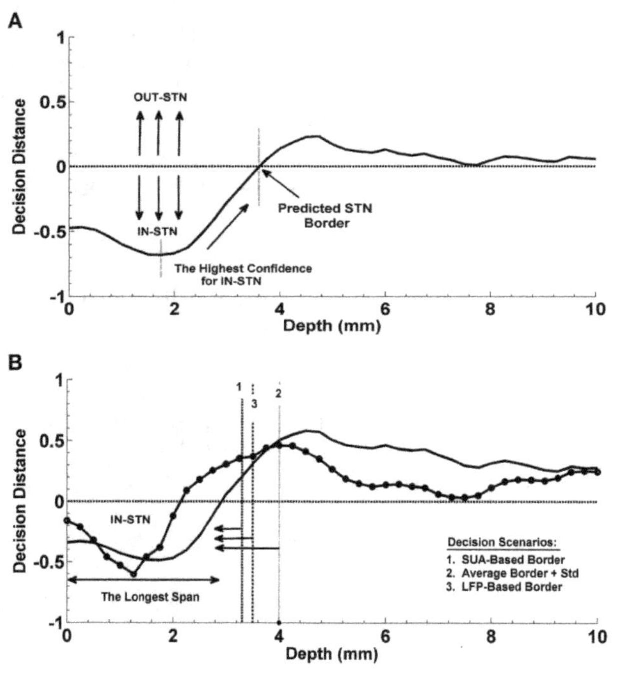

FIGURE 3 | Prediction of the dorsal border of STN and prediction of optimal track. (A) Decision strategy in the prediction of dorsal border of STN. The classifier trained by contrasting the LFP sub-band features coming from inside and outside of STN gives a decision at each depth from top to bottom. These decision distances were used as a measure of confidence. Depth with the highest confidence for IN-STN decisions was marked. Then decisions were traced back where the LDA classifier voted for OUT-STN. This point where the classifier made IN vs. OUT decision transition was chosen as the predicted dorsal border of STN. **(B)** Decision strategy in the optimal track prediction. Classifier trained by contrasting the LFP subband features of selected track vs. un-selected tracks below the dorsal border of STN returned decision distances at all depths. The decision distances were used in three different scenarios: (1) Below the SUA-based STN border, (2) below the one standard deviation from the average of STN border, and (3) below the LFP-based STN border obtained from prediction of dorsal border of STN. The decision distance with the longest span was used as a decision criterion to predict the optimal track.

was used in three different scenarios for final decision making (See **Figure 3B**). In the first scenario, the optimal track was predicted below the STN border provided by the neurosurgeon for that specific test subject based on the SUA interpretation. This represents the setup in which we fuse SUA- and LFP-based information. In the second scenario, no SUA information about the STN border of the test subject was used, and the decisions were given below the one standard deviation from the average of STN border estimated from all training subjects. In the third scenario, the optimal track decisions were made below the STN border which was derived solely from the LFP data. Specifically, here we explored whether or not the LFP could predict the optimal track without any SUA-based interpretation. We studied the classification performance below and above the STN border in these three different scenarios. A schematic diagram related to this process is given in **Figure 3B**. Depth-varying LFP subband features of each track were classified using the trained LDA and a label and related decision distance were generated by the classifier for each depth. We classified one of the tracks as the optimal one based on the longest span of decision distances voting for optimal track within the STN. Note that the longest span is a common approach used intraoperatively by neurosurgeons for MER-SUA-based optimal track selection. Also note that, if the track selected by neurosurgeon in the operating room did not match with the decision of the algorithm, the decision was counted as a misclassification.

The prediction of optimal trajectory was investigated using individual sub-band powers, beta and HFO, and their combination. To explore the benefit of the LMS algorithm over monopolar signals (raw signals), the same classification procedure was carried out with the raw data.

Finally, in order to assess the efficiency and reproducibility of the classification, a leave-one-subject-out method was used. In each step, one subject was used for testing, whereas the other subjects were used for training the LDA classifiers for STN dorsal border and optimal track prediction. The procedure was repeated until the whole sample was classified. In addition, this procedure was performed separately for individual beta and HFO sub-bands of LFP and their combinations to examine their efficacy in classification performance.

In order to explore a relationship between classification results and post-operative simulation parameters used for the initial programming 6 months after the surgery were compared in correctly classified and misclassified groups. The distribution of stimulation amplitude was investigated by box and whisker plots. Student's t-test with two-sample was used to check if the distribution of simulation amplitude, frequency, and pulse width were significantly different or not.

RESULTS

De-Correlation of LFP Data from Multiple Tracks

We analyzed LFP data derived from 75 MER tracks in patients with PD who were undergoing STN DBS electrode placement. Typical raw SUA and LFP data coming from various depths were shown in **Figure 4**. The red dashed line indicates the dorsal border of STN. The correlation between the two modalities is clearly seen. When the electrode enters the STN, both single cell firing and oscillatory activity increase.

In **Figures 5A,B**, the mean correlation matrices of raw LFP data filtered in beta band (11–32 Hz) and HFO band (200–450 Hz) were shown. The correlation matrix in the beta band (**Figure 5A**) explicitly shows that the spatial correlation between tracks is high whereas the correlation between tracks in HFO range is small (**Figure 5B**). The small amount of correlation at HFO band in raw data also shows that oscillations at higher frequencies are more localized than the oscillations at lower frequencies. For these reasons, the LFP data were de-correlated with LMS separately in these frequency bands. It was found that the correlation between tracks is reduced after the LMS-based preprocessing step (**Figure 5C**) which helped more to distinguish the tracks.

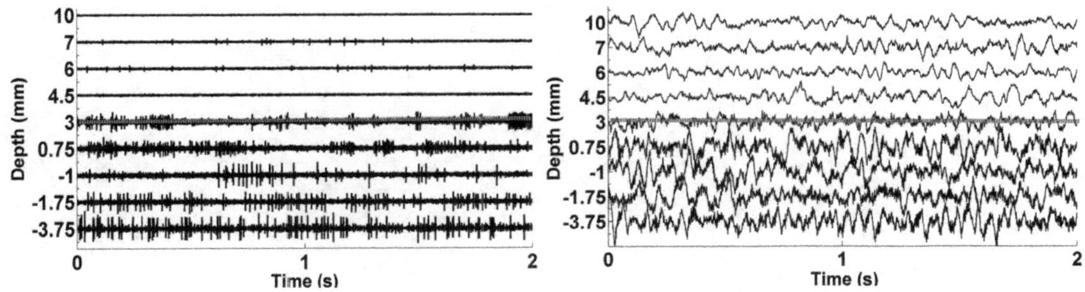

FIGURE 4 | The plots of raw SUA and LFP signals. The graphic on the left shows the single neuron activity lasting 2 s while the graphic on the right indicates the aggregate activity of neuron populations at the same depths with the same duration. The dorsal border of STN shown as red dashed lines is 3 mm for this representative subject.

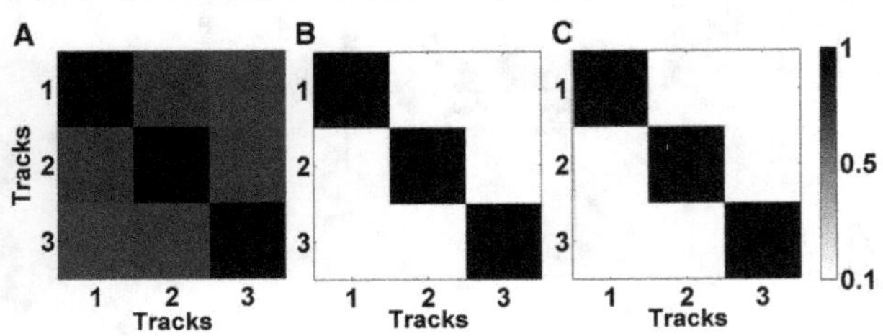

FIGURE 5 | Correlation matrices of raw and de-correlated data. (A) The correlation matrix of raw data in beta band (11–32 Hz). All three tracks show high correlation. **(B)** The correlation matrix of raw data in HFO band (200–450 Hz). Small correlation between tracks indicate spatially more localized HFOs. **(C)** The correlation matrix of subband-decorrelated data. All three tracks demonstrate a small correlation indicating spatio-spectrally distinguished LFPs.

Figure 6 demonstrates the effect of LMS algorithm by :omparing it to the raw LFP signals. As it can be seen n **Figures 6A–C**, the raw LFP data have a high amount of ommon activity across all tracks at various depths which nasks the spatially and temporally distinguishing patterns during argeting. In **Figure 6B**, DFMs indicate that the high-energy ow band activity among tracks masks other oscillations. The ommon activity across three tracks and the high energy low and oscillations can be also seen in the power spectrum hown in **Figure 6C** which was generated from the LFP data elow the dorsal border of STN. On the other hand, target pecific oscillations are clearly seen on de-correlated LFP data **Figure 6D**). In particular, the energy in the first track is much igher than the other two tracks and it is easier to observe ne track differences and the estimated STN border depth for ne target localization. The DFMs of these tracks shown in **igure 6E** demonstrate that the first track contains LFPs with igher energy in low and high frequency bands below the orsal border of the STN which is marked with a white dashed ne. Furthermore, the power spectrum shown in **Figure 6F** emonstrates that not all three tracks show excessive beta activity. There is an increase in the gamma band (35–55 Hz) and great enhancement in HFO range (200–400 Hz) in the first track compared to other tracks. The LMS algorithm not only reveals the pathological beta oscillations but also the HFOs having lower energy.

Spatio-Spectral Patterns of Multitrack LFP

In order to provide a sense of the depth-varying frequency content of multitrack LFPs, we demonstrated representative normalized DFMs of de-correlated LFP data of all three tracks from four patients in **Figure 7**. In each map, the dorsal STN border is marked with a white dashed line. The excessive beta oscillations can be clearly seen in the first subject dominantly in the center track and localized to certain depths (**Figure 7A**). The power of beta oscillations in the posterior and medial track is weak, yet it can be still observed. Furthermore, there is a strong and track-specific HFO around 350 Hz which is well aligned with the low band activity. On the other hand, in the subject presented in **Figure 7B**, beta oscillations are observed in all tracks along with HFOs. Although the excessive LFP activity occurs below the STN dorsal border as for the patient presented in the **Figure 7A**, the excessive depth varying spectral patterns are pretty track and region specific. The HFO in the center track sits at 350 Hz while it is located at 250 Hz in the posterior track. The lateral track shows wider but weaker oscillations. DFMs in **Figure 7C** demonstrate similar LFP characteristics to the first subject (**Figure 7A**) with dominant beta oscillations and HFOs in the center track. Similarly, these oscillations are well aligned below the dorsal border and highly stronger than the beta oscillations in the other two tracks. Distinctly, strong oscillations at higher depths are observed above the dorsal border in the posterior track which might be related to thalamic activity. Note that we observed high frequency activity localized at higher depths above the dorsal border of STN in at least one of the un-selected tracks in 56% of recordings. The number of the un-selected tracks with the observed oscillations were: 8 posterior, 5 center, and 1 medial. Similar to the HFO activity seen in **Figure 7C**, these oscillations were noted from 11.5 ±

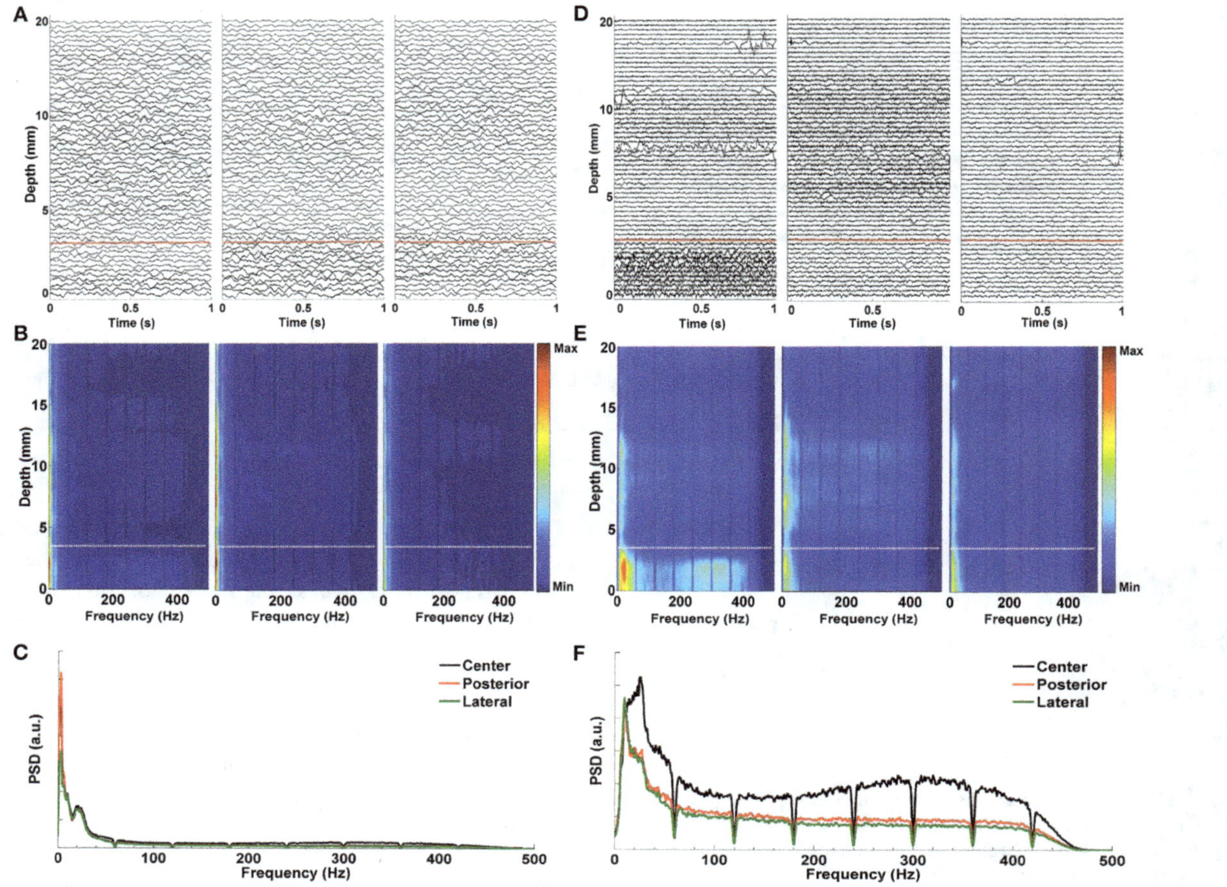

FIGURE 6 | Effect of LMS algorithm by comparing it to the raw LFP signals. (A) Raw LFP distribution. Raw LFPs were recorded from 20 mm above the estimated target down to 0 mm. Distribution of raw LFPs in each depth shows no visible difference between tracks. Red dashed line indicates the dorsal border of STN. **(B)** Depth frequency map (DFM) generated from raw LFPs. Neither pathological beta oscillations nor HFOs are visible in tracks. The high-energy and low band common activity masks other oscillations. White dashed line indicates the dorsal border of STN. **(C)** Power spectrum of raw LFPs. It was generated from the LFP data below the dorsal border of STN. The high correlation between tracks in low frequencies can be clearly seen. Since HFOs are masked by these low frequency oscillations, it is not possible to distinguish them in the spectrum. **(D)** De-correlated LFP distribution. Effect of LMS algorithm on the raw LFPs is clearly seen. Target specific oscillations are visible on de-correlated LFP data. The red dashed line shows the dorsal border of STN determined by MER-SUA. **(E)** DFM of de-correlated LFPs in each microelectrode track. The high energy oscillations in distinct low and high frequency bands inside the STN (below the white dashed line) can be clearly seen in the first track. **(F)** Power spectrum of de-correlated LFPs. Tracks do not show excessive and correlated beta activity anymore. There is an increase in the gamma band (35–55 Hz) and great enhancement in HFO range (200–400 Hz) in the first track compared to other tracks.

2.6 to 5.7 ± 2.4 mm (average values) above the estimated final location of the electrode tip. The tracks having higher-depth HFOs do not include strong beta activity. These oscillations have a longer spatial span with lower power. It is likely that these oscillations rise from thalamic structures (Hutchison et al., 1998; Falkenberg et al., 2006), and given their spatial distribution in relation to the beta band activity, they might be used as markers for STN localization. The fourth representative subject shown in **Figure 7D** introduces a different LFP characteristic compared to others. None of the tracks are associated with strong, long span of beta oscillations. Specified border is not aligned with weak beta oscillations but the short lasting excessive one in the lateral track. All tracks demonstrate spatially different weak-to-minor HFOs. The overlap in the LFP activity between tracks, the weak activity across tracks and thalamic oscillations are some of the factors contributing to the challenges to the prediction of dorsal border of STN and selection of optimal track.

Intra-Track and Inter-Track Differences of LFP Spectra

For the neurosurgeon selected track, the distribution of beta and HFO subband powers above and below the dorsal border of STN are given in **Figure 8A**. The analysis shows that there is a significant difference between the power inside and outside the STN region (above the STN dorsal border) ($t = 44.72, p < 0.001$; $t = 34.89, p < 0.001$) in the selected track. As seen from the box-plot in **Figure 8A**, the sub-band power is much higher

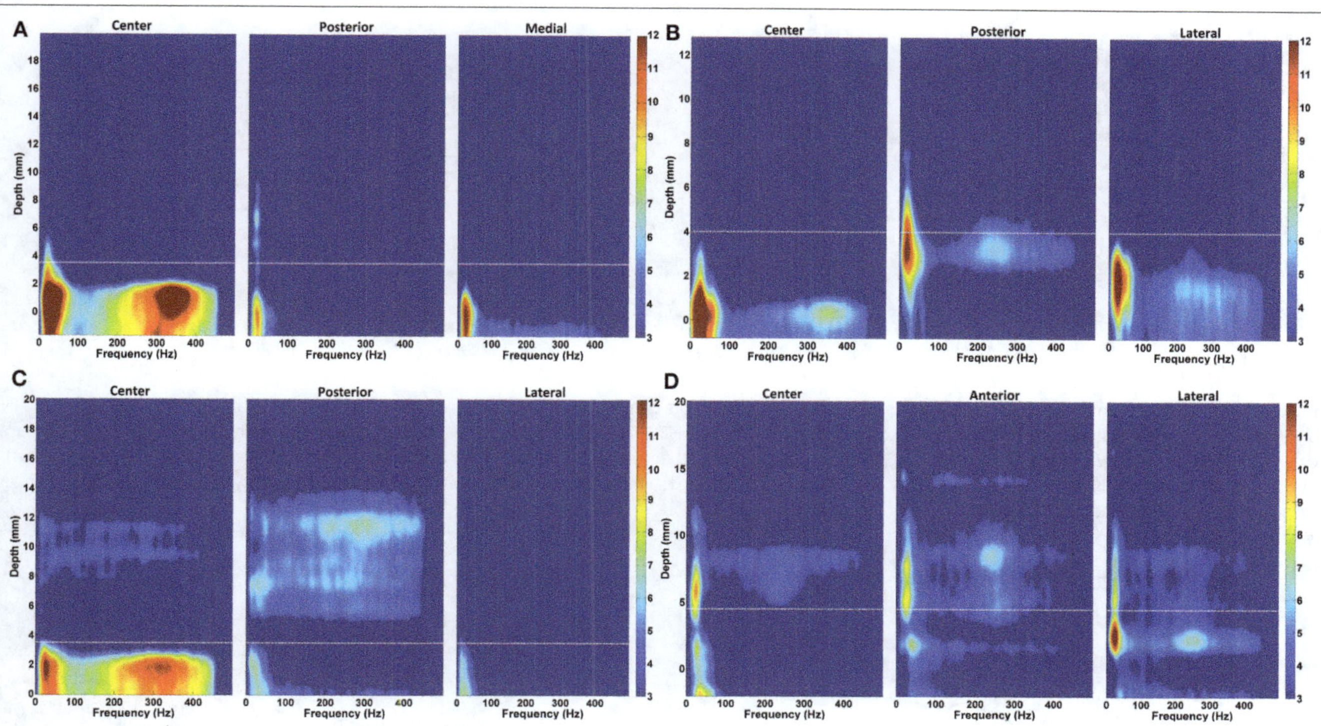

FIGURE 7 | Normalized depth-frequency maps. Representative normalized DFMs of de-correlated LFP data of all three tracks from four representative patients are shown. **(A)** The excessive beta oscillations can be clearly seen in the first subject dominantly in the center track and localized to certain depths. There is a strong and track-specific HFO around 350 Hz which is well aligned with the low band activity. In this subject, selected track by neurosurgeon for the DBS electrode implantation is center track. **(B)** Beta oscillations are observed in all tracks along with HFOs. The HFO in the center track sits at 350 Hz while it is located at 250 Hz in the posterior track. The lateral track shows wider but weaker oscillations. The selected track by neurosurgeon is lateral. **(C)** A similar LFP characteristics to the first subject (shown in **A**) with dominant beta oscillations and HFOs in the center track can be seen. Similarly, these oscillations are well aligned below the border and highly stronger than the beta oscillations in the other two tracks. Center track is selected for DBS electrode implantation. **(D)** These DFMs show different LFP characteristic compared to others. None of the tracks shows strong, long span beta oscillations. Specified border is not aligned with beta oscillations. All three tracks demonstrate spatially different weak-to-minor HFOs. The white dashed line indicates the dorsal STN border. In this subject, the selected track is anterior.

inside the STN. When the subband power was compared between the optimal and other tracks (**Figure 8B**), the distributions were found significant as well ($t = 16.47$, $p < 0.001$; $t = 15.17$, $p < 0.001$). The significance is consistent at the beta band and HFO band in both distributions. The variance of HFO power in the un-selected tracks is higher than the variance in the selected track. Based on our previously mentioned findings, we postulate that thalamic activity in un-selected tracks might contribute to increased variance of HFO power when the distribution includes entire track.

Localization of the Dorsal Border of STN

The progression of prediction of STN dorsal border for representative subjects and the average results estimated from the entire patient population is shown in **Figure 9**. In **Figures 9A,B**, decision distances returned by the classifier voting either for IN-STN or OUT-STN are shown for two representative subjects. The decision distance curves were obtained from the fused beta and HFO features. Note that the predicted STN border is shown with an arrow corresponds to the position where we find the maximum confidence point associated with IN-STN and trace back to the depth crossing zero. The dorsal border of STN provided by the neurosurgeon based on SUA interpretation is shown with a dashed vertical line. **Figure 9A** shows a late prediction of the dorsal border ($e = -0.75$ mm) while **Figure 9B** indicates an early border prediction ($e = +1$ mm). **Figure 9C** demonstrates the average border decisions with the standard deviation coming from all test subjects by using individual sub-band powers, beta and HFO, and fused features. The overall localization error of the dorsal border of STN was quantified by calculating RMS of the error between target values and LFP predictions across all subjects. The red and blue lines show the decisions obtained with beta and HFO band features indicating an RMS error of 1.98 mm and 1.18 mm, respectively. The mean value of prediction error for beta band features was 0.83 ± 1.84 mm while the mean of error for HFO band features was -0.23 ± 1.18 mm. The decisions obtained through the fused beta and HFO band features had an RMS error of 1.22 mm with mean of 0.24 ± 1.22 mm. In **Figure 9D**, the distribution of prediction errors are shown for each studied subband and their fusion. Student's two sample t-test analysis indicated that the difference between mean values of beta-based prediction error and HFO-based prediction error was significantly different ($t = 2.22$, $p = 0.0322$) while no statistically significant difference

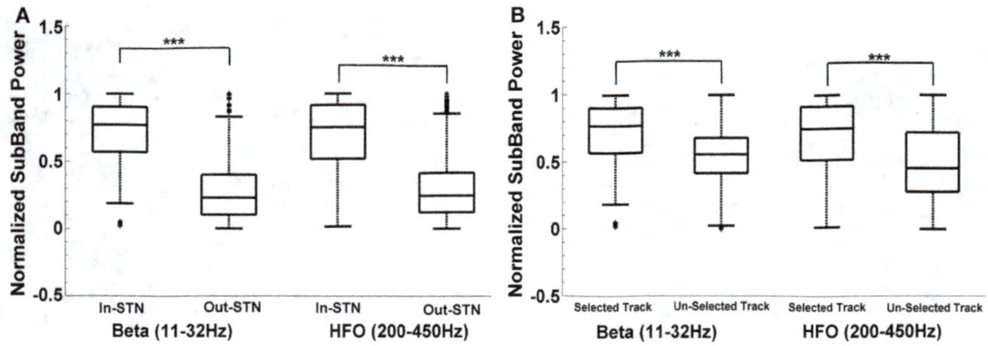

FIGURE 8 | Intra-track and inter-track differences of LFP spectra. Box plots demonstrate the normalized subband power of all subjects. Panel **(A)** shows the IN and OUT of STN power distribution in the selected track in beta (11–32 Hz) and HFO (200–450 Hz) bands. The sub-band power is much higher inside the STN. The difference between the power inside and outside the STN region (above the STN dorsal border) is statistically significant in each specified frequency band ($p < 0.001$). Panel **(B)** shows the IN-STN power in the selected vs. un-selected tracks. Both distributions are statistically significant in each frequency bands. ***Statistically significant difference between distributions ($\alpha = 0.01$).

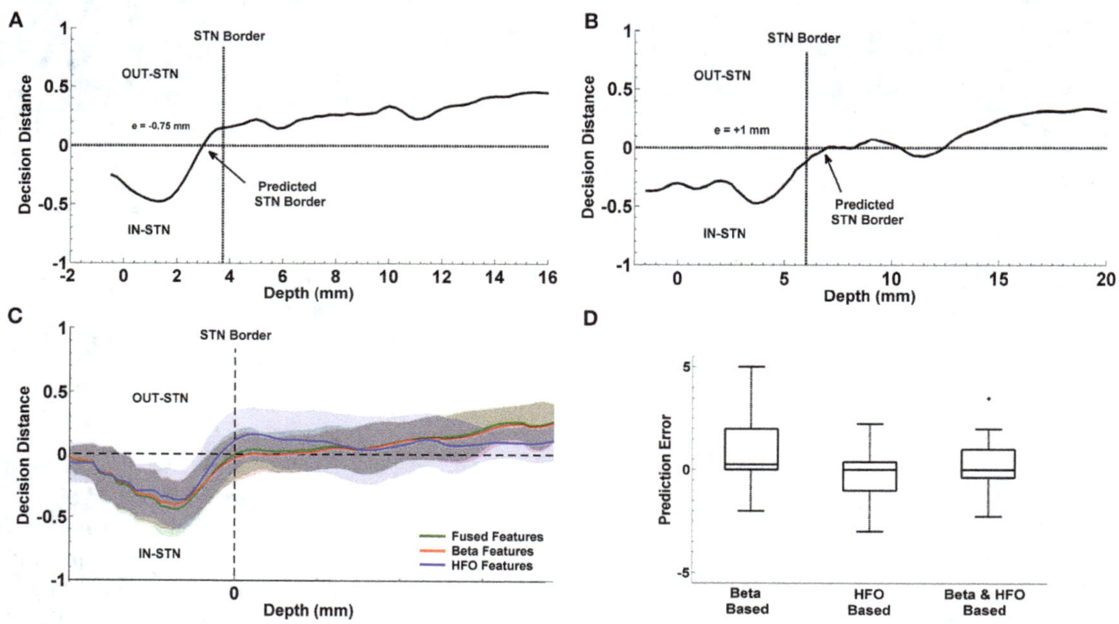

FIGURE 9 | Localization of dorsal border of STN. Panels **(A,B)** show the decision distances returned by the classifier voting either for IN-STN or OUT-STN for two representative subjects. Predicted STN border is shown with an arrow corresponds to the position where we find the maximum confidence point voted for IN-STN and trace back to the depth crossing zero. The black dashed lines indicate the dorsal border of STN obtained by MER/SUA. The predicted border is 0.75 mm lower than the SUA-based border in the first subject **(A)** and 1 mm higher in the second **(B)**. Panel **(C)** demonstrates the average border decisions with the standard deviation coming from all test subjects by using individual sub-band powers, beta (red) and HFO (blue), and fused features (green). **(D)** Comparison of prediction errors. The error (RMS) of the predictions obtained with beta and HFO band features are 1.98 and 1.18 mm. The RMS of the error in predictions obtained from fused features is 1.22 mm. The variance of RMS values were compared by *F-test*. The difference between beta-based and HFO-based prediction error is marginally significant ($p = 0.054$) with $\alpha = 0.05$. +indicates the outlier error value.

was found neither between beta-based prediction error and the error of fused features ($t = 1.23$, $p = 0.2244$) nor HFO-based prediction error and the error of fused features ($t = -1.25$, $p = 0.2185$). When the variances of these distributions were compared by using an *F-test*, the analysis showed that the difference between beta-based and HFO-based border prediction was only marginally significant [$F_{(1,2)} = 2.42$, $p = 0.054$] while there was no statistically significant difference between the variance of individual sub-band powers (beta and HFO) anc fused power [$F_{(1,3)} = 2.26$, $p = 0.075$; $F_{(2,3)} = 0.94$, $p = 0.88$ respectively].

Prediction of the Optimal Track

We studied the optimal track classification in three differen scenarios using the LFP data: (i) below the SUA-based ST border, (ii) below one standard deviation from the average ST border obtained from training data, and (iii) the LFP-based STN border. We trained the LDA classifier using individual subband powers and their combination. Our results toward the prediction of optimal track from LFP data is given in **Table 2**. We note that the best results were obtained from the combined subband power features and consistently in all these scenarios, the optimal track prediction accuracy was 80% (shown in bold type) indicating that the classifier can predict the track targeted to the STN in 20/25 recordings. These results show that prediction of optimal track can be performed independently from single unit recordings. When the beta and HFO subband features were used individually, the classification accuracy dropped to 72 and 68% respectively. When the procedure was repeated with the raw data, the prediction rate was poor. In particular, the classification accuracy was 64% for beta band power and 68% for the HFO and fused features which supports the observation that HFOs obtained in monopolar configuration are already highly de-correlated among different tracks.

Despite the spatially localized thalamic oscillations, the classification results obtained above the STN border were quite poor. The prediction accuracy was found to be 40% when the classification was computed above SUA-based or LFP-based STN border. Decision accuracy with average STN border was even lower at 36% by using fused sub-band power. The results indicate that the LDA classifier trained with the LFP features above the STN does cannot predict the optimal track with a reasonable accuracy and was close to chance level.

The progression of classification over depths for three representative subjects are shown in **Figures 10A–C**. In each plot, the STN border location provided by the neurosurgeon based on the SUA interpretation is also represented with a vertical dashed line. The decision distances in both selected and un-selected tracks returned by the classifier are close to each other down to the dorsal border of STN. Since the spectral characteristics of LFPs change inside the STN compared to higher depths, we observe a sudden change between the decision distances as well. If only one of the tracks deviates from the others and reaching the highest confidence level, it is easily determined as the optimal track by the classifier. If more than one track are voted for the optimal track (below the zero line in **Figure 10**) with high confidence levels, algorithm gives the optimal track decision by computing the longest span of the selected track votes. The progression of the classification for a misclassified subject is given in **Figure 10C**. The average decisions for the optimal track of all subjects with the associated standard deviation are given in **Figure 10D**. A clear separation is observed in decision distances between selected and un-selected tracks indicating a high percentage of correct prediction among the subjects.

Distribution of Selected Tracks

Table 3 shows the frequency of selected tracks based on MER-SUA interpretation and LFP processing. As per standard clinical protocol, the initial trajectory to target STN is determined by preoperative stereotactic imaging. Three tracks are selected by the neurosurgeon based on the initial planning for microelectrode recordings. The initial expectation is that the center track will hit the STN while other tracks account for possible targeting error. Then based on the MER-SUA recordings the optimal track is selected among these three trajectories. Although the image based planning aims to hit the STN with the center track, **Table 3** demonstrates that intraoperative MER-SUA-based decisions among 25 recordings is not biased toward the center track. We note that the selection frequency is higher in anterior track based on MER-SUA mapping. In addition, the posterior track is not selected at all. When the selection frequency based on LFPs is studied, it can be seen that both MER-SUA and LFP decisions (shown in bold) match with a high percentage but LFP based prediction was more in favor of the center track. Overall, our results indicate that stereotactic planning does not perfectly correlate with intraoperative electrophysiology based track selection and highlight the variance in track selection.

TABLE 2 | Prediction rates of classifier.

Power of IN STN in all tracks	LMS data	Raw data
Beta	0.72	0.64
HFO	0.68	0.68
Beta & HFO	**0.80**	0.68

TABLE 3 | Frequency of track selection in the present study.

Comparison of SUA-based and LFP-based track selection		
	Anterior: 10/**9**	
Medial: 2/**1**	Center: 8/**10**	Lateral: 5/**4**
	Posterior: **0/1**	

The selection frequency based on LFPs are shown in bold type.

Post-Operative Programming Parameters

We explored whether there exist any difference in programming parameters between the correctly classified and misclassified patients. In particular we investigated the post-operative simulation parameters such as voltage, frequency and pulse width which were selected during the programming 6 months after the surgery. The distribution of selected stimulation voltages are presented in **Figure 11**. We note that the average stimulation voltage used in correctly classified group is 1.72 $\pm$ 0.63 V while it is 2.12 $\pm$ 0.69 V in misclassified group. Student's two sample t-test analysis indicates that the difference in voltages between two groups is not statistically significant ($t = -1.16$, $p = 0.2595$). However, one of the misclassified subjects we observed has high level beta and HFO activity in both selected and un-selected track and this patient is stimulated with 1 V. This indicates that both tracks could be viable. When this subject is removed from the misclassified group, we note that the mean post-operative stimulation voltage increases to 2.4 V $\pm$ -0.46 for the misclassified population. The difference in post-operative stimulation voltages between correctly classified and misclassified groups without this outlier becomes marginally significant ($t = -1.92$ $p = 0.0685$). No significant difference is found either in the frequency (183.1 $\pm$ 5.8 Hz) or in the pulse width (90 $\pm$

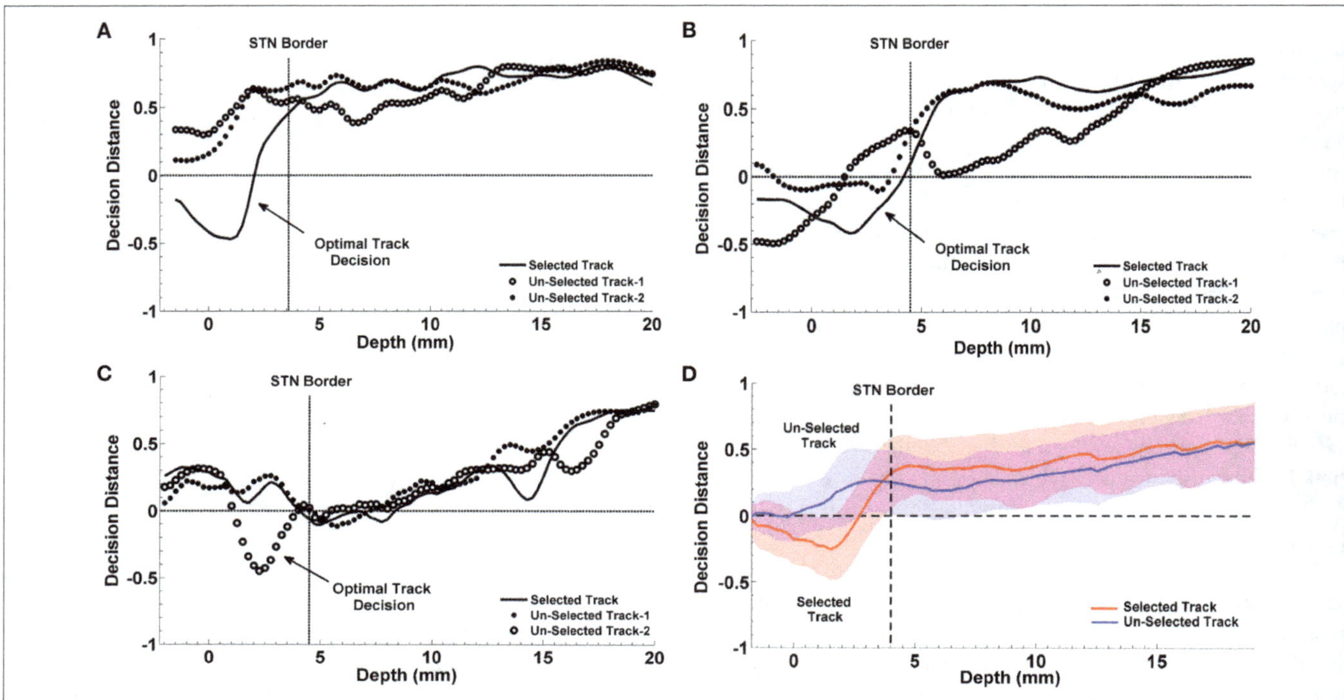

FIGURE 10 | Progression of classification in optimal track prediction. The progression of classification over depths for three representative subjects are shown in **(A–C)**. The black dashed lines show the STN border provided by the neurosurgeon based on the SUA interpretation. The decision distances with the highest confidence and the longest span below the STN border indicate the optimal track. Panel **(A)** shows that decision distance is reaching the highest confidence level only in selected track which is determined as the optimal track by the algorithm. Panel **(B)** shows that all tracks pass the zero line however, only the selected track points the longest span of decisions. So, the selected track is determined as the optimal track by the classifier. Panel **(C)** demonstrates a misclassified subject. Since only the un-selected track-2 is passing zero line and reaching the highest confidence level, it is determined as the optimal track by the algorithm. Panel **(D)** shows the average optimal track decisions with the standard deviation coming from all test subjects. It shows a clear separation in decision distances between selected (red) and un-selected tracks (blue) indicating a high percentage of correct prediction among the subjects.

26.5 μs) between groups ($t = -0.74$, $p = 0.4692$ and $t = 0.96$, $p = 0.3477$, respectively).

DISCUSSION

Significant variability exists in the axial and coronal orientation of the STN in humans (Patel et al., 2008), and the motor territory of the STN is small, measuring ~4–6 mm extent from dorsal to ventral. These factors combined with brain shift between preoperative stereotactic imaging and intraoperative electrode brain penetration can lead to targeting errors in the operating room. Pre- and intra-operative clinical imaging methods alone are suboptimal for accurate placement of a DBS electrode; they are subject to distortion, and visualization of a clear differentiation between the STN and surrounding structures can be difficult. In this regard, our study also indicates a considerable amount of variance in track selection. Under the assumption of hitting the STN through center track by image based planning, track selection was not found to be biased toward the center track in the intraoperative MER/SUA-based decisions indicating that stereotactic planning does not perfectly correlate with intraoperative electrophysiology based track selection.

Accurate localization of STN motor territory through intraoperative electrophysiology is a crucial step for DBS electrode implantation (Zonenshayn et al., 2000; Gross et al., 2006). As recently as 2013, an international survey of high-volume DBS implanting sites revealed that 83% of centers use microelectrode recording indicating that the most commonly used electrophysiological mapping method remains MER-SUA recordings (Abosch et al., 2013). However, the method has several limitations in practice as subjective interpretation o complex signal patterns to localize the anatomical borders of the STN, being less stable and more "susceptible to technical (e.g., impedance) and physiological (e.g., cerebrospinal fluid and blood) fluctuations" (Thompson et al., 2014). As Gross et al. indicated, the number of groups using solely macroelectrode/DBS mapping to target the STN without any microelectrode recording is high (Chen et al., 2006; Gross et al. 2006; Telkes et al., 2014). Although there are advantages o using macroelectrode/DBS technique alone in STN targeting lik carrying less amount of risk for intracranial hemorrhage sinc there is no multiple trajectories and due to the blunt-tip o the macroelectrode (Xiaowu et al., 2010), the drawbacks lik microlesion effect which might limit the clinician's ability t test or therapeutic effectiveness in the operating room and poo spatial resolution should be taken into consideration (Rezai e al., 2006; Wang et al., 2014). Although asleep, MRI-based non-MER-guided surgery is gaining sway (Starr et al., 2014), th possibility of clinically testing a DBS electrode prior to permaner

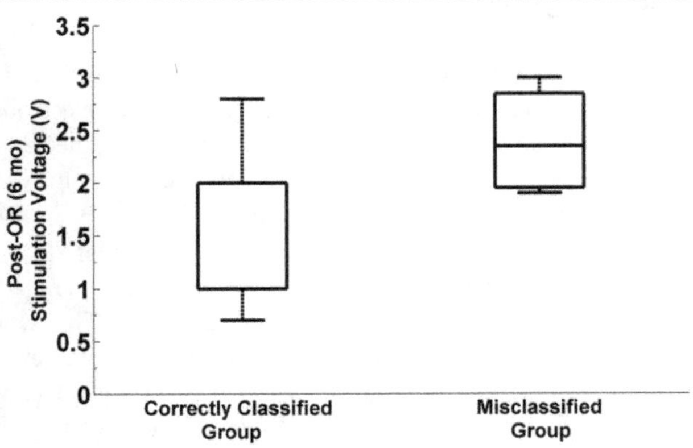

FIGURE 11 | Distribution of post-operative stimulation voltages in correctly classified and misclassified groups. Box plots show the stimulation voltages which were used in two groups during the programming 6 months after the surgery. The box plot on the right indicates the distribution of post-operative stimulation voltages in misclassified group by excluding the outlier subject with 1V stimulation. The difference between stimulation voltages in the correctly classified and misclassified group is marginally significant ($p = 0.068$, $\alpha = 0.05$).

implantation does not exist as yet in the context of such a procedure.

Earlier investigations have documented that excessive beta oscillations in certain basal ganglia structures, especially the STN, represent a pathophysiological feature of PD (Weinberger et al., 2006; Kane et al., 2009; Lopez-Azcarate et al., 2010; Oswal et al., 2013). Excessive beta band (8–30 Hz) activity is detected when the electrodes enter into the STN (Levy et al., 2002; Kühn et al., 2008; Brittain and Brown, 2014). Similarly, excessive oscillations at very high frequency ranging from 200–400 Hz are also observed (Priori et al., 2004; Lopez-Azcarate et al., 2010; Özkurt et al., 2011). Even though these high frequency oscillations are considered to represent a pro-kinetic state, and appear with dopaminergic medication and/or induced movement (Foffani et al., 2003, 2006; Trottenberg et al., 2006), others have demonstrated that HFOs (>200 Hz) can still be observed in the STN during the medication OFF state or at rest (Lopez-Azcarate et al., 2010). In our study, all patients discontinued with their short and long acting medication before the surgery and were in OFF state. As others, we observed HFOs in the resting state and increased band power along with entry into the STN. Existence of excessive beta band and HFOs within the STN in PD can be used in target localization. However, the variability and patient-specific characteristics of spatial distribution of excessive beta and HFOs should be taken into consideration (Chen et al., 2006; Weinberger et al., 2006; Wang et al., 2014).

Despite a few publications using intraoperative microelectrode LFPs for STN localization (Michmizos et al., 2008; Holdefer et al., 2010; Wang et al., 2014), to our knowledge, no studies exist on the functional use of LFPs recorded from multiple microelectrodes for the selection of the optimal trajectory targeting the STN in PD. The present study demonstrates that using spectral features of LFP to identify the optimal track without any decorrelation technique provide sub-optimal results due to widely distributed neural signals and/or artifacts masking the spatially and temporally distinguishing patterns during targeting. Therefore, the LMS algorithm is used as an efficient technique to decorrelate the tracks by keeping localized activities in each. The adaptive LMS algorithm is widely used in the biosignal processing field since early 80s for signal enhancement due to its efficiency and low complexity (Widrow et al., 1975; Ferrara and Widrow, 1982; Chen et al., 1990). Since the decorrelation is being done recursively without violating the causality constraint, where each channel is predicted by the current samples of other data channels, the algorithm can be easily executed on standard PC architectures in real-time. Since it is an adaptive technique, the time and depth varying parameters allows tracking time and depth varying LFP activity and does not suffer from the cross talk as much as in the common average based derivation. It should be noted that since it estimates current signal by using a linear combination of other signals, the LMS algorithm cannot fully eliminate the high amplitude artifacts if they are not distributed among the tracks, which constitutes a major drawback of the algorithm. One way of reducing the effect of large artifacts and keep the system stable is to use an error threshold with upper and lower boundaries. Another important factor influencing the benefit of the algorithm is the learning parameter μ. It should be investigated by considering signal properties such that adaptation of the system should be neither very slow nor very fast.

Spectral analysis showed that beta oscillations are getting stronger as the electrodes approach the STN. Not only beta oscillations but also strong HFOs can be observed in the STN area well aligned with beta oscillations. This strong relation is noted in the tracks selected by neurosurgeons in 17 recordings out of 25. In rest of the eight recordings, HFO was either weak or fully absent or they were noted only in one of the un-selected tracks. The energy changes above and in the STN were used to localize the dorsal border. The RMS error of prediction for the dorsal border of STN is obtained from 1.18 to 1.98 mm when the different features are used. The minimum prediction error is found with the power of HFOs (1.18 mm) indicating that, despite the unknown functional role of these high frequency components, they can still be eligible in STN targeting. The LFP is a continuous process and does not suffer from SUA isolation challenge while the target variable is a SUA driven information which is also prone to interpretation error and isolation challenge. Considering the dorsa-ventral size of STN, 1.22 mm prediction error in depth with the fused features may represent 11% in DBS electrode 3387 or 16% in 3389 difference which can be easily compensated with the multiple contacts of the DBS electrode.

The features computed above the STN border provided poor results in prediction of optimal track. We note that the optimal track can be predicted with higher accuracy with the features obtained below the dorsal border of STN. Analysis manifest that 14 recordings out of 25 (56% of entire dataset) indicate spatially distinct HFOs together with beta activity above the dorsal border of STN (see **Figures 7C,D**) in at least one of the un-selected tracks. It can be assumed that these relatively weak oscillations located away from the dorsal border of STN are recorded from thalamic structures. To our knowledge, this considerable amount of thalamic oscillations in PD are not well studied phenomena. These findings presented here might be used as spatial markers in STN localization and might form the basis of further investigation into PD pathophysiology from a spatio-spectral perspective.

It should be noted that our classification technique could not predict the selected track in 20% of the subjects. We did not observe a gender difference between these five misclassified subjects. Specifically, three of them were men and two of them were women. None of the misclassified patients were tremor dominant. Three of these patients were typical PD and the other two were bradykinetic/rigid. The mean age and disease duration were 62.2 ± 13.6 and 12 ± 4.6, respectively and were not significantly different from other correctly classified patients (62.1 ± 8.3 and 10.1 ± 4.6, respectively). The misclassification in the 20% of the patients occurred due to many different factors in LFP signal including weak activity or similar activity between tracks. During these recordings, we did not use any sedation. Therefore, weak activity cannot be related to anesthesia. In one patient with typical PD phenotype, the LFP signal was weak across all tracks. We noted that the beta and HFO activity started to develop toward the bottom border of the planned target deeper than the other patients. We believe that in this particular patient the weak activity across all tracks can be described with the electrode positions. Our observations indicate that the three tracks just started to enter the STN and did not fully went through it. In another misclassified case, the LFP activity was quite strong and similar in two out of three tracks. Therefore, the classifier output was very close for these two tracks. In the other three patients, the HFO activity in the SUA selected track was weak compared to LFP selected track. Studies hypothesize that maximum beta band (13–32 Hz) and gamma band (48–220 Hz) power is highly correlated with stimulation programming parameters in DBS chronic electrode (Ince et al., 2010). When a particular contact pair on the electrode shows strong beta and gamma oscillations, it's assumed that the electrode is closer to the source so that lower stimulation would provide better symptom improvement and less side effects. The present study supports these results. We observed higher stimulation voltages in those patients where the LFPs did not correlate with MER/SUA selected tracks. Despite the lack of statistical significance, the stimulation voltages in the 6-mo-programming of implantable pulse generator (IPG) indicate lower values in the patient group having stronger LFPs in beta and/or HFO bands. A study with larger sample size would be needed to test the validity of this observation.

CONCLUSION

The present study describes an automated approach for electrophysiological localization of STN, using microelectrode-recorded LFPs acquired during DBS surgery simultaneous to MER. This work is novel, in that it is the first study to combine different sub-band features derived from beta (11–32 Hz) and HFOs (150–450 Hz) of LFPs in order to (1) estimate the optimal track for DBS implantation, and (2) identify the dorsal STN border, with high accuracy. This work also contributes to knowledge about the neurophysiology of PD by describing the spatial localization of HFOs. Because recording LFPs *simultaneous* with MER/SUA does not prolong the total duration of surgery, using this technique online in the operating room would increase the chance of optimal placement of the DBS macroelectrode within the motor sub-territory of the STN, without an appreciable downside. Fused with existing mapping techniques, automated online LFP analysis may increase the accuracy of the DBS macroelectrode placement. This might contribute to the efficacy of DBS by reducing the stimulation voltage and associated side effects. Since the electrode placement is guided by LFP activity, the current technique could also be useful to monitor the LFP events which are capable to fine tune the future DBS settings in a closed loop paradigm (Ince et al., 2010; Rouse et al., 2011; Priori et al., 2013).

Further prospective investigations regarding the clinical outcomes using this technique of optimal track selection are warranted.

AUTHOR CONTRIBUTIONS

NI and IT designed the study, collected the data, wrote the manuscript, and conducted the analyses. AA and AV performed the surgeries, contributed to data collection, and interpretation of the results. JJ performed the behavioral tests during surgery, evaluated the condition of subjects, and contributed to interpretation of the results. All authors reviewed the manuscript and approved the final version of the manuscript.

ACKNOWLEDGMENTS

We wish to thank all the patients who participated in this study. We are grateful to Akshay Gupte for his help with clinical data collection. We are also thankful to Ibrahim Onaran, Anish Sen, and Jiang Tianxiao for their help with data collection and visualization. This research was supported by National Science Foundation, award CBET-1343548.

REFERENCES

Abosch, A., Hutchison, W. D., Saint-Cyr, J. A., Dostrovsky, J. O., and Lozano, A. M. (2002). Movement-related neurons of the subthalamic nucleus in patients with Parkinson disease. *J. Neurosurg.* 97, 1167–1172. doi: 10.3171/jns.2002.97.5.1167

Abosch, A., Timmermann, L., Bartley, S., Rietkerk, H. G., Whiting, D., Connolly, P. J., et al. (2013). An international survey of deep brain stimulation procedural steps. *Stereotact. Funct. Neurosurg.* 91, 1–11. doi: 10.1159/000343207

Alpaydin, E. (2010). *Introduction to Machine Learning, 2nd Edn.* Cambridge, MA: The MIT Press.

Benabid, A. L., Chabardes, S., Mitrofanis, J., and Pollak, P. (2009). Deep brain stimulation of the subthalamic nucleus for the treatment of Parkinson's disease. *Lancet Neurol.* 8, 67–81. doi: 10.1016/S1474-4422(08)70291-6

Brittain, J. S., and Brown, P. (2014). Oscillations and the basal ganglia: motor control and beyond. *Neuroimage* 85, 637–647. doi: 10.1016/j.neuroimage.2013.05.084

Chen, C. C., Pogosyan, A., Zrinzo, L. U., Tisch, S., Limousin, P., Ashkan, K., et al. (2006). Intra-operative recordings of local field potentials can help localize the subthalamic nucleus in Parkinson's disease surgery. *Exp. Neurol.* 198, 214–221. doi: 10.1016/j.expneurol.2005.11.019

Chen, J., Vandewalle, J., Sansen, W., Vantrappen, G., and Janssens, J. (1990). Multichannel adaptive enhancement of the electrogastrogram. *IEEE Trans. Biomed. Eng.* 37, 285–294. doi: 10.1109/10.52329

Falkenberg, J. H., McNames, J., Favre, J., and Burchiel, K. J. (2006). Automatic analysis and visualization of microelectrode recording trajectories to the subthalamic nucleus: preliminary results. *Stereotact. Funct. Neurosurg.* 84, 35–45. doi: 10.1159/000093721

Ferrara, E. R., and Widrow, B. (1982). Fetal electrocardiogram enhancement by time-sequenced adaptive filtering. *IEEE Trans. Biomed. Eng.* 29, 458–460. doi: 10.1109/TBME.1982.324973

Foffani, G., Ardolino, G., Egidi, M., Caputo, E., Bossi, B., and Priori, A. (2006). Subthalamic oscillatory activities at beta or higher frequency do not change after high-frequency DBS in Parkinson's disease. *Brain Res. Bull.* 69, 123–130. doi:10.1016/j.brainresbull.2005.11.012

Foffani, G., Priori, A., Egidi, M., Rampini, P., Tamma, F., Caputo, E., et al. (2003). 300-Hz subthalamic oscillations in Parkinson's disease. *Brain* 126, 2153–2163. doi: 10.1093/brain/awg229

Gross, R. E., Krack, P., Rodriguez-Oroz, M. C., Rezai, A. R., and Benabid, A. L. (2006). Electrophysiological mapping for the implantation of deep brain stimulators for Parkinson's disease and tremor. *Mov. Disord.* 21, S259–S283. doi: 10.1002/mds.20960

Hariz, M. (2012). Twenty-five years of deep brain stimulation: celebrations and apprehensions. *Mov. Disord.* 27, 930–933. doi: 10.1002/mds.25007

Hayes, M. (1996). *Statistical Digital Signal Processing and Modeling, 2006th Edn.* New York, NY: John Wiley & Sons.

Herzog, J., Fietzek, U., Hamel, W., Morsnowski, A., Steigerwald, F., Schrader, B., et al. (2004). Most effective stimulation site in subthalamic deep brain stimulation for Parkinson's disease. *Mov. Disord.* 19, 1050–1054. doi: 10.1002/mds.20056

Holdefer, R. N., Cohen, B. A, and Greene, K. A. (2010). Intraoperative local field recording for deep brain stimulation in Parkinson's disease and essential tremor. *Mov. Disord.* 25, 2067–2075. doi: 10.1002/mds.23232

Hutchison, W. D., Allan, R. J., Opitz, H., Levy, R., Dostrovsky, J. O., Lang, A. E., et al. (1998). Neurophysiological identification of the subthalamic nucleus in surgery for Parkinson's disease. *Ann. Neurol.* 44, 622–628.

Ince, N. F., Gupte, A., Wichmann, T., Ashe, J., Henry, T., Bebler, M., et al. (2010). Selection of optimal programming contacts based on local field potential recordings from subthalamic nucleus in patients with Parkinson's disease. *Neurosurgery* 67, 390–397. doi: 10.1227/01.NEU.0000372091.64824.63

Kane, A., Hutchison, W. D., Hodaie, M., Lozano, A. M., and Dostrovsky, J. O. (2009). Dopamine-dependent high-frequency oscillatory activity in thalamus and subthalamic nucleus of patients with Parkinson's disease. *Neuroreport* 20, 1549–1553. doi: 10.1097/WNR.0b013e32833282c8

Kühn, A. A., Kempf, F., Brücke, C., Gaynor Doyle, L., Martinez-Torres, I., Pogosyan, A., et al. (2008). High-frequency stimulation of the subthalamic nucleus suppresses oscillatory beta activity in patients with Parkinson's disease in parallel with improvement in motor performance. *J. Neurosci.* 28, 6165–6173. doi: 10.1523/JNEUROSCI.0282-08.2008

Levy, R., Ashby, P., Hutchison, W. D., Lang, A. E., Lozano, A. M., and Dostrovsky, J. O. (2002). Dependence of subthalamic nucleus oscillations on movement and dopamine in Parkinson's disease. *Brain* 125(Pt 6), 1196–1209. doi: 10.1093/brain/awf128

Lopez-Azcarate, J., Tainta, M., Rodriguez-Oroz, M. C., Valencia, M., Gonzalez, R., Guridi, J., et al. (2010). Coupling between beta and high-frequency activity in the human subthalamic nucleus may be a pathophysiological mechanism in Parkinson's disease. *J. Neurosci.* 30, 6667–6677. doi: 10.1523/JNEUROSCI.5459-09.2010

Michmizos, K. P., Tagaris, G. L., Sakas, D. E., and Nikita, K. S. (2008). "Automatic intra-operative localization of STN using the beta band frequencies of microelectrode recordings," in *8th IEEE International Conference on BioInformatics and BioEngineering, 2008 (BIBE 2008)* (Athens), 1–6. doi: 10.1109/BIBE.2008.4696820

Novak, P., Przybyszewski, A. W., Barborica, A., Ravin, P., Margolin, L., and Pilitsis, J. G. (2011). Localization of the subthalamic nucleus in Parkinson disease using multiunit activity. *J. Neurol. Sci.* 310, 44–49. doi: 10.1016/j.jns.2011.07.027

Okun, M. S., Tagliati, M., Pourfar, M., Fernandez, H. H., Rodriguez, R. L., Alterman, R. L., et al. (2005). Management of referred deep brain stimulation failures. *Arch. Neurol.* 62, 1250–1255. doi: 10.1001/archneur.62.8.noc40425

Oswal, A., Brown, P., and Litvak, V. (2013). Synchronized neural oscillations and the pathophysiology of Parkinson's disease. *Curr. Opin. Neurol.* 26, 662–670. doi: 10.1097/WCO.0000000000000034

Patel, N. K., Khan, S., and Gill, S. S. (2008). Comparison of atlas- and magnetic-resonance-imaging-based stereotactic targeting of the subthalamic nucleus in the surgical treatment of Parkinson's disease. *Stereotact. Funct. Neurosurg.* 86, 153–161. doi: 10.1159/000120427

Priori, A., Foffani, G., Pesenti, A., Tamma, F., Bianchi, A. M., Pellegrini, M., et al. (2004). Rhythm-specific pharmacological modulation of subthalamic activity in Parkinson's disease. *Exp. Neurol.* 189, 369–379. doi:10.1016/j.expneurol.2004.06.001

Priori, A., Foffani, G., Rossi, L., and Marceglia, S. (2013). Adaptive deep brain stimulation (aDBS) controlled by local field potential oscillations. *Exp. Neurol.* 245, 77–86. doi: 10.1016/j.expneurol.2012.09.013

Rouse, A, G., Stanslaski, S. R., Cong, P., Jensen, R. M., Afshar, P., Ullestad, D., et al. (2011). A chronic generalized bi-directional brain-machine interface. *J. Neural Eng.* 8:036018. doi: 10.1088/1741-2560/8/3/036018

Rezai, A. R., Kopell, B. H., Gross, R. E., Vitek, J. L., Sharan, A. D., Limousin, P., et al. (2006). Deep brain stimulation for Parkinson's disease: surgical issues. *Mov. Disord.* 21, S197–S218. doi: 10.1002/mds.20956

Richardson, R. M., Ostrem, J. L., and Starr, P. (2009). Surgical repositioning of misplaced subthalamic electrodes in Parkinson's disease: location of effective and ineffective leads. *Stereotact. Funct. Neurosurg.* 87, 297–303. doi: 10.1159/000230692

Sanghera, M., and Grossman, R. (2004). "Techniques in data analysis: general principles," in *Microelectrode Recording in Movement Disorder Surgery*, eds Z. Israel and K. Burchiel (New York, NY: Thieme Medical Publisher), 111–118.

Starr, P. A., Markun, L. C., Larson, P. S., Volz, M. M., Martin, A. J., and Ostrem, J. L. (2014). Interventional MRI-guided deep brain stimulation in pediatric dystonia: first experience with the clearpoint system. *J. Neurosurg. Pediatr.* 14, 400–408. doi: 10.3171/2014.6.PEDS13605

Özkurt, T. E., Butz, M., Homburger, M., Elben, S., Vesper, J., Wojtecki, L., et al. (2011). High frequency oscillations in the subthalamic nucleus: A neurophysiological marker of the motor state in Parkinson's disease. *Exp. Neurol.* 229, 324–331. doi: 10.1016/j.expneurol.2011.02.015

Telkes, I., Ince, N. F., Onaran, I., and Abosch, A. (2014). "Localization of subthalamic nucleus borders using macroelectrode local field potential recordings," in *36th Annual International Conference of the IEEE Engineering in Medicine and Biology Society* (Chicago, IL), 2621–2624. doi: 10.1109/EMBC.2014.6944160

Thompson, J. A., Lanctin, D., Ince, N. F., and Abosch, A. (2014). Clinical implications of local field potentials for understanding and treating movement disorders. *Stereotact. Funct. Neurosurg.* 92, 251–263. doi: 10.1159/000364913

Trottenberg, T., Fogelson, N., Kühn, A., Kivi, A., Kupsch, A., Schneider, G.-H., et al. (2006). Subthalamic gamma activity in patients with Parkinson's disease. *Exp. Neurol.* 200, 56–65. doi: 10.1016/j.expneurol.2006.01.012

Wang, J., Hirschmann, J., Elben, S., Hartmann, C. J., Vesper, J., Wojtecki, L., et al. (2014). High-frequency oscillations in Parkinson's disease: spatial distribution and clinical relevance. *Mov. Disord.* 29, 1265–1272. doi: 10.1002/mds.25962

Weinberger, M., Mahant, N., Hutchison, W. D., Lozano, A. M., Moro, E., Hodaie, M., et al. (2006). Beta oscillatory activity in the subthalamic nucleus and its relation to dopaminergic response in Parkinson's disease. *J. Neurophysiol.* 96, 3248–3256. doi: 10.1152/jn.00697.2006

Widrow, B., Williams, C. S., Glover, J. R., McCool, J. M., Hearn, R. H., Zeidler, J. R., et al. (1975). Adaptive noise cancelling: principles and applications. *Proc. IEEE* 63, 1692–1716. doi: 10.1109/PROC.1975.10036

Wong, S., Baltuch, G. H., Jaggi, J. L., and Danish, S. F. (2009). Functional localization and visualization of the subthalamic nucleus from microelectrode recordings acquired during DBS surgery with unsupervised machine learning. *J. Neural Eng.* 6:026006. doi: 10.1088/1741-2560/6/2/026006

Xiaowu, H., Xiufeng, J., Xiaoping, Z., Bin, H., Laixing, W., Yiqun, C., et al. (2010). Risks of intracranial hemorrhage in patients with Parkinson's disease receiving deep brain stimulation and ablation. *Parkinsonism Relat. Disord.* 16, 96–100. doi: 10.1016/j.parkreldis.2009.07.013

Zonenshayn, M., Rezai, A. R., Mogilner, A. Y., Beric, A., Sterio, D., and Kelly, P. J. (2000). Comparison of anatomic and neurophysiological methods for subthalamic nucleus targeting. *Neurosurgery* 47, 282–292; discussion 292–294. doi: 10.1097/00006123-200008000-00005

7

Detection of Movement Related Cortical Potentials from EEG Using Constrained ICA for Brain-Computer Interface Applications

*Fatemeh Karimi[1], Jonathan Kofman[1], Natalie Mrachacz-Kersting[2], Dario Farina[3] and Ning Jiang[1]**

[1] Department of Systems Design Engineering, Faculty of Engineering, University of Waterloo, Waterloo, ON, Canada,
[2] Department of Health Science and Technology, Aalborg University, Aalborg, Denmark, [3] Neurorehabilitation Engineering Department of Bioengineering, Imperial College London, London, United Kingdom

Edited by:
Paolo Bonifazi,
Tel Aviv University, Israel

Reviewed by:
Ricardo Chavarriaga,
École Polytechnique Fédérale de Lausanne, Switzerland
Jianjun Meng,
University of Minnesota, United States

***Correspondence:**
Ning Jiang
ning.jiang@uwaterloo.ca

The movement related cortical potential (MRCP), a slow cortical potential from the scalp electroencephalogram (EEG), has been used in real-time brain-computer-interface (BCI) systems designed for neurorehabilitation. Detecting MPCPs in real time with high accuracy and low latency is essential in these applications. In this study, we propose a new MRCP detection method based on constrained independent component analysis (cICA). The method was tested for MRCP detection during executed and imagined ankle dorsiflexion of 24 healthy participants, and compared with four commonly used spatial filters for MRCP detection in an offline experiment. The effect of cICA and the compared spatial filters on the morphology of the extracted MRCP was evaluated by two indices quantifying the signal-to-noise ratio and variability of the extracted MRCP. The performance of the filters for detection was then directly compared for accuracy and latency. The latency obtained with cICA (−34 ± 29 ms motor execution (ME) and 28 ± 16 ms for motor imagery (MI) dataset) was significantly smaller than with all other spatial filters. Moreover, cICA resulted in greater true positive rates (87.11 ± 11.73 for ME and 86.66 ± 6.96 for MI dataset) and lower false positive rates (20.69 ± 13.68 for ME and 19.31 ± 12.60 for MI dataset) compared to the other methods. These results confirm the superiority of cICA in MRCP detection with respect to previously proposed EEG filtering approaches.

Keywords: brain-computer interface (BCI), movement related cortical potential (MRCP), constrained independent component analysis (cICA), electroencephalogram (EEG), spatial filters

INTRODUCTION

The movement-related cortical potential (MRCP) is a low frequency (0–5 Hz) negative shift in the electroencephalogram (EEG) signal, which has recently been used as an EEG modality for real-time brain computer interface (BCI) applications, particularly in neuromodulation systems (Mrachacz-Kersting et al., 2016). The ability to detect MRCPs with high accuracy and short latency (usually shorter than 300 ms) on a single trial basis is crucial for these applications. Specifically, the high demand on temporal precision has been shown to be fundamental in efficiently inducing plasticity in neurorehabilitation applications (Mrachacz-Kersting et al., 2012). Improvement in accuracy and latency of single-trial MRCP detection is therefore a relevant challenge. The amplitude of the MRCP is typically between 5 and 30 μV and therefore easily masked by other brain activities (Wright et al., 2011). Moreover, low frequency motion artifacts and the electrooculogram (EOG) have frequency bandwidths similar to the MRCP, but with much greater magnitudes. Thus, extracting a single trial MRCP from an EEG signal with high accuracy and minimal latency in real-time is a challenging task.

Spatial filtering is one of the most commonly used EEG signal processing approaches for artifact removal and improving the detection accuracy of cortical potentials. The MRCP has a well-defined spatial distribution, being located directly over the scalp area of the corresponding primary motor cortex region. For example, the MRCP accompanying an ankle dorsiflexion task is most pronounced over the apex (Cz of 10–20 montage). The most common spatial filters used in EEG-based BCI systems are the Common Spatial Pattern (CSP) (Blankertz et al., 2008), Laplacian spatial filter (LAP) (McFarland et al., 1997; Xu et al., 2014a,b), and Independent Component Analysis (ICA) (Bell and Sejnowski, 1995; Cardoso, 1999). CSP decomposes multi-channel EEG signals into distinct spatial patterns by solving a generalized eigenvalue problem. This method has been widely used to extract motor imagery-based BCIs, particularly in sensory-motor rhythm (SMR) (Ramoser et al., 2000; Blankertz et al., 2008) and has also been tested preliminarily in MRCP detection (Niazi et al., 2011). However, the performance of CSP is very sensitive to outliers, which are inevitable in real-time BCI applications (Blankertz et al., 2008). LAP calculates the second derivative of the instantaneous spatial voltage distribution for each electrode location, and thereby emphasizes the activity originating in radial sources immediately below the electrode (McFarland et al., 1997). LAP has been applied in MRCP detection (Xu et al., 2014a,b). ICA-based spatial filters have been also successfully used in a variety of EEG signal processing applications, such as artifact reduction and source localization (Xu et al., 2004; Jiang et al., 2015). However, there are limitations associated with the implementation of ICA, especially for real-time applications, as it requires manual selection of the desired components from the estimated sources.

The constrained ICA (cICA), also known as one-unit ICA (Zhang, 2008), is a recent approach introduced to overcome the manual intervention limitation of ICA. cICA is a spatial filter extended from ICA that uses a reference signal to automatically extract only the desired source, without requiring the manual selection procedure of traditional ICA-based methods. cICA has recently been applied for EEG signal processing applications (James and Gibson, 2003; Joshua and Rajapakse, 2005) and has been shown to be successful in extracting event-related cortical potentials (ERP), such as the P300 (Spyrou and Sanei, 2006; Lee et al., 2013), as well as removing ocular artifacts (Huang et al., 2011); however, cICA has not been used previously for the detection of MRCPs. In this paper, we present for the first time, the application of cICA for MRCP detection, including a systematic investigation of the efficacy of cICA in single-trial MRCP detection, and comparison of cICA performance with the previously proposed CSP, LAP, Infomax (Bell and Sejnowski, 1995), and JADE (Cardoso, 1999). The performance of these filters was evaluated both with metrics based on the morphology of the MRCP and on the detection accuracy. For quantifying detection accuracy, the filtered EEG was classified with the previously proposed Locality Preserved Projection (LPP) followed by Linear Discriminator Analysis (LDA) (Xu et al., 2014a).

MATERIALS AND METHODS

Data Acquisition

Participants

The data used in the current study are part of the dataset previously reported in Jochumsen et al. (2015). In the following, the experimental protocol is briefly described for clarity. The full details of the experimental procedure can be found in Jochumsen et al. (2015). Twenty-four healthy participants (7 female and 17 male 27 ± 4 years old) without any prior BCI experience participated in the experiment. All procedures were approved by the local ethics committee (N-20130081), and the participants gave their written informed consent before the experiment.

Experimental Procedures

The participants were seated in a chair, relaxed and with their foot fixed to a pedal. During the experimental session, the participants were instructed to perform ankle dorsiflexion following a visual cue display on a computer screen that was located at a distance of 1.5 m in front of them. The cue was presented with a custom-made program (Knud Larsen, SMI, Aalborg University) which provides the instructions by displaying *Ready*, *Focus*, and *Task* commands in 8–10 s intervals. The 24 participants were divided into two groups. The first 12 participants (Group 1) were asked to perform actual dorsiflexion (motor execution, ME), while the remaining 12 participants (Group 2) were asked to perform only motor imagery (MI) of the movement. Four contraction types were performed: fast contraction targeted at 20% maximum voluntary contraction (MVC), fast contraction targeted at 60%, slow contraction targeted at 20%, and slow contraction targeted at 60% MVC. In the visual cue, a moving cursor showed when and how fast the subject should perform the task. For each of the four contraction types, each participant performed approximately 50 trials of the ankle dorsiflexion task (ME or MI). The order of contraction types was randomized for both ME and MI sessions. The motor tasks were separated randomly between 8 to 10 s. For the purpose of this study, we only analyzed and report the results using the trials of fast 20% MVC, for both ME and MI tasks. For this particular task, the instruction shown on the screen for Ready, Focus, and Task commands lasted between 4–6, 3, and 1 s, respectively. The subjects focused for 3 s, followed by the execution phase 0.5 s to reach 20% MVC, and the contraction was maintained for 0.5 s, after which a rest period was given (between 4 to 6 s).

EEG Recording

A multichannel EEG electrode system (32 Channel Quick-Cap, Neuroscan) and an EEG Amplifier (Numaps Express, Neuroscan) were used according to the international 10–20 system to obtain EEG signals. Ten electrodes placed at standard 10–20 positions FP1, F3, Fz, F4, C3, Cz, C4, P3, Pz, and P4 were used to collect EEG data at a sampling rate of 500 Hz. The reference electrode was located on the right ear lobe. All analyses presented below were performed offline.

Data Processing

Since zero-phase non-causal IIR filters have been shown to perform well on Slow Cortical Potentials (SCPs) related to anticipatory behavior (Garipelli et al., 2011), the EEG data in the current paper were non-causally bandpass filtered between 0.05 to 3 Hz using a zero-phase second-order Butterworth bandpass filter prior to further processing. The choice of the filter was consistent with prior studies that used MRCP for real-time detection of motor intentions (Xu et al., 2014a) and similar to the recommendations of (Garipelli et al., 2011). All data were analyzed without rejecting segments with artifacts.

cICA for MRCP Detection

The cICA approach is briefly explained in the following.

Suppose that a N-dimensional observed sensor signal $x(t) = [x_1(t), x_2(t), \ldots, x_N(t)]^T$ can be expressed as:

$$x(t) = As(t), \tag{1}$$

where $s(t) = [s_1(t), s_2(t), \ldots, s_M(t)]^T$ is a M-dimensional mutually-independent latent source vector, and A is an unknown non-singular mixing matrix. The objective of cICA is to find a separating or de-mixing vector w without knowing the source vector and mixing matrix, such that:

$$y(t) = w^T x(t) = w^T As(t), \tag{2}$$

where $y(t)$ is the desired independent component (desired source signal). To determine this de-mixing vector, the cICA algorithm consists of the following steps. First, a linear whitening transformation is applied to the time series so that each column of $z(t)$ has unit variance and the columns are uncorrelated, i.e., the covariance matrix of $z(t)$ becomes the identity matrix:

$$z(t) = Vx(t), \tag{3}$$

where V is a whitening matrix (Zhang, 2008). Next, according to the negentropy maximum criterion (Hyvärinen et al., 2001), the objective function of the next step is defined by:

$$J(y) \approx \gamma[E\{G(y(t))\} - E\{G(\nu)\}]^2, \tag{4}$$

where $E\{\}$ indicates expectation of the signal and $y(t) = w^T z(t)$ is the output of the algorithm, γ is a positive constant, ν is a Gaussian variable having zero mean and unit variance, and $G(\cdot)$ can be any non-quadratic function. For traditional ICA methods, which have several independent components at the output, all columns of the output will be independent of each other by maximizing (4). To obtain one specific source signal, *a priori* information about the particular desired source needs to be incorporated into the cost function. In order to achieve this goal, the cICA problem is formulated as:

$$J(w) \approx \gamma[E\{G(w^T z)\} - E\{G(v)\}]^2$$
$$\text{Subject to}: g(w) = \varepsilon(y, r) - \xi,\ h(w) = E\{y^2\} - 1 = 0, \tag{5}$$

where $\varepsilon(y,r)$ is the similarity measure between the independent component y and the reference signal r, and ξ is a the similarity threshold. Therefore, $g(\omega)$ is the similarity constraint for the ICA optimization criterion, and $h(\omega)$ constrains y to have unit variance. Assuming that the desired IC is the one and only one closest to the reference r, one can get the following inequality relationship:

$$\varepsilon(w^{*T} z, r) < \varepsilon(w_1{}^T z, r) < \ldots \varepsilon(w_{N-1}{}^T z, r), \tag{6}$$

where the optimum vector ω^* is the optimum demixing vector corresponding to the desired IC, and $w_i (i = 1, \ldots, N-1)$ corresponds to other unwanted ICs. The value of the similarity threshold lies in $[\varepsilon(w^{*T} z, r), \varepsilon(w_1{}^T z, r)]$. The Lagrange multipliers method is used to solve the optimization problem of (5) (Lu and Rajapakse, 2005, 2006; Zhang, 2008):

$$\begin{aligned} w_{t+1} &= w_t - \eta R_z^{-1} \Gamma_1 / \Gamma_2 \\ \Gamma_1 &= \bar{\gamma} E\{zG'_y(y)\} - 1/2\mu E\{g'_y(y)\} - \lambda E\{zy\} \\ \Gamma_2 &= \bar{\gamma} E\{zG''_{y^2}(y)\} - 1/2\mu E\{g''_{y^2}(y)\} - \lambda, \end{aligned} \tag{7}$$

where t represents the iteration number. $R_z = E\{zz^T\}$, $\bar{\gamma} = \gamma \cdot sign(E\{G(y)\} - E\{G(v)\})$; and $G'_y(y), g'_y(y)$, $G''_{y^2}(y), g''_{y^2}(y)$, are respectively, the first and second derivatives of $G(y)$, $g(y)$ with respect to y. The optimum multipliers μ and λ are found by iteratively updating them based on a gradient-ascent method:

$$\begin{aligned} \mu_t &= \text{Max}\{0, \mu_{t-1} + \eta g(w_{t-1})\} \\ \lambda_t &= \lambda_{t-1} + \gamma_{t-1} h(w_{t-1}) \end{aligned} \tag{8}$$

Designing the reference signal plays a crucial role in cICA. The reference signal should be closely related to the desired source signal in terms of shape and phase (Zhang and Zhang, 2006; Zhang, 2008). For example, it is possible to use one of the observed channels as a reference signal (Mi, 2014). We propose the use of the average MRCP from Cz (for dorsiflexion) over all trials of a training set to build a subject-specific reference signal. Details of the training sets and construction of the reference signal using the training sets are discussed below.

Movement Detection Analysis

"Go" epochs and "No-go" epochs were extracted from the recorded signals according to the onset of the performed dorsiflexion task. Go epochs were the time intervals containing the MRCP whereas No-go epochs contained only noise. The effect of the filters on the MRCP morphology was quantified by two indices: the Signal to Noise Ratio (SNR) and the Go epoch variability (ρ). Moreover, three additional indices were calculated from the dataset of each subject to evaluate the performance of spatial filters in MRCP detection: True Positive

Rate (TPR), False Positive Rate (FPR), and Detection Latency (DL). This was done using an offline evaluation framework, as described next. Following the extraction of Go epochs and No-go epochs, cross validation was implemented, and in each fold of the cross-validation, two thirds of the Go epochs and No-go epochs were randomly selected as the training set, and the remaining third of the Go and No-go epochs formed the testing set. Cross validation was performed whereby two thirds of the trials from the entire data set were randomly selected as a training set and the remaining one third as the testing set, and this was repeated ten times. The training set was used to generate the weights for spatial filters, and by assuming that the characteristics of the MRCP signals did not change across sessions, the demixing vector obtained from the training phase was applied to the test data. This offline evaluation over a number of folds allows a systematic evaluation of each method's performance by obtaining the receiver operating characteristics (ROC) curve of each method through cross-validation.

The SNR was calculated for each subject by extracting Go and No-go epochs, respectively, from [−2, 2] s and [2, 6] s with respect to the task onset (the turning point of the cue, see (Jochumsen et al., 2015)). Denoting the lth Go epoch and No-go epoch by $x_S^l(t)$ and $x_N^l(t)$, respectively, each containing T samples, the SNR can be expressed as:

$$SNR = \frac{\sum_{l=1}^{L}\sum_{t=0}^{T}\left[x_S^l(t)\right]^2}{\sum_{l=1}^{L}\sum_{t=0}^{T}\left[x_N^l(t)\right]^2}. \tag{9}$$

The Go epoch variability ρ was defined as:

$$\rho = \frac{\frac{1}{LT}\sum_{l=1}^{L}\sum_{t=0}^{T}\left|x_S^l(t) - \overline{x_S(t)}\right|}{\max\left[\overline{x_S(t)}\right] - \min\left[\overline{x_S(t)}\right]}, \tag{10}$$

where $\overline{x_S(t)}$ is the average of the L Go epochs. The lower the value of ρ, the more consistent the Go epochs are. It should be noted that the two indices are calculated for all spatial filter outputs.

TPR, FPR, and DL were calculated on Go and No-go epochs, respectively extracted from [−3, 1] s and [2, 6] s with respect to the task onset, for each subject. TPR and FPR for each fold of the testing set were defined as:

$$TPR = \frac{\text{Total number of correctly detected Go epochs}}{\text{Total number of Go epochs}}, \tag{11}$$

and

$$FPR = \frac{\text{Total number of incorrectly detected No-go epochs}}{\text{Total number of No-go epochs}}$$

The Go epoch interval used to calculate the measures of detection performance was chosen to be different from the Go-epochs used for SNR calculation because, considering the length of the moving window, the time interval [−2 2] s, which perfectly covers all MRCP components, cannot be used if one would expect negative detection latencies where detection happens before the movement execution ($t = 0$). It should be noted that since the time interval [−3, 1] covers most parts of MRCP, this choice does not affect the TPR values.

To train Infomax and JADE, the training sets were built by concatenating all Go epochs and all No-go epochs of the training set. This means that all concatenated Go epochs (randomly selected) formed the first half of the training set signals; and the corresponding second half of the training set signals was formed by the concatenation of randomly selected No-go epochs in each channel. This approach was chosen as it provided a consistent training process for each method, and furthermore, it enabled us to perform the cross validation process. A similar approach was used for cICA, with an additional reference signal for the EEG signals. The reference signal for cICA was constructed using two steps: first, a subject-specific MRCP template was generated by averaging all Go-epochs of the Cz epochs in the training set ([−2, 2] s with respect to the task onset). Next, considering that the training sets were concatenated Go and No-go epochs for the other methods (Infomax and JADE), the reference signal of cICA was built by repeating the MRCP template corresponding to the signal epochs and using zero for the No-go epochs. By knowing the actual occurrence time of the executed or imagined movements, this approach could be implementable in the training phase of an online application as well. To train CSP, No-Go epochs and Go epochs were provided to the algorithm in two different matrices built by placing Go epochs in the rows of the signal matrix and each No-Go epoch in the rows of the noise matrix. LAP is not a supervised method; therefore, no training was required.

A LPP-LDA classifier was used for classification of the Go and No-go epochs (Xu et al., 2014a). A sliding window with length 2 s and 50 ms shift was applied to each Go and No-go epoch. A detection occurred when n consecutive sliding windows resulted in detection at the output of the LPP-LDA classifier. The choice for n determines the sensitivity of the overall system. Therefore by varying n from 1 to 10, the average (over subjects) ROC curve was derived through cross-validation on the testing dataset of all subjects. TPR is defined as the ratio of the number of correctly detected Go epochs to the total number of Go epochs in the testing set. Similarly, FPR is defined as the ratio of the number of false detections of No-go epochs to the total number of No-go epochs in the testing set. The detection latency is defined as the time difference between detection and movement onset for the executed movements, and between detection and task onset for the imagined movements, in each Go epoch.

Statistical Analysis

To investigate the effect of the spatial filtering method on SNR and ρ, Friedman's Two-way ANOVA was performed, where the factor was Methods with five levels (LAP, CSP, Infomax, JADE, and cICA). When a significant difference was observed a multiple comparison (Bonferroni) was carried out to identify which methods were significantly different. The significance level

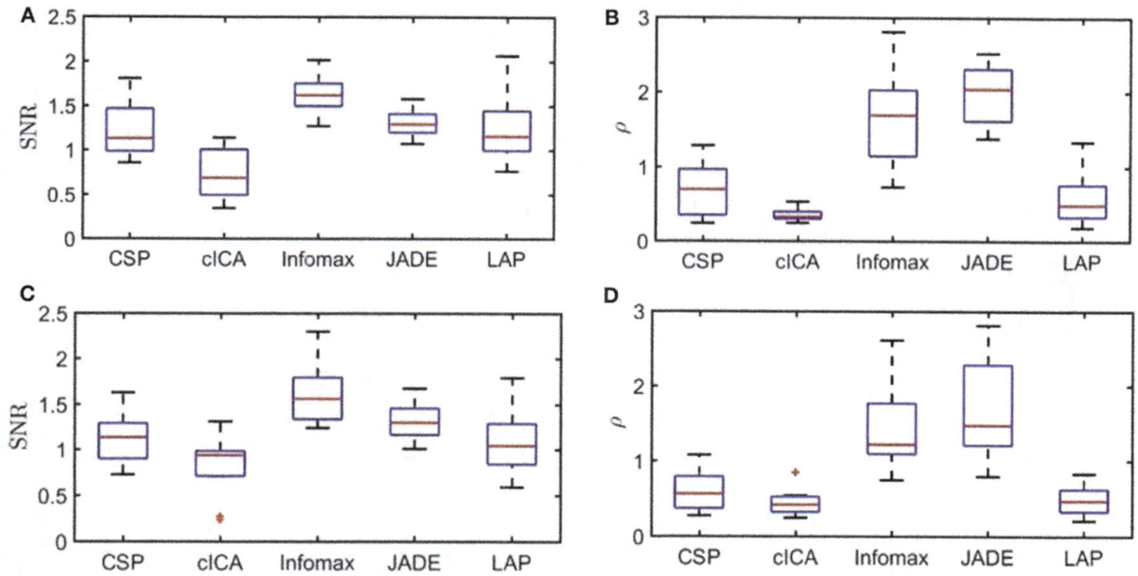

FIGURE 1 | Boxplots of SNR and ρ-values for ME and MI datasets: **(A)** SNR values for ME dataset, **(B)** ρ-values for ME dataset, **(C)** SNR values for MI dataset, and **(D)** ρ-values for MI dataset.

of all tests was set at $p < 0.05$. Furthermore, in order to investigate the effect of the five methods on MRCP detection, two-way repeated measure ANOVA was performed on the ME and MI datasets, with fixed factor the spatial filtering algorithms (LAP, CSP, Infomax, JADE, and cICA) and random factor the subject (SUB, 12 levels). The main null hypothesis was that Methods was not a significant factor on TPR, FPR, and DL. When the null hypothesis was rejected, a multiple comparison (Tukey with Bonferroni correction) followed.

RESULTS

The boxplot for the average values of SNR and ρ for the output of the spatial filters over folds from the testing sets, and for all subjects are presented in **Figure 1**. Direct observation indicates that, in this offline study, Infomax is able to suppress the noise better than other methods (highest SNR) in both the ME and MI datasets. In contrast, cICA had the lowest SNR values compared to other methods. However, in both the ME and MI datasets, cICA resulted in the lowest values for ρ among all methods. For the ME dataset, results from the Friedman's Two-way ANOVA showed that Methods had a significant effect on ρ and SNR ($p < 0.001$). The multiple comparison tests found that the SNR was smaller for cICA than LAP, Infomax, and JADE. Moreover, cICA, LAP, and CSP led to significantly lower variability compared to JADE and Infomax. For the MI dataset, the factor Methods again had a significant effect on ρ and SNR ($p < 0.001$). Post-hoc comparisons showed that SNR for cICA was significantly lower than Infomax, and JADE; and Infomax had significantly greater SNR values than LAP. For ρ, similar to the ME dataset, cICA, LAP, and CSP led to significantly lower variability than JADE and Infomax.

Figure 2 represents the algorithm used to calculate the detection latency when 5 consecutive windows result in detection at the output of the LPP-LDA classifier ($n = 5$). The average of the ROC curves of MRCP detection over all subjects for both ME and MI (testing) datasets is provided in **Figure 3** for all spatial filters and 10 decision thresholds ($n = 1, 2, \ldots, 10$). The area under the ROC curves is provided in **Table 1**. For both datasets, the area under the ROC curve of cICA has the highest value confirming that for each n, cICA provides the best combination of TPRs and FPRs (high TPR and low FPR). Therefore, the accuracy of cICA is superior compared to other spatial filters. As seen from the ROC curves, five decision windows are located at the midpoint of the convex part of the ROC curve, meaning that five consecutive detections could be a good balance between TPR and FPR for all filters. Therefore, the results presented next were calculated for five as the decision threshold.

The detection performance is presented in **Table 2** for both ME and MI datasets. The highest TPRs and lowest FPRs and DLs were obtained for cICA for both datasets. The detection latency for cICA (-34 ± 29 ms for ME and 28 ± 16 ms for MI dataset) was significantly smaller than for the other spatial filters.

For the ME dataset, the ANOVA test showed that Methods has a significant effect on TPR, FPR, and DL ($p < 0.001$). Multiple comparisons found that TPR for cICA (87.11 ± 11.73) was significantly higher than with all other methods. LAP (74.65 ± 13.13) had significantly greater TPRs than CSP (67.14 ± 13.99) and Infomax (67.27 ± 7.69). FPR for cICA (20.69 ± 13.68) was significantly lower than for Infomax (31.70 ± 9.94) and JADE (30.44 ± 10.26); and FPR for Infomax (31.70 ± 9.94) was significantly higher than for CSP (24.55

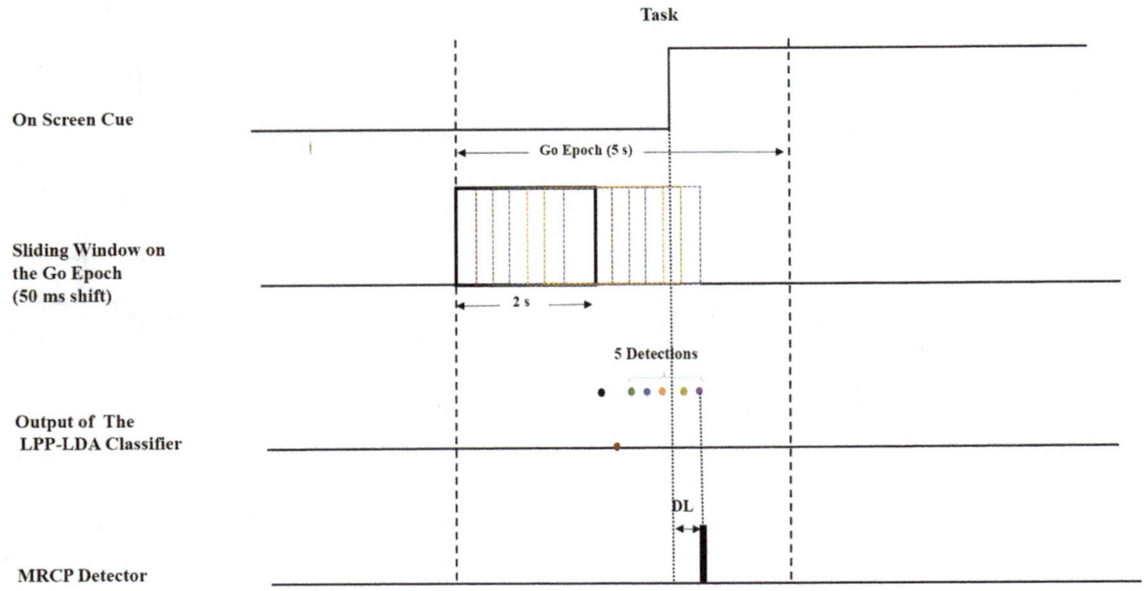

FIGURE 2 | Offline implementation of movement detection.

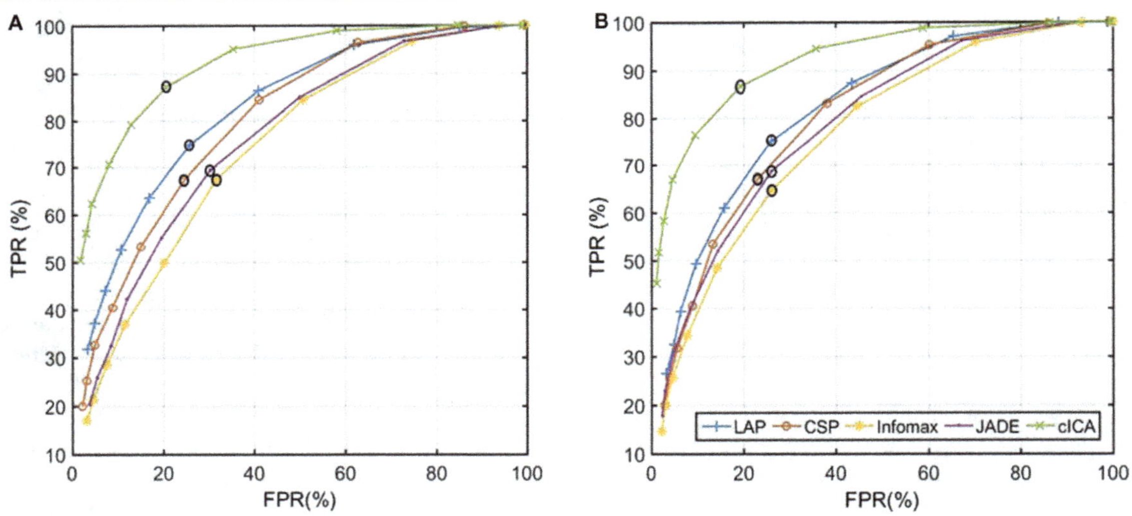

FIGURE 3 | Average of the ROC curves of five spatial filters across all subjects: **(A)** ME dataset **(B)** MI dataset (black circle represents the value of each ROC curve when $n = 5$ in both graphs).

± 11.31) and cICA (20.69 ± 13.68). Regarding the detection latencies, the statistical analysis showed that cICA (−34 ± 29 ms) had significantly lower detection latencies compared with all other methods. In contrast, the detection latencies with CSP (295 ± 13 ms) were significantly greater than for Infomax (245 ± 9 ms), LAP (197 ± 15 ms), and cICA (−34 ± 29 ms).

Results for the MI dataset were similar to those for the ME dataset. Methods influenced significantly TPR, FPR, and DL ($p = 0.00$ for TPR and DL, and $p = 0.02$ for FPR). Multiple comparisons indicated that TPR from cICA (86.66 ± 6.96) was significantly greater than for all other methods and TPR for LAP (75.06 ± 12.94) was significantly higher than for CSP (66.87 ± 10.13) and Infomax (64.69 ± 9.42) FPR of cICA (19.31 ± 12.60) was significantly lower than for LAP (25.99 ± 17.04), Infomax (26.19 ± 7.78), and JADE (26.12 ± 10.25), but not significantly different from CSP (23.02 ± 10.56). The detection latency obtained with cICA (28 ± 16) was significantly lower than for all other methods.

The average TPR, FPR, and DL over the 10 folds are reported for each subject from both datasets in **Figure 4**. For 11 of the

12 subjects, cICA has the highest TPR and lowest FPR and DL among all spatial filters.

DISCUSSION

The MRCP has recently been implemented as a control signal in a variety of BCI applications (Xu et al., 2014a,b; Jiang et al., 2015; Mrachacz-Kersting et al., 2016). The reliable and efficient detection of MRCPs enables the design of accurate and fast brain switches. Depending on the application of BCI systems, the importance of accuracy and latency of the system may vary. To be more specific, while large DL may not be ideal for BCI applications developed to induce brain plasticity, slightly lower TPR may not greatly affect the performance of the BCI system. On the other hand, high TPR are required for the control of exoskeletons for replacement rather than restoration of function, and for this application, a low DL is not so imperative. Accuracy and latency of detection of the MRCP highly relies on the signal processing method used to extract features from raw EEG. Spatial filters are one of the most efficient and successful feature extraction methods in EEG signal processing due to the spatial distribution of the signal features. In this study, the performance of cICA, a newly introduced ICA-based spatial filter, was compared with four other spatial filters in an offline experiment for MRCP detection from multi-channel EEG recordings, during execution and imaginary dorsiflexion of healthy subjects.

The performance of each spatial filtering algorithm in the detection of MRCPs was initially evaluated based on clarity and consistency of the extracted MRCP, quantified by SNR and ρ, respectively. Moreover, TPR, FPR, and DL were investigated through cross-validation in an offline experiment. The reported TPRs in this study are in agreement with the previous similar studies (Xu et al., 2014a,b). However, since, in this study, it was intended to evaluate the performance of the detector and determine the optimum parameters for movement detection using ROC, the values of FPR were calculated with a different measure than previous similar studies. In the previous studies, FPR was defined as the number of false detections per minute. Such approach for calculating FPRs caused the values of FPRs to be biased by the experiment protocol and inconsistent with TPRs. In this paper, the approach used to calculate FPR values makes the values independent of the experimental protocol, in which parameters such as the refractory period of the MI/ME can affect the accuracy of the definition of FPR used in previous studies (Niazi et al., 2011, 2013): false positive per unit time. Also, this approach is consistent with the approach used to calculate TPRs, enabling us to obtain ROC curves for the detector. The calculation of DL in this study is also in agreement with previous studies. It should be noted that a non-causal filter was used in the current study. In a real online experiment, a causal filter should be used. In order to investigate the effect of type of the bandpass filtering method (causal vs. non-causal), we performed an additional analysis to compare the performance of a causal second-order Butterworth bandpass filter with the bandwidth of 0.05–3 Hz with the same non-causal filter. The average signal of all causally and non-causally filtered Go-epochs (MRCPs) from the Cz channel for Subject 1 are provided in **Figure 5**. The observations indicate that there is a smaller amplitude in the negative peak of MRCP when the causal filter is used. We also compared the detection performance for causally and non-causally filtered signals for all subjects in the ME group. The causal filtering resulted in slightly higher FPR and lower TPRs compared to using non-causally filtered data, and the change was consistent in overall detection accuracy for all spatial filters investigated (the change of the averaged TPR values from causally to non-causally filtered signals was: 0.87, −0.19, −3.87, −5.89, −4; and the corresponding change of the averaged FPR values was: −7.69, 9.95, 7.46, 10.86, 13.47 for LAP, CSP, Infomax, JADE, and cICA respectively). This consistent change in overall detection accuracy is expected given the results shown in the figure, as the causal filter resulted in a less pronounced MRCP. However, causal filtering had no significant effect on the detection latencies (the difference between the averaged DL values for causally and non-causally filtered signals was: −0.07, −0.03, −0.06, −0.02, 0.00 s for LAP, CSP, Infomax, JADE, and

TABLE 1 | Average of the ROC curves of movement detection for ME and MI datasets.

Spatial filter	Area under the ROC curve				
	LAP	CSP	Infomax	JADE	cICA
ME dataset	0.81	0.79	0.73	0.75	0.90
MI dataset	0.80	0.79	0.76	0.78	0.91

TABLE 2 | Average TPR, FPR, and DL for movement detection for ME and MI datasets.

Spatial filter	Motor execution			Motor imagery		
	TPR	FPR	DL (ms)	TPR	FPR	DL (ms)
AP	74.65 ± 13.13	25.83 ± 16.91	197 ± 15	75.06 ± 12.94	25.99 ± 17.04	216 ± 14
SP	67.14 ± 13.99	24.55 ± 11.31	295 ± 13	66.87 ± 10.13	23.02 ± 10.56	246 ± 15
fomax	67.27 ± 7.69	31.70 ± 9.94	245 ± 9	64.69 ± 9.42	26.19 ± 7.78	286 ± 11
ADE	69.33 ± 8.56	30.44 ± 10.26	256 ± 16	68.68 ± 10.35	26.12 ± 10.25	250 ± 13
CA	87.11 ± 11.73	20.69 ± 13.68	−34 ± 29	86.66 ± 6.96	19.31 ± 12.60	28 ± 16

e results are presented (mean ± standard deviation across subjects) for each spatial filter.

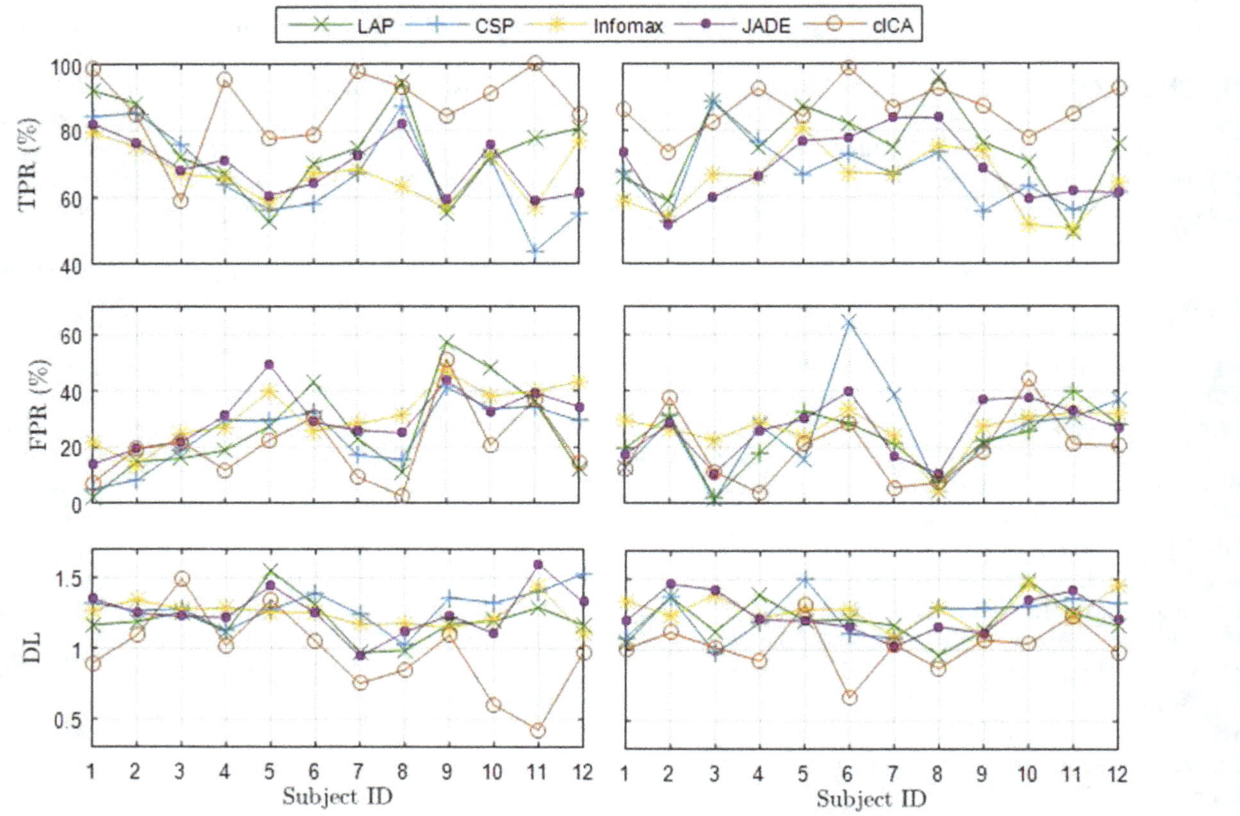

FIGURE 4 | Average TPR, FRP, and DL for all subjects for both ME **(left)** and MI datasets **(right)**.

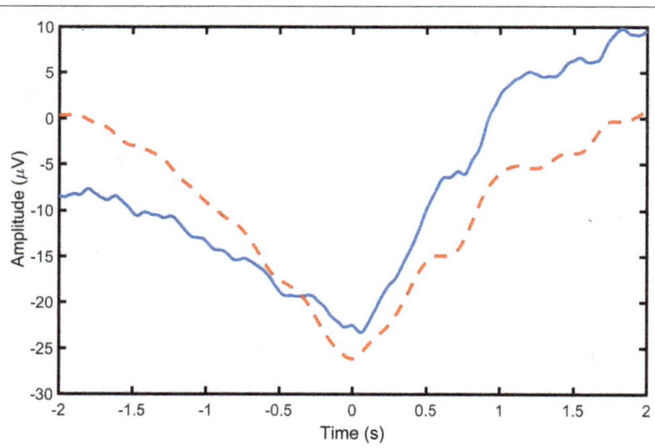

FIGURE 5 | Average signal of all causally (___) and non-causally (- - - - -) filtered Go-epochs (MRCPs) from the Cz channel for Subject 1.

cICA, respectively). Therefore, it is highly possible that the choice of causal or non-causal filtering has a slight effect on the overall detection accuracy, but there was no effect on DL values. However, this needs to be verified in a subsequent dedicated online study, which is beyond the scope of the current study with the objective of introducing cICA for MRCP detection.

The cICA requires the choice of a threshold that weights the relative importance of similarity with the reference signal in the optimization (Zhang, 2008). The suitable value of threshold depends on both the designed reference signal and the similarity measure. An effective way to determine the threshold given a reference signal, which was also used in this paper, is to use a small threshold initially, and then gradually increase the threshold (Lu and Rajapakse, 2006). For the reference signal based on the average of the Go epochs of the Cz channel, the value of the threshold was set to 0.9. On the other hand, as mentioned earlier, the shape of the designed reference signal plays an important role in the performance of cICA. Therefore investigation of the effect of other types of reference signals such as the common rectangular pulse, smoothed MRCPs (Garipelli et al., 2013), and discriminative-based reference signal (Lee et al., 2016) will be done in the future in attempt to improve detection performance.

With the selected parameters, the area under the ROC curve for cICA was greater than for the other methods and cICA outperformed all the other filters for TPR and DL. Moreover FPR was lower for cICA than for three of the other investigated methods. Overall, this indicates an improved performance of cICA with respect to previously proposed filtering methods. Considering that the detection of MRCP can be affected by hyper parameters such as the overlap of the sliding windows and the number of detections required, further investigation will be done in the future to optimize the cICA algorithm based on these and other aspects. The averaged SNR values for the tested methods were not well associated with the detection performance. Indeed, cICA provided high TPRs and low FPRs compared to other methods but resulted in the lowest SNR values. One reason for the low SNR of cICA may be the optimization criteria of the method and the way SNR values were calculated in this study. The reference signal for cICA requires the algorithm to optimize the weights such that the desired signal can be obtained. As a result, the trial-by-trial consistency of the signal was improved by cICA. On the other hand, the results for the average ρ-values were more consistent with those obtained for TPRs. This is one of the findings of the current study: SNR does not necessarily correlate very well with detection performance, and the consistency of the Go epochs is equally (if not more) important for achieving a high detection performance. This likely stems from the fact that MRCP is a rather deterministic waveform, compared to other motor imagery BCI signal modalities, such as ERD/ERS. It can be concluded that, considering the shape of the reference signal applied in the current study, cICA seems to allow a more accurate modeling of the class of the Go epochs, and consequently a more pronounced effect on the sensitivity of the detector. This is because the choice of the reference signal can affect the ability of the cICA in modeling each class and separability of the classes. Therefore, cICA in the current study has limited effect on the specificity of the detector due to the choice of reference signal. It is possible that other types of reference signals can tune the algorithm to focus on other aspects of performance, such as specificity, which will be explored in future studies.

Regression analysis and template matching are also methods that have been used to extract desired EEG features and for EEG artifact removal (Wallstrom et al., 2004; Niazi et al., 2013; Urigüen and Garcia-Zapirain, 2015). Regression algorithms estimate the influence of the reference signal on the desired signal either in the frequency or time domain. Linear regression assumes that each EEG channel is the sum of the non-noisy source signal and a fraction of the source artifact that is available through a reference channel. Then, the goal of regression is to estimate the optimal value for the factor that represents such a fraction. Regression approaches need a reference channel to be able to operate automatically. In comparison, cICA is more flexible because although it uses a reference signal to extract features of the EEG signal or artifacts, the reference signal does not have to be a good estimation of the source(s). In fact, the reference signal can be very general, as long as it provides some reasonable constraint to ICA. For example, in Lee et al. (2016), a rectangular reference signal, which was not similar to the underlying source, was successfully implemented. In addition, since the regression methods are based on the time and frequency characteristics of the signals, they do not take into account the spatial information of the sources. Template matching techniques such as matched filter, which uses a template to maximize the SNR of the extracted signal, are also methods used for MRCP extraction (Niazi et al., 2013). Similar to regression, such methods only depend on the temporal features of the template and do not consider the spatial distribution of different sources. Also, matched filters are only optimal with additive Gaussian noise, so they are sensitive to other types of noise and artifacts.

In the current manuscript, we only used data from one of the four tasks for the purpose of introducing cICA for the first time in MRCP detection. Subsequent studies will be performed to investigate the generalizability of cICA when presented with data from different types of tasks.

CONCLUSION

We have proposed a new spatial filter for MRCP detection. The proposed cICA extracts the desired signal by utilizing additional prior (spatial) information with respect to classic ICA, while exploiting higher order statistical structures as the CSP does. The results indicated that cICA did not enhance the extracted MRCP from multi-channel EEG significantly better than several commonly used spatial filters, including CSP, LAP, and ICA. However, cICA significantly outperformed these spatial filters in single-trial MRCP detection, with higher TPRs, lower FPRs, and shorter latency, both for ME and MI tasks. These results indicate that cICA is a promising new algorithm for detecting MRCP from multi-channel EEG. Following the promising results of the current study, we will conduct online experiments in a future study, in which cICA will be compared with LAP and CSP.

AUTHOR CONTRIBUTIONS

Inception of ideas for the manuscript was by FK, NJ, JK, DF, and NM; conceptualization, methodology, validation, investigation, writing (review and editing) by FK, NJ, JK, DF, and NM; data acquisition/curation by NJ, DF, and NM; formal data analysis by FK and NJ; manuscript first draft by FK; manuscript revisions by FK, NJ, JK, NM, and DF; resources, supervision, administration, funding acquisition by NJ, JK, DF, and NM.

REFERENCES

Bell, A. J., and Sejnowski, T. J. (1995). An information-maximization approach to blind separation and blind deconvolution. *Neural Comput.* 7, 1129–1159. doi: 10.1162/neco.1995.7.6.1129

Blankertz, B., Tomioka, R., Lemm, S., Kawanabe, M., and Muller, K. (2008). Optimizing spatial filters for robust EEG single-trial analysis. *IEEE Signal Process. Mag.* 25, 41–56. doi: 10.1109/MSP.2008.4408441

Cardoso, J. F. (1999). High-order contrasts for independent component analysis. *Neural Comput.* 11, 157–192. doi: 10.1162/089976699300016863

Garipelli, G., Chavarriaga, R., and Millan, J. D. R. (2011). "Single trial recognition of anticipatory slow cortical potentials: the role of spatio-spectral filtering," in *2011 5th International IEEE/EMBS Conference on Neural Engineering, Vol. 1* (Cancun: IEEE), 408–411. doi: 10.1109/NER.2011.5910573

Garipelli, G., Chavarriaga, R., and Millan, J. D. R. (2013). Single trial analysis of slow cortical potentials: a study on anticipation related potentials. *J. Neural Eng.* 10:036014. doi: 10.1088/1741-2560/10/3/036014

Huang, L., Wang, H., and Wang, Y. (2011). Removal of ocular artifact from EEG using constrained ICA. *Adv. Eng. Forum* 105–110.

Hyvärinen, A., Karhunen, J., and Oja, E. (2001). *Independent Component Analysis.* New York, NY: Wiley.

James, C. J., and Gibson, O. J. (2003). Temporally constrained ica: an application to artifact rejection in electromagnetic brain signal analysis. *IEEE Trans. Biomed. Eng.* 50, 1108–1116. doi: 10.1109/TBME.2003.816076

Jiang, N., Gizzi, L., Mrachacz-Kersting, N., Dremstrup, K., and Farina, D. (2015). A brain–computer interface for single-trial detection of gait initiation from movement related cortical potentials. *Clin. Neurophysiol.* 126, 154–159. doi: 10.1016/j.clinph.2014.05.003

Jochumsen, M., Niazi, I. K., Mrachacz-Kersting, N., Jiang, N., Farina, D., and Dremstrup, K. (2015). Comparison of spatial filters and features for the detection and classification of movement-related cortical potentials in healthy individuals and stroke patients. *J. Neural Eng.* 12:056003. doi: 10.1088/1741-2560/12/5/056003

Joshua, L. K. L., and Rajapakse, J. C. (2005). "Extraction of event-related potentials from EEG signals using ICA with reference," in *Proceedings 2005 IEEE International Joint Conference on Neural Networks, Vol. 4* (Montreal, QC: IEEE), 2526–2531. doi: 10.1109/IJCNN.2005.1556300

Lee, W. L., Tan, T., and Leung, Y. H. (2013). "An improved P300 extraction using ICA-R for P300-BCI speller," in *2013 35th Annual International Conference of the IEEE Engineering in Medicine and Biology Society (EMBC)* (Osaka: IEEE), 7064–7067. doi: 10.1109/EMBC.2013.6611185

Lee, W. L., Tan, T., Falkmer, T., and Leung, Y. H. (2016). Single-trial event-related potential extraction through one-unit ICA-with-reference. *J. Neural Eng.* 13:066010. doi: 10.1088/1741-2560/13/6/066010

Lu, W., and Rajapakse, J. C. (2005). Approach and applications of constrained ICA. *IEEE Trans. Neural Netw.* 16, 203–212. doi: 10.1109/TNN.2004.836795

Lu, W., and Rajapakse, J. C. (2006). ICA with reference. *Neurocomputing* 69, 2244–2257. doi: 10.1016/j.neucom.2005.06.021

McFarland, D. J., McCane, L. M., David, S. V., and Wolpaw, J. R. (1997). Spatial filter selection for EEG-based communication. *Electroencephalogr. Clin. Neurophysiol.* 103, 386–394. doi: 10.1016/S0013-4694(97)00022-2

Mi, J. X. (2014). A novel algorithm for independent component analysis with reference and methods for its applications. *PLoS ONE* 9:e93984. doi: 10.1371/journal.pone.0093984

Mrachacz-Kersting, N., Jiang, N., Stevenson, A. J. T., Niazi, I. K., Kostic, V., Pavlovic, A., et al. (2016). Efficient neuroplasticity induction in chronic stroke patients by an associative brain-computer interface. *J. Neurophysiol.* 115, 1410–1421. doi: 10.1152/jn.00918.2015

Mrachacz-Kersting, N., Kristensen, S. R., Niazi, I. K., and Farina, D. (2012). Precise temporal association between cortical potentials evoked by motor imagination and afference induces cortical plasticity. *J. Physiol.* 590, 1669–1682. doi: 10.1113/jphysiol.2011.222851

Niazi, I. K., Jiang, N., Jochumsen, M., Nielsen, J. F., Dremstrup, K., and Farina, D. (2013). Detection of movement-related cortical potentials based on subject-independent training. *Med. Biol. Eng. Comput.* 51, 507–512. doi: 10.1007/s11517-012-1018-1

Niazi, I. K., Jiang, N., Tiberghien, O., Nielsen, J. F., Dremstrup, K., and Farina, D. (2011). Detection of movement intention from single-trial movement-related cortical potentials. *J. Neural Eng.* 8:066009. doi: 10.1088/1741-2560/8/6/066009

Ramoser, H., Muller-Gerking, J., and Pfurtscheller, G. (2000). Optimal Spatial filtering of single trial EEG during imagined hand movement. *IEEE Trans. Rehabil. Eng.* 8, 441–446. doi: 10.1109/86.895946

Spyrou, L., and Sanei, S. (2006). "A robust constrained method for the extraction of P300 subcomponents," in *2006 IEEE International Conference on Acoustics Speed and Signal Processing Proceedings, Vol. 2* (Toulouse: IEEE), 1184–1187. doi: 10.1109/ICASSP.2006.1660560

Urigüen, J. A., and Garcia-Zapirain, B. (2015). EEG artifact removal—state-of-the-art and guidelines. *J. Neural Eng.* 12:031001. doi: 10.1088/1741-2560/12/3/031001

Wallstrom, G. L., Kass, R. E., Miller, A., Cohn, J. F., and Fox, N. A. (2004). Automatic correction of ocular artifacts in the EEG: a comparison of regression-based and component-based methods. *Int. J. Psychophysiol.* 53, 105–119. doi: 10.1016/j.ijpsycho.2004.03.007

Wright, D. J., Holmes, P. S., and Smith, D. (2011). Using the movement-related cortical potential to study motor skill learning. *J. Mot. Behav.* 43, 193–201. doi: 10.1080/00222895.2011.557751

Xu, N., Gao, X., Hong, B., Miao, X., Gao, S., and Yang, F. (2004). BCI competition 2003—data set IIb: enhancing P300 wave detection using ICA-based subspace projections for BCI applications. *IEEE Trans. Biomed. Eng.* 51, 1067–1072. doi: 10.1109/TBME.2004.826699

Xu, R., Jiang, N., Lin, C., Mrachacz-Kersting, N., Dremstrup, K., and Farina, D. (2014a). Enhanced low-latency detection of motor intention from EEG for closed-loop brain-computer interface applications. *IEEE Trans. Biomed. Eng.* 61, 288–296. doi: 10.1109/TBME.2013.2294203

Xu, R., Jiang, N., Mrachacz-Kersting, N., Lin, C., Prieto, G. A., Moreno, J. C., et al. (2014b). A closed-loop brain-computer interface triggering an active ankle-foot orthosis for inducing cortical neural plasticity. *IEEE Trans. Biomed. Eng.* 61, 2092–2101. doi: 10.1109/TBME.2014.2313867

Zhang, Z. L. (2008). Morphologically constrained ICA for extracting weak temporally correlated signals. *Neurocomputing* 71, 1669–1679. doi: 10.1016/j.neucom.2007.04.004

Zhang, Z. L., and Zhang, L. Q. (2006). A two-stage based approach for extracting periodic signals. *Independent Component Anal. Blind Signal Sep. Proc.* 3889, 303–310. doi: 10.1007/11679363_38

8

EEG-Based Quantification of Cortical Current Density and Dynamic Causal Connectivity Generalized across Subjects Performing BCI-Monitored Cognitive Tasks

Hristos Courellis [1,2], Tim Mullen [1], Howard Poizner [3], Gert Cauwenberghs [2,3] and John R. Iversen [1]*

[1] *Swartz Center for Computational Neuroscience, University of California, San Diego, San Diego, CA, United States,* [2] *Department of Bioengineering, University of California, San Diego, San Diego, CA, United States,* [3] *Institute for Neural Computation, University of California, San Diego, San Diego, CA, United States*

Edited by:
Timothée Levi,
University of Bordeaux 1, France

Reviewed by:
David Thomas Bundy,
Kansas University of Medical Center Research Institute, United States
Alireza Mousavi,
Brunel University London, United Kingdom

***Correspondence:**
Hristos Courellis
hcourellis@gmail.com

Quantification of dynamic causal interactions among brain regions constitutes an important component of conducting research and developing applications in experimental and translational neuroscience. Furthermore, cortical networks with dynamic causal connectivity in brain-computer interface (BCI) applications offer a more comprehensive view of brain states implicated in behavior than do individual brain regions. However, models of cortical network dynamics are difficult to generalize across subjects because current electroencephalography (EEG) signal analysis techniques are limited in their ability to reliably localize sources across subjects. We propose an algorithmic and computational framework for identifying cortical networks across subjects in which dynamic causal connectivity is modeled among user-selected cortical regions of interest (ROIs). We demonstrate the strength of the proposed framework using a "reach/saccade to spatial target" cognitive task performed by 10 right-handed individuals. Modeling of causal cortical interactions was accomplished through measurement of cortical activity using (EEG), application of independent component clustering to identify cortical ROIs as network nodes, estimation of cortical current density using cortically constrained low resolution electromagnetic brain tomography (cLORETA), multivariate autoregressive (MVAR) modeling of representative cortical activity signals from each ROI, and quantification of the dynamic causal interaction among the identified ROIs using the Short-time direct Directed Transfer function (SdDTF). The resulting cortical network and the computed causal dynamics among its nodes exhibited physiologically plausible behavior, consistent with past results reported in the literature. This physiological plausibility of the results strengthens the framework's applicability in reliably capturing complex brain functionality, which is required by applications, such as diagnostics and BCI.

Keywords: brain-computer interface (BCI), electroencephalography (EEG), causality analysis, source localization, LORETA, independent component analysis, motor activity, spatial reach and saccade

INTRODUCTION

Dynamic intra-cortical interactions offer a wealth of information that can be used to develop an understanding of brain functionality and quantify the effects of brain pathologies on brain functionality. Traditional static functional characteristics of individual brain regions, and dynamic interactions within a network of brain regions (Moeller et al., 2015) offer limited insight into brain function as they typically do not examine the causality among these interactions. The advent of Granger-causal analysis provided a framework to quantify the asymmetric causal interactions between regions of the cortex through specific frequency bands, which hold functional significance for those regions (Barnett and Seth, 2014; Seth et al., 2015), and has shed light on a large number of network-related disorders, such as Alzheimer's and Parkinson's Disease (Pievani et al., 2014). However, this connectivity information is not limited in use to diagnostics, as an increasing number of brain-computer interface (BCI) applications are utilizing connectivity features for intent discrimination when conducting BCI-related tasks (Zhang et al., 2012; Kabbara et al., 2016).

While a potential wealth of information is available in intra-cortex interactions, a systematic algorithmic approach that allows for reliable generalization of cortical network dynamics across test subjects in a subject group is not readily available. Many sophisticated tools exist (Linder et al., 2011; Niso et al., 2013; Barnett and Seth, 2014), which allow for both parametric and non-parametric estimation of dynamic causal interactions among neural activity signals within an individual. However, these tools exhibit various limitations, such as strict channel-space applicability or lack of accounting of common sources, thus, giving rise to spurious causal interactions within the chosen cortical network (Trongnetrpunya et al., 2015). Additional limitations exist in the source-localization algorithms applied to reconstruct cortical-source activity from the measured channel space data. Many popular algorithms stemming from Independent Component Analysis (ICA) are not able to achieve reproducible source localization outcomes across test subjects (Bell and Sejnowski, 1995). The inability to control where these algorithms localize the sources for decomposition on separate subjects presents a large problem since the sources represent nodes in a cortical network, and an ICA-based algorithm could localize a different network for every subject in a group, making group-level network comparisons difficult. Independent Component (IC) ordering is a highly non-trivial task (Hyvärinen and Oja, 2000) for which very few automated approaches exist barring manual selection, a prohibitively tedious and time consuming task for increasingly large datasets.

In this paper, we develop an algorithmic and computational framework that addresses the aforementioned issues through a multi-step, open-source pipeline of analytic tools (Delorme et al., 2011; Iversen et al., 2014). The pipeline combines the deconvolution power of ICA; the systematic modeling of the geometry of gray matter, thereby creating a common source space across subjects with the use of individually warped boundary element models (BEMs); the selectivity afforded by Cortical Low Resolution Electromagnetic Tomography (cLORETA)—a source-space based, distributed source localization algorithm; and the robustness of the Short-time direct Directed Transfer Function (SdDTF)—a causality measure, computed from Multivariate Autoregressive (MVAR) model coefficients, that addresses the spurious connectivity affecting Granger Causal methods (Korzeniewska et al., 2003).

A similar approach to source localization and connectivity analysis was proposed by Mullen et al. (2015) as a means of demonstrating that the connectivity features considered in this framework can be applied with great success in real-time brain state identification. In order to demonstrate the power afforded by this framework in group-level analysis, a BCI-related task originally introduced by Park et al. (2014) was employed, requiring subjects to reach and saccade to presented visual targets while their cortical activity was recorded using electroencephalography (EEG) as the neuroimaging modality. The approach utilized for BCI-related task is a passive-BCI approach, also described as an implicit human-computer interaction, wherein passive EEG equipment that senses the user is used to evaluate cognitive states of the user (Schmidt, 2000; George and Lecuyer, 2010). While, in this case, the closed-loop feedback elements of the task simply involve auditory and visual confirmation of reach/saccade task completion, the applicability of this approach to more active real-time closed-loop feedback BCI systems is also discussed. Although the motor activity present in the human cortex during simple planned motor actions has been carefully documented with respect to the activity of individual cortical regions (Johnson et al., 1996; Filimon, 2010; Heider et al., 2010; Glover et al., 2012), the dynamic interactions among these cortical regions during planning and execution of the task have not been documented as extensively. Park et al. were able to differentiate between spatial movement of the arm and eye by employing channel-space empirical mode decomposition, but did not characterize connectivity between cortical regions underlying these processes. The algorithmic approach implemented in this paper was first described by Iversen et al. (2014), where the method was applied to a smaller subject group. In this paper, we introduce modifications to the original pipeline in Iversen et al. (2014) including a new maximum-power heuristic that captured previously undetected connectivity involving the Supplementary Motor Area and Precuneus, regions expected to exhibit connectivity given the motor-related BCI task and non-parametric statistical thresholding of the computed causal connectivity values. Through application of our new pipeline, described fully in the Methods section that follows, we demonstrate in the Results section the strength and specificity of the inference that can be made regarding the dynamic causal interactions present among regions of the cortex during reach/saccade planning and execution. The Discussion section illustrates the physiological plausibility of the findings reported in the Results section with reference to previous findings reported in the literature. The Conclusion section summarizes the features, the scalability, extensibility, and the applicability of the proposed algorithmic and computational framework.

METHODS

Overview

Electrophysiological data were collected from human participants conducting a BCI-monitored task, and processed according to the methodology and computational tools outlined in **Figure 1**, using MATLAB as the computational platform. The workflow in **Figure 1** was employed to extract cortical source information from a cortical network defined for all of the participants, and, subsequently, identify statistically significant spectro-temporal interactions among the nodes (sources) of this network.

Participants and Task

Ten healthy, right-handed individuals (age: 20.8 ± 2.6 years) participated in this study. The study was approved by the

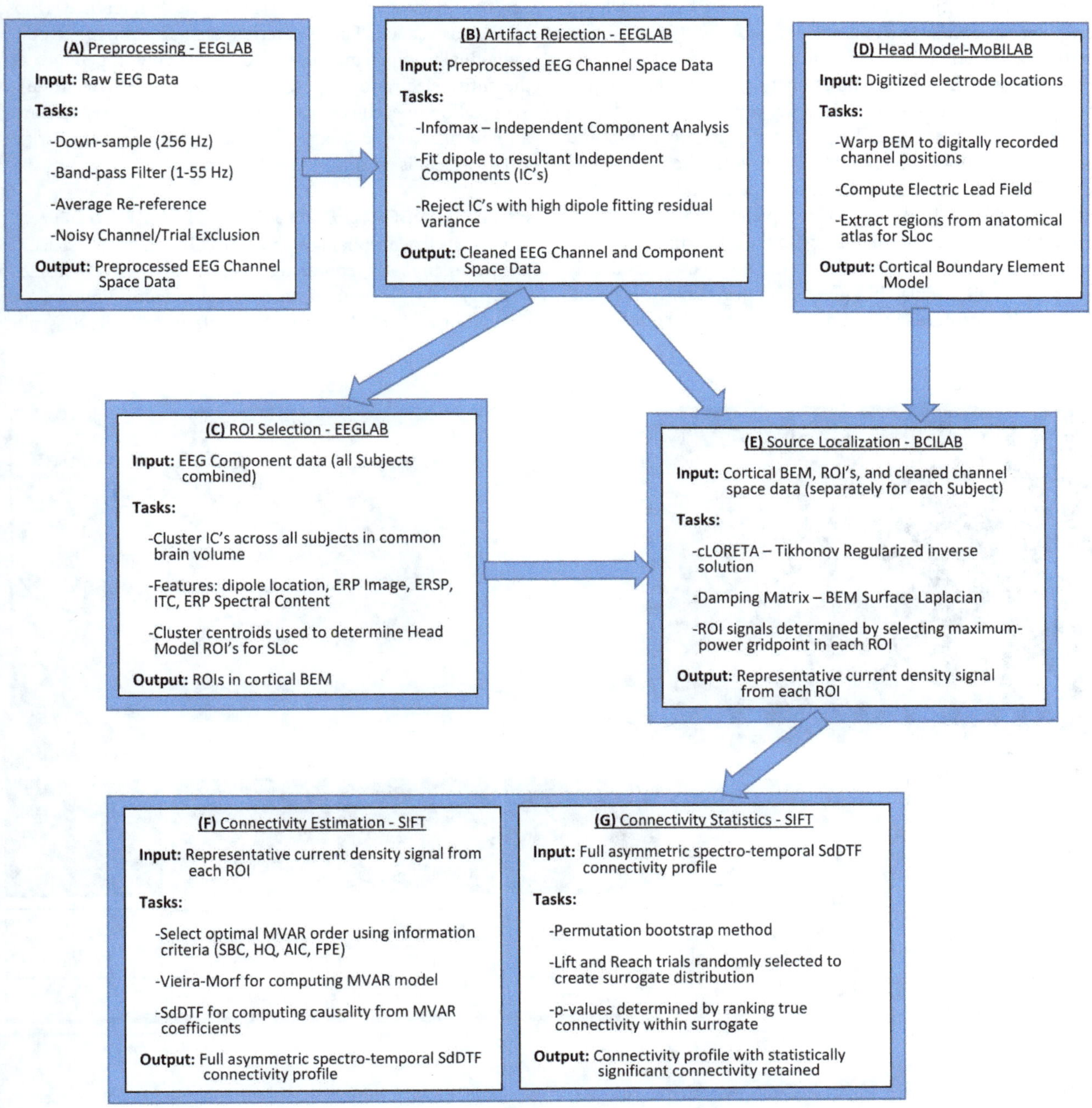

FIGURE 1 | General outline for cross-subject quantification of cortical connectivity. Initial data processing and artifact rejection is conducted in EEGLAB (Delorme and Makeig, 2004) **(A,B)**. ROIs are selected through IC clustering, also conducted in EEGLAB **(C)**. Head model construction and Electric Lead Field calculation are conducted in MoBILAB (Ojeda et al., 2014) **(D)**. Source localization is conducted in BCILAB (Delorme et al., 2011) through an implementation of cLORETA that iteratively estimates regularization hyperparameters **(E)**. Connectivity estimation is conducted using SIFT, an extension of EEGLAB (Delorme et al., 2011) **(F,G)**. All of the above software and their internal dependencies are run in MATLAB.

Human Subjects Institutional Review Board of the University of California, San Diego. Written informed consent was obtained from all subjects prior to the start of the experiment.

The task involved a time-constrained eye movement and reach using the subject's dominant hand (right) from a target in the center of a touch-screen to a laterally-offset target as depicted in **Figure 2** (Park et al., 2014). Each trial was either a control condition (lift), where the participant moved the stylus off of the central fixation dock after a brief target onset period (500–700 ms), or a test condition (reach/saccade), where the participant shifted their visual focus on and reached with the stylus to a new target that appeared in the upper right or lower left of the screen. Trials were defined as a combination of the planning period, 0 to 500 ms after the end of the target onset window, during which the subject planned either the reach/saccade or lift, and subsequent execution from 500 to 1000 ms after the target onset window, during which the subject moved their hand and reached for the new target. Each subject completed 256 trials, 96 of which were control condition trials, with the remaining 192 being test condition trials. The position of the new target randomly varied by a small angular amount (± 5 degrees) about a 30-degree direction centered at the position of the initial target—the center of the screen. Detailed description of the cognitive task performed by the participants can be found in Park et al. (2014).

EEG Recording

Scalp electroencephalographic (EEG) activity was recorded with a sampling rate of 512 Hz from 64 electrodes positioned on the scalps of the participants in an extended International 10–20 system configuration. The electrode array was grounded/referenced on a standard Driven Right Leg/Common Mode Sense (DRL/CMS) reference (Biosemi Inc., Amsterdam, The Netherlands), and each electrode was individually impedance-tested to ensure low impedance across the entire electrode array (below 5 kΩ for each electrode). The 3D position of each electrode was digitized in order to construct individualized head models for each participant (see Park et al., 2014 for details on the digitization system).

Preprocessing and Artifact Rejection

Scalp electroencephalographic (EEG) channel space data preprocessing was conducted using EEGLAB (Delorme and Makeig, 2004) through a procedure outlined in **Figure 1A**. EEG data from each of the 10 participants were band-pass filtered,

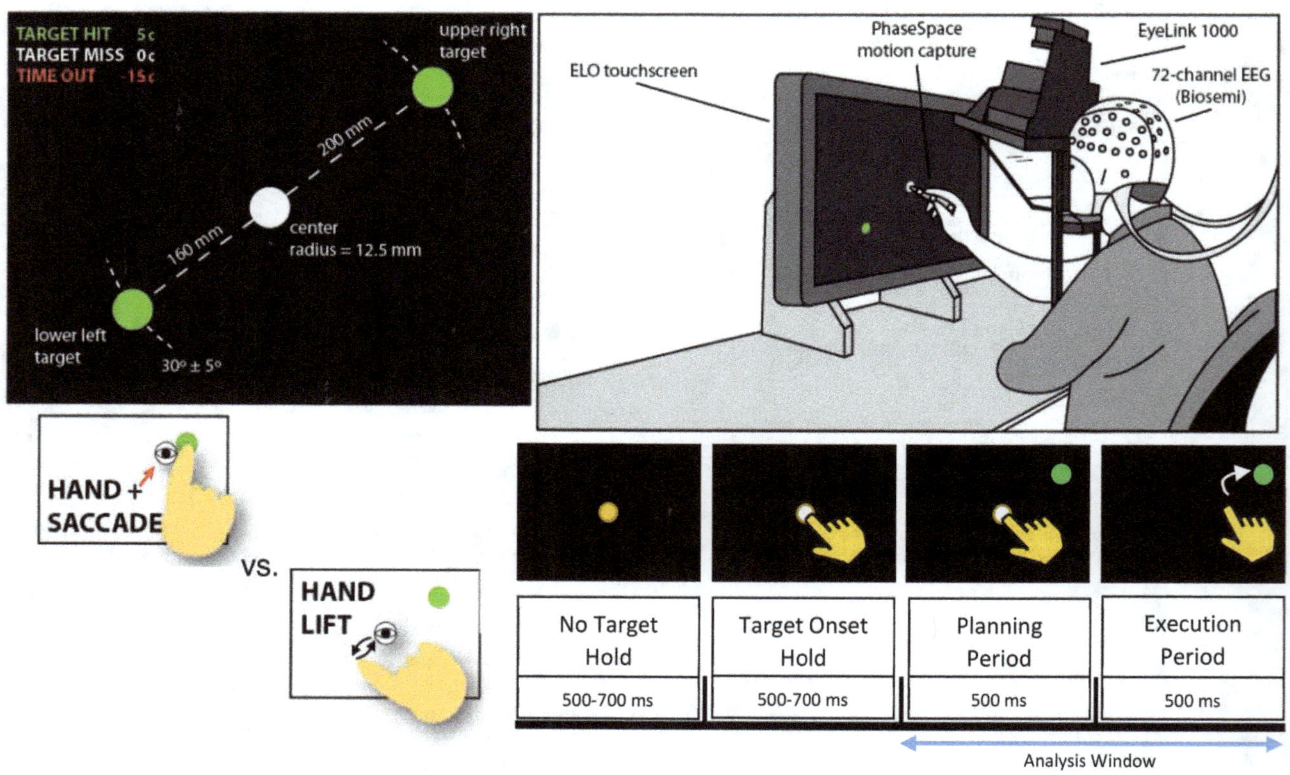

FIGURE 2 | Depiction of experimental setup from Hyvärinen and Oja (2000). Participants (Top Right) were placed in front of a touchscreen while brain activity was monitored by 64-channel EEG. Participants held stylus over a white fixation point in the center of the screen (Top Left) and were prompted for each trial to either lift and retouch the stylus (Control Condition) or to reach and saccade (Test Condition) to a randomly generated green target (Bottom Left). Epoch structure (Bottom Right) was identical for control and test conditions, with planning conducted while the participants remained on the fixation point with the green target present, and execution beginning when the fixation point was removed. Analysis window includes both planning and execution periods of reach/saccade or lift. Direction of the reach (upper right vs. lower left) was not discriminated since our focus was on the general causal dynamics involved in reaching rather than the encoding of spatial directionality.

retaining frequencies from 1 to 55 Hz, and re-referenced to the channel average since the data was recorded reference-free. The data were epoched, extracting the time period of interest, which encompassed both the planning phase and the execution phase of every trial. No distinction was made between reach directions since the emphasis for this analysis was placed on the general process of reach/saccade planning and execution rather than directional discrimination and, as such, both upward and downward angled reach trials were pooled and analyzed together. The control trials (Lift) and test trials (Reach/Saccade) were analyzed separately, using a cortical network defined over the same ROIs. Differences between the control and test conditions were examined by considering differences in network dynamics between the control and test conditions during the planning and execution phases. Noise and artifact laden trials and channels were identified and removed in a semi-automated manner. The kurtosis of each channel or trial was used as the identification metric, with channels or trials exhibiting a kurtosis Z-score $> +5$ or < -5 being flagged and subsequently visually inspected before removal.

The epoched channel space data were decomposed into sets of maximally independent components, where independence was achieved by minimizing mutual information between components using Infomax ICA (Bell and Sejnowski, 1995) (process outlined in **Figure 1B**). These components represented a combination of putative effective cortical sources, muscular artifacts, ocular artifacts, and electrical activity from the heart, among other noise sources. Through a semi-automated procedure, cortical sources were defined by employing independent components that both visually, by identifying power spectra and topographical maps with dipolar cortical source character, and computationally, through dipole-fitted residual variance, corresponded to dipoles (each fitted to a dipole with low residual variance). This procedure is particularly well suited for EEG artifact removal since the electrophysiological activity of interest present in the cortex manifests detectably in the form of an electrical dipole. The linear mixing of the electric fields generated by these dipoles, and corresponding unmixing through ICA allows for very precise retention of cortical data and rejection of non-cortical artifacts. Using the weight matrix computed during ICA, the retained cortical independent components were re-projected to channel space, creating cleaned channel space electrical signals that were further downsampled to 128 Hz for use in subsequent processing.

ROI Selection Methods-Clustering

Cortical regions of interest (ROIs) for source localization were determined by spatially and functionally clustering the ICs aggregated across all datasets/participants into a common cortical volume, as outlined in **Figure 1C**. The clustering feature vector for each IC was constructed by combining information from: the topographical scalp map of the IC, the event related potential (ERP) associated with the IC and its power spectrum, the spectral power content of a rolling window Fourier transform (FT) across the IC time-series data before ERP-type averaging, known as the Event-Related Spectral Perturbation (ERSP) of the IC, the associated phases from this rolling FT window that give the Inter-Trial Coherence (ITC) of the IC, the ERP-image constructed from concatenation of all trials for the epoched event, and the three dimensional location of the equivalent current dipole fitted to the IC (Makeig, 1993). These features were selected to ensure that the IC clusters were both spatially tight and functionally homogeneous, thus promoting the creation of clusters from the same cortical region that demonstrated similar spectro-temporal dynamics during the conducted task. PCA was used to reduce both the dimensionality of each of the above features, as well as the final feature vector for each IC to 10 dimensions corresponding to the 10 highest-eigenvalues, and, subsequent, K-means clustering of the ICs was conducted with $K = 14$ groups, whose clustering outcome yielded more spatially tight and functionally homogeneous clusters than the outcomes for $K = 9$ and $K = 16$ groups. The centroid of each cluster was computed and anatomically labeled using the Talairach atlas (Lancaster et al., 2000).

Head Model Construction

The (BEMs) that defined the geometry of the cortical source space for current localization were constructed using MoBILAB (Ojeda et al., 2014), as outlined in **Figure 1D**. The BEM approximation for the cortex of each participant included a standardized head model—the MRI MNI Colin27 three-layer BEM comprised of scalp, skull, and cortical layers. The cortical layer, where the source localization n occurs, was discretized into a triangular mesh containing 4825 vertices, which were automatically aggregated into anatomical regions based on the MNI standard gray matter atlas, used for ROI selection. A customized head model was constructed for each of the 10 participants based on the digitized electrode positions on EEG cap conforming to the participant's scalp during the experiment. Using standard electrical conductance values for the three BEM layers (0.33 S/m Scalp, 0.022 S/m Skull, 0.33 S/m Cortex Oostendorp et al., 2000), an electrical lead field matrix was derived, relating the conduction of electric fields generated by current dipoles from the cortical mesh (bottom layer) to the top of the skin (outer layer) where the field potential is recorded by scalp electrodes. This lead field matrix, along with the discrete surface Laplacian of the cortex layer of the BEM, were computed using the OpenMEEG toolbox (Gramfort et al., 2010) which was also used later for computing the current density during source localization.

Source Localization-Cloreta

Cortically Constrained Low Resolution Electromagnetic Tomography (cLORETA) (Pascual-Marqui et al., 1994) was used for source localization due to the fixed source-space it required for current localization, allowing for cross-participant ROI consistency. The source-space was the cortical BEM constructed in the previous section that accounted for the conduction of electric fields generated in the cortex and projected to the surface of the scalp where they were detected by EEG. The cortical constraint placed on the BEM was also necessary due to the inability of EEG to reliably resolve electrophysiological activity in subcortical regions of the brain. Source localization (procedure outlined in **Figure 1E**) was conducted independently for every epoch in each dataset in order to prevent regularization parameters and current activations from being computed by concatenating temporally non-contiguous epochs. The solution to the minimum-norm Lagrange multiplier problem for cLORETA is the Tikhonov regularized pseudoinverse solution for cortical current density expressed as follows:

$$J = T\Phi \tag{1}$$

$$T = (K^T K + \lambda^2 H^T H)^{-1} K^T \tag{2}$$

where J is the current density on the cortex, Φ is the channel space data, $\boldsymbol{T}$ is the optimal transformation matrix from channel space to current density space, $\boldsymbol{K}$ is the discrete electrical lead field matrix, and $\boldsymbol{H}$ is the 2D spatial Laplacian of the cortical head model, introduced to spatially regularize the localized current on the head model grid points. λ is a regularization parameter initialized on a log-space, using generalized cross validation (GCV), and subsequently inferred using an iterative EM formulation derived from the Bayesian structure of the original current localization problem (Trujillo-Barreto et al., 2004). The cLORETA implementation in BCILAB (Delorme et al., 2010) was used for source localization.

Since the regularization parameter λ was recomputed for every epoch, a new transformation matrix ($\boldsymbol{T}$) was also computed, leading to dynamic increases and decreases of spatial regularization in the final current solution as needed. This prevented both over-regularization in cases where current density ramped quickly between grid points, and under-regularization when channel space, and therefore current density magnitudes, were lower. A representative signal was extracted from each ROI by computing the signal power of the current localized at each gridpoint within a given ROI and selecting the gridpoint that exhibited the maximum power.

Based on this max-power selection heuristic, representative current signals were generated for the ROIs—a process which was applied to each of the 10 subjects individually, greatly simplifying network-level comparisons across test subjects since the nodes of the cortical network (the ROIs) were localized in the same location every time. This approach differs from traditional ROI determination methods involving ICs because the latter rely heavily on the common spatial localization of ICA outcomes, which is not guaranteed for multiple separate runs of ICA on different data, and, thus, may lead to inconsistencies for group level connectivity analysis (Thompson et al., 2011).

Connectivity Analysis–Sift

Application of the maximum power heuristic on the results of cLORETA created a single time series that represented cortical current dynamics for each ROI selected through clustering. These time series representing ROIs (ROI signals) were used to construct linear (MVAR) models from which spectro-temporal causal interactions between ROIs were computed using the Source Information Flow Toolbox (SIFT) (procedure outlined in **Figure 1F**) (Delorme et al., 2011). Specifically, for each participant, the ROI signals were preprocessed by employing detrending and normalization across time and ensemble. The MVAR models were constructed by applying the Vieira-Morf lattice algorithm to the ROI signals, using a sliding window with a length of 550 ms and a window step size of 10 ms, leveraging the window size to decrease the number of the estimated MVAR coefficients (ratio of data points to parameters > 10:1)—a necessary provision arising from the lack of regularization in the Vieira-Morf algorithm. The optimal order for the MVAR model was determined automatically by averaging the optimal orders estimated by six different information criteria: Akaike Information Criterion, corrected Akaike Information Criterion, Hannan-Quinn Criterion, Schwarz-Bayes Criterion, Rissanen Prediction Error, and logarithm of Akaike's Final Prediction Error (Rissanen, 1978; Tu and Xu, 2012). Each of these information criteria was computed for the range of possible model orders between 1 and 30, and the optimal model order for each participant was automatically determined by identifying the minimum value for each of the six generated curves, computing the average, and rounding down to the nearest integer. The model order for the Lift and Reach/Saccade conditions were determined independently. After model order determination, tests of stability and consistency were performed for each MVAR model in order to validate the ability of the model to capture the dynamics of the ROI signal. The autocorrelation function and three different portmanteau tests were used to determine the whiteness of the model residuals. The percent consistency of the model was evaluated for every sliding window within the epoch, indicating, as a percentage, the relative amount of correlational structure within the data that had been captured by the model. A stability test was conducted on every window within the epoch the MVAR coefficient matrix was evaluated.

Pairwise causal relationships between ROIs were computed from the validated MVAR models by employing the (SdDTF) (Korzeniewska et al., 2008). The SdDTF connectivity $\eta^2_{ij}(f,t)$ at a given spectro-temporal point (f,t) between ROI-i and ROI-j is computed as follows:

$$\eta^2_{j\to i}(f,t) = \frac{|H_{ij}(f,t)|\,|P_{ij}(f,t)|}{\sum_f \sum_{kl} |H_{kl}(f,t)|^2 |P_{kl}(f,t)|^2} \tag{3}$$

where $H_{mn}(f,t)$ is the MVAR transfer matrix between network nodes (ROIs) m and n, and $P_{mn}(f,t)$ is the partial coherence of the signals for nodes m and n. The SdDTF connectivity metric is similar to conditional spectral Granger Causality but only reports direct causal relationship between signals removing spurious or indirect relationships caused by upstream network topology, particularly common inputs. Unlike Granger Causality, which utilizes AR model residuals to determine causal influence, SdDTF utilizes the AR transfer functions themselves (see Equation 3) allowing for straightforward generalization of the metric to multivariate systems, in this case a network with more than two cortical nodes. To control for the potentially large and unregularized AR transfer functions, DTF normalization is conducted across incoming and outgoing signals, and across frequencies. This normalized term is weighted by the partial coherence in order to incorporate the direct relationship between source nodes, thus mitigating the phantom source problem present in Granger causal metrics and yielding th full form of the direct Directed Transfer Function. This metric is further developed by evaluating it over a short sliding window across the epoch, an additional feature which serves to promote local stationarity of the ROI source signals and observe changes in connectivity dynamics between signals as the epoch progresses. The SdDTF measure was computed separately across epochs and frequencies of interest in this way, yielding a spectro-temporal asymmetrical causal connectivity matrix of SdDTFs with causal source nodes (FROM) defining the columns and sink nodes (TO) defining the rows of the connectivity matrix. Note that the diagonal elements of this matrix do not have relevant physical meaning for the purposes of this network analysis, and were, therefore, omitted.

A permutation-bootstrap approach was employed to determine the statistical significance of each SdDTF value within the asymmetric connectivity matrix (outlined in **Figure 1G**). The permutations were created by randomly mixing ROI-current density epochs from the control and test conditions with equal representation, generating an epoch ensemble on which connectivity analysis was conducted. The resulting ROI connectivity matrices from each permutation were accumulated to create a surrogate distribution. The values of each spectro-temporal position in this distribution were, then, sorted in ascending order, allowing for the associated *p*-value of the tested connectivity value to be computed in a non-parametric manner through its place in the ranked connectivity values at that spectro-temporal position of the surrogate distribution. This process was applied to both the Lift and Reach/Saccade conditions, where the null hypothesis (H_0) was the lack of significant increase or decrease in connectivity between the evaluated condition and the case of randomly mixed ROIs. The alternative hypothesis (H_1) was that the evaluated condition individually exhibited connectivity structure that was significantly different from the structure acquired by randomly intermixing the two conditions. The *p*-value for each spectro-temporal point was determined by using an averaged surrogate distribution computed across all 10 participants. A surrogate distribution for each of the 10 participants was computed by conducting connectivity analysis on 300 permutations of the original data, yielding 300 SdDTF values for each spectro-temporal position. The average surrogate distribution was computed by applying spectro-temporal position-wise averages across all 10 surrogate distributions for each of the 300 values and, subsequently, sorting in ascending order the resulting average values at each spectro-temporal position. With 300 permutations computed for each subject, there was sufficient *p*-value resolution to establish which time-frequency points passed the $\alpha = 0.05$ threshold. This threshold was automatically adjusted since the statistical significance of each spectro-temporal point was evaluated independently by applying the False Detection Rate (FDR) control method as a means of accounting for the multiple comparisons problem (Benjamini and Hochberg, 1995).

The difference between statistically significant values of average connectivity matrices corresponding to the Lift condition and Reach/Saccade condition was computed in order to determine the statistically significant changes in the cortical network between the two conditions.

RESULTS

IC Clustering Outcome

The ROIs selected for source localization based on the cluster centroids were: bilateral (left/right) inferior occipital (Occ), superior parietal (Par), and precentral gyrus motor (Mot) cortices, as well as, anterior cingulate cortex (ACC), supplementary motor area (SMA), and precuneus, whose left and right hemisphere grid point regions were combined and treated as a single anatomical region during source localization and ROI collapse.

Figure 3 depicts the clustering outcome for the reach/saccade condition, showing the dipole cluster and average scalp projection for the eight clusters from which ROIs were determined. The 3D dipole maps plotted on a standard MNI MRI volume demonstrate the spatial tightness of the clusters selected as candidates for ROIs, while the average composite topographical maps indicate that there is consistency in both the orientation and di-polarity of the ICs in each cluster. All of the selected clusters feature a relatively tight positive spike in electric potential over the cortical area where the equivalent dipoles are placed; suggesting that the collection of dipoles within the cluster originate from similarly oriented pyramidal cells in gray matter, generating electrical dipoles whose resultant field produces the positive potential present in the scalp maps. Were the IC clusters not as spatially tight, or comprised of dipoles oriented in different directions, the average scalp maps would have electric potential much lower in magnitude and dispersed over a much wider area of the brain. The spatial tightness of the dipoles and the scalp maps suggests that a robust clustering outcome was achieved, and the associated ROIs were reliably utilized with this data in subsequent analysis.

The determination of ROIs from ICs is not necessarily a one-to-one mapping. A single cluster can provide evidence for inclusion of multiple ROIs, as is the case with cluster 5, for example, whose dipole locations span across both hemispheres. So, when identified with the Talairach atlas, the ROIs fall in bilateral regions of the Occipital Cortex (Inferior gyri) that are too far from each other to be grouped across the medial longitudinal fissure, as was the case with all of the other midline ROIs.

All nine ROIs selected for the cortical network are displayed in **Figure 4**, with color-coded grid-points associated with each ROI as follows: midline ROIs are colored Red (ACC, SMA, Precuneus), and bilaterally (left and right) situated ROIs away from the midline (Mot, Par, and Occ) are dark blue, light blue, and yellow respectively.

MVAR Model Construction and Validation

Model order selection was conducted with an average MVAR parameter-to-datapoint ratio of 0.096 for the Lift condition and 0.034 for the Reach/Saccade condition. The window size was selected so that, in all cases, this ratio never exceeded 0.1, as is recommended for a well-posed MVAR model computed via the Vieira-Morf Lattice Algorithm. For the Lift condition, the average model order across all subjects was 7.4 with a standard deviation of 1.35, and for the Reach/Saccade condition, the model order

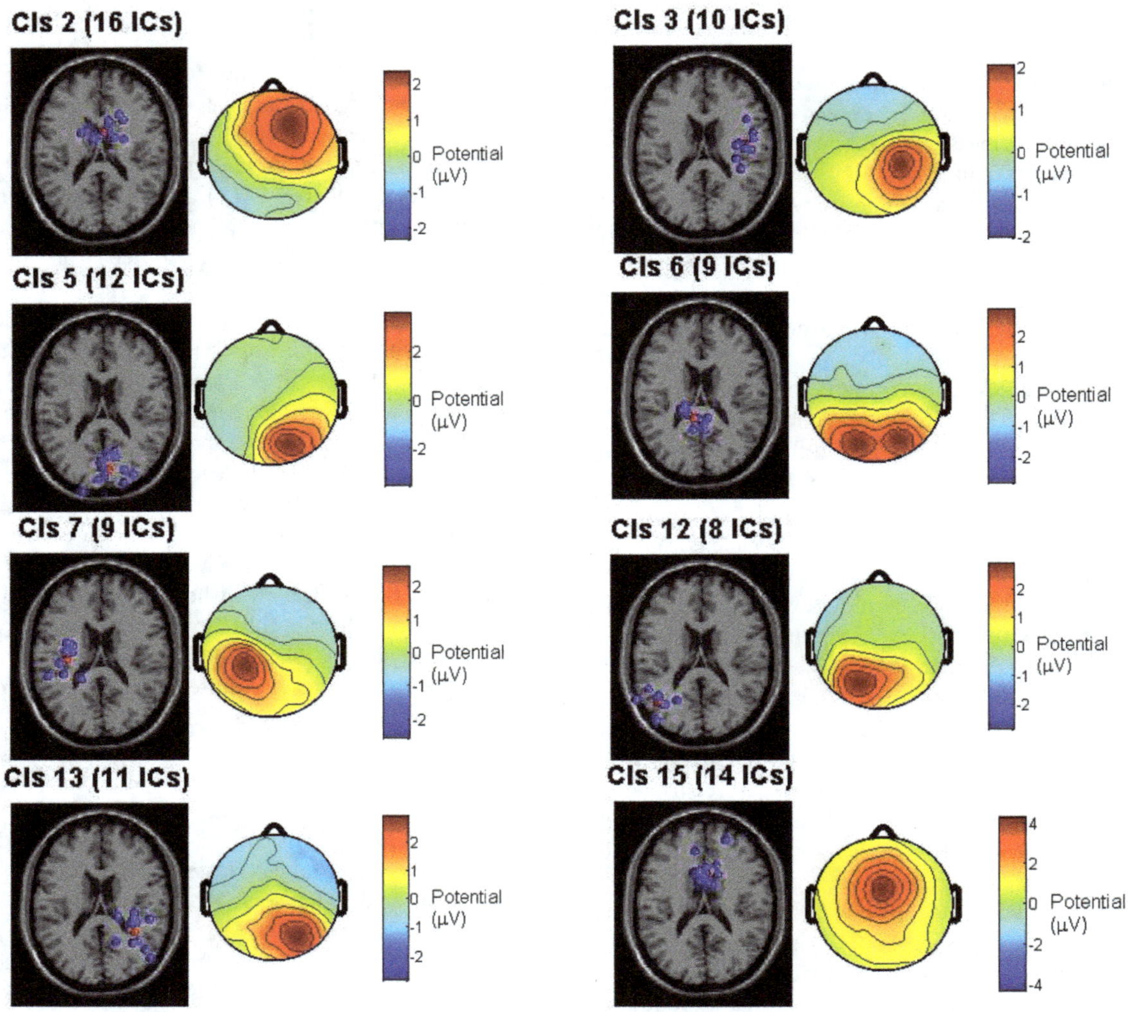

Cluster Number	Associated Region of Interest (ROI)	Abbreviation
Cls 2	Anterior Cingulate Cortex	ACC
Cls 3	Right Precentral Gyrus	R-Mot
Cls 5	Left/Right Inferior Occipital Gyrus	L/R-Occ
Cls 6	Precuneus	Prec
Cls 7	Left Precentral Gyrus	L-Mot
Cls 12	Left Superior/Inferior Parietal Gyri	L-Par
Cls 13	Right Superior/Inferior Parietal Gyri	R-Par
Cls 15	Supplementary Motor Area	SMA

FIGURE 3 | Clustering outcome across all test subjects for the Reach/Saccade condition. IC dipole locations in each cluster are displayed in blue on a standard MRI volume, with the cluster centroid in red (centroid itself is not an IC, interpolated from other dipoles in cluster). The scalp maps are composites displaying the average electric potential on the scalp arising from the equivalent IC-dipoles within each cluster. The cluster centroids provide the foundation for subsequent ROI selection by association with the anatomical structure(s) the cluster occupies. The associated ROIs for each cluster are shown in table y. Note that for non-bilaterally separated ROIs, the areas in the left and right hemispheres were combined due to close proximity across the medial longitudinal fissure.

average was 7.2 with a standard deviation of 1.03. **Figure 5** shows the output of the model order selection criteria pertaining to the MVAR model order of the Lift condition for a single participant. The top graph shows the average (across epochs and sliding windows) value of each criterion over model orders from 1 to 30. The histograms that follow show the order distribution using each of the criteria.

The MVAR model validation results averaged across all subjects and both conditions are shown in **Figure 6**. The average model performance was highly representative of the individual

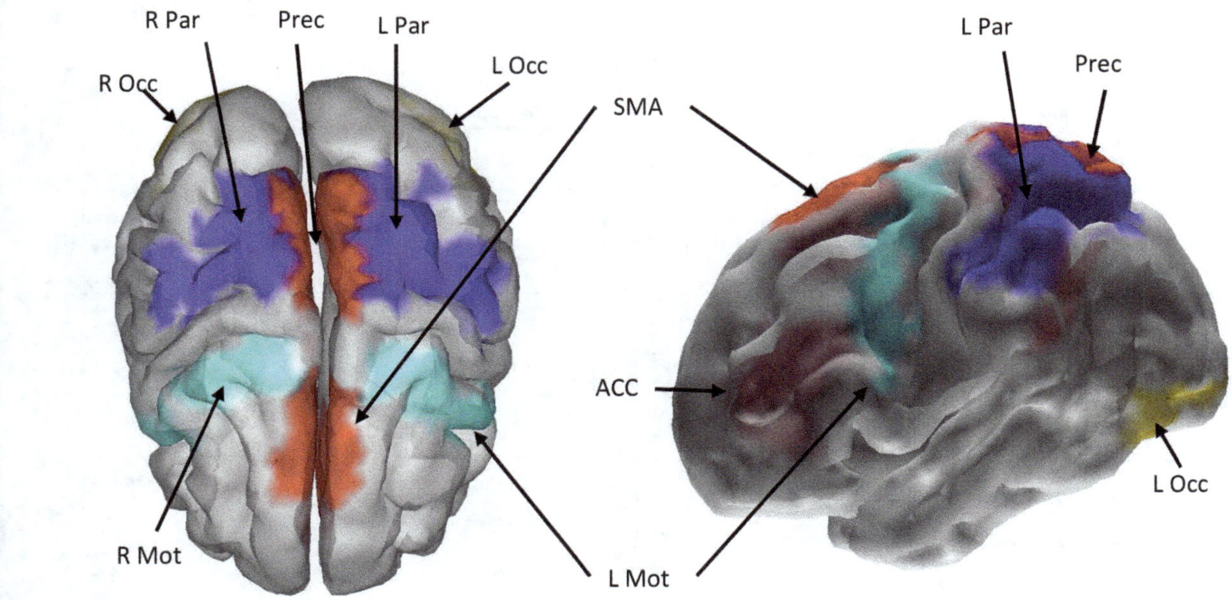

FIGURE 4 | Cortical boundary element head model with the nine selected ROIs marked with color. Red color indicates that the left and right hemispheres of the ROI were merged and treated as a single ROI during source localization and signal extraction. Other colors indicate that bilateral cortices were selected across the hemispheres. ROI abbreviations are: Mot, Precentral Gyrus; ACC, Anterior Cingulate Cortex; SMA, Supplementary Motor Area; Prec, Precuneus; Occ, Inferior Occipital Gyrus; Par, Superior and Inferior Parietal Gyri.

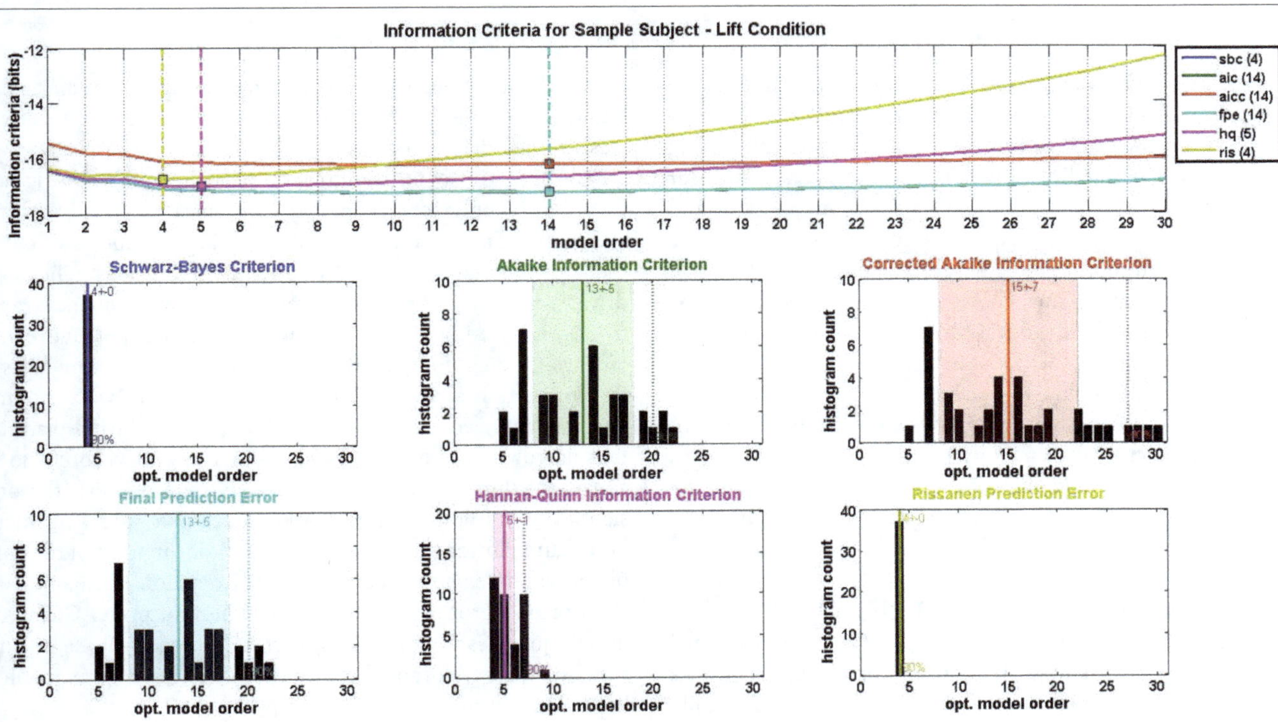

FIGURE 5 | MVAR model order selection for the lift condition of a single test subject. Each of six information criteria (Schwarz-Bayes Criterion, Akaike Information Criterion, Corrected Akaike Information Criterion, Final Prediction Error, Hannan-Quinn Information Criterion, and Rissanen Prediction Error Rissanen, 1978; Tu and Xu, 2012) were evaluated for model orders 1–30 and averaged across all condition trials. Optimal model order corresponds to the minimum of each information criterion curve. Distributions of optimal model order for all trials are shown in histograms for each of the six information criteria used. Center lines and shaded regions in each histogram indicate the mean and standard deviation respectively for each information criterion.

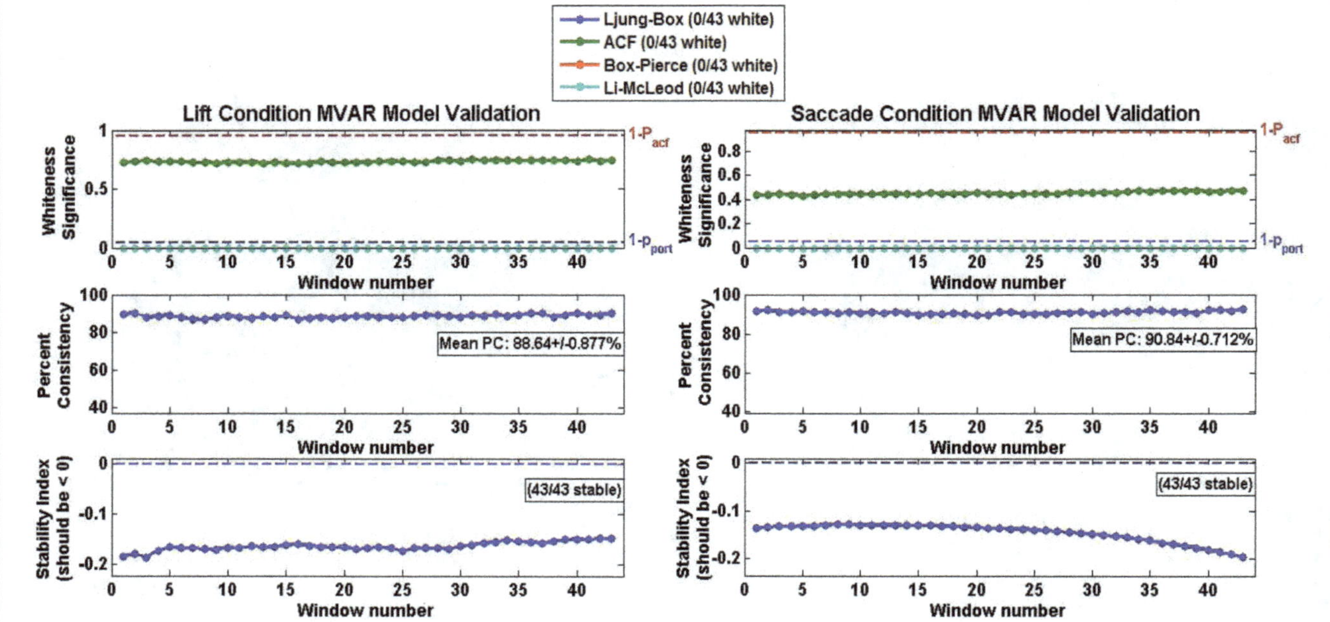

FIGURE 6 | Model validation criteria for Lift (left) and Reach/Saccade (right) Conditions averaged across all 10 subjects. Whiteness of AR model residuals (top row) evaluated using Autocorrelation function (ACF) and three different Portmanteau tests. None of the MVAR models passed any of the whiteness tests, suggesting that none of the models captured adequately the modeled temporal dynamics. Percent consistency (middle row) indicates percent of correlational structure of original data captured by the model. Percent consistency was uniformly high as its values were in the order of 90% with small standard deviations. Stability index (bottom row) is log of largest eigenvalue of AR model. Negative index implies that largest eigenvalue is less that one, and thus, the MVAR models were stable. Note, that all tests were conducted individually for every sliding window (43 in total) across the epoch, hence the 43 data points in each graph.

performance of each subject's MVAR model since, in all cases, the MVAR model was stable across the entirety of the epoch, as indicated by the natural logarithm of the largest eigenvalue being negative (**Figure 6** Stability Panel). The percent consistency for both Lift and Reach/Saccade conditions was above 90% and the standard deviation in the percent consistency was <1.0% (0.877% for Lift and 0.712% for Reach/Saccade), indicating that the high consistency of the MVAR model with respect to the data was maintained for the duration of the epoch (all 43 sliding windows within each epoch). None of the computed MVAR models passed the residual-whiteness tests at any point during the epoch, suggesting that there was statistically significant correlational structure exhibited by the MVAR model residuals, and that the MVAR modeling did not succeed in capturing the entirety of the temporal dynamics exhibited by the network nodes during the epoch.

Spectro-Temporal Connectivity

The connectivity computed between the ROIs in the defined cortical network is displayed in **Figure 7** for the lift condition and **Figure 8** for the reach/saccade condition, with statistically significant spectro-temporal connectivity ($p < 0.05$) thresholded for each matrix respectively.

The difference between the p-value thresholded connectivity matrices for Lift and Reach/Saccade, shown in **Figures 7**, **8** respectively, was computed and shown in **Figure 9**. Since the lift (control) condition was subtracted from the reach/saccade (test) condition, the warmer (brighter red) regions of the matrix indicate that connectivity was stronger during the reach/saccade and the cooler (brighter blue) regions indicate that connectivity was stronger during the lift.

The majority of lift-dominant causal interactions originate from the supplementary motor area, parietal areas and the Precuneus. During Lift, the SMA exhibits notable outflow to the Left Parietal Area (L Par) and the Precuneus. The SMA drives activity in the L Par over a constant frequency range (8–15 Hz) during both planning and execution (**Figure 9A**). However, a dichotomy between planning and execution exists in the connection form the SMA to the Precuneus, with sporadic low-frequency connectivity (3–14 Hz) present during planning that narrows in frequency band (8–14 Hz) and becomes more consistent during execution (**Figure 9B**). From L Par, the only significant outflow of information occurs to the Precuneus dominating lower frequencies (3–14 Hz) during part of the early planning phase and the entirety of the execution phase of the lift (**Figure 9C**). From R Par, information flows to the ACC across low frequencies (3–14 Hz) during the planning phase and for some of the execution phase, though the causal connection is limited to a narrow frequency band (10–14 Hz) by the end of the epoch (**Figure 9D**). Similar connectivity is present with the SMA although in the case of information flow from R Par to SMA, the connectivity does not subside as late in the execution phase as is the case with the ACC (**Figure 9E**). The R Par exhibits another connectivity motif, providing strong causal influence on both the Left Parietal Area and the Precuneus during the planning phase of the lift over a low frequency band (3–10 Hz), and wit

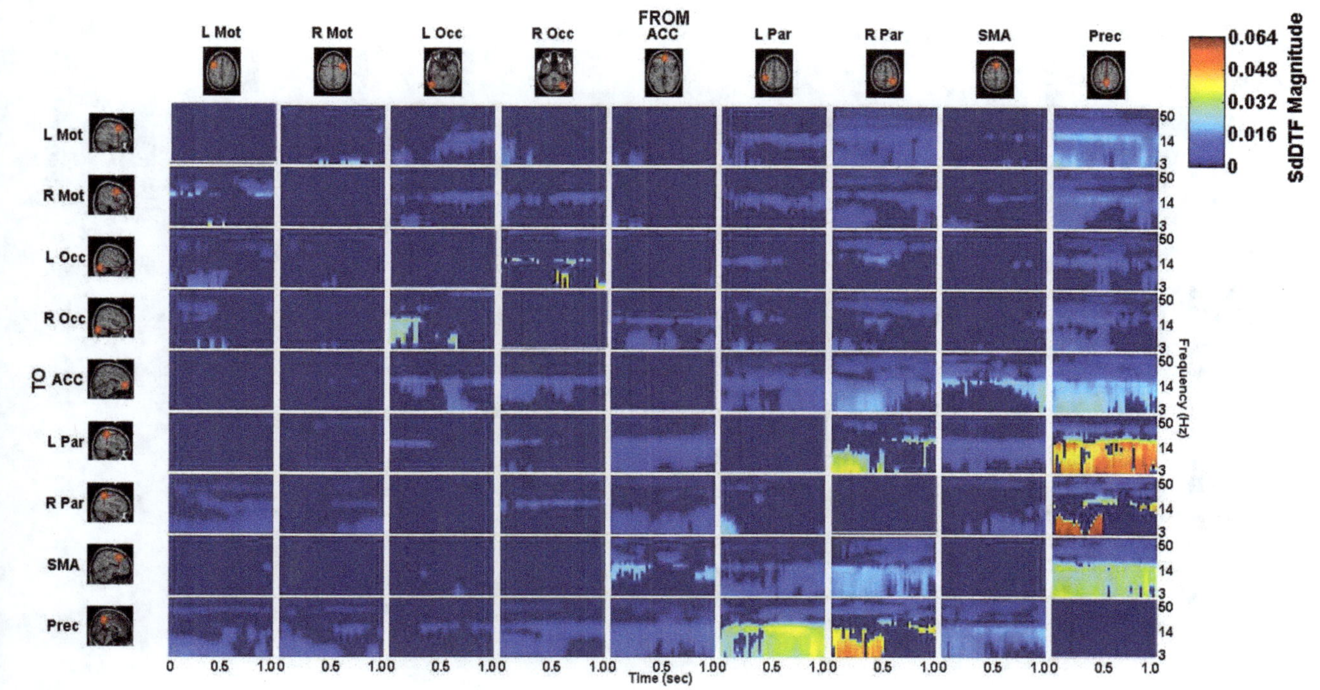

FIGURE 7 | *p*-value thresholded spectro-temporal asymmetric cortical connectivity matrix for the lift condition. Network sources are tabulated at the columns and sinks at the rows. The dynamic causal relationship between each source and sink is expressed by the corresponding SdDTF. Non-zero connectivity is displayed only at spectro-temporal points with $p < 0.05$, thus only displaying statistically significant connectivity in the cortical network for the Lift condition. Note the frequency axis is plotted on a logarithmic scale to more clearly show lower frequency band connectivity, where the majority of causal flow occurs in this network.

relatively higher power compared to its other causal influences (**Figure 9F**). The Precuneus exhibits the greatest amount of causal outflow during lift, acting as an information source for the majority of the other ROIs in the network. The Precuneus has relatively lower-power (lighter blue shading) influence on both precentral gyri, during both planning and execution, with the band of active connectivity narrowing when transitioning from planning to execution (**Figure 9G**). The Precuneus sends information with a similar spatiotemporal structure to the ACC, but with slightly greater causal power, hence the brighter shading of the connectivity during the planning period (**Figure 9H**). The influence the Precuneus has on the SMA is stronger still (even darker shade of blue), and now occupies the entire duration of the epoch and maintains signal bandwidth (3–14 Hz) (**Figure 9H**). The Precuneus influences both parietal areas very strongly during lift, with R Par receiving information only during the planning phase across a low frequency band (3–10 Hz) (**Figure 9I**), and L Par receiving information across a slightly larger band (3–14 Hz) and for both planning and execution. During execution, however, the connectivity is limited to the higher end of that frequency band (10–14 Hz) (**Figure 9J**).

Within reach/saccade-dominant activity regions, which are defined by the red spectro-temporal regions of **Figure 9**, greater connectivity is present in the frontal regions of the cortex. Specifically, both the left and right precentral gyri exhibit stronger connectivity to the left parietal composite area during the planning phase of the epoch across lower frequencies (3–14 Hz), with this connectivity decreasing in power relative to lift during the execution phase (**Figure 9K**). Additionally, the anterior cingulate cortex (ACC) exhibits increased outflow of information across lower frequencies (3–14 Hz) to both precentral gyri again during the planning phase (**Figure 9L**). The ACC also appears to feed information to the left and right visual cortices across a narrower frequency band (8–14 Hz) during the planning phase (**Figure 9M**), with the bandwidth of information flow encompassing lower frequencies from ACC to R Occ as the epoch progresses from planning to execution. For the reach/saccade condition, the SMA exhibits a greater amount of causal influence on the ACC than any other cortical node, with a strong 14–40 Hz communication band present during the planning phase that dips down to lower frequencies (3–8 Hz) as the subject transitions from planning to execution (**Figure 9N**). The ACC reciprocates some of this activity to the SMA, with higher frequency (15–40 Hz) communication during the planning phase that dies down during the execution phase (**Figure 9N**). The SMA also exhibits some information outflow to the visual cortices, with the L Occ flow subsiding by the end of the planning period, and the R Occ flow remaining constant in both frequency band and relative amplitude over the entire epoch (**Figure 9O**). The right parietal composite area (R Par) exhibits causal influence on the Precuneus in higher frequencies (20–25 Hz) during the planning phase, and significantly stronger lower frequency (3–13 Hz) influence during reach/saccade execution in comparison to the lift execution (**Figure 9F**). The

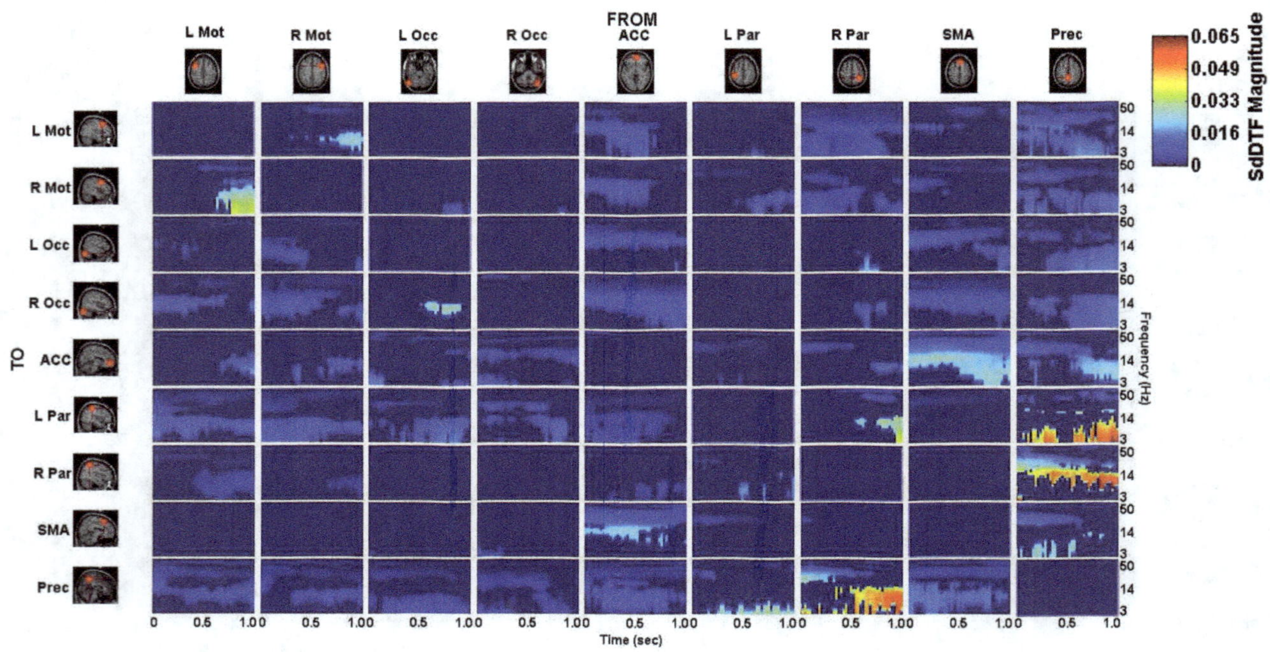

FIGURE 8 | *p*-value thresholded spectro-temporal asymmetric cortical connectivity matrix for the reach/saccade condition. Network sources are tabulated at the columns and sinks at the rows. The dynamic causal relationship between each source and sink is expressed by the corresponding SdDTF in the pertinent location in the connectivity matrix. Non-zero connectivity is displayed only at spectro-temporal points with $p < 0.05$, thus only displaying statistically significant connectivity in the cortical network for the Reach/Saccade condition. Note the frequency axis is plotted on a logarithmic scale to more clearly show lower frequency band connectivity, where the majority of causal flow occurs in this network.

last of the significant communication motif that is strong during the reach/saccade conditions originates from the Precuneus. The influence of Prec on L/R Occ is most prevalent during the execution phase (**Figure 9P**). In both cases, however, the precuneus predominantly drives lower frequency activity (3–14 Hz), with a significant decrease in connectivity magnitude above 14 Hz. There is also evidence of temporally localized higher power bursts of connectivity across low frequency from the Precuneus to the right parietal area, beginning early in the planning period in the 14–20 Hz band and terminating at the end of the epoch after drifting down to 8–13 Hz (**Figure 9I**).

DISCUSSION

Neurophysiological Connectivity

A cortical network associated with the Lift and the Reach/Saccade conditions was identified across 10 subjects, involving distinct ROIs, and the dynamic causal interactions between pairs of ROIs were computed for each condition. The cortical network, the ROIs, and the dynamic causal connections between pairs of ROIs exhibited physiological plausibility consistent with previous results reported in the literature, although some important differences were noted as outlined further below. The bilateral Inferior Occipital Gyri coupled with adjacent Occipital regions, known to form the Visual ROIs, represent primary processing of the visual stimuli present in the reaching task (Blumberg and Kreiman, 2010) . The various motor regions, including bilateral Precentral Gyri (housing the Left and Right Motor Cortices) and the bilaterally grouped Supplementary Motor Area, have been implicated in the planning and execution of the physical movement, e.g., in this case of the participant's arm to reach the presented target as well as the saccade of the eyes to focus on the target (Johnson et al., 1996; Nachev et al., 2008; Wang et al., 2010). Parietal activity is largely implicated by existing literature in guiding action directed at visual targets (Blangero et al., 2009; Filimon, 2010). The Anterior Cingulate Cortex, a grouped ROI consisting of the Left and Right cortices merged across the longitudinal fissure, is thought to be involved in higher level decision making and, of particular interest in this case, the translation of intentions to actions (Kennerley et al., 2006). The Precuneus, also bilaterally grouped across the longitudinal fissure, has been shown to be directly involved in both visual and non-visual reaching tasks in both macaque monkeys and humans, being responsible for the processing of both visual and proprioceptive sensory information during the task (Filimon et al., 2009).

Though entirely possible to treat the three grouped ROIs (SMA, Prec, and ACC) as distinct, the close proximity of the bilateral ROIs to each other within the longitudinal fissure and the spatially-regularized source localization can lead to significant overlap of posterior current density between the ROIs, generating spurious causal interhemispheric coupling, which is avoided by considering those three ROIs to be trans-hemispheric.

Inspection of the connectivity during the lift and reach/saccade condition, shown in **Figure 9**, reveals that the cortical network exhibits relatively lower strength, bu

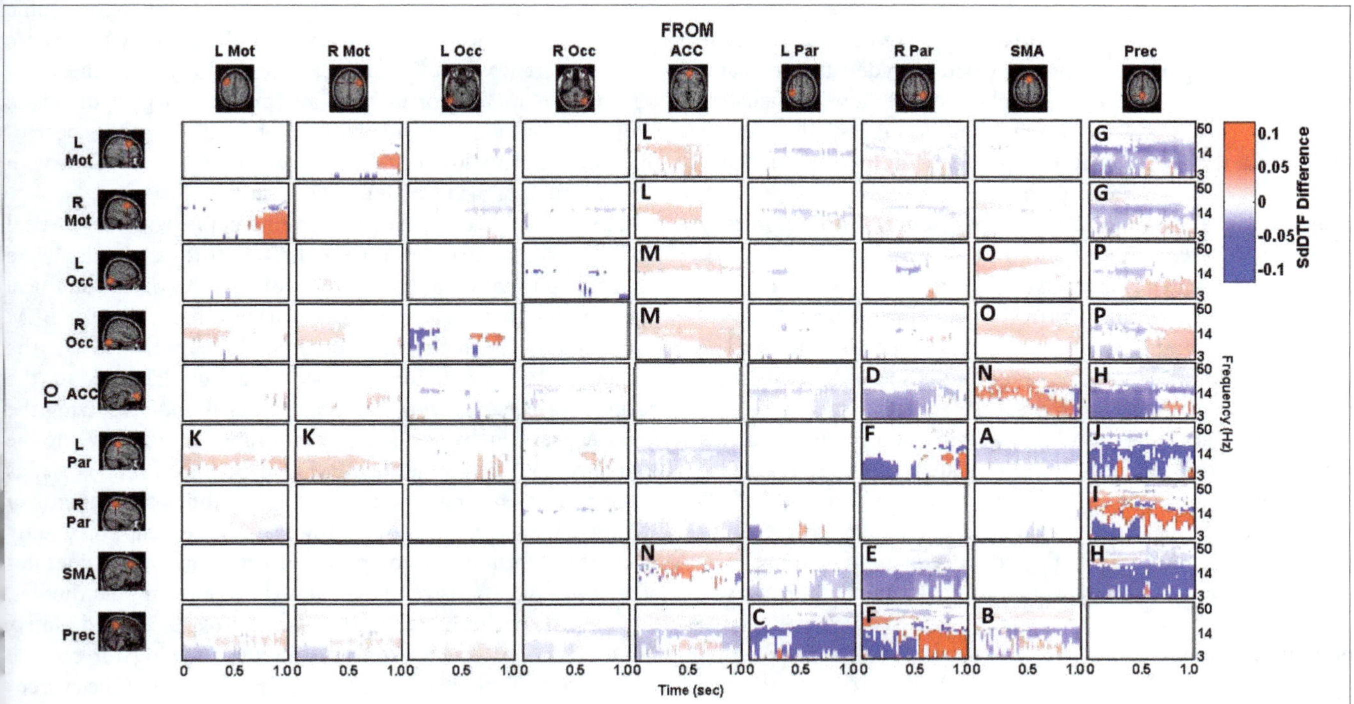

FIGURE 9 | Difference of statistically significant values ($p < 0.05$) of the connectivity matrix between the Reach/Saccade and Lift condition. Warmer colors indicate Reach/Saccade > Lift, cooler colors indicate Lift > Reach/Saccade. Note, that during Reach/Saccade, information flow is facilitated from both precentral gyri (L/R Mot) to left parietal area **(K)** and ACC exhibits greater influence on precentral gyri during planning (0–0.5 s) as well as the visual cortices (L/R Occ) during both planning and execution **(L,M)**; during Lift, Precuneus is much more active both inflow **(B,C,F)** and outflow **(G,H,J,P)** except when communicating with the right parietal area **(I)**, especially during the execution phase (0.5–1.0 ms) of the task. The SMA also drives activity in the visual cortices **(O)**, as well as displaying outflow to the ACC **(N)** and L Par **(A)** during Reach/Saccade and Lift respectively. Also during Reach/Saccade, the parietal region ipsilateral to the moving arm (R Par) demonstrates reduced outflow to both ACC and SMA **(D,E)** relative to Lift. Brighter red and brighter blue show stronger Reach/Saccade and Lift connectivity respectively.

widespread effective connectivity during the reach/saccade condition, and more focal, higher-strength connectivity during the lift condition. In the case of the reach/saccade condition, the ACC exemplifies this widespread, low-power connectivity profile, driving activity in both Left and Right Precentral Gyri during the planning period, and driving activity in both visual cortices for both planning and execution of the reach. The connection from the ACC to L/R Mot (**Figure 9L**) suggests a causal influence of a decision making center in the frontal cortex onto regions directly involved in the planning and execution of a reach and saccade, a connectivity motif that has been observed before using other neuroimaging modalities (Asemi et al., 2015). Furthermore, this causal influence is shown only to exceed lift-connectivity magnitude during the planning period, indicated by the lack of ACC to L/R Motor interaction after 0.5 s, suggesting that after the movement is planned, execution no longer requires direct influence of the ACC onto the Motor cortices. On the other hand, the ACC to L/R Visual connections (**Figure 9M**) remain elevated for the entirety of the epoch during the reach/saccade condition, indicating a possible involvement of the cognitive-control and error detection functions of the ACC (Stevens et al., 2011) in visual processing during execution. The task-positive connections formed by the ACC exhibit higher frequency connectivity (**Figures 9 L–N**), with the lower end of these connectivity bands lying in the α (8–13 Hz) wave range, which is expected considering the motor-relevance of the α-band to indicate inactivation of motor regions (Brinkman et al., 2014), and the higher end of these connectivity bands stretching into the 30–50 Hz range, consistent with the generally higher-frequency content of cognitive cortical processes (Buzsáki and Silva, 2012).

However, this does not seem to be the case for the information flow from the SMA to the ACC (**Figure 9N**), wherein a high α/low β band connection (10–20 Hz) present during the planning period migrates down to lower frequencies (3–8 Hz), occupying the θ band by the end of execution. A possible explanation for this exception stems from the suggested involvement of the SMA in the real-time control of actions during execution, by which it might provide feedback to the ACC regarding the accuracy of the conducted reach (Nachev et al., 2008). The connections from L and R Mot to L Par (**Figure 9K**) exhibit a connectivity profile similar to the ACC → L/R Mot interaction, with lower-power, reach/saccade-dominant connectivity during planning that is absent during execution. While both the composite parietal regions and the precentral gyri have been implicated in visuo-spatial processing and reaching to identified targets, the analysis indicates that their interaction is limited during the planning phase of a reach, and is not required in order for the reach to be executed after planning. A strong, sharply divided connection is also observed from the Right Composite Parietal Region to the Precuneus (**Figure 9F**)—a connection which is facilitated during lift-planning and reach/saccade-execution, and suppressed during reach/saccade-planning (for low frequencies) and lift-execution. The connectivity profile suggests that during reach/saccade planning, R Par predominantly communicates with the Precuneus through higher frequencies (14–30 Hz), which is of great significance to the Precuneus since it normally communicates with other nodes in the Default Mode Network through this frequency band (Neuner et al., 2014). The transition to lower frequency connectivity (3–14 Hz) during Reach/Saccade execution may simply be a feature of task demands, since similar communication was seen in **Figures 9H,I,M,N,P**, suggesting a generalized tendency for visuo-spatial and motor related cortical regions to communicate through lower frequency bands when the reach/saccade is being executed. The reach/saccade-dominant dynamics of the connection from the Precuneus to R Par (**Figure 9I**) also exhibit characteristics similar to the other motor regions, where the high-frequency planning connectivity gives way to lower frequency execution connectivity. However, during the epoch, the frequency range of the connectivity varies periodically, dipping to lower frequencies and, subsequently, returning to higher frequencies (**Figure 9I**, red profile) at the rate of 5 Hz. This behavior suggests that the Precuneus dynamically alters the frequencies over which it communicates with R Par in a periodic manner. The persistence of this behavior through both planning and execution suggests that the behavior is associated with generalized motor-reach information processing, though the decrease (**Figure 9I**, red profile) at the transition between planning and execution at 0.5 s supports the involvement of this periodicity in the motor task being executed by the subject.

Connectivity present in the cortical network is summarized in **Figure 10**, where the Reach/Saccade condition is shown in a 3D (BrainMovie3D) rendering of a cortical volume (Delorme et al., 2011). The ROIs are represented by labeled spheres of varying size and color, with the magnitude of causal information in-flow indicated by color and the magnitude of causal information out-flow indicated by size. Larger size spheres indicate larger information out-flow and warmer colored spheres (brighter red) indicate larger information in-flow. Connections between ROIs are represented by tapered cylinders with varying color and diameter. Cylinder tapering indicates the direction of information flow, while cylinder width indicates flow magnitude, and cylinder color represents the dominant frequency of communication, with cooler colors for lower frequencies and warmer colors for higher frequencies. Causal information flow is integrated across all computed frequencies (2–50 Hz), and is shown here (**Figure 10**) for $t = 250$ ms, that is, during the planning period. The 3D rendering demonstrates the dominant role of the Precuneus as an information source, indicated by its large size, the higher power/frequency coupling of frontal regions (ACC, SMA, L/R Mot), indicated by warmer colored and larger connecting cylinders, and the higher frequency communication present in the network during reach planning.

Framework Limitations

The above discussion of neurophysiologically relevant findings serves to demonstrate the nature of the conclusions that can be drawn through the application of this algorithmic framework. Application of this method yields findings that are both consistent with existing literature, and reveal connectivity information in the cortex with an immense degree of detail, allowing for the documentation of source-space spectro-temporal information flow. There are, however, limitations with the current approach which must be considered.

The source orientation assumptions applied to the cortical BEM for the source space held that all cortical dipoles were oriented normally to the surface of the BEM, a canonical assumption that has been previously employed for BEM construction (Fuchs et al., 2002), and is motivated by the perpendicular orientation of cortical pyramidal cells to the cortical surface. Applying this assumption simplifies solving the inverse problem by reducing the number of variables to be estimated to N_g (number of BEM grid-points) from $3 * N_g$, as is the case when accounting for the x, y, and z components of the current at each grid-point. However, this assumption greatly restricts the form of the computed current density, and does not allow for any data-driven flexibility with the computed dipoles. Utilizing the position-free BEM and associated Lead Field Matrix would allow for much greater flexibility, allowing for cortical dipole orientation to be computed either jointly with the current density, or after source localization using the current density, and thus identifying orientations through observed data instead of through a prior model.

Another potential drawback of the current source-localization algorithm is the Laplacian regularization utilized by cLORETA. The smoothing features of the discrete Laplacian when used as a Tikhonov matrix cause the estimated current density to be blurred over large regions of the cortical surface. This blurring can cause current density from a single source to spill over into multiple adjacent ROIs and potentially skew causal interactions between these ROIs in a manner that is not corrected by using the SdDTF connectivity metric. Preliminary investigations using this data suggest that this spill-over does not have a significant effect on causal analysis in this proposed framework, but further investigation would be prudent to ensure that the computed connectivity dynamics are not skewed by the choice of cLORETA as the source localization algorithm.

The validity of the presented connectivity dynamics is supported by the statistical analysis of the SdDTF connectivity matrix and the validation conducted on the fitted MVAR models. Though a large amount of the computed connectivity was statistically significant, the residuals of the computed MVAR models failed the whiteness tests because not all correlational structure of the localized current was captured by the models, suggesting the existence of non-linear dynamics. These non-linear dynamics are readily visible in the model prediction error and suggest that non-linear AR modeling is required to effectively capture these dynamics in the MVAR coefficients. However, all models exhibited a large Percent Consistency in the order of 90%, indicating that a very large percentage of the correlational structure of the localized current in each node was captured by the MVAR. The high percent consistency of the models indicates that these nonlinearities constitute a small portion of the localized current, and the computed MVAR models are able to account for the vast majority of the observed dynamics.

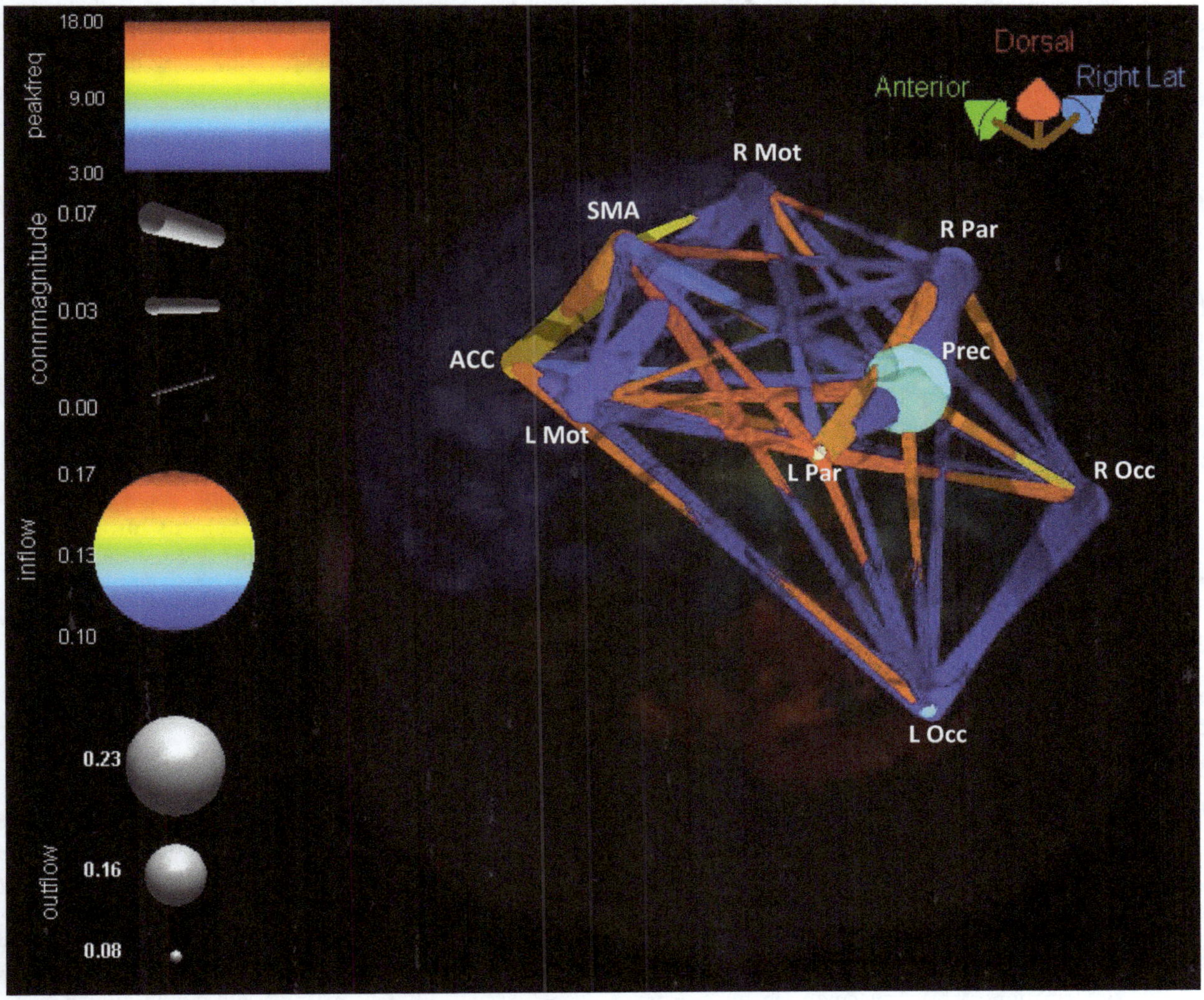

FIGURE 10 | Cortical connectivity present during the planning phase of the Reach/Saccade condition, shown in a 3D (BrainMovie3D) rendering of a cortical volume (Delorme et al., 2011). ROIs are represented by labeled spheres of varying size and color, with the magnitude of causal information in-flow indicated by color and the magnitude of causal information out-flow indicated by size. Connections between ROIs are represented by tapered cylinders with varying color and diameter. Cylinder tapering indicates the direction of information flow, cylinder width indicates flow magnitude, and cylinder color represents the dominant frequency of communication, with cooler colors for lower frequencies and warmer colors for higher frequencies. Causal information flow was integrated across all computed frequencies (2–50 Hz), and is shown here for $t = 250$ ms, during the planning period. The 3D rendering demonstrates the dominant role of the Precuneus as an information source, indicated by its large size, the higher power/frequency coupling of frontal regions (ACC, SMA, L/R Mot) indicated by warmer colored and larger connecting cylinders, and higher frequency communication present in the network during reach planning.

Extensions to Real-Time BCI Applications

In spite of the potential limitations discussed in the previous section, the proposed algorithmic framework has great potential as a means for extracting connectivity features in real time that can be used for brain state identification and BCI control. While in its current form, the framework is designed for off-line processing, Mullen et. al have demonstrated in Mullen et al. (2015) that elements of this framework can be applied in a real-time BCI setting and, with high accuracy, decode brain states using the spectro-temporal connectivity features computed through the use of this framework. The linear nature of the inverse problem formulated through cLORETA allows for rapid localization of current density in the cortex by application of the closed-form solution given in equation 2. Furthermore, the lattice algorithm used for MVAR coefficient estimation, while well suited for off-line analysis where all data is available for fitting, can be replaced by alternative estimation algorithms which take advantage of the convexity of MVAR model-fitting to compute robust models quickly and with relatively few data-points. In addition, the development of online recursive ICA (Hsu et al., 2014) allows for robust online artifact rejection, source identification, and lends to the overall feasibility of this approach in real-time BCI applications. There are other elements of the pipeline, such as the data-driven identification of ROI's for connectivity analysis, which must be adapted to account for the lack of all data present, or meet the computational demands in real-time analysis. Nevertheless, there is great potential use for this framework in both a clinical and research settings for real-time BCI control.

CONCLUSION

The presented algorithmic and computational framework successfully identified a cortical network, across several subjects, associated with a cognitive task, using EEG signals recorded from individuals performing the task with the aid of a BCI. It also computed statistically significant causal dynamic connectivity profiles among the ROIs comprising the nodes of the identified cortical network. The modular nature of the presented framework allows for flexibility and scalability. The algorithm computing the cortical network can easily scale up to include a greater number of participants without compromising the reliability or accuracy. The ease of incorporating large amounts of data comes as a consequence of utilizing a distributed source localization method with a BEM-defined source space. The flexible-yet-fixed source space geometry allows for warping head models to align with a realistic 3D representation of each participant's cortex by way of the digitized electrode positions, while retaining the identity of anatomical ROIs and their associated gray matter grid points in the head model. Should the user deem it necessary, the modular nature of this framework allows for substitutions of preprocessing algorithms, source localization methods, and connectivity analysis tools as is seen fit. As long as a source-space based localization algorithm is utilized to maintain consistent anatomical regions across subjects, the user is free to create a customized pipeline that best suits their needs, and is not strictly limited to usage of the algorithmic pipeline with the proposed software and algorithms. The proposed analytical approach allows for extraction of information rich connectivity features which account for spectro-temporal connectivity dynamics during the performance of a cognitive task. This feature extraction is made possible by coupling the segmentation-MVAR modeling of cortical signals with the SdDTF—a connectivity metric that is evaluated independently for different frequencies, leading to the asymmetric spectro-temporal connectivity dynamics displayed in **Figures 7–9**. The presented framework also includes a non-parametric statistical test to assess the statistical significance of the extracted features—the spectro-temporal connectivity dynamics. The physiological plausibility of the cortical network and the causal dynamic features characterizing interaction among the nodes of the network computed by employing this framework strengthens the framework's applicability in reliably capturing complex brain functionality, which is required by applications, such as diagnostics and BCI.

ETHICS STATEMENT

This study was carried out in accordance with the recommendations of the Human Subjects Institutional Review Board of the University of California, San Diego with written informed consent from all subjects. All subjects gave written informed consent in accordance with the Declaration of Helsinki. The protocol was approved by the Human Subjects Institutional Review Board of the University of California, San Diego.

AUTHOR CONTRIBUTIONS

HC introduced improvements to the pipeline, conducted re-processing and analysis of data, and wrote the manuscript. TM assisted with data processing on the first iteration of the pipeline. HP and GC contributed in an advisory manner with strategy and direction of the paper and the underlying computational methods. HP also directed the original project in which the data was collected, and GC assisting with editing the manuscript. JI (senior author) conducted processing and analysis on the first iteration of the pipeline, contributed in an advisory manner more closely than GC and HP, and assisted with editing the manuscript.

REFERENCES

Asemi, A., Ramaseshan, K., Burgess, A., Diwadkar, V., and Bressler, S. (2015). Dorsal anterior cingulate cortex modulates supplementary motor area in coordinated unimanual motor behavior. *Front. Hum. Neurosci.* 9:309. doi: 10.3389/fnhum.2015.00309

Barnett, L., and Seth, A., K. (2014). The MVGC Multivariate Granger Causality Toolbox: a new approach to granger-causal inference. *J. Neurosci. Methods* 223, 50–68. doi: 10.1016/j.jneumeth.2013.10.018

Bell, A. J., and Sejnowski, T. J. (1995). An information-maximisation approach to blind separation and blind deconvolution. *Neural Comput.* 7, 1004–1034.

Benjamini, Y., and Hochberg, Y. (1995). Controlling the false discovery rate: a practical and powerful approach to multiple testing. *J. R. Stat. Soc.* 57, 289–300.

Blangero, A., Menz, M. M., McNamara, A., and Binkofski, F. (2009). Parietal modules for reaching. *Neuropsychologia* 47, 1500–1507. doi: 10.1016/j.neuropsychologia.2008

Blumberg, J., and Kreiman, G. (2010). How cortical neurons help us see: visual recognition in the human brain. *J. Clin. Invest.* 120, 3054–3063. doi: 10.1172/JCI42161

Brinkman, L., Stolk, A., Dijkerman, H. C., de Lange, F. P., and Toni, I. (2014). Distinct roles for alpha- and beta-band oscillations during mental simulation of goal-directed actions. *J. Neurosci.* 34, 14783–14792. doi: 10.1523/JNEUROSCI.2039-14.2014

Buzsáki, G., and Silva, F. L. (2012). High frequency oscillations in the intact brain. *Prog. Neurobiol.* 98, 241–249. doi: 10.1016/j.pneurobio.2012.02.004

Delorme, A., Kothe, C., Vankov, A., Bidgley-Shamlo, N., Oostenveld, R., Zander, T., et al. (2010). "MATLAB-based tools for BCI research," in *Proceedings Fourth International Brain-Computer Interface Meeting*, eds D. S. Tan and A. Nijhol (London: Springer), 241–259.

Delorme, A., and Makeig, S. (2004). EEGLAB: an open source toolbox for analysis of single-trial EEG dynamics including independent component analysis. *J. Neurosci. Methods* 134, 9–21. doi: 10.1016/j.jneumeth.2003.10.009

Delorme, A., Mullen, T., Kothe, C., Akalin Acar, Z., Bigdely-Shamlo, N., Vankov, A., et al. (2011). EEGLAB, SIFT, NFT, BCILAB, and ERICA: new tools for advanced EEG processing. *Comput. Intell. Neurosci.* 2011:130714. doi: 10.1155/2011/130714

Filimon, F. (2010). Human cortical control of hand movements: parietofrontal networks for reaching, grasping, and pointing. *Neuroscientist* 16, 388–407. doi: 10.1177/1073858410375468

Filimon, F., Nelson, J. D., Huang, R. S., and Sereno, M. I. (2009). Multiple parietal reach regions in humans: cortical representations for visual and proprioceptive feedback during on-line reaching. *J. Neurosci.* 29, 2961–2971. doi: 10.1523/JNEUROSCI.3211-08.2009

Fuchs, M., Kastner, J., Wagner, M., Hawes, S., and Ebersole, J. S. (2002). A standardized boundary element method volume conductor model. *Clin. Neurophysiol.* 113, 702–712. doi: 10.1016/S1388-2457(02)00030-5

George, L., and Lecuyer, A. (2010). "An overview of research on "passive" brain-computer interfaces for implicit human-computer interaction," in *Presented at the IEEE ICABB* (Venice).

Glover, S., Wall, M. B., and Smith, A. T. (2012). Distinct cortical networks support the planning and online control of reaching-to-grasp in humans. *Eur. J. Neurosci.* 35, 909–915. doi: 10.1111/j.1460-9568.2012.08018.x

Gramfort, A., Papadopoulo, T., Olivi, E., and Clerc, M. (2010). OpenMEEG: opensource software for quasistatic bioelectromagnetics. *BioMed. Eng. Online* 9:45. doi: 10.1186/1475-925X-9-45

Heider, B., Karnik, A., Ramalingam, N., and Siegel, R. M. (2010). Neural representation during visually guided reaching in macaque posterior parietal cortex. *J. Neurophysiol.* 104, 3494–3509. doi: 10.1152/jn.01050.2009

Hsu, S. H., Mullen, T., Jung, T. P., and Cauwenberghs, G. (2014). "Online recursive independent component analysis for real-time source separation of high-density EEG," in *Presented at the Conference Proceedings IEEE EMBS* (Chicago, IL).

Hyvärinen, A., and Oja, E. (2000). Independent component analysis: algorithms and applications. *Neural Netw.* 13, 411–430. doi: 10.1016/S0893-6080(00)00026-5

Iversen, J. R., Ojeda, A., Mullen, T., Plank, M., Snider, J., Cauwenberghs, G., et al. (2014). "Causal analysis of cortical networks involved in reaching to spatial targets. Engineering in Medicine and Biology Society (EMBC)," in *36th Annual International Conference of the IEEE, 2014* (Chicago, IL).

Johnson, P. B., Ferraina, S., Bianchi, L., and Caminiti, R. (1996). Cortical networks for visual reaching: physiological and anatomical organization of frontal and parietal lobe arm regions. *Cereb. Cortex* 6, 102–119. doi: 10.1093/cercor/6.2.102

Kabbara, A., Khalil, M., El-Falou, W., Eid, H., and Hassan, M. (2016). Functional brain connectivity as a new feature for P300 speller. *PLoS ONE* 11:e0146282 doi: 10.1371/journal.pone.0146282

Kennerley, S. W., Walton, M. E., Behrens, T. E. J., Buckley, M., and Rushworth, M. (2006). Optimal decision making and the anterior cingulate cortex. *Nat. Neurosci.* 9, 940–947. doi: 10.1038/nn1724

Korzeniewska, A., Crainiceanu, C. M., Kus, R., Franaszczuk, P. J., and Crone, N. E. (2008). Dynamics of event-related causality in brain electrical activity. *Hum. Brain Mapp.* 29, 1170–1192. doi: 10.1002/hbm.20458

Korzeniewska, A., Mańczak, M., Kamiński, M., Blinowska, K. J., and Kasicki, S. (2003). Determination of information flow direction among brain structures by a modified directed transfer function (dDTF) method. *J. Neurosci. Methods* 125, 195–207. doi: 10.1016/S0165-0270(03)00052-9

Lancaster, J. L., Woldorff, M. G., Parsons, L. M., Liotti, M., Freitas, C. S., Rainey, L., et al. (2000). Automated Talairach Atlas labels for functional brain mapping. *Hum. Brain Mapp.* 10, 120–131. doi: 10.1002/1097-0193(200007)10:3<120::AID-HBM30>3.0.CO;2-8

Lindner, M., Vicente, R., Priesemann, V., and Wibral, M. (2011). TRENTOOL: a Matlab open source toobox to analyse information flow in time series data with transfer entropy. *BMC Neurosci.* 12:119. doi: 10.1186/1471-2202-12-119

Makeig, S. (1993). Auditory Event-Related dynamics of the EEG spectrum and effects of exposure to tones. *Electroencephalogr. Clin. Neurophysiol.* 86, 282–293. doi: 10.1016/0013-4694(93)90110-h

Moeller, K., Willmes, K., and Klein, E. (2015). A review on functional and structural brain connectivity in numerical cognition. *Front. Hum. Neurosci.* 9:227. doi: 10.3389/fnhum.2015.00227

Mullen, T., Kothe, C., Chi, Y. M., Ojeda, A., Kerth, T., Makeig, S., et al. (2015). Real-time neuroimaging and cognitive monitoring using wearable dry EEG. *IEEE Trans. Biomed. Eng.* 62, 2533–2567. doi: 10.1109/tbme.2015.2481482

Nachev, P., Kennard, C., and Husain, M. (2008). Functional role of the supplementary and pre-supplementary motor areas. *Nat. Rev. Neurosci.* 9, 856–869. doi: 10.1038/nrn2478

Neuner, I., Arrubla, J., Werner, C. J., Hitz, K., Boers, F., Kawohl, W., et al. (2014). The default mode network and EEG regional spectral power: a simultaneous fMRI-EEG study. *PLoS ONE* 9:e88214. doi: 10.1371/journal.pone.0088214

Niso, G., Bruna, R., Pereda, E., Gutierrez, R., Bajo, R., Maestú, F., et al. (2013). HERMES: towards an integrated toolbox to characterize functional and effective brain connectivity. *Neuroinformatics* 11, 405–434. doi: 10.1007/s12021-013-9186-1

Ojeda, A., Bigdely-Shamlo, N., and Makeig, S. (2014). MoBILAB: an open source toolbox for analysis and visualization of mobile brain/body imaging data. *Front. Hum. Neurosci.* 8:121. doi: 10.3389/fnhum.2014.00121

Oostendorp, T. F., Delbeke, J., and Stegeman, D. F. (2000). The conductivity of the human skull: results of *in vivo* and *in vitro* measurements. *IEEE Trans. Biomed. Eng.* 47, 1487–1492. doi: 10.1109/TBME.2000.880100

Park, C., Plank, M., Snider, J., Kim, S., Huang, H. C., Gepshtein, S., et al. (2014). EEG gamma band oscillations differentiate the planning of spatially directed movements of the arm versus eye: multivariate empirical mode decomposition analysis. *IEEE Trans. Neural Syst. Rehabil. Eng.* 22, 1083–1096. doi: 10.1109/TNSRE.2014.2332450

Pascual-Marqui, R. D., Michel, C. M., and Lehmann, D. (1994). Low resolution electromagnetic tomography: a new method for localizing electrical activity in the brain. *Int. J. Psychol.* 18, 49–65. doi: 10.1016/0167-8760(84)90014-x

Pievani, M., Filippini, N., van den Heuvel, M. P., Cappa, S. F., and Frisoni, G. B. (2014). Brain connectivity in neurodegenerative diseases – from phenotype to proteinopathy. *Nat. Rev. Neurol.* 10, 620–633. doi: 10.1038/nrneurol.2014.178

Rissanen, J. (1978). Modeling by shortest data description. *Automatica* 14, 465–471. doi: 10.1016/0005-1098(78)90005-5

Schmidt, A. (2000). Implicit human computer interaction through context. *Personal. Technol.* 4, 191–199. doi: 10.1007/BF01324126

Seth, A. K., Barrett, A. B., and Barnett, L. (2015). Granger causality in neuroscience and neuroimaging. *J. Neurosci.* 35, 3293–3297. doi: 10.1523/JNEUROSCI.4399-14.2015

Stevens, F. L., Hurley, R. A., and Taber, K. H. (2011). Anterior cingulate cortex: unique role in cognition and emotion. *J. Neurospsychiatry Clin. Neurosci.* 23, 120–125. doi: 10.1176/jnp.23.2.jnp121

Thompson, W., Mullen, T., Onton, J., and Makeig, S. (2011). "A bayesiabn spatiotemporal model for multi-subject EEG source dynamics and effective connectivity," in *Front Hum Neurosci Conference: XI International Conference on Cognitive Neuroscience* (Palma, Majorca).

Trongnetrpunya, A., Nandi, B., Kang, D., Kocsis, B., Schroeder, C. E., and Ding, M. (2015). Assessing granger causality in electrophysiological data: removing the adverse effects of common signals via bipolar derivations. *Front. Syst. Neurosci.* 9:189. doi: 10.3389/fnsys.2015.00189

Trujillo-Barreto, N. J., Aubert-Vázquez, E., and Valdés-Sosa, P. A. (2004). Bayesian model averaging in EEG/MEG imaging. *Neuroimage* 21, 1300–1319. doi: 10.1016/j.neuroimage.2003.11.008

Tu, S., and Xu, L. (2012). A theoretical investigation of several model selection criteria for dimensionality reduction. *Pattern Recognit. Lett.* 33, 1117–1126. doi: 10.1016/j.patrec.2012.01.010

Wang, W., Sudre, G. P., Xu, Y., Kass, R. E., Collinger, J. L., Degenhart, A. D., et al. (2010). Decoding and cortical source localization for intended movement direction with MEG. *J. Neurophysiol.* 104, 2451–2461. doi: 10.1152/jn.00239.2010

Zhang, H., Chavarriaga, R., Goel, M. K., Gheorghe, L., and Millan Jdel, R. (2012). Improved recognition of error related potentials through the use of brain connectivity features. *Conf. Proc. IEEE Eng. Med. Biol. Soc.* 2012, 6740–6743. doi: 10.1109/EMBC.2012.6347541

9

Factors of Influence on the Performance of a Short-Latency Non-Invasive Brain Switch: Evidence in Healthy Individuals and Implication for Motor Function Rehabilitation

Ren Xu[1,2]*, Ning Jiang*[3]*, Natalie Mrachacz-Kersting*[4]*, Kim Dremstrup*[4] *and Dario Farina*[1*]

[1] *Department of Neurorehabilitation Engineering, Bernstein Center for Computational Neuroscience, University Medical Center, Göttingen, Germany,* [2] *Institute of Computer Science, Faculty of Mathematics and Computer Secience, Georg-August University, Göttingen, Germany,* [3] *Department of Systems Design Engineering, University of Waterloo, Waterloo, ON, Canada,* [4] *Center for Sensory-Motor Interaction, Department of Health Science and Technology, Aalborg University, Aalborg, Denmark*

Edited by:
Michela Chiappalone, Istituto Italiano di Tecnologia, Italy

Reviewed by:
Jose Luis Contreras-Vidal, University of Houston, USA
Dingguo Zhang, Shanghai Jiao Tong University, China

***Correspondence:**
Dario Farina
dario.farina@bccn.uni-goettingen.de

Brain-computer interfacing (BCI) has recently been applied as a rehabilitation approach for patients with motor disorders, such as stroke. In these closed-loop applications, a brain switch detects the motor intention from brain signals, e.g., scalp EEG, and triggers a neuroprosthetic device, either to deliver sensory feedback or to mimic real movements, thus re-establishing the compromised sensory-motor control loop and promoting neural plasticity. In this context, single trial detection of motor intention with short latency is a prerequisite. The performance of the event detection from EEG recordings is mainly determined by three factors: the type of motor imagery (e.g., repetitive, ballistic), the frequency band (or signal modality) used for discrimination (e.g., alpha, beta, gamma, and MRCP, i.e., movement-related cortical potential), and the processing technique (e.g., time-series analysis, sub-band power estimation). In this study, we investigated single trial EEG traces during movement imagination on healthy individuals, and provided a comprehensive analysis of the performance of a short-latency brain switch when varying these three factors. The morphological investigation showed a cross-subject consistency of a prolonged negative phase in MRCP, and a delayed beta rebound in sensory-motor rhythms during repetitive tasks. The detection performance had the greatest accuracy when using ballistic MRCP with time-series analysis. In this case, the true positive rate (TPR) was ~70% for a detection latency of ~200 ms. The results presented here are of practical relevance for designing BCI systems for motor function rehabilitation.

Keywords: brain-computer interface, motor intention detection, ballistic and repetitive task, movement-related cortical potential, sensory-motor rhythm

INTRODUCTION

In the past decade, non-invasive brain-computer interfacing (BCI) based assistive technology has been proposed as a novel rehabilitation tool for people suffering of motor disorders (Daly and Wolpaw, 2008; Shih et al., 2012), such as stroke (Ramos-Murguialday et al., 2013) and spinal cord injury (Enzinger et al., 2008). In BCI systems for neurorehabilitation, the volition of subjects i detected from brain signals. Such a brain switch is used to control a neuroprosthetic device, such as an electrical stimulator (Niazi et al., 2012; King et al., 2014) or a robotic system (Xu et al., 2014b), to close the sensory-motor loop for either restoring motor function or modulating neural pathways (Shih et al., 2012).

As the first step of these closed-loop systems, accurate online detection of motor intention is a crucial and challenging task for non-invasive neural recordings such as scalp electroencephalography (EEG), mainly due to its low spatial resolution and poor signal-to-noise ratio. For neuroprosthesis control in general, the acceptable delay between intention and action is ~200 ms (Lauer et al., 2000). In particular, the detection latency is crucial in inducing Hebbian associative neural plasticity for rehabilitation purposes (Hebb, 1949). The efficiency of plasticity induction would be extremely slow, if at all possible, when the artificially afferent triggered by the brain switch arrived at the cortical level either too early or too late relative to motor intention (Mrachacz-Kersting et al., 2012).

Several signal processing approaches have been proposed for motor intention detection from EEG (Venkatakrishnan et al., 2014). Among these methods, two main EEG signal modalities have been explored for the purpose of motor rehabilitation: sensory motor rhythms (SMRs; Yuan and He, 2014) and movement related cortical potentials (MRCPs; Xu et al., 2014a), a type of slow cortical potential.

SMR corresponds to an increase or decrease in power at various subbands of EEG signals recorded over the sensory motor cortex (e.g., *Cz* for foot movements), prior to, during and after movement, or movement imagination (Yuan and He, 2014). The increase of subband power implies that the neurons in the corresponding cortical area discharge more synchronously than at baseline and therefore it is referred to as event-related synchronization (ERS; Pfurtscheller and Lopes Da Silva, 1999). Conversely, the decrease of subband power corresponds to less synchronous neural activity, termed event-related desynchronization (ERD; Pfurtscheller and Lopes Da Silva, 1999). Immediately after movement imagination, an ERS is usually observed in the beta-band (~20 Hz; Pfurtscheller and Solis-Escalante, 2009). This is also referred to as beta-rebound. In most SMR-based BCI studies for neurorehabilitation, the movement imagery that the subjects were instructed to perform was repetitive movement, such as foot tapping, with a few exceptions (Pfurtscheller and Solis-Escalante, 2009).

MRCP is another EEG signal modality observable on the sensory motor cortex prior to, during and after movement or movement imagery. It is characterized by a slow negative deflection of the near-DC component in the EEG signal before movement or movement imagery, reaching its peak of negativity near the onset of movement or movement imagination, and followed by a positive rebound before the signal returns back to its reference level (Jahanshahi and Hallett, 2003). MRCP is characterized by a time-series change at a very narrow low frequency content (0.05–3 Hz; Jahanshahi and Hallett, 2003). In MRCP-based BCI studies, the movement or imagined movement is usually executed once, often as a brisk or ballistic task, as opposed to the repetitive movement used in SMR-based studies. More recently, a combined approach of subband SMR and time-series MRCP has been proposed (Ibáñez et al., 2014). This fusion approach yielded improved performance for the detection of ballistic reaching movement (Ibáñez et al., 2014).

Due to the low signal-to-noise ratio of EEG, spatial filtering is usually used as a pre-processing step to enhance the desired feature. Among them, common spatial pattern (CSP) has been very successful in processing SMRs (Ang et al., 2008; Blankertz et al., 2008), particularly when the channels are more than 20. When the channels are less (typically <10), the Laplacian filter has been widely used for both signal modalities (Müller-Putz and Kaiser, 2010; Niazi et al., 2011).

The above survey indicates that a motor imagery based short-latency brain switch is predominantly influenced by three factors: the type of motor task (ballistic or repetitive), the frequency band (e.g., MRCP, alpha or beta band) of EEG, and the corresponding processing technique (subband power estimation or time-series analysis). In previous studies, the effect of some of these factors was partly investigated, e.g., SMR in brief and sustained movement (Cassim et al., 2000; Alegre et al., 2003) or MRCP vs. SMR in real movements (Toro et al., 1994; Babiloni et al., 1999; Filipovic et al., 2001). More recently, there have been studies on the analyses of the frequency band in motor intention detection (Garipelli et al., 2013; Ibáñez et al., 2014; López-Larraz et al., 2014). However, to date, there has been no direct comparison of advantages and disadvantages of all the above factors in the context of a short-latency brain switch for rehabilitation purposes. In this study on healthy subjects, these factors are directly compared in their influence on the low latency detection of movement intention, in an attempt to provide a guideline for BCI researchers working toward closed-loop neuroprosthetic applications.

METHODS

Subjects

Ten healthy volunteers (seven male and three female, age: 26.5 ± 4.6 years) participated in the study. Informed consent was obtained from all participants, and ethical approval was provided by the local ethics committee in accordance with the Declaration of Helsinki.

Experimental Setup

- EEG

Nine channels of EEG were acquired with an active electrode system (ActiCap, Brain Products, Germany) and 16-channel EEG amplifier (g.USBamp, gTec GmbH, Austria). The electrodes were placed in the standard 10–20 locations at Cz, Fz, F3, F4, C3, C4, P3, P4, and Pz. The ground and reference located on AFz and the left earlobe, respectively. Sampling frequency was 1200 Hz, with no hardware filter. During all experiments, the impedances of all channels were monitored regularly to ensure that they were below the recommended values indicated by the manufacturers of the active electrode system.

- EMG

Surface electromyography (EMG) signals were collected from the tibialis anterior (TA) muscle of the right foot with disposable electrodes (Neuroline 720, Ambu). EMG was acquired by the last channel of the g.USBamp amplifier, with separate ground and reference electrode from the EEG channels. A monopolar electrode was placed on the mid-belly of the right TA muscle while the reference and ground electrodes were placed on the bony surface of the right knee and right ankle, respectively.

Experimental Procedure

During an experimental session, the subject was comfortably seated in a chair, ~1 m from a computer screen. Participants were instructed to look at the center of the screen and to follow the cue presented, minimizing eye movements. During the experiment, the cue on the screen indicated four states (**Figure 1**): idle, focus, preparation, and task. Each trial started from the 5-s idle phase, during which the subjects could adjust their position as they wished. In the second phase, the subjects were asked to focus on the screen without moving. This was followed by the preparation phase, where the subjects were instructed to follow the 3-s backwards counting presented on the screen, and to start imagining the movement immediately when it turned to the task phase, which lasted for 4 s. One trial ended with the next idle phase before the next trial commenced.

Each experimental session was divided into six runs, which consisted of three ballistic and three repetitive runs. The ballistic and repetitive runs were identical, except in the task phase. For ballistic runs, the subjects were instructed to imagine performing ballistic dorsiflexions at the beginning of the 4-s task phase; in repetitive runs, they were continuously repeating motor imagery for the whole 4-s task phase. The subjects were instructed to perform the repetitive task at a moderate speed, i.e., around once per second. The TA muscle activity was monitored through the EMG recording, and those trials with visible EMG signal were not included in further analysis. Each run comprised approximately 20 trials of ballistic or repetitive imaginary movements. The duration of each run was ~6 min. The order of ballistic and repetitive runs was randomized.

EEG Processing Algorithm

MRCP and SMR Morphology Analysis

The nine channels of EEG were band-pass filtered (2nd order Butterworth) at 0.05–3 Hz for MRCP analysis, (Xu et al., 2014a) and 4–40 Hz for SMR analysis (Planelles et al., 2014). Then a large Laplacian spatial filter centered at *Cz* (see Equation 1) was used to enhance the signal-to-noise ratio of the "virtual" *Cz* channel, which was then processed in subsequent steps.

$$virtual\_Cz = Cz - \sum_i CH_i/8 \tag{1}$$

Where CH_i stands for the eight channels around *Cz*.

In subsequent data segmentation, the data from $t = -3$ to $t = 6$ s, w.r.t. the task onset, of the filtered virtual *Cz* were extracted for each trial. For both SMR and MRCP, the reference interval, from which the baseline value was calculated, was -3 to -2 s (3 to 2 s before motor imagery onset).

1. MRCP morphology analysis

For each subject and each movement type, a statistical comparison was performed on the characteristics of the morphorlogy of the MRCP (see details in the Section of Statistical Methods below).

2. SMR morphology analysis

The power spectral density (PSD) of each trial was calculated over 1 s windows overlapped for 0.5 s using Hamming windows (Matlab function pwelch). For each subject and each movement type, a Bootstrap test was performed between the PSD of the SMR at each time-frequency point and the reference PSD of the SMR in a baseline window. The time-frequency SMR characterization was quantified as follows (Pfurtscheller and Lopes Da Silva, 1999):

$$SMR_{f,t}\% = \frac{A_{f,t} - R_f}{R_f} \tag{2}$$

where $SMR_{f,t}\%$ is the relative power of the SMR at time *t* and frequency *f*, $A_{f,t}$ is the absolute power of the SMR at the same time-frequency point, and R_f is the power of the reference interval for the frequency f. A positive $SMR_{f,t}\%$ value indicates an ERS, while a negative value of SMR indicates an ERD.

Time-Series Feature Extraction and Motor Imagery Detection

In order to analyze the information content in EEG for motor intention detection, six types of time-series features were extracted with band-pass filters at MRCP (0.05–3 Hz), Theta (4–7 Hz), Alpha (8–15 Hz), Beta (16–30 Hz), lower Gamma (31–40), and the full frequency band (0.05–40 Hz), followed by a large Laplacian filter centered at *Cz*. In order to evaluate the BCI performance, a three-fold cross-validation was used, in which two runs of the virtual *Cz* (either ballistic or repetitive) were taken

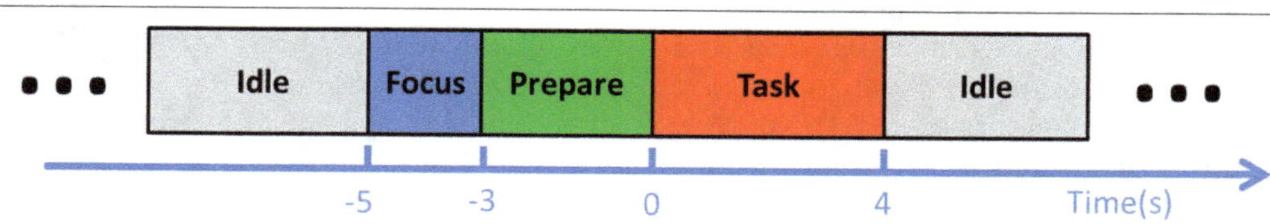

FIGURE 1 | Experimental procedure. Each trial began with an idle phase, followed by a 2-s focus phase and a 3-s preparation phase. In the consequential task phase, the subject was instructed to perform ballistic or repetitive imagination of dorsiflexion.

as the training set, while the remaining ballistic or repetitive run was used as the testing set. For the training set, the virtual *Cz* was segmented into portions of 2-s segments with 0.1-s increments. The segments between −1 to 1 s with respect to the task onset were labeled as "signal" portion, while all the remaining segments were labeled as "noise" portion. The testing set was treated in a pseudo-online way, mimicking the real online processing, where the data arrives continuously with a 2 s-length window and a refresh step of 0.1 s.

For the time-series feature, a manifold-learning based method called Locality Preserving Projection (LPP; He and Niyogi, 2003), followed by a Linear Discriminant Analysis (LDA) classifier was trained and used for detection. LPP-LDA has previously been implemented for MRCP detection with good performance (Xu et al., 2014a). The procedure is described briefly here. The "signal" and "noise" portions were first projected to a lower dimension using LPP, which maintained the intrinsic structure in the original manifold with high dimension (He and Niyogi, 2003). A LDA classifier was trained using the LPP projected training data. Once the LPP-LDA classifier was trained, the testing segments were projected by the obtained LPP projection, and the trained LDA was used to classify the testing data into either "signal" or "noise." A detection of motor intention would be registered when a number of continuous windows [referred to window number (WN)] were classified as "signal." One detection would be determined either as a true or false detection according to the detection latency (DL), i.e., the time difference between the detection and the task cue. If the DL was between -1 and 1 s, the detection was considered a true detection, otherwise a false detection. It should be emphasized here that the target of this study is a short-latency brain switch. Therefore, we only considered these detections within a few hundreds microseconds, even though signals outside this range may improve the accuracy for modalities such as Beta rebound. The true positive rate (TPR), false positive (FP) per minute, and DL were calculated to quantify the BCI performance. Compared with false positive rate (or specificity) which is generally used for evaluating binary classification (Hashimoto and Ushiba, 2013; Jochumsen et al., 2013) FP/min is more suitable for quantifying the performance of continuous detection in a (pseudo-) online paradigm, as was done in Niazi et al. (2011) and Xu et al. (2014a). As any detector, there is a trade-off between TPR and FP. Both TPR and FP are constrained by WN, whose increment would make the detection stricter (more difficult), leading to lower TPR and smaller FP. In order to objectively compare the BCI performance, we chose the WN value for which the FP was smaller than or equal to 8/min for all comparisons. Thus, only the TPR and DL were statistically compared.

Subband Power Estimation and Motor Imagery Detection

The subband power was also used as a direct feature for classification. For this purpose, the powers of the virtual *Cz* channel at the six frequency bands were estimated using the Welch periodogram with a resolution of 1 Hz. As for the time-series features, the window duration was of 2 s, with increments of 0.1 s. "Signal" and "noise" portions were the same as for the time-series features, and the same three-fold cross-validation method was used to test performance.

Since the dimensions of the subband power features are small, no dimension reduction method was used. The "signal" and "noise" portions were directly used to train a LDA classifier, which was used for detection of motor intention from the testing set. All BCI performance criteria were calculated with the same steps as in the time-domain processing, and analyzed using the statistical methods described in the following.

Statistical Methods

A paired *t*-test was performed for MRCP morphology analysis. The comparison was between the amplitude of the MRCP for the reference interval (i.e., mean value of −3 to −2 s w.r.t. task onset) and the magnitude of each 0.1 s-length segments of the virtual *Cz* outside the reference interval. A Holm-Bonferroni correction was performed for this multiple comparison, and the significance level was set to 0.05.

Three-way repeated ANOVA was used to investigate the effect of the three factors on BCI performance. The independent variables were TPR and DL. The three main factors were motor task (ballistic and repetitive imagination), frequency band (MRCP, Theta, Alpha, Beta, Gamma, and full frequency bands), and processing technique (time-series analysis and subband power estimation). A full model ANOVA with all interaction terms was performed first and, when significant interactions were detected, *post-hoc* tests (Tukey simultaneous test with significance level of 0.05) were performed.

RESULTS

Signal Morphology

MRCP Morphology

The MRCPs of a typical subject performing the two types of motor imageries are shown in **Figures 2A,B**. For the ballistic task (**Figure 2A**), the MRCP started to decrease approximately 2 s prior to the task onset, reached the negative peak around $t = 0$ s, and returned to the baseline in approximately 2 s after the task onset. In the repetitive task, the MRCP (**Figure 2B**) had a similar shape to that of the ballistic case before $t = 0$ s but the rebound phase was much longer in duration. Before task onset, both the ballistic and repetitive MRCP showed significant differences to the baseline starting from −1 s. However, the characteristics of the two motor tasks were different for the rebound part. No significant difference was found between the ballistic MRCP and the baseline from the time of 1 s, indicating it already returned back to the baseline. On the other hand, the repetitive MRCP still showed significance as late as 4 s after the task onset.

The above difference between ballistic and repetitive tasks was consistent across all subjects, as shown in **Figure 2C**. These results indicate a strong predictive power of MRCPs in detection of movement intention of the subjects for both types of motor imageries.

SMR Mapping

The SMR maps for three representative subjects for the two types of movement imageries are shown in **Figure 3**. For subject

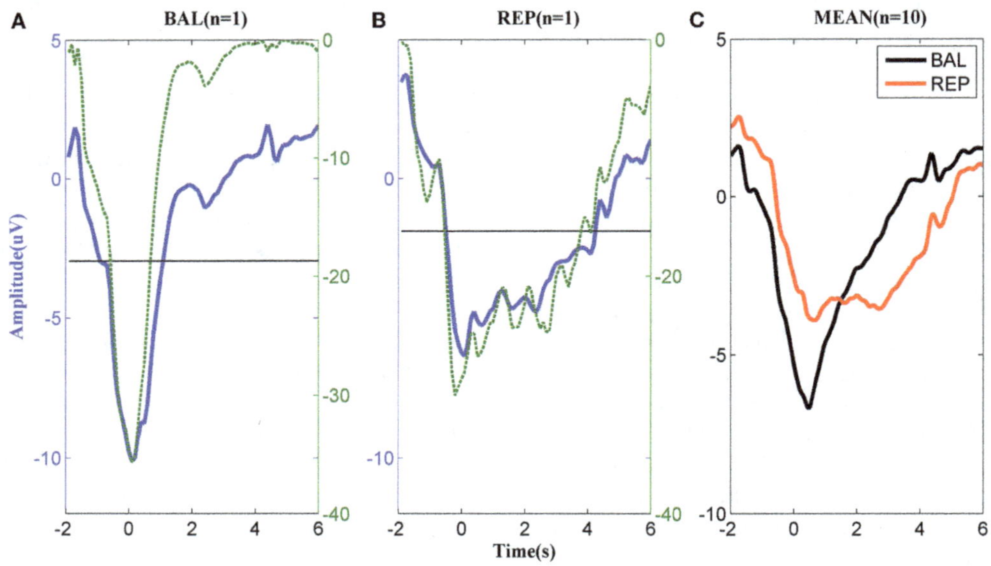

FIGURE 2 | MRCP corresponding to (A) ballistic (BAL) and (B) repetitive (REP) motor imagery from a typical subject. The dashed lines indicate the logarithmic *p*-value of the paired *t*-test between the MRCP (either ballistic or repetitive) and its reference between −3 and −2 s., while the solid horizontal line indicates significance level. **(C)**: The average MRCP over the 10 subjects. The black line corresponds to ballistic imagery and the red line to the repetitive motor imagery.

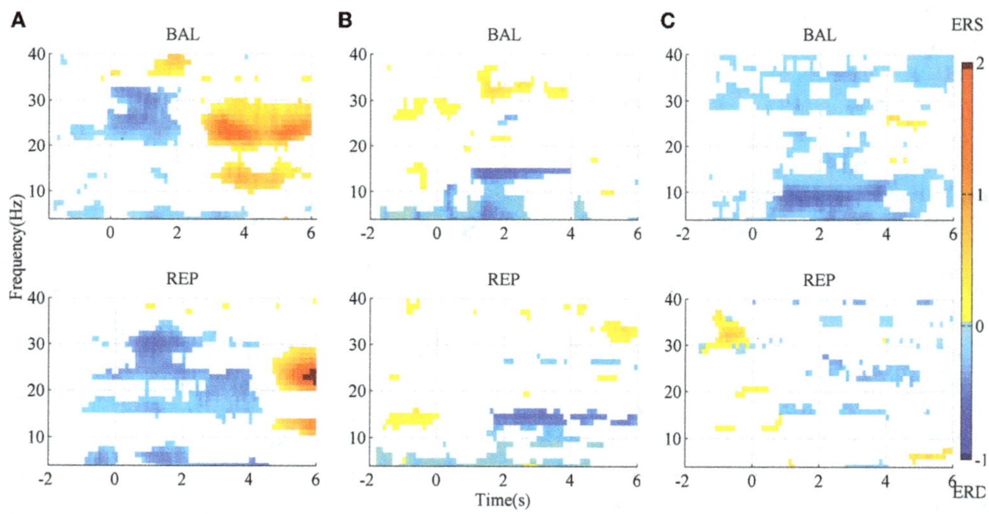

FIGURE 3 | SMR mapping from three representative subjects. (A) subject A; **(B)** subject B; **(C)** subject C. BAL and REP stand for ballistic and repetitive task, respectively. Only those points with significance in bootstrap test are presented. Red area indicates ERS, while blue area is ERD.

A, there was an evident ERD starting slightly earlier than the task onset, between the Beta and the lower Gamma band (above ~20 Hz) for the ballistic imagery, while it corresponded to a larger bandwidth for repetitive imagery. There was also an evident ERS in the Alpha and Beta bands for both tasks, but the repetitive ERS occurred much later than the ballistic one. However, the SMR landscape was very different for subject B, whose ERD and ERS mainly appeared in the Alpha and lower Gamma band, respectively. Subject C showed still other characteristics. The ERD occurred over almost the full band for the ballistic imagery, whereas it did not present a clear pattern in the repetitive imagery. Moreover, for all subjects, both the ERD and ERS occurred earlier in case of ballistic imagery with respec to repetitive imagery. ERS appeared before imagery onset in bot ballistic and repetitive tasks of subject B, and also in the repetitiv task of subject C.

In summary, the SMR mapping differed substantially amon the subjects, thus a general average across the subjects would nc be meaningful and therefore is not reported.

BCI Performance

The BCI performance in detection of motor imagery i summarized in **Table 1**. The WN is shown in **Figure 4**. Th ballistic MRCP with time-series analysis reached the highest TP

TABLE 1 | BCI performance.

Frequency band	Time-series analysis				Subband power estimation			
	BAL		REP		BAL		REP	
	TPR%	DL/ms	TPR%	DL/ms	TPR%	DL/ms	TPR%	DL/ms
MRCP	**70 ± 20**	267 ± 121	44 ± 13	197 ± 201	47 ± 18	389 ± 113	47 ± 25	239 ± 228
Theta	41 ± 8	64 ± 151	41 ± 9	132 ± 127	47 ± 21	369 ± 128	43 ± 20	204 ± 230
Alpha	32 ± 8	37 ± 138	28 ± 8	83 ± 180	48 ± 18	260 ± 218	48 ± 16	230 ± 176
Beta	32 ± 10	106 ± 144	32 ± 9	36 ± 113	57 ± 19	282 ± 198	50 ± 16	142 ± 243
Gamma	37 ± 8	40 ± 97	36 ± 10	37 ± 161	53 ± 16	256 ± 121	48 ± 16	210 ± 111
Full	54 ± 18	224 ± 108	30 ± 7	185 ± 202	51 ± 19	192 ± 195	46 ± 11	254 ± 174

BAL and REP stand for ballistic and repetitive imagery, respectively. True positive rate (TPR) is the ratio between true detection and the total number of trials in the testing set. Detection latency (DL) is the timing difference between the detection point and the task onset. The TPR and DL were chosen where false positive ≤8 min−1. The positive DL indicates that the detection happened after the task onset. The best accuracy is indicated in bold.

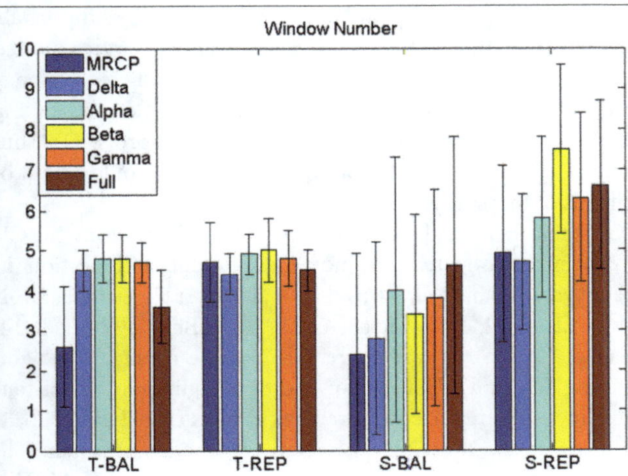

FIGURE 4 | Window number (WN). WN is chosen where false positive $\leq 8\,\text{min}^{-1}$. T-BAL and T-REP represent ballistic and repetitive task with time serial analysis, while S-BAL and S-REP stand for these two motor task with subband power estimation.

(70 ± 20%), followed by ballistic Beta band with subband power estimation (57 ± 19%). SMRs with time-series analysis yielded shorter DL (<100 ms), however the corresponding detection accuracy was extremely low (~30%). For each frequency band of either motor task (except the full band of the ballistic task), the time-domain technique resulted in shorter DL than the frequency-domain technique.

A representative segment of detecting ballistic MRCP with time-serial analysis was shown in **Figure 5**. Three black stars stand for the onsets of three consecutive tasks. For the first two, the detector successfully identifies them, which were labeled as Green stars. Moreover, this method demonstrated its robustness again moderate variation which appeared after the second trial (~25 s). In spite of this, there is still a false detection (labeled as a red star) when huge noise was introduced during the third trial.

Analysis of True Positive Rate

For a meaningful comparison between methods, the TPR is reported in all cases for the same level of false positives (≤8 min−1). The Three-way ANOVA on TPR found no three-way interaction ($p = 0.074$). Neither was the interaction between motor task and processing technique ($p = 0.283$). However, there was a significant interaction between motor task and frequency band ($p = 0.015$), as well as between processing technique and frequency band ($p < 0.001$). Therefore, we performed *post-hoc* tests on the significant interactions.

Focusing on the interaction between motor task and frequency band, the post-hoc comparison revealed that the MRCP of the ballistic task yielded the highest TPR (60 ± 22%). This was comparable to the full band of the same task, and significantly better than all other combinations (no significance was found among them). In addition, for both the MRCP and the full band, the ballistic task significantly outperformed the repetitive task.

For the other significant interaction between processing technique and frequency band, the difference depended on each factor. MRCP with time-series analysis provided the highest TPR (57 ± 22%), which was significantly better than all other frequency bands with the same processing technique. For the other processing technique, i.e., subband power analysis, there was no significant difference among frequency bands. Furthermore, it was observed that, for Alpha and Beta band, subband power analysis outperformed time-series analysis.

Analysis of Detection Delay

There was no three-factor interaction ($p = 0.451$), nor two-factor interactions ($p = 0.197, 0.532, 0.081$). Both the processing technique and frequency band were significantly different ($p < 0.001$ and $p = 0.004$, respectively). The *post-hoc* comparison revealed that the time-domain technique had lower DL than the frequency-domain technique (117 ± 169 vs. 252 ± 194 ms), while the MRCP resulted in longer DL than Alpha, Beta, and Gamma band (265 ± 185 vs. 145 ± 205, 129 ± 193, and 125 ± 159 ms, respectively).

Summary

Based on the above statistical analysis of TPR and DL, we summarize the influence of the three factors here. The ballistic task, is preferable over the repetitive task, as it yielded higher TPR for both MRCP and full band. Even though MRCP's DL

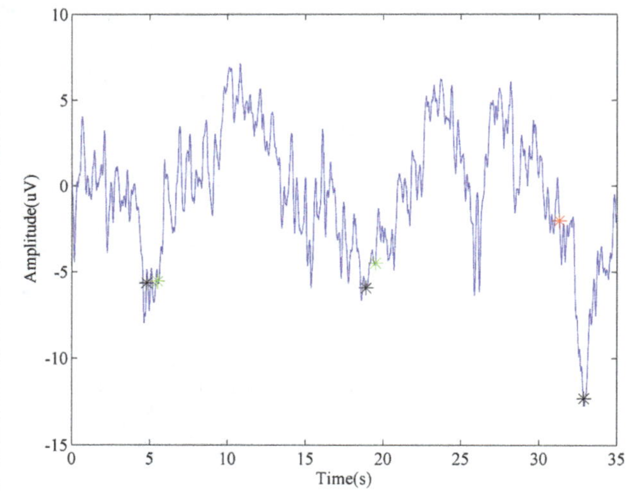

FIGURE 5 | Representative detection of MRCP. The blue line is a segment of virtual *Cz* from ballistic task. Black stars stand for the task onsets. Green stars represent true detections, while the red star is a false detection.

was slightly larger than for some SMRs, MRCP was still the best choice among all six frequency bands, given its highest TPR for both tasks and for the time-series processing technique. Time-series analysis outperformed subband power analysis, mainly due to a significantly shorter DL.

In summary, this comprehensive comparison on motor intention detection with two motor tasks (ballistic and repetitive), six frequency bands (MRCP, Theta, Alpha, Beta, Gamma, and full band), and two processing techniques (time-series analysis and subband power estimation) showed that the combination of ballistic, MRCP and time-series analysis significantly is preferred among all the considered options.

DISCUSSION

As a crucial aspect of closed-loop rehabilitation systems, the detection of the motor intention from scalp EEG is a central challenge in motor imagery based BCI. In recent years, there has been an increasing number of publications of clinical studies using SMR-based BCI (Ramos-Murguialday et al., 2013; Ang et al., 2014a,b; Li et al., 2014; Mukaino et al., 2014; Ono et al., 2014). On the other hand, MRCPs have also been proven as a promising signal type, particularly for neuromodulation purposes due to its short detection latency (Mrachacz-Kersting et al., 2012; Niazi et al., 2012; Xu et al., 2014b). Preliminary studies of MRCP-based BCI applied to chronic stroke patients have also been reported (Mrachacz-Kersting et al., 2015).

According to the Hebbian principle of associative plasticity (Hebb, 1949), neuroplasticity would only be induced when the motor intention and the task specific afferent feedback, e.g., passive movement delivered by an orthosis, occur synchronously in a cause-and-effect fashion. Therefore, an effective neuromodulation system requires not only accurate algorithms, but also algorithms that present short detection latencies, ideally shorter than 300 ms.

In the past decades, SMR has been the main signal modality used for detection purposes. TPRs above 80% were reported with Beta ERS (Müller-Putz and Kaiser, 2010; Wang et al., 2012), while the performance of ERD was also demonstrated to be above 70% (Planelles et al., 2014; Yang et al., 2014). However, the issue of detection latency was largely overlooked in these studies, with only one exception which reported a latency in the range of seconds (Hashimoto and Ushiba, 2013). In this study, the best TPR using SMR was 57%, for the beta band in the ballistic task using subband power estimation. Compared with previous studies, the performance here decreased obviously, mainly due to the limited range of latency. In these previous studies using SMR, detection latency was rarely reported. Its average latency can be more than one second if we take into consideration those detections which occur several seconds after the task onset (Hashimoto and Ushiba, 2013). On the contrary, in the current study, short latency detection is essential, as it is mandatory for the purpose of plasticity induction (Mrachacz-Kersting et al., 2012). As such, those detections occurring after 1 s were counted as false detections rather than true ones, resulting in a latency of several hundred milliseconds as shown in **Table 1**. Taking later windows into consideration would likely improve TPR, but would lead to a long-latency brain switch, which would be out of the focus of this study.

On the other hand, slow cortical potentials, such as MRCP, have been investigated for movement intention detection in recent years (Qian et al., 2010; Bai et al., 2011; Niazi et al., 2011; Lew et al., 2012; Bulea et al., 2013, 2014; Bhagat et al., 2014; Xu et al., 2014a). In the current study, the average TPR and DL was 70% and <300 ms for motor imagination, consistent with the results reported in previous studies (Niazi et al., 2011, 2012; Xu et al., 2014a,b). The relatively good performance in TPR (>70%) is essential for the high efficiency of MRCP-based BCI system. In particular, the detection latency of a few hundred milliseconds was demonstrated to be crucial for plasticity induction (Mrachacz-Kersting et al., 2012).

In this study, we demonstrated that ballistic motor imagery task, frequency band of MRCP, and time-series analysis is the optimal combination in terms of detection performance. Other options investigated are sub-optimal, mainly due to a trade-off between TPR and DL.

We also observed that repetitive SMR with subband power estimation was significantly better in accuracy than the ballistic one. This is in accordance with the discussion by Pfurtscheller & Solis-Escalante that SMR in repetitive task is easier to classify (Pfurtscheller and Solis-Escalante, 2009).

The different EEG features between the ballistic and repetitive task may be attributed to the difference in their afferent input (Cassim et al., 2000). As explained by Bear (Bear et al., 2007), compared to the repetitive task which has sufficient time for the sensory-motor loop to feedback, the ballistic movement, once initialized, is too fast to adjust. In addition, this difference may also be explain by the fact that there is an inhibitory process immediate following the ballistic task (Alegre et al., 2003), while this is not the case for the repetitive task.

The morphological difference between ballistic and repetitive tasks may mainly contribute to the differences in the detection performance of the two motor tasks. The prolonged negative phase in repetitive MRCP (in **Figure 2**) makes its rebound feature after task onset not as distinct as the ballistic one. That is why the accuracy of repetitive MRCP with time-series analysis is much lower than the ballistic one. On the other hand, in the case of subband power analysis, the frequency band did not have a significant influence on accuracy. This is likely explained due to the observed variability in the optimal frequency bands among individual subjects (see **Figure 3**).

Limitations

The above comparison was performed only on healthy subjects. Previous findings mostly support the similarity in slow EEG waves (e.g., MRCP) between healthy and stroke or spinal cord injured patients (Castro et al., 2007; Mattia et al., 2009; Niazi et al., 2011; Xu et al., 2014c), despite their non-negligibly distinct features such as onset and amplitude (Yilmaz et al., 2014), whereas SMRs trend to have greater difference on patients with central neural injury (Tran et al., 2004; Gourab and Schmit, 2010; Müller-Putz et al., 2014). Other different factors such as medication and mental status in patients could be challenging for clinical measurements. Therefore, further investigation on the target patient population is necessary.

In addition, the combination of several features with different processing techniques, such as those presented in Ibáñez et al. (2014) and López-Larraz et al. (2014), was not investigated in the current study. This study focused exclusively on a general comparison without subject-specific optimization, the combined features, e.g., SMR and MRCP, would be worthy to investigate in future work.

CONCLUSION

In this study, we performed a comprehensive comparison of motor task, frequency band, and processing technique, to investigate their influence on the performance of a short-latency brain switch. The morphological investigation found cross-subject consistency in MRCP, which supports its advantage for a subject-independent use. The BCI detection performance was maximized by using the ballistic imagery task, the DC bandwidth (MRCP), and the time-series analysis.

AUTHOR CONTRIBUTIONS

Conceived and designed the experiments: RX, NJ, NM, KD, DF. Performed the experiments: RX, NJ. Analyzed the data: RX, NJ, DF. Wrote the paper: RX, NJ, NM, DF.

ACKNOWLEDGMENTS

This work was supported financially by the China Scholarship Council (Contract Nr. 201204910155).

REFERENCES

Alegre, M., Labarga, A., Gurtubay, I. G., Iriarte, J., Malanda, A., and Artieda, J. (2003). Movement-related changes in cortical oscillatory activity in ballistic, sustained and negative movements. *Exp. Brain Res.* 148, 17–25. doi: 10.1007/s00221-002-1255-x

Ang, K. K., Chin, Z. Y., Zhang, H., and Guan, C. (2008). "Filter Bank Common Spatial Pattern (FBCSP) in brain-computer interface," in *2008 IEEE International Joint Conference on Neural Networks* (Hong Kong: IEEE World Congress on Computational Intelligence), 2390–2397.

Ang, K. K., Chua, K. S. G., Phua, K. S., Wang, C., Chin, Z. Y., Kuah, C. W. K., et al. (2014a). A randomized controlled trial of eeg-based motor imagery brain-computer interface robotic rehabilitation for stroke. *Clin. EEG Neurosci.* 46, 310–320. doi: 10.1177/1550059414522229

Ang, K. K., Guan, C., Phua, K. S., Wang, C., Zhou, L., Tang, K. Y., et al. (2014b). Brain-computer interface-based robotic end effector system for wrist and hand rehabilitation: results of a three-armed randomized controlled trial for chronic stroke. *Front. Neuroeng.* 7:30. doi: 10.3389/fneng.2014.00030

Babiloni, C., Carducci, F., Cincotti, F., Rossini, P. M., Neuper, C., Pfurtscheller, G., et al. (1999). Human movement-related potentials vs desynchronization of EEG alpha rhythm: a high-resolution EEG study. *Neuroimage* 10, 658–665. doi: 10.1006/nimg.1999.0504

Bai, O., Rathi, V., Lin, P., Huang, D., Battapady, H., Fei, D.-Y., et al. (2011). Prediction of human voluntary movement before it occurs. *Clin. Neurophysiol.* 122, 364–372. doi: 10.1016/j.clinph.2010.07.010

Bear, M. F., Connors, B. W., and Paradiso, M. A. (2007). *Neuroscience.* Philadelphia, PA: Lippincott Williams & Wilkins.

Bhagat, N. A., French, J., Venkatakrishnan, A., Yozbatiran, N., Francisco, G. E., O'Malley, M. K., et al. (2014). Detecting movement intent from scalp EEG in a novel upper limb robotic rehabilitation system for stroke. *Conf. Proc. IEEE Eng. Med. Biol. Soc.* 2014, 4127–4130. doi: 10.1109/EMBC.2014.6944532

Blankertz, B., Tomioka, R., Lemm, S., Kawanabe, M., and Muller, K.-R. (2008). Optimizing spatial filters for robust EEG single-trial analysis. *Signal Process. Mag. IEEE* 25, 41–56. doi: 10.1109/MSP.2008.4408441

Bulea, T. C., Prasad, S., Kilicarslan, A., and Contreras-Vidal, J. L. (2013). Classification of stand-to-sit and sit-to-stand movement from low frequency EEG with locality preserving dimensionality reduction. *Conf. Proc. IEEE Eng. Med. Biol. Soc.* 2013, 6341–6344. doi: 10.1109/embc.2013.6611004

Bulea, T. C., Prasad, S., Kilicarslan, A., and Contreras-Vidal, J. L. (2014). Sitting and standing intention can be decoded from scalp EEG recorded prior to movement execution. *Front. Neurosci.* 8:376. doi: 10.3389/fnins.2014.00376

Cassim, F., Szurhaj, W., Sediri, H., Devos, D., Bourriez, J.-L., Poirot, I., et al. (2000). Brief and sustained movements: differences in event-related (de)synchronization (ERD/ERS) patterns. *Clin. Neurophysiol.* 111, 2032–2039. doi: 10.1016/S1388-2457(00)00455-7

Castro, A., Díaz, F., and Van Boxtel, G. J. M. (2007). How does a short history of spinal cord injury affect movement-related brain potentials? *Eur. J. Neurosci.* 25, 2927–2934. doi: 10.1111/j.1460-9568.2007.05532.x

Daly, J. J., and Wolpaw, J. R. (2008). Brain–computer interfaces in neurological rehabilitation. *Lancet Neurol.* 7, 1032–1043. doi: 10.1016/S1474-4422(08)70223-0

Enzinger, C., Ropele, S., Fazekas, F., Loitfelder, M., Gorani, F., Seifert, T., et al. (2008). Brain motor system function in a patient with complete spinal cord injury following extensive brain-computer interface training. *Exp. Brain Res.* 190, 215–223. doi: 10.1007/s00221-008-1465-y

Filipovic, S., Jahanshahi, M., and Rothwell, J. (2001). Uncoupling of contingent negative variation and alpha band event-related desynchronization in a go/no-go task. *Clin. Neurophysiol.* 112, 1307–1315. doi: 10.1016/S1388-2457(01)00558-2

Garipelli, G., Chavarriaga, R., and Millán, J. (2013). Single trial analysis of slow cortical potentials: a study on anticipation related potentials. *J. Neural Eng.* 10:036014. doi: 10.1088/1741-2560/10/3/036014

Gourab, K., and Schmit, B. D. (2010). Changes in movement-related β-band EEG signals in human spinal cord injury. *Clin. Neurophysiol.* 121, 2017–2023. doi: 10.1016/j.clinph.2010.05.012

Hashimoto, Y., and Ushiba, J. (2013). EEG-based classification of imaginary left and right foot movements using beta rebound. *Clin. Neurophysiol.* 124, 2153–2160. doi: 10.1016/j.clinph.2013.05.006

He, X., and Niyogi, P. (2003). Locality preserving projections. *Adv. Neural Inf. Process. Syst.* 16, 153–160.

Hebb, D. O. (1949). *The Organization of Behavior: A Neuropsychological Theory.* Mahwah, NJ: Lawrence Erlbaum Associates.

Ibáñez, J., Serrano, J. I., del Castillo, M. D., Monge-Pereira, E., Molina-Rueda, F., Alguacil-Diego, I., et al. (2014). Detection of the onset of upper-limb movements based on the combined analysis of changes in the sensorimotor rhythms and slow cortical potentials. *J. Neural Eng.* 11:056009. doi: 10.1088/1741-2560/11/5/056009

Jahanshahi, M., and Hallett, M. (2003). *The Bereitschaftspotential: Movement-Related Cortical Potentials.* New York, NY: Springer Science & Business Media.

Jochumsen, M., Niazi, I. K., Mrachacz-Kersting, N., Farina, D., and Dremstrup, K. (2013). Detection and classification of movement-related cortical potentials associated with task force and speed. *J. Neural Eng.* 10, 056015. doi: 10.1088/1741-2560/10/5/056015

King, C. E., Dave, K. R., Wang, P. T., Mizuta, M., Reinkensmeyer, D. J., Do, A. H., et al. (2014). Performance assessment of a brain-computer interface driven hand orthosis. *Ann. Biomed. Eng.* 42, 2095–2105. doi: 10.1007/s10439-014-1066-9

Lauer, R. T., Peckham, P. H., Kilgore, K. L., and Heetderks, W. J. (2000). Applications of cortical signals to neuroprosthetic control: a critical review. *IEEE Trans. Rehabil. Eng.* 8, 205–208. doi: 10.1109/86.847817

Lew, E., Chavarriaga, R., Silvoni, S., and Millán, J. (2012). Detection of self-paced reaching movement intention from EEG signals. *Front. Neuroeng.* 5:13. doi: 10.3389/fneng.2012.00013

Li, M., Liu, Y., Wu, Y., Liu, S., Jia, J., and Zhang, L. (2014). Neurophysiological substrates of stroke patients with motor imagery-based brain-computer interface training. *Int. J. Neurosci.* 124, 403–415. doi: 10.3109/00207454.2013.850082

López-Larraz, E., Montesano, L., Gil-Agudo, A., and Minguez, J. (2014). Continuous decoding of movement intention of upper limb self-initiated analytic movements from pre-movement EEG correlates. *J. Neuroeng. Rehabil.* 11:153. doi: 10.1186/1743-0003-11-153

Mattia, D., Cincotti, F., Astolfi, L., de Vico Fallani, F., Scivoletto, G., Marciani, M. G., et al. (2009). Motor cortical responsiveness to attempted movements in tetraplegia: evidence from neuroelectrical imaging. *Clin. Neurophysiol.* 120, 181–189. doi: 10.1016/j.clinph.2008.09.023

Mrachacz-Kersting, N., Jiang, N., Stevenson, A. J. T., Niazi, I. K., Kostic, K., Pavlovic, A., et al. (2015). Efficient neuroplasticity induction in chronic stroke patients by an associative brain-computer interface. *J. Neurophysiol.* doi: 10.1152/jn.00918.2015. [Epub ahead of print].

Mrachacz-Kersting, N., Kristensen, S. R., Niazi, I. K., and Farina, D. (2012). Precise temporal association between cortical potentials evoked by motor imagination and afference induces cortical plasticity. *J. Physiol.* 590, 1669–1682. doi: 10.1113/jphysiol.2011.222851

Mukaino, M., Ono, T., Shindo, K., Fujiwara, T., Ota, T., Kimura, A., et al. (2014). Efficacy of brain-computer interface-driven neuromuscular electrical stimulation for chronic paresis after stroke. *J. Rehabil. Med.* 46, 378–382. doi: 10.2340/16501977-1785

Müller-Putz, G., and Kaiser, V. (2010). Fast set-up asynchronous brain-switch based on detection of foot motor imagery in 1-channel EEG. *Med. Biol. Eng. Comput.* 48, 229–233. doi: 10.1007/s11517-009-0572-7

Müller-Putz, G. R., Daly, I., and Kaiser, V. (2014). Motor imagery-induced EEG patterns in individuals with spinal cord injury and their impact on brain-computer interface accuracy. *J. Neural Eng.* 11, 035011. doi: 10.1088/1741-2560/11/3/035011

Niazi, I. K., Jiang, N., Tiberghien, O., Nielsen, J. F., Dremstrup, K., and Farina, D. (2011). Detection of movement intention from single-trial movement-related cortical potentials. *J. Neural Eng.* 8, 066009. doi: 10.1088/1741-2560/8/6/066009

Niazi, I. K., Mrachacz-Kersting, N., Jiang, N., Dremstrup, K., and Farina, D. (2012). Peripheral electrical stimulation triggered by self-paced detection of motor intention enhances motor evoked potentials. *IEEE Trans. Neural Rehabil. Syst. Eng.* 20, 595–604. doi: 10.1109/TNSRE.2012.2194309

Ono, T., Shindo, K., Kawashima, K., Ota, N., Ito, M., Ota, T., et al. (2014). Brain-computer interface with somatosensory feedback improves functional recovery from severe hemiplegia due to chronic stroke. *Front. Neuroeng.* 7:19. doi: 10.3389/fneng.2014.00019

Pfurtscheller, G., and Lopes Da Silva, F. H. (1999). Event-related EEG/MEG synchronization and desynchronization: basic principles. *Clin. Neurophysiol.* 110, 1842–1857. doi: 10.1016/S1388-2457(99)00141-8

Pfurtscheller, G., and Solis-Escalante, T. (2009). Could the beta rebound in the EEG be suitable to realize a "brain switch"? *Clin. Neurophysiol.* 120, 24–29. doi: 10.1016/j.clinph.2008.09.027

Planelles, D., Hortal, E., Costa, A., Ubeda, A., Iáez, E., and Azorín, J. M. (2014). Evaluating classifiers to detect arm movement intention from EEG signals. *Sensors (Basel)* 14, 18172–18186. doi: 10.3390/s141018172

Qian, K., Nikolov, P., Huang, D., Fei, D.-Y., Chen, X., and Bai, O. (2010). A motor imagery-based online interactive brain-controlled switch: paradigm development and preliminary test. *Clin. Neurophysiol.* 121, 1304–1313. doi: 10.1016/j.clinph.2010.03.001

Ramos-Murguialday, A., Broetz, D., Rea, M., Läer, L., Yilmaz, O., Brasil, F. L., et al. (2013). Brain-machine interface in chronic stroke rehabilitation: a controlled study. *Ann. Neurol.* 74, 100–108. doi: 10.1002/ana.23879

Shih, J. J., Krusienski, D. J., and Wolpaw, J. R. (2012). Brain-computer interfaces in medicine. *Mayo Clin. Proc.* 87, 268–279. doi: 10.1016/j.mayocp.2011.12.008

Toro, C., Deuschl, G., Thatcher, R., Sato, S., Kufta, C., and Hallett, M. (1994). Event-related desynchronization and movement-related cortical potentials on the ECoG and EEG. *Electroencephalogr. Clin. Neurophysiol. Potentials Sect.* 93, 380–389. doi: 10.1016/0168-5597(94)90126-0

Tran, Y., Boord, P., Middleton, J., and Craig, A. (2004). Levels of brain wave activity (8–13 Hz) in persons with spinal cord injury. *Spinal Cord* 42, 73–79. doi: 10.1038/sj.sc.3101543

Venkatakrishnan, A., Francisco, G. E., and Contreras-Vidal, J. L. (2014). Applications of brain–machine interface systems in stroke recovery and rehabilitation. *Curr. Phys. Med. Rehabil. Reports* 2, 93–105. doi: 10.1007/s40141-014-0051-4

Wang, P. T., King, C. E., Chui, L. A., Do, A. H., and Nenadic, Z. (2012). Self-paced brain-computer interface control of ambulation in a virtual reality environment. *J. Neural Eng.* 9, 056016. doi: 10.1088/1741-2560/9/5/056016

Xu, R., Jiang, N., Lin, C., Mrachacz-Kersting, N., Dremstrup, K., and Farina, D. (2014a). Enhanced low-latency detection of motor intention from EEG for closed-loop brain-computer interface applications. *IEEE Trans. Biomed. Eng.* 61, 288–296. doi: 10.1109/TBME.2013.2294203

Xu, R., Jiang, N., Mrachacz-Kersting, N., Lin, C., Asín, G., Moreno, J. C., et al. (2014b). A closed-loop brain-computer interface triggering an active ankle-foot orthosis for inducing cortical neural plasticity. *IEEE Trans. Biomed. Eng.* 61 2092–2101. doi: 10.1109/TBME.2014.2313867

Xu, R., Jiang, N., Vuckovic, A., Hasan, M., Mrachacz-Kersting, N., Allan, D., et al. (2014c). Movement-related cortical potentials in paraplegic patients: abnormal patterns and considerations for BCI-rehabilitation. *Front. Neuroeng.* 7:35. doi: 10.3389/fneng.2014.00035

Yang, H., Guan, C., Wang, C. C., and Ang, K. K. (2014). Detection of motor imagery of brisk walking from electroencephalogram. *J. Neurosci. Methods* 244, 33–44. doi: 10.1016/j.jneumeth.2014.05.007

Yilmaz, O., Birbaumer, N., and Ramos-Murguialday, A. (2014). Movement related slow cortical potentials in severely paralyzed chronic stroke patients. *Front. Hum. Neurosci.* 8:1033. doi: 10.3389/fnhum.2014.01033

Yuan, H., and He, B. (2014). Brain-computer interfaces using sensorimotor rhythms: current state and future perspectives. *IEEE Trans. Biomed. Eng.* 61, 1425–1435. doi: 10.1109/TBME.2014.2312397

10

Generation of Locomotor-Like Activity in the Isolated Rat Spinal Cord Using Intraspinal Electrical Microstimulation Driven by a Digital Neuromorphic CPG

*Sébastien Joucla[1,2], Matthieu Ambroise[3,4], Timothée Levi[3,4], Thierry Lafon[1,2], Philippe Chauvet[1,2], Sylvain Saïghi[3,4], Yannick Bornat[3,5], Noëlle Lewis[3,4], Sylvie Renaud[3,5] and Blaise Yvert[1,2,6,7]**

[1] Centre National de la Recherche Scientifique, Institute for Cognitive and Integrative Neuroscience (INCIA), UMR 5287, Talence, France, [2] Institute for Cognitive and Integrative Neuroscience (INCIA), UMR 5287, University of Bordeaux, Talence, France, [3] Laboratoire de l'Intégration du Matériau au Système, UMR 5218, University of Bordeaux, Talence, France, [4] Centre National de la Recherche Scientifique, Laboratoire de l'Intégration du Matériau au Système, UMR 5218, Talence, France, [5] Bordeaux INP, Laboratoire de l'Intégration du Matériau au Système, UMR 5218, Talence, France, [6] Institut National de la Santé et de la Recherche Médicale, Clinatec-Lab, U1205, Grenoble, France, [7] Université Grenoble Alpes, Clinatec-Lab, U1205, Grenoble, France

Edited by:
Mikhail Lebedev,
Duke University, USA

Reviewed by:
Wolfgang Stein,
Illinois State University, USA
Johnny Padulo,
eCampus University, Italy
Shawn B. Frost,
University of Kansas Medical Center, USA

***Correspondence:**
Blaise Yvert
blaise.yvert@inserm.fr

Neural prostheses based on electrical microstimulation offer promising perspectives to restore functions following lesions of the central nervous system (CNS). They require the identification of appropriate stimulation sites and the coordination of their activation to achieve the restoration of functional activity. On the long term, a challenging perspective is to control microstimulation by artificial neural networks hybridized to the living tissue. Regarding the use of this strategy to restore locomotor activity in the spinal cord, to date, there has been no proof of principle of such hybrid approach driving intraspinal microstimulation (ISMS). Here, we address a first step toward this goal in the neonatal rat spinal cord isolated *ex vivo*, which can display locomotor-like activity while offering an easy access to intraspinal circuitry. Microelectrode arrays were inserted in the lumbar region to determine appropriate stimulation sites to elicit elementary bursting patterns on bilateral L2/L5 ventral roots. Two intraspinal sites were identified at L1 level, one on each side of the spinal cord laterally from the midline and approximately at a median position dorso-ventrally. An artificial CPG implemented on digital integrated circuit (FPGA) was built to generate alternating activity and was hybridized to the living spinal cord to drive electrical microstimulation on these two identified sites. Using this strategy, sustained left-right and flexor-extensor alternating activity on bilateral L2/L5 ventral roots could be generated in either whole or thoracically transected spinal cords. These results are a first step toward hybrid artificial/biological solutions based on electrical microstimulation for the restoration of lost function in the injured CNS.

Keywords: hybrid neural networks, neural prostheses, neuromorphic hardware, rehabilitation

INTRODUCTION

Following spinal cord injury, neural prosthesis using electrical stimulation of the spinal circuitry below the lesion can be considered to restore functional locomotor capabilities (Giszter, 2008; Borton et al., 2013; Nishimura et al., 2013). These approaches rely on the ability of intraspinal central pattern generators (CPGs) to generate locomotor rhythms even when isolated from descending inputs, as first assessed *ex vivo* (Brown, 1911; Grillner et al., 1981; Grillner and Wallén, 1985; Cazalets et al., 1992, 1995; Kjaerulff and Kiehn, 1996), and then confirmed *in vivo* in animals and humans (Dimitrijevic et al., 1998; Ichiyama et al., 2005; Minassian et al., 2007). Based on this property, very promising rehabilitation results have been achieved in rodents using epidural stimulation of lumbar segments combined with pharmacological drug applications and rehabilitation training (Courtine et al., 2008, 2009; Musienko et al., 2009; van den Brand et al., 2012). Such approach also allowed a paraplegic patient to achieve assisted standing and stepping movements with full-weight bearing (Harkema et al., 2011).

Because epidural stimulations can activate large networks from the surface of the spinal cord including proprioceptive fibers, a higher degree of control in the activation of the spinal circuitry may be expected using intraspinal microstimulation (ISMS). It has been found in cats that different stereotyped hindlimb mouvements could be elicited by ISMS delivered on single microelectrodes, depending on the position of the microelectrode. Microstimulations delivered in dorsal L5-S1 segments generally elicit hindlimb flexions, while ventral stimulation mostly evokes hindlimb extension (Tai et al., 2003; Lemay and Grill, 2004). More rostral stimulations delivered in the dorsal half of L3-L5 segments also elicit ipsilateral flexion (Barthélemy et al., 2006). Combining ISMS delivered on the dorsal surface of L3-L7 segments with intraveneous injection of the noradrenergic agonist clonidine could further elicit bilateral locomotion (Barthélemy et al., 2006, 2007). Yet, producing sustained locomotion by intraspinal ISMS solely in absence of drugs remains unachieved. Toward this goal, tonic ISMS delivered at 20–50 Hz on microwires implanted in the lumbar ventral horn to target motoneurons of spinalized cats could elicit episodes of hindlimb flexion, extension, and even alternating sequences (Saigal et al., 2004; Guevremont et al., 2006; Lau et al., 2007).

These encouraging results open the way to the design of autonomous neural prosthesis, where coordinated sequences of ISMS control sustained locomotion. For this purpose, artificial neural networks can be used to drive coordinated ISMS sequences, a method recently used to control intramuscular stimulations to restore locomotor behavior (Vogelstein et al., 2008; Mazurek et al., 2012). Here we address this question in the neonatal rat spinal cord isolated *ex-vivo* and interfaced with a penetrating microelectrode array. This preparation can indeed generate locomotor-like activity under pharmacological activation while offering a direct access to intraspinal networks. Here, our goal was to achieve a proof of principle that an artificial neural network can control ISMS to drive locomotor-like activity in this preparation. Two intraspinal sites were identified at L1 level, the alternated stimulation of which generated locomotor-like activity on bilateral L2/L5 ventral roots. An artificial CPG was then implemented on FPGA to control ISMS on these two sites. This hybrid connection could successfully be used to generate lumbar locomotor-like rhythms in a whole and a transected spinal cord.

METHODS

Ethics Statement

All experimental protocols conformed to recommendations of the European Community Council Directive of November 24, 1986 (86/609/EEC) and local French legislation for care and use of laboratory animals. They were approved by the local ethical committee of Bordeaux under recommendation No A5012083.

Experimental Preparation and Recording

Whole spinal cord and medulla from newborn Sprague Dawley rats at postnatal stage between P1 and P3 (**Figure 1A**) were dissected in a cooled artificial CSF (aCSF) solution (pH 7.5) gassed with carbogen (95% O_2 and 5% CO_2) and composed of (in mM): 113 NaCl, 4.5 KCl, 2 $CaCl_2 2H_2O$, 1 $MgCl_2 6H_2O$, 25 $NaHCO_3$, 1 $NaH_2PO_4H_2O$, and 11 D-Glucose. Bilateral L2 and L5 ventral roots were recorded using succion glass electrodes. Ventral root signals were amplified with a gain of 750, band-pass filtered between 0.08 Hz and 3 kHz, and then sampled at a rate of 20 kHz using the previously developed NeuroPXI system (Bonnet et al., 2012), which is an extended version of the former BioMEA system (Charvet et al., 2010). As shown in **Figure 1B**, this preparation exhibits locomotor-like activity under the application of 5-HT (5 μM), NMA (10 μM), and Dopamine (50 μM), and is thus a good model to explore rehabilitation strategies *in vitro* with an easy access to intraspinal networks. The cords were superfused for 10 min with this cocktail to check that locomotor-like activity could be elicited pharmacology in each preparation prior to hybrid experiments. The drugs were rinsed for at least 60 min to let ventral root activity return to baseline before hybrid experiments started.

Data Processing

Raw ventral root signals were processed as follows to extract spiking activity (see also Heim et al., 2012): for each data sample, a moving average of the signal computed over a 10-ms window centered on this sample was first subtracted from the raw data (DC-removing), and then the obtained value was replaced by the average of the signal computed over a 1-ms time window centered on this sample (smoothing). Signals were then integrated to assess alternating patterns using polar representations and statistics. For this purpose, the signals were first blanked over a period ranging from 15 ms before the stimulation to 150 ms after, and then integrated with a time constant of 0.2 s (see gray traces superimposed on spiking activity in **Figure 1B**) and finally smoothed with a window of 1 s. The statistical significance of the phase relationship between bursting activity recorded on two different ventral roots was

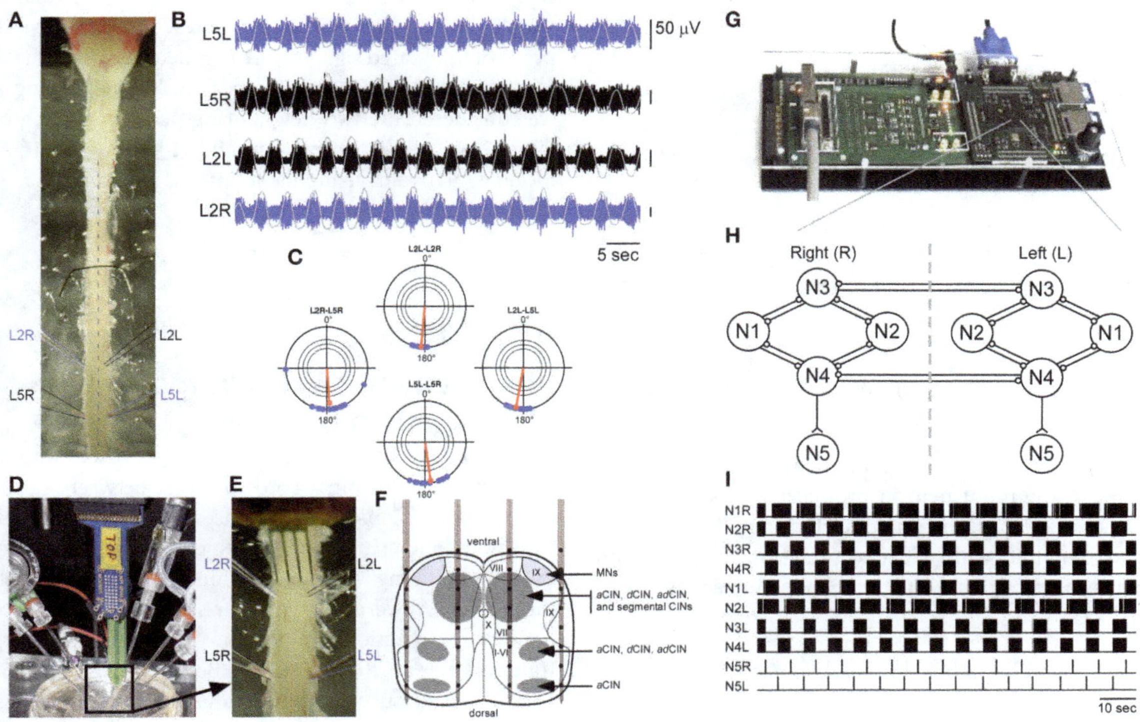

FIGURE 1 | Experimental paradigm. (A) Neonatal rat preparation. **(B)** Example of locomotor-like activity on bilateral L2 and L5 ventral roots. Integrated and smoothed traces are superimposed in gray. **(C)** This rhythm can be represented as four polar plots showing the antiphase relationship (180° angle in the plot) between two recordings of same level ipsi and contralateral ventral roots, as well as between two levels on the same side. In each plot, the three concentric circles indicate significance levels of the Rayleigh test at $P < 0.05$, $P < 0.01$, and $P < 0.001$. **(D,E)** View of the experimental setup showing simultaneous ventral root recordings and a 4-shank multichannel neural probe inserted at L1 level for ISMS. **(F)** Schematic representation of the neural probe in the transverse plane of the lumbar spinal cord adapted from Kiehn and Butt (2003). MNs, Motoneurons; CINs, Commissural interneurons; a, ascending; d, descending. **(G)** The multimed platform housing the artificial CPG implemented in an FPGA. **(H)** Structure of the artificial CPG ("o" connections are inhibitory, "<" connections are excitatory). **(I)** Example of the activity of all neurons of the artificial CPG. Neurons N5L and N5R were used to trigger ISMS at the time of every of their spikes.

ıssessed using a Rayleigh test on the delays between the peaks ›f both integrated signals normalized to 360°. **Figure 1C** shows he typical polar representation of a locomotor-like activity licited pharmacologically, with antiphase locking between L2 ınd L5 ventral roots on each side and left-right L2 or L5 ›airs.

:lectrical Stimulation

ıs shown in **Figures 1D–F**, electrical microstimulations were elivered on single microelectrodes of Neuronexus neural probes ıade of four shanks separated by 400 µm, each containing ight 30-µm-diameter microelectrodes separated by 100 µm ›robe model A4x8-5 mm-100-400-703-A32). Based on earlier :udies showing the localization of rat CPGs (Cazalets et al., 995; Antri et al., 2011), the neural probe was inserted at the 1 level of the spinal cord. Depending on the preparation, etween 15 and 26 sites of the probe were individually tested ›r stimulation. Each stimulation consisted of a train of 10 iphasic pulses separated by 1 ms. Each pulse was charge-alanced with an initial cathodic phase of 500 µs and an nplitude of typically 150–300 µA, immediately followed by a) times longer anodic phase of 10 times smaller amplitude. Stimulations were monopolar with respect to a distant electrode in the bath.

Artificial CPG

An artificial CPG neural network inspired from Hill et al. (2001) was implemented onto a configurable digital integrated circuit (FPGA), supported by an electronic platform designed at IMS (**Figure 1G**). The implementation of this network is fully described in Ambroise et al. (2013). In brief, the core CPG network shown in **Figure 1H** consisted of two symmetric sub-networks of four regular spiking neurons (N1L-N4L and N1R-N4R in **Figure 1H**). These eight neurons have identical biomimetic dynamics following the Izhikevich model (Izhikevich, 2003) and are interconnected by reciprocal inhibitory $GABA_A$-like synapses. Synaptic efficiency was governed by activity-dependent depression (Tabak et al., 2000). The dynamics of each neuron was thus governed by four parameters a, b, c, and d according to the following differential equations:

$$\frac{dv}{dt} = \frac{v^2}{32} + 4v + 109.375 - u + I_{bias} + \sum_{i=1}^{Nsynapses} I_{syn}^{i}$$

$$\frac{du}{dt} = a(bv - u)$$

with the after-spike resetting condition:

$$\text{if } v \geq 30mV \text{ then } \begin{cases} v \leftarrow c \\ u \leftarrow u + d \end{cases}$$

where the other parameter I_{bias} is a constant bias current and I^{isyn} is the synaptic current received from the ith input neurons. For each input, the synaptic current I_{syn} is governed by the following equation:

$$\frac{dI_{syn}}{dt} = -\frac{I_{syn}}{\tau_{syn}} + (1 - \lambda_{syn}) \cdot W_{syn} \cdot \delta(t - t_{spike}),$$

where τ_{syn} is the synaptic current decay time constant, $\delta(t - t_{spike}) = 1$ if the input neuron produces a spike at time t and 0 otherwise, and λ_{syn} is the synaptic efficiency. The synaptic efficiency was dynamic with a decay time constant τ_{reg} and synaptic depression modeled through the following equations:

$$\frac{d\lambda_{syn}}{dt} = -\frac{\lambda_{syn}}{\tau_{reg}} \cdot (1 - \delta(t - t_{spike})) + P \cdot (1 - \lambda_{syn})\delta(t - t_{spike}),$$

where P is a dissipation percentage parameter decreasing synaptic efficiency after each spike.

The design was optimized to cost few digital resources on the FPGA while running in real-time at the ms resolution (Ambroise et al., 2013). Both sub-networks of the CPG produced alternating rhythmic bursting activity (**Figure 1I**). The resulting bursting activity was integrated for each sub-network by a fifth spiking neuron (N5L and N5R in **Figure 1H**), producing only one spike per burst, and representing the CPG output neurons. In the current system version, each parameter change in the neural network model requires a new synthesis of the FPGA configuration, which is done by the implementation of a new configuration file (bit file) from the computer to the FPGA, a procedure taking several seconds. Further versions will allow dynamic reconfiguration of the FPGA, thus allowing online synaptic adaptation for example.

Hybridization of the Artificial CPG to the Spinal Cord

The CPG output neurons produced a rhythmic left-right alternating activity made of 1 spike per cycle on each network side. These output spikes were used to trigger intraspinal electrical microstimulations on two different microelectrodes of the neural probe, one on each side of the spinal cord.

Statistical Analysis

The statistical significance of alternating patterns of bursting activity recorded on two ventral roots VR1 and VR2 was assessed by a circular Rayleigh test performed on the angular values of individual bursts. The amplitude of the Rayleigh statistics was compared to three significance levels ($P < 0.05$, $P < 0.01$, and $P < 0.001$) represented as different circles on the polar representations in **Figures 1C, 3C, 4C**. The angular values on which the test was performed were computed as follows. The peaks of integrated signals were first detected on each ventral root for each burst. Then, for each peak of VR2 occurring at time t2, we considered the two neighboring peaks occurring before and after t2 on VR1 (t1_prev ≤ t2 and t1_after ≥ t2) to compute a local angular value using the following relation:

$$\phi = \frac{\pi}{2} + 2\pi \frac{t_2 - t_{1prev}}{t_{1after} - t_{1prev}}$$

RESULTS

Identification of Two Intraspinal Microstimulation Sites

An initial set of 10 preparations were used to identify the best levels of the spinal cord to target between T11 and L5 in order to elicit consistent responses on the L2/L5 ventral roots. This was done using either a single glass pipette microelectrode or a penetrating shank. We found that ISMS delivered at the L1 level were the most reliable. We then considered 6 other preparations in which we inserted a 4 × 8 probe transversally at the L1 level. Between 15 and 26 contacts were scanned successfully at different current intensity levels between 40 and 800 μA. We initially tested classical symmetrical biphasic pulses (cathodic-first with a cathodic phase of 500 μs), and found that they were less efficient than balanced but non-symmetrical pulses where the anodic phase was twice weaker and longer. Cathodic current intensities above 150 μA were generally required to obtain reliable responses on the ventral roots. As shown in **Figure 2**, we found that ISMS at L1 level elicited different burst responses on bilateral L2/L5 ventral roots depending on the location of the stimulation site. ISMS delivered dorsolaterally elicited a burst on the ipsilateral L2 ventral root (**Figures 2A,B**). Stimulations delivered dorsomedially typically elicited a response on both ipsilateral L2 and L5 ventral roots (as in **Figure 2C**), and occasionally also on the contralateral L5 ventral root. Consistently across preparations, we identified two intraspinal sites, one on each side of the spinal cord located about 200 μm laterally from the midline and approximately at a median position dorso ventrally near the central canal (about 400 μm from the dorsal surface). We found that a stimulation delivered on either site elicited a burst response simultaneously on the ipsilateral L2 and contralateral L5 motor outputs (**Figures 2D,E**). This result thus opened the possibility to generate locomotor-like activity using coordinated stimulation between these two stimulation sites.

Generation of Alternating Patterns Using the Artificial CPG

The eight neurons of the core network had the following identical parameters that were found to lead to a robust alternating activity on the output neurons of the CPG: $a = 0.02$, $b = 0.2$, $c = -65$, $d = 8$, and $I_{bias} = 8$. The time constant τ_{syn} of the exponential decay of synaptic current was set to 100 ms. For output synapses from neurons N2R and N2L, w

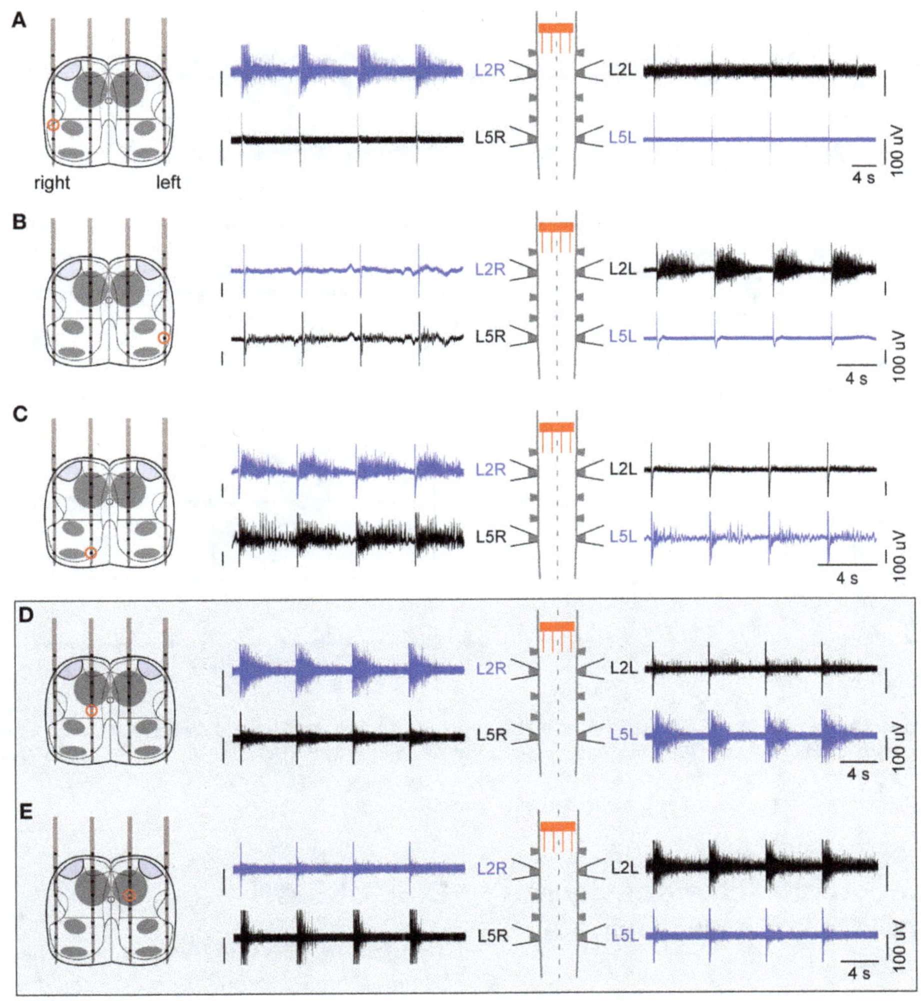

FIGURE 2 | Ventral root responses to ISMS at L1 level. ISMS elicited different responses depending on the site of stimulation. **(A,B)** Dorsolateral stimulations elicited a burst response mainly on the ipsilateral L2 ventral root. **(C)** Example of a more medial stimulation eliciting a response on ipsilateral L2 and L5 ventral roots. **(D,E)** Importantly, ISMS delivered medially on either side of the central canal elicited a burst response on the diagonal L2 ipsilateral and L5 contralateral. These specific intraspinal locations were found consistently across preparations and thus further used for the hybrid experiments. For all panels, a sequence of four stimulations is illustrated.

ısed $W_{syn} = -1.26$ and $P = 0.1\%$; for input synapses onto ıeurons N2R and N2L, we used $W_{syn} = -3$ and $P = 0.03\%$. For all other inhibitory synapses, we used $W_{syn} = -3.8$ and $P = 0.03\%$. The output layer neurons N5R and N5L received excitatory AMPA-like connections respectively from N4R and N4L, both defined by $W_{syn} = 30$ and $P = 90\%$. The initial conditions were $v = -20$ and $u = -4$ for N1R, N3L, N4L, N2R neurons, $v = 0$ and $u = 0$ for N1L, N3R, N4R, N2L, and $v = -65$ and $u = -13$ for N5R and N5L. With these parameters, each CPG bursting activity pattern generated one spike on N5L and one spike on N5R, used as trigger for delivering microstimulation to the spinal cord. The stimulation is only triggered by the CPG output and consisted of a short train of 10 stimuli (see Methods). By changing τ_{reg} (from 4 to 12 s), the artificial CPG alternating period could be modulated between 2 and 7 s.

Generation of Locomotor-Like Activity in a Whole *Ex-vivo* Spinal Cord Using a Hybrid Connection

In a first step, we made a hybrid connection between the artificial CPG and a whole spinal cord. The output neuron of each side of the artificial CPG controlled intraspinal stimulations on one of the intraspinal stimulation site (**Figure 3A**). Each spike of an artificial output neuron triggered one stimulation on the corresponding intraspinal site. Using this strategy, clear locomotor-like activity could be obtained on bilateral L2 and L5 ventral roots (**Figures 3B,C**). Once the artificial CPG was turned on, this activity established at the first or second stimulation, remained robust with a 1:1 correspondence to the artificially imposed pace as long as the artificial CPG was ON, and then vanished as soon as the CPG was turned off.

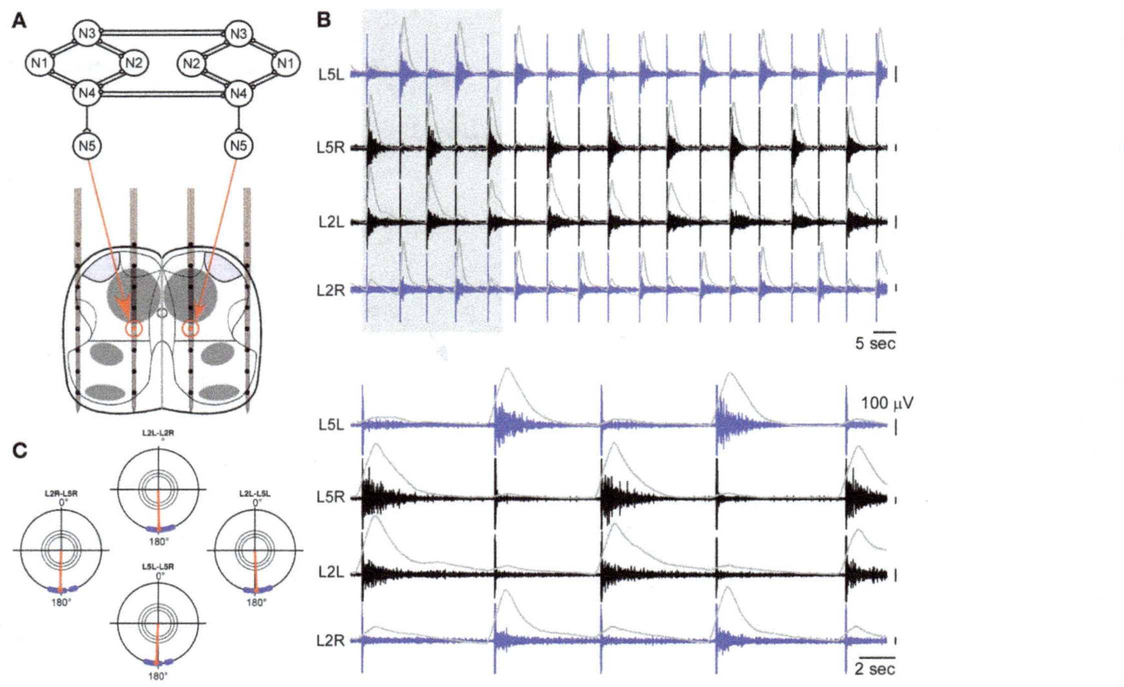

FIGURE 3 | Hybrid experiment in the case of a whole spinal cord. (A) Schematic representation of the hybrid connection between the output neurons of the artificial CPG and the two intraspinal stimulation sites. **(B)** Ventral root responses to a sequence of ISMS (150 and 200 μA for the cathodic phase on the left and right sites, respectively) driven by the artificial CPG at a cycle frequency of 6.7 s (integrated traces shown in gray), showing clear left-right and ipsilateral alternating patterns (top: 2 min, bottom 30 s). **(C)** Polar representation of this induced rhythm as in **Figure 1C**.

Generation of Locomotor-Like Activity in a Transected Spinal Cord *Ex-vivo* Using a Hybrid Connection

In a second step, we tested whether this result could also be obtained in a lumbar spinal cord fully isolated from descending inputs to mimic a lesion situation. We thus considered another preparation, which was transected at the T7 level (**Figure 4A**). The same type of hybrid connection was used between the artificial CPG and the intraspinal stimulation sites. As shown in **Figures 4B,C**, this strategy could also successfully elicit locomotor-like activity on bilateral L2 and L5 ventral roots. The locomotor pattern could be maintained for more than 7 min as long as the artificial CPG was ON. Moreover, several periods of alternating cycle were tested in this preparation spanning the range allowed by the artificial CPG (2.6, 3.1, 4, 5.2, and 6.7 s between successive left and right stimulations). We found that the spinal cord could follow the imposed rhythm in an exact 1:1 correspondence at these different frequencies for the whole durations of the hybrid connection tested: 560 s at of 6.7 s (84 left+right stimulations), 430 s at 5.2 s (85 stimulations), 369 s at 4 s (97 stimulations), 392 s at 3.1 s (123 stimulations), and 363 s at 2.6 s (217 stimulations). The artificial CPG was limited to these period values and we thus could not test higher speeds to see when the spinal cord would stop following the artificial network. Nevertheless, the tested frequencies covered the pace of a pharmacologically-evoked rhythm with inter-burst period around 5 s on each ventral root (as shown in **Figure 1B**).

DISCUSSION

The goal of this study was to test whether ISMS controlled by an artificial neural network could in principle be used to restore locomotor-like activity in a transected spinal cord. This proof of principle was achieved here in the neonatal rat spinal cord isolated *ex vivo*, using the advantage that this preparation can display locomotor rhythms while offering a direct access to intraspinal networks. This paradigm allowed identifying appropriate intraspinal sites for stimulation, which were localized on either side of the central canal at L1 level. Efficient stimulations could be obtained for current levels of the order of 150–300 μA. These current amplitudes were higher than those generally used in previous *in vivo* studies to elicit limb movements using ISMS in cats (Guevremont et al., 2006) and rats (Shahdoost et al., 2014). One possibility could be the difference in the frequency of the pulse train between these studies and our paradigm. Here we used only 1 ms between two successive pulses of the same train, while *in vivo* ISMS typically used lower frequency 40–50-Hz trains, likely to be more efficient. Moreover the level of excitability of the CPGs might be different between our *ex vivo* situation at room temperature and the *in vivo* context where the complete network including sensory feedbacks remain present. Also, the activity elicited here on the ventral roots did not result from a direct activation of the motoneurons since a stimulation delivered on a precise site in L1 elicited activity simultaneously on the ipsilateral L2 and the contralateral L5. Thus, we created an indirect activation of the motoneurons, likely

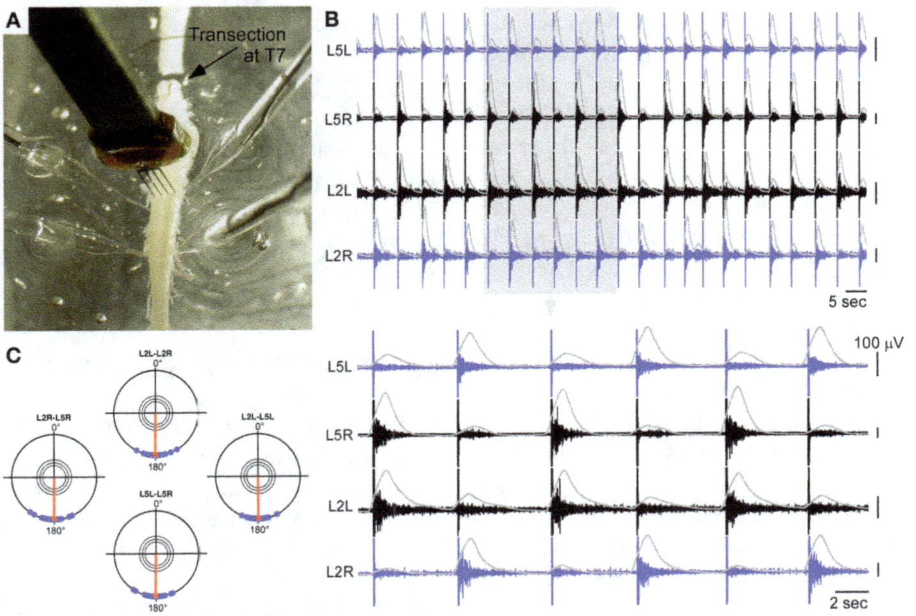

FIGURE 4 | Hybrid experiment in the case of a spinal cord transected at T7. (A) Picture of the experiments showing the transection, the 4 ventral root recordings, and the neural probe used to deliver ISMS. **(B)** Ventral root responses to a sequence of ISMS (300 μA for the cathodic phase on each site) driven by the artificial CPG at a cycle frequency of 5.2 s (integrated traces shown in gray), showing clear left-right and ipsilateral alternating patterns (top: 2 min, bottom 30 s). **(C)** Polar representation of this induced rhythm as in **Figure 1C**.

›y activating a group of interneurons participating in the lumbar ⊐PG. It is possible that higher stimulation intensities are required ›o robustly activate the whole CPG rather than generating more liscrete muscle contractions. As a result and based on previous ;tudies (Ranck, 1975; Yeomans et al., 1986; Joucla et al., 2012), t is likely that the currents we used typically activated neurons within a distance of about 250–500 μm from the electrode. Nevertheless, we could verify experimentally the specificity of our SMS. Indeed, many electrode positions of the same probe were ested for stimulation and, as illustrated in **Figure 2**, the response o ISMS on the four ventral roots greatly depended on the site ›f stimulation. In particular, there was a clear dissociation of the esponse for the two stimulation sites that we identified on each ide of the central canal, which were separated by typically only 00 μm and yet triggered completely different output patterns opposite L2-L5 diagonals). Using adjacent sites of the same hanks distant by only 100 μm from the optimal stimulation ites did not produce consistent activation of the L2-L5 diagonal. ctually, the fact that we were able to reproduce locomotor-like ctivity patterns by coordinating ISMS on these two sites was recisely based on this dissociation.

The localization of the two intraspinal sites was in the region f the lumbar CPGs, which have previously been localized at ie upper lumbar region within T13 and L2 segments (Cazalets al., 1995; Kjaerulff and Kiehn, 1996). The ISMS positions lentified here fall in this region and are close to several asses of projecting commissural interneurons (Kiehn and Butt,)03). Moreover, these locations are also consistent with a high ensity of neurons involved in alternating locomotor activity, entified between L1 and L2 levels with calcium imaging (Antri et al., 2011). Altogether this suggests that ISMS may activate elements of the lumbar CPGs responsible for the coordination of opposite L2 and L5 motoneuronal pools, maybe through the direct activation of commissural interneurons. It should be noted that each stimulation typically triggered only one burst episode on output roots (as clearly seen in **Figures 2–4**). Thus, all bursts were followers of the stimulation pulses. In particular, no wind-up was observed since bursts disappeared as soon as the stimulation stopped, and the frequency of the locomotor pattern could be imposed by the frequency of the artificial CPG. For these reasons, it is possible that each stimulation activated a group of interneurons participating in the lumbar CPG, and that the coordination of two stimulation sites could allow reproducing locomotor-like activity by the coordinated activation of these groups.

The quest for fully autonomous neural prosthesis based on hybrid connections between the CNS and artificial neural networks is a tremendous challenge. Here, we only performed a first step toward this goal by making a unidirectional (open-loop) connection between an artificial CPG and the spinal cord circuitry. In this work, the artificial network was initially configured with proper parameters to exhibit adequate alternating rhythmic activity. In particular, modifying the frequency of the rhythm required a manual reconfiguration and re-synthesis of the network in the FPGA. Further versions of the CPG hardware implementation will offer the possibility to modulate its dynamics in real time. This will then open the possibility to build bidirectional hybrid connections, where supralesional activity can be used to control the artificial network dynamically in order to achieve a close loop artificial connection over the lesion. In particular, future developments could include paradigms where the artificial network would be dynamically controlled and/or modulated by inputs from supraspinal and/or intraspinal supralesional information, and possibly modulated in real time by sensory feedbacks produced after ISMS in preparations preserving whole hindlimbs attached to the spinal cord.

As a further perspective, such hybrid approach will also need to be extended *in vivo* in order to assess whether it can also help recover locomotion capabilities in adult animals subject to chronic spinal cord lesions. While this has started to be addressed using ISMS in spinal cats (Guevremont et al., 2006; Mazurek et al., 2012), little ISMS work has yet been obtained in rats (Shahdoost et al., 2014). Previous lesion results in adult rats showed that destruction of the gray matter at T13-L2 level induce severe locomotor deficits, while more caudal lesions have more limited influence (Magnuson et al., 2005), suggesting a localization of neonatal lumbar CPGs consistent with those of adult animals. Yet, whether the two stimulation sites identified in this study remain conserved in adulthood to elicit locomotor movements in spinal animals remain to be tested. Moreover, in the case of chronic animal models of paralysis, lesions may induce remodeling of intraspinal circuits on the long term (Dietz and Müller, 2004), which may change the way networks could be activated. However, previous studies indicate that despite such plastic changes, lumbar CPG circuitry remain present and can be reactivated below the lesion with training to recover functional locomotion (Barrière et al., 2008; van den Brand et al., 2012). An open question is whether such rehabilitation perspective can also be obtained using active neural prosthesis solely based on ISMS. Chronical experiments will thus be necessary to determine if the spinal circuitry below the lesion may also be exploited through hybrid connections with artificial neural networks to recover locomotor functions with autonomous spinal neural prosthesis.

CONCLUSION

In conclusion, the present study is a first demonstration of a hybrid interconnexion between a living spinal cord and an artificial neural network driving ISMS to restore functional activity. These results are a first step toward intelligent neural prostheses based on hybrid live/artificial connections for the restoration of lost function in the injured CNS.

AUTHOR CONTRIBUTIONS

SJ, SR, and BY designed the study. MA, TLe, SS, YB, NL, and SR designed the artificial CPG and associated electronics (Multimed system). SJ, MA, TLa, PC, and BY developed the experimental setup. SJ and MA performed the experiments. SJ and BY analyzed the data. SJ, TL, SS, NL, SR, and BY wrote the manuscript.

ACKNOWLEDGMENTS

This work was supported by the French National Research Agency (ANR) under the Hyrene project No ANR-BLAN-0316 and by the European Union's Seventh Framework Programme (ICT-FET FP7/2007-2103, FET Young Explorers scheme) under the grant agreement n°284772 BRAINBOW. The funders had no role in study design, data collection and analysis, decision to publish, or preparation of the manuscript. The authors also wish to thank Nathalie Argenta and Dominique Panzeri (INCIA) for taking care of the animals, Eric Basier (INCIA) and Gilles N'Kaoua (IMS) for technical help, and Lionel Rousseau and Gaëlle Lissorgues from ESIEE-Paris for constructive discussions.

REFERENCES

Ambroise, M., Levi, T., Joucla, S., Yvert, B., and Saïghi, S. (2013). Real-time biomimetic central pattern generators into FPGA for hybrid experiments. *Front. Neurosci.* 7:215. doi: 10.3389/fnins.2013.00215

Antri, M., Mellen, N., and Cazalets, J. R. (2011). Functional organization of locomotor interneurons in the ventral lumbar spinal cord of the newborn rat. *PLoS ONE* 6:e20529. doi: 10.1371/journal.pone.0020529

Barrière, G., Leblond, H., Provencher, J., and Rossignol, S. (2008). Prominent role of the spinal central pattern generator in the recovery of locomotion after partial spinal cord injuries. *J. Neurosci.* 28, 3976–3987. doi: 10.1523/JNEUROSCI.5692-07.2008

Barthélemy, D., Leblond, H., Provencher, J., and Rossignol, S. (2006). Nonlocomotor and locomotor hindlimb responses evoked by electrical microstimulation of the lumbar cord in spinalized cats. *J. Neurophysiol.* 96, 3273–3292. doi: 10.1152/jn.00203.2006

Barthélemy, D., Leblond, H., and Rossignol, S. (2007). Characteristics and mechanisms of locomotion induced by intraspinal microstimulation and dorsal root stimulation in spinal cats. *J. Neurophysiol.* 97, 1986–2000 doi: 10.1152/jn.00818.2006

Bonnet, S., Bêche, J.-F., Gharbi, S., Abdoun, O., Bocquelet, F., Joucla, S., et al. (2012). A real-time multi-electrode array system for recording, processing and stimulation of neural networks and the control of high-resolution neural implants for rehabilitation. *IRBM* 33, 55–60. doi: 10.1016/j.irbm.2012.01.013

Borton, D., Micera, S., Millán, J. D. R., and Courtine, G. (2013). Personalized neuroprosthetics. *Sci. Transl. Med.* 5:210rv2. doi: 10.1126/scitranslmed.3005968

Brown, G. T. (1911). The intrinsic factors in the act of progression in the mammal. *Proc. R. Soc. Lond. B Biol. Sci.* 84, 308–319. doi: 10.1098/rspb.1911.0077

Cazalets, J. R., Borde, M., and Clarac, F. (1995). Localization and organization of the central pattern generator for hindlimb locomotion in newborn rat. *J. Neurosci.* 15, 4943–4951.

Cazalets, J. R., Sqalli-Houssaini, Y., and Clarac, F. (1992). Activation of the central pattern generators for locomotion by serotonin and excitatory amino acids in neonatal rat. *J. Physiol.* 455, 187–204. doi: 10.1113/jphysiol.1992.sp019296

Charvet, G., Rousseau, L., Billoint, O., Gharbi, S., Rostaing, J. P., Joucla, S., et al. (2010). BioMEA: A versatile high-density 3D microelectrode array system using integrated electronics. *Biosens. Bioelectron.* 25, 1889–1896. doi: 10.1016/j.bios.2010.01.001

Courtine, G., Gerasimenko, Y., van den Brand, R., Yew, A., Musienko, P., Zhong, H., et al. (2009). Transformation of nonfunctional spinal circuits into functional states after the loss of brain input. *Nat. Neurosci.* 12, 1333–1342 doi: 10.1038/nn.2401

Courtine, G., Song, B., Roy, R. R., Zhong, H., Herrmann, J. E., Ao, Y., et al. (2008). Recovery of supraspinal control of stepping via indirect propriospinal relay connections after spinal cord injury. *Nat. Med.* 14, 69–74. doi: 10.1038/nm168

Dietz, V., and Müller, R. (2004). Degradation of neuronal function following spinal cord injury: mechanisms and countermeasures. *Brain* 127, 2221–223 doi: 10.1093/brain/awh255

Dimitrijevic, M. R., Gerasimenko, Y., and Pinter, M. M. (1998). Evidence for a spinal central pattern generator in humans. *Ann. N.Y. Acad. Sci.* 860, 360–376. doi: 10.1111/j.1749-6632.1998.tb09062.x

Giszter, S. F. (2008). Spinal cord injury: present and future therapeutic devices and prostheses. *Neurotherapeutics* 5, 147–162 doi: 10.1016/j.nurt.2007.10.062

Grillner, S., McClellan, A., Sigvardt, K., Wallén, P., and Wilén, M. (1981). Activation of NMDA-receptors elicits "fictive locomotion" in lamprey spinal cord *in vitro*. *Acta Physiol. Scand.* 113, 549–551. doi: 10.1111/j.1748-1716.1981.tb06937.x

Grillner, S., and Wallén, P. (1985). Central pattern generators for locomotion, with special reference to vertebrates. *Annu. Rev. Neurosci.* 8, 233–261. doi: 10.1146/annurev.ne.08.030185.001313

Guevremont, L., Renzi, C. G., Norton, J. A., Kowalczewski, J., Saigal, R., and Mushahwar, V. K. (2006). Locomotor-related networks in the lumbosacral enlargement of the adult spinal cat: activation through intraspinal microstimulation. *IEEE Trans. Neural Syst. Rehabil. Eng.* 14, 266–272. doi: 10.1109/TNSRE.2006.881592

Harkema, S., Gerasimenko, Y., Hodes, J., Burdick, J., Angeli, C., Chen, Y., et al. (2011). Effect of epidural stimulation of the lumbosacral spinal cord on voluntary movement, standing, and assisted stepping after motor complete paraplegia: a case study. *Lancet* 377, 1938–1947 doi: 10.1016/S0140-6736(11)60547-3

Heim, M., Rousseau, L., Reculusa, S., Urbanova, V., Mazzocco, C., Joucla, S., et al. (2012). Combined macro/mesoporous microelectrode arrays (MEAs) for low noise extracellular recording of neural networks. *J. Neurophysiol.* 108, 1793–1803 doi: 10.1152/jn.00711.2011

Hill, A. A., Lu, J., Masino, M. A., Olsen, O. H., and Calabrese, R. L. (2001). A model of a segmental oscillator in the leech heartbeat neuronal network. *J. Comput. Neurosci.* 10, 281–302 doi: 10.1023/A:1011216131638

Ichiyama, R. M., Gerasimenko, Y. P., Zhong, H., Roy, R. R., and Edgerton, V. R. (2005). Hindlimb stepping movements in complete spinal rats induced by epidural spinal cord stimulation. *Neurosci. Lett.* 383, 339–344 doi: 10.1016/j.neulet.2005.04.049

Izhikevich, E. M. (2003). Simple model of spiking neurons. *IEEE Trans. Neural Netw.* 14, 1569–1572. doi: 10.1109/TNN.2003.820440

Joucla, S., Branchereau, P., Cattaert, D., and Yvert, B. (2012). Extracellular neural microstimulation may activate much larger regions than expected by simulations: a combined experimental and modeling study. *PLoS ONE* 7:e41324. doi: 10.1371/journal.pone.0041324

Kiehn, O., and Butt, S. J. (2003). Physiological, anatomical and genetic identification of CPG neurons in the developing mammalian spinal cord. *Prog. Neurobiol.* 70, 347–361. doi: 10.1016/S0301-0082(03)00091-1

Kjaerulff, O., and Kiehn, O. (1996). Distribution of networks generating and coordinating locomotor activity in the neonatal rat spinal cord *in vitro*: a lesion study. *J. Neurosci.* 16:5777–5794.

Lau, B., Guevremont, L., and Mushahwar, V. K. (2007). Strategies for generating prolonged functional standing using intramuscular stimulation or intraspinal microstimulation. *IEEE Trans. Neural Syst. Rehabil. Eng.* 15, 273–285. doi: 10.1109/TNSRE.2007.897030

Lemay, M. A., and Grill, W. M. (2004). Modularity of motor output evoked by intraspinal microstimulation in cats. *J. Neurophysiol.* 91, 502–514. doi: 10.1152/jn.00235.2003

Magnuson, D. S. K., Lovett, R., Coffee, C., Gray, R., Han, Y., Zhang, Y. P., et al. (2005). Functional consequences of lumbar spinal cord contusion injuries in the adult rat. *J. Neurotrauma* 22, 529–543. doi: 10.1089/neu.2005.22.529

Mazurek, K. A., Holinski, B. J., Everaert, D. G., Stein, R. B., Etienne-Cummings, R., and Mushahwar, V. K. (2012). Feed forward and feedback control for over-ground locomotion in anaesthetized cats. *J. Neural Eng.* 9, 26003. doi: 10.1088/1741-2560/9/2/026003

Minassian, K., Persy, I., Rattay, F., Pinter, M. M., Kern, H., and Dimitrijevic, M. R. (2007). Human lumbar cord circuitries can be activated by extrinsic tonic input to generate locomotor-like activity. *Hum. Mov. Sci.* 26, 275–295. doi: 10.1016/j.humov.2007.01.005

Musienko, P., van den Brand, R., Maerzendorfer, O., Larmagnac, A., and Courtine, G. (2009). Combinatory electrical and pharmacological neuroprosthetic interfaces to regain motor function after spinal cord injury. *IEEE Trans. Biomed. Eng.* 56, 2707–2711. doi: 10.1109/TBME.2009.2027226

Nishimura, Y., Perlmutter, S. I., and Fetz, E. E. (2013). Restoration of upper limb movement via artificial corticospinal and musculospinal connections in a monkey with spinal cord injury. *Front. Neural Circuits* 7:57. doi: 10.3389/fncir.2013.00057

Ranck, J. B. Jr., (1975). Which elements are excited in electrical stimulation of mammalian central nervous system: a review. *Brain Res.* 98, 417–440. doi: 10.1016/0006-8993(75)90364-9

Saigal, R., Renzi, C., and Mushahwar, V. K. (2004). Intraspinal microstimulation generates functional movements after spinal-cord injury. *IEEE Trans. Neural Syst. Rehabil. Eng.* 12, 430–440 doi: 10.1109/TNSRE.2004.837754

Shahdoost, S., Frost, S., Acker, G., Van Dejong, S., Barbay, S., Nudo, R., et al. (2014). "Towards a miniaturized brain-machine-spinal cord interface (bmsi) for restoration of function after spinal cord injury," in *36th Annual International Conference of the IEEE Engineering in Medicince and Biology Society* (Chicago, IL), 486–489.

Tabak, J., Senn, W., O'Donovan, M. J., and Rinzel, J. (2000). Modeling of spontaneous activity in developing spinal cord using activity-dependent depression in an excitatory network. *J. Neurosci.* 20, 3041–3056.

Tai, C., Booth, A. M., Robinson, C. J., de Groat, W. C., and Roppolo, J. R. (2003). Multi-joint movement of the cat hindlimb evoked by microstimulation of the lumbosacral spinal cord. *Exp. Neurol.* 183, 620–627. doi: 10.1016/S0014-4886(03)00210-3

van den Brand, R., Heutschi, J., Barraud, Q., DiGiovanna, J., Bartholdi, K., Huerlimann, M., et al. (2012). Restoring voluntary control of locomotion after paralyzing spinal cord injury. *Science* 336, 1182–1185. doi: 10.1126/science.1217416

Vogelstein, R. J., Tenore, F., Guevremont, L., Etienne-Cummings, R., and Mushahwar, V. K. (2008). A silicon central pattern generator controls locomotion *in vivo*. *IEEE Trans. Biomed. Circuits Syst.* 2, 212–222. doi: 10.1109/TBCAS.2008.2001867

Yeomans, J., Prior, P., and Bateman, F. (1986). Current-distance relations of axons mediating circling elicited by midbrain stimulation. *Brain Res.* 372, 95–106. doi: 10.1016/0006-8993(86)91462-9

11

Proceedings of the Third Annual Deep Brain Stimulation Think Tank: A Review of Emerging Issues and Technologies

P. Justin Rossi[1], Aysegul Gunduz[1], Jack Judy[1], Linda Wilson[2], Andre Machado[3], James J. Giordano[4], W. Jeff Elias[5], Marvin A. Rossi[6], Christopher L. Butson[7], Michael D. Fox[8], Cameron C. McIntyre[9], Nader Pouratian[10], Nicole C. Swann[11], Coralie de Hemptinne[11], Robert E. Gross[12], Howard J. Chizeck[13], Michele Tagliati[14], Andres M. Lozano[15], Wayne Goodman[16], Jean-Philippe Langevin[17], Ron L. Alterman[8], Umer Akbar[18], Greg A. Gerhardt[19], Warren M. Grill[20], Mark Hallett[21], Todd Herrington[22], Jeffrey Herron[13], Craig van Horne[19], Brian H. Kopell[16], Anthony E. Lang[15], Codrin Lungu[21], Daniel Martinez-Ramirez[1], Alon Y. Mogilner[23], Rene Molina[1], Enrico Opri[1], Kevin J. Otto[1], Karim G. Oweiss[1], Yagna Pathak[24], Aparna Shukla[1], Jonathan Shute[1], Sameer A. Sheth[24], Ludy C. Shih[8], G. Karl Steinke[25], Alexander I. Tröster[26], Nora Vanegas[24], Kareem A. Zaghloul[21], Leopoldo Cendejas-Zaragoza[6], Leonard Verhagen[6], Kelly D. Foote[1] and Michael S. Okun[1]*

[1] Department of Neuroscience, Center for Movement Disorders and Neurorestoration, University of Florida, Gainesville, FL, USA, [2] Formerly affiliated with the International Technology Roadmap for Semiconductors (ITRS), Washington, USA, [3] Neurological Institute Cleveland Clinic, Cleveland, OH, USA, [4] Neuroethics Studies Program, Department of Neurology, Georgetown University Medical Center, Washington, DC, USA, [5] Neurological Surgery and Neurology, Stereotactic and Functional Neurosurgery, Department of Neurosurgery, University of Virginia Health Science Center, Charlottesville, VA, USA, [6] Department of Neurology, Rush University Medical Center, Chicago, IL, USA, [7] Scientific Computing and Imaging Institute, University of Utah, Salt Lake City, UT, USA, [8] Beth Israel Deaconess Medical Center, Harvard Medical School, Boston, MA, USA, [9] Department of Biomedical Engineering, School of Medicine, Case Western Reserve University, Cleveland, OH, USA, [10] Department of Neurosurgery, University of California, Los Angeles, Los Angeles, CA, USA, [11] University of California, San Francisco, San Francisco, CA, USA, [12] The Emory Clinic, Emory University, Atlanta, GA, USA, [13] Department of Electrical Engineering, University of Washington, Seattle, WA, USA, [14] Movement Disorders Program, Department of Neurology, Cedars-Sinai Medical Center, Los Angeles, CA, USA, [15] Department of Neurosurgery, University of Toronto, Toronto, ON, Canada, [16] The Icahn School of Medicine at Mount Sinai, New York, NY, USA, [17] Greater Los Angeles Veterans Affairs Healthcare System, Los Angeles, CA, USA, [18] Department of Neurology, Alpert Medical School, Brown University, Providence, RI, USA, [19] University of Kentucky Medical Center, Lexington, KY, USA, [20] Department of Biomedical Engineering, Duke University, Durham, NC, USA, [21] National Institute of Neurological Disorders and Stroke, National Institutes of Health, Bethesda, MD, USA, [22] Massachusetts General Hospital, Harvard Medical School, Boston, MA, USA, [23] Department of Neurosurgery-Center for Neuromodulation, NYU Langone Medical Center, New York, NY, USA, [24] Neurological Institute, Columbia University Medical Center, New York, NY, USA, [25] Boston Scientific Neuromodulation, Valencia, CA, USA, [26] Department of Clinical Neuropsychology, Barrow Neurological Institute, Phoenix, AZ, USA

Edited by:
Paolo Massobrio, University of Genoa, Italy

Reviewed by:
Fritz A. Henn, Mt. Sinai Medical Center, USA
Daniela S. Andres, ETH Zurich & University of Zurich, Switzerland

***Correspondence:**
P. Justin Rossi
pjrossi@ufl.edu

The proceedings of the 3rd Annual Deep Brain Stimulation Think Tank summarize the most contemporary clinical, electrophysiological, imaging, and computational work on DBS for the treatment of neurological and neuropsychiatric disease. Significant innovations of the past year are emphasized. The Think Tank's contributors represent a unique multidisciplinary ensemble of expert neurologists, neurosurgeons, neuropsychologists, psychiatrists, scientists, engineers, and members of industry. Presentations and discussions covered a broad range of topics, including policy and advocacy considerations for the future of DBS, connectomic approaches to DBS targeting, developments in electrophysiology and related strides toward responsive DBS systems, and recent developments in sensor and device technologies.

Keywords: deep brain stimulation, local field potentials, neuromodulation, closed-loop, electrodes

INTRODUCTION

The Third Annual Deep Brain Stimulation (DBS) Think Tank convened at the University of Florida's Research and Academic Center in Orlando, FL, on March 18-20, 2015. This report provides a summary of the conference sessions, which addressed the most current research, clinical, ethical and policy work on DBS for the treatment of neurological and psychiatric disease. DBS research and its clinical translation incur wide ranging, complex issues that necessitate ongoing frank discourse and exchange of ideas among the multi-disciplinary group of neurologists, neurosurgeons, neuropsychologists, psychiatrists, scientists, engineers, and ethicists developing and engaging DBS in research and clinical practice. The DBS Think Tank aims to provide an annual forum where contemporary issues, innovations, and challenges of the research and use of DBS are shared, discussed, and debated. Presentations and discussions addressed policy and advocacy considerations for the continued advancement of DBS, connectomic approaches to DBS targeting, developments in electrophysiology and related progress in responsive DBS systems, and recent innovation in sensor- and stimulation-device technologies.

The field continues to advance at an impressive pace. Our hope is that this meeting promotes awareness among stakeholders in DBS of currently unresolved and newly emerging issues, so as to ultimately strengthen the field and better serve patients. As in previous years, the meeting was conducted in a "think tank" style; speakers presented analyses of critical issues to foster dialog in subsequent discussions. The nature of this think tank format implies that this is not an evidence-based overview of developments in DBS; rather, it is a report of on-going developments that have been advancing this dynamic field and discussion of obstacles hindering further advancement and potential solutions. This summary includes key points of both the presentations and the follow-up discussions.

POLICY AND ADVOCACY FOR THE FUTURE OF DBS

Viability of a DBS Industry Roadmap and Consortium

An industry roadmap process, organization, success factors, and typical and expected outcomes were discussed, using the semiconductor technology roadmap as a prior example of successful effort (Spencer and Seidel, 1995; Schaller, 2001). Industry roadmaps provide a dynamic and evolving collaborative technology management process for determining critical needs and drivers, identifying technology and manufacturing targets, and assessing and modeling potential solutions to focus an industry community. They can also provide direction toward consensus-based resolution of needs and problems within specific timeframes (Rathore, 2009; Cartreine et al., 2010; Qattan et al., 2012; Finch et al., 2014). Such "road mapping" has existed within corporations and organizations for decades. Industry-wide roadmaps are versions of the corporate process that can effectively be used to identify gaps in solutions for common precompetitive challenges; suggest methods and programs to resolve those gaps, and address lead-time issues by indicating timeframes of opportunities for facilities, materials, and equipment development within a supply chain community (Garcia and Bray, 1997). Implementation can occur within organizations in the competitive space, thereby contributing to the growth of industry, by generating positive outcomes inclusive of strategic and tactical partnerships throughout the industry.

DBS is being used to mitigate signs and symptoms of an increasing range of neuropsychiatric disorders. In this way, DBS has attained considerable success in treating a greater number of patients, and in turn, fostered increased public awareness, receptivity and demand for this technology.

The investment and success of DBS has fortified the viability of key technological, commercial, and clinical aspects of neurotechnology and are contributing to the continued expansion, development, and success of the field of neurotechnology in general and the use of DBS in medical practice in particular. As a result, there is substantial energy and investment to broaden the applications of DBS and to increase the capability and complexity of DBS systems. The question of whether and how the DBS industry would be best served by a technology roadmap and/or consortium may reflect the nature and extent of the common challenges presently impeding technology advancement and deployment. The field is laden with numerous issues, including increasing system complexity (e.g., increasing interfaces and channel count, telemetry bandwidth, recording and stimulation capability, etc.), variable biocompatibility, packaging challenges (i.e., demands for smaller size units with greater power efficiency and battery capacity), a proliferation of potential brain targets and indications, and these are reflected in—and foster—increasing regulatory requirements. **Figure 1** presents an overview of expert perceptions of the state of maturity of DBS relative to other neurotechnologies, solicited from participants at the think tank in an anonymous poll.

Implementation of industry-wide standards can evoke both positive and negative effects for different stakeholders. For example, on one hand growing mandated regulatory standards can result in longer development times and higher development costs. On the other hand, such standards can fortify the integrity, efficacy, and safety of DBS technology in use, particularly now as the applications of DBS are expanding tremendously. In addition, the use of standards could actually lower barriers to market entry as certain components of DBS systems become more common commodities (e.g., the implanted pulse generator,

Abbreviations: DBS, deep brain stimulation; FDA, Food and Drug Administration; IIR, investigator-initiated research; IDE, investigational device exemption; NIH, National Institutes of Health; RoR, right of reference; SEEG, stereoencephalography; MRI, magnetic resonance imaging; DTI, diffusion tensor imaging; FA, fractional anisotropy; MCT, modulated circuit tractography; SAS, subtraction activated SPECT; fcMRI, functional connectivity magnetic resonance imaging; TAM, tractography activation models; PD, Parkinson's disease; IPG, implantable pulse generator; MICC, multiple independent current control; HIFU, high intensity focused ultrasound; LFP, local field potential; ECoG, electrocorticography; STN, subthalamic nucleus; ViM, ventralis intermedius; TS, Tourette's syndrome; CM-PF, centromedian parafascicular nucleus of the thalamus; SVM, support vector machine; SC, subcallosal cingulate gyrus; TRD, treatment resistant depression; PFG, prefrontal gyrus; EEG, electroencephalography; LHb, lateral habenula; ECT, electroconvulsive therapy; CSF, cerebrospinal fluid; PTSD, post-traumatic stress disorder; CAPS, clinican-administered PTSD scale; BLn, basolateral nucleus of the amygdala.

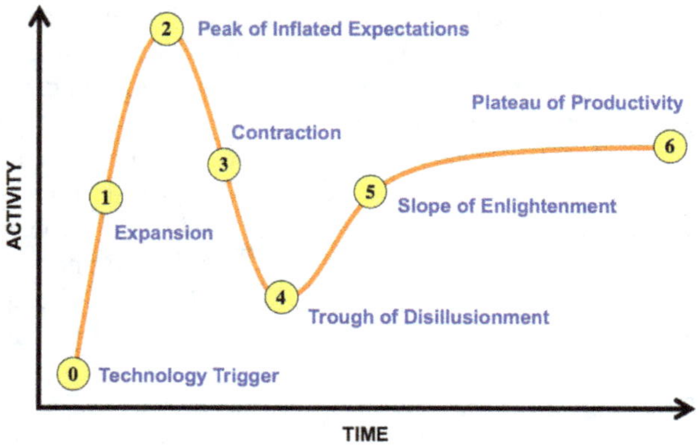

Technology Development →

Maturity	Neurotechnology	Survey
Plateau of Productivity	Cochlear Implant	5.91
	DBS for Parkinson's	5.70
Slope of Enlightenment	DBS for Essential Tremor	5.35
	Spinal Cord Stimulation for Pain Management	4.91
Trough of Disillusionment	FES for Foot Drop	4.09
	DBS for Depression	4.08
	FES for SCI - Limb Control	3.75
	Imaging Post DBS Implant	3.63
	FES for SCI - Bladder Control	3.63
	DBS for Epilepsy	3.55
Contraction Slope	EEG for Decoding Limb Movement (Chronic Use)	3.31
	DBS for Chronic Pain	3.28
	DBS for OCD	3.28
	DBS for Tourette's	3.13
	MRI Safety of Neurotechnology Implants	3.03
	Imaging to Guide Surgical Targeting	3.03
	Transcranial Magnetic Stimulation	2.85
	ECoG for Decoding Limb Movement (Chronic Use)	2.79
	Retinal Implant	2.70
	Microelectrodes in the CNS for Decoding Limb Movement (Chronic Use)	2.69
Peak of Inflated Expectations	Modeling to Guide Surgical Targeting	2.50
	Closed-Loop Feedback	2.25
	Neural Stimulation for Stroke Symptoms	2.21
	Microelectrodes in the PANS for Decoding Limb Movement (Chronic Use)	1.79
	ECoG for Encoding Sensory Feedback (Chronic Use)	1.69
	Reliable Implantable High-Channel Count Connectors (>= 100 Channels)	1.68
	DBS for Alzheimer's	1.68
	Microelectrodes in the CNS for Encoding Sensory Feedback (Chronic Use)	1.65
Expansion Slope	Bi-Directional Wireless Telemetry	1.26
	Wireless Power for Implants	1.24
	DBS for TBI	1.21
	Microelectrodes in the PNS for Encoding Sensory Feedback (Chronic Use)	1.13
	Low-Intensity Focused Ultrasound	1.12
	Optogenetics for Clinical Neural Interfaces	1.12
	DBS for PTSD	1.11
	DBS for Obesity	1.05
	Neuromagnetic Interfaces	1.03
Technology Trigger	DBS for Addiction	0.82

FIGURE 1 | (A) A conceptual model of stages in technology development. **(B)** Results of survey evaluating participants' perceptions of neurotechnology development. Participants in the Think Tank were asked to submit examples of current or emerging neurotechnologies. A list was subsequently compiled and participants were asked to indicate where they believed each of the items ranked in terms of the six stages shown in **(B)**. Survey responses were averaged and the item was subsequently placed in the category corresponding to the nearest whole number.

wireless telemetry). If regulatory processes at the Food and Drug Administration (FDA) related to DBS systems evolve to approve key target-agnostic DBS system blocks or components, rather than entire systems designed for specific anatomical targets, it could significantly increase the rate of neurotechnology innovation. Specifically, such new regulatory processes would support the efforts of smaller companies, with novel algorithmic, anatomical target, and neural-interface concepts, to more quickly deliver solutions to an increasing diversity of patient populations, including those that are smaller and thus less economically appealing to the existing medical-design manufacturers. More attention is required to assess the potential viability of industry-wide roadmaps and consortia to resolve these issues.

Policy to Support Physician Initiated Research and Innovation

Physician investigator-initiated research (IIR) is generally regarded as conferring considerable advantages to DBS research compared to industry-sponsored studies. Physicians are more likely than industry to sponsor research focused on orphan and small disease populations, and increasing IIR in DBS would diversify and broaden ideas focusing upon the current challenges—and opportunities—in the field (Rossi P. J. et al., 2014). Moreover, as a group, physician researchers also have a longer time horizon for assessing outcomes and adding knowledge than most industry sponsors, which can lead to different and uniquely valuable types of studies. However, anecdotal evidence from physician researchers performing DBS trials suggests that significant regulatory burdens are slowing the pace of IIR research, and could be discouraging physicians from participating in such efforts (Rossi P. J. et al., 2014).

A case study providing an overview of the timeline and resources required to meet regulatory requirements for a DBS clinical trial was presented (Kelly et al., 2014). Financial costs for FDA-compliant data management were estimated at $100,000 USD for a 10 patient pilot study. Appropriate data management is critically important for both enabling maximum use of any and all information, and for protecting the privacy of patients and the integrity of the research. However, the costs of FDA-compliant data management substantially reduced funds available for performing the study. Regulatory consultants and support staff to interface with the FDA and to insure that all necessary requirements for the investigational device exemption (IDE) were met also contributed to overall regulatory costs which in the case study were ~$75,000 per year. It was noted that such costs are prohibitive to many "stand-alone" investigators without federal funding or institutional resource sharing.

While industry-sponsorship of a study is possible for certain indications, such support is unlikely for research involving orphan disease populations that represent a small market share of potential consumers. Time costs were also significant; in the case study presented, it took three (3) years from approval of the NIH funding to the time that the first patient was enrolled in the trial. Time costs to the investigator also include dedicated effort preparing regulatory paperwork. For example, it was estimated that the amount of hours required to prepare documentation for submission of an IDE was equivalent to the time required to prepare three (3) NIH R-01 grant proposals.

Even given these barriers to physician-initiated DBS research it was emphasized that physicians are not seeking "less regulation" but instead are calling for regulatory reform. In this light, it was recommended that practices such as data review, process auditing, and unannounced site visits would be welcomed and could be increased, while processes relate to documentation could be streamlined. Specifically, it was recommended that a FDA-approved template for DBS-related IDEs could guide investigators to more efficiently dedicate time and resources to the components definitively required for this type of research. In addition, it was recommended that the right of reference (RoR) process be reformed. Currently, RoR requires that industry partners approve studies that use their devices; this approval is a means of protecting commercial intellectual property and corporate assets and providing protection from litigation. It was suggested that this process could be reformed by indemnifying companies from the consequences of an investigator's FDA-approved off-label use of corporate intellectual property. This reform would center responsibility for the scope and conduct of research upon the physician, rather than the industrial sponsor. In turn, this would enable physicians' control over clinical studies and, at the same time, incur benefits to industry by no longer holding industry partners accountable for reviewing (and ultimately deciding upon) research proposals. Still, this reform may not resolve device manufacturers' concerns about a potential loss of confidence in their brand should a poor outcome occur.

The DBS field is becoming increasingly competitive, with potentially sizeable prizes, and sizeable risks. Achieving a leftward shift in the time course for IIR will require, attention to the benefits and burdens incurred in biomedical, ethical, and legal domains. Toward this end, a multi-step paradigm for comprehensively addressing critical issues and, importantly, guide forward progress in DBS research and its clinical translation was described and recommended. First, an overall "6-R" stance was advocated, which encourages responsibility for: assessment of capabilities and limitations of DBS in treatment of particular neuropsychiatric conditions, research to evaluate DBS effects in practice, regulation, responsivity to incurred burdens and harms and revision of DBS technology and techniques, and regulatory process, as necessary. Meeting these responsibilities invokes a "6-W" set of questions that can be used to define the parameters of use, and "6-Cs" that must be addressed in order to establish ethical probity in use (Giordano, 2015). Details of the "6-R, 6-W, 6-C" model for the ethical development of DBS technology are presented in **Figure 2**.

While the need for continuity of care for patients involved in experimental DBS interventions is clear from ethical and clinical perspectives, the actual provision of such longitudinal care has proven to be challenging in practice (Rossi P. et al., 2014). One vexing recurrent issue is that insurance providers occasionally decline reimbursing costs for off-label DBS, despite granting "pre-approval" in a peer-to-peer review process with the insurance company's medical directors.

Given the increasing diversity of DBS approaches, cumulative data aggregation, sharing, assimilation and synthesis will be increasingly important to the iterative assessment and improvement of the field. Toward these ends recommendation was made to establish a common database for DBS research and clinical outcomes, although the question was posed how—and through which entity or institution—such a common database would be established, hosted and curated (Giordano, 2012, 2014). Modification of extant systems, and development of new information management frameworks will be required to collect and integrate, support and sustain the wide distribution of many types and levels of data. Such approaches should: establish a common data format, optimize harvesting, aggregation and synthesis, establish checking systems to assess and characterize the type and quality of data, maximize accessibility and ensure the source of data, and enable retraction of data that are inaccurate or in need of revision for currency. In light of the increasing number and internationality of IIR DBS studies, it will also be important to address issues and questions of intellectual property and proprietary use (Brindley and Giordano, 2014). To fortify IP, provenance, attribution (and relative indemnities), and data use and sharing agreements will need to be implemented to achieve a dynamic repository that supports the range of intended uses for these data (clinical care, training, and research).

Highlights

1. The DBS industry may be served by a roadmap and/or consortium to address common challenges that are impeding novel technology development and deployment at present and in the near future.
2. Valuable investigator initiated research (IIR) could be strengthened by regulatory reform emphasizing data review, process auditing, and unannounced site visits while streamlining processes related to documentation.
3. FDA-approved template(s) for DBS-related investigational device exemptions (IDEs) could guide investigators to more efficiently dedicate time and resources.
4. There is an urgent need to establish databases for DBS research-related purposes.
5. Continuity of care concerns for patients involved in investigational DBS procedures must be considered.

INNOVATIVE TECHNIQUES AND TECHNOLOGIES IN DBS

Functional Connectivity Tools to Guide Stimulation for Epilepsy

A critical step toward optimizing direct modulation of refractory focal-onset epilepsy is to effectively interface depth electrodes with complex epileptogenic brain circuits. Some novel approaches are currently being exploited to achieve this goal.

It was recently shown that a correlation-based measure of functional connectivity could be used to identify epileptogenic zones from intracranial stereoencephalography (SEEG) signals and that this information can be used to predict the outcome of lobectomy in intractable temporal lobe epilepsy (Antony et al., 2013). Indeed, patients with weakly connected, homogenous networks responded less favorably to temporal lobectomy. These findings suggest the value of such SEEG-based functional connectivity modeling in predicting the outcomes of depth electrode placement for epilepsy (Gonzalez-Martinez et al., 2013).

In addition, the FDA recently approved a depth electrode system as an adjunctive therapy for individuals with refractory focal-onset epilepsy with two epileptogenic sources. A novel

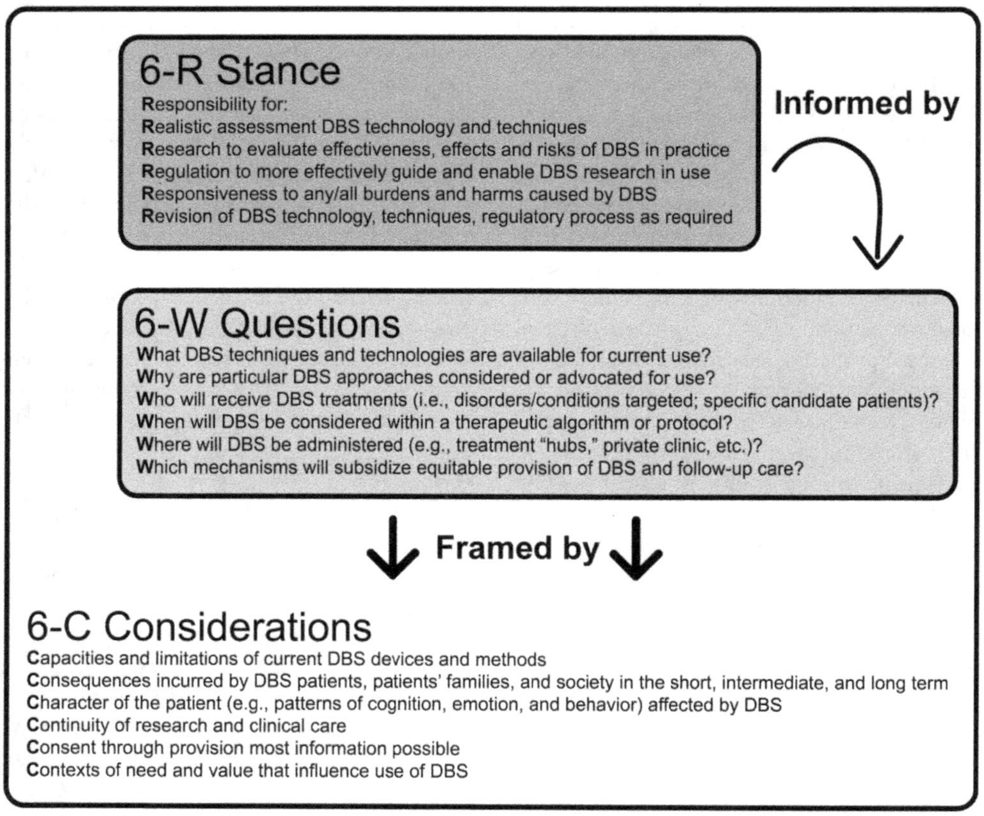

FIGURE 2 | Overview of the "6-R, 6-W, 6-C" model for the ethical development of DBS technology.

pre-implant depth electrode placement planning system has been shown to enable the propagation of therapeutic current to communicating distant epileptogenic sources. The pre-implantation planning process consisted of several components: (1) structural magnetic resonance imaging (MRI) and diffusion tensor imaging (DTI) datasets; (2) computation of the induced electric potential surrounding the electrode contacts using a finite element method; (3) analysis of the effect of the electric field-dependent FA (fractional anisotropy) model on depolarizing axon bundles as identified by high-resolution DTI; and (4) predicting distant cortical activation by strategically placing the FA volume seeds to create a modulated circuit tractography (MCT) map. The pre-implant MCT map was then used as a targeting template for placing up to two depth leads intra-operatively. This planning system was validated via subtraction activated SPECT (SAS), which is a perfusion imaging technique that captures stimulation induced transient changes in cerebral blood flow. SAS was utilized post-implantation to validate *in vivo*, the maximal extent of epileptogenic regions influenced by stimulation therapy.

Functional Connectivity Tools Enable Personalized DBS

The effect of focal brain stimulation is not limited to the region targeted and a DBS current can propagate through anatomical connections to influence distributed neural networks in the brain. Emerging techniques that can help DBS practitioners visualize these networks are likely to prove valuable for understanding and guiding brain stimulation. One imaging technique particularly well suited to visualizing brain networks is resting state functional connectivity magnetic resonance imaging (fcMRI) (Fox and Raichle, 2007). This technique has already been demonstrated to (1) identify thalamic DBS targets based on connectivity to brain regions implicated in tremor (Anderson et al., 2011), (2) link invasive and non-invasive brain stimulation sites across 14 different neurological and psychiatric diseases (Fox et al., 2014), and (3) be safely applied in patients implanted with DBS electrodes using special low-energy MRI sequences (Kahan et al., 2014).

Another method that has emerged with considerable promise is patient-specific tractography-activation models (TAMs), which can enable the identification and visualization of white matter pathways activated by brain stimulation. TAMs essentially predict action potential generation in specific pathways. They combine anatomical imaging data, probabilistic tractography from the brain region surrounding the implanted DBS electrode, models of the electrical fields generated by DBS parameter settings, and cable models of axons (Lujan et al., 2013). TAM may lead to improved personalized surgical targeting and stimulation parameter selection. TAM may also facilitate identification of new DBS targets (Downes and Pouratian, 2014), and deeper understanding of the mechanisms underlying both the therapeutic and off-target effects of DBS (Riva-Posse et al., 2014; Sweet et al., 2014).

Harnessing advances in neuroimaging techniques may also play a role in re-evaluating conventional thinking in the field. For example, with probabilistic diffusion tensor tractography, the four anatomical targets for DBS in cluster headache described as hypothalamic in literature were shown to be localized to the midbrain tegmentum posterior to the hypothalamus. Importantly, tractography also revealed common tracts across these targets, which included projections to the ipsilateral hypothalamus, reticular formation, and cerebellum (Clelland et al., 2014). Collectively, these results can motivate a shift from stimulation of specific brain targets to stimulation of specific brain networks.

Investigating Lead Placement Variability

There can be considerable variability in DBS outcomes, and some clinical trials have failed recently because of profound variability in response rate across the patient cohort. This is evident even in successful clinical trials. For example, in one of the larger DBS trials in PD the standard deviation in clinical outcome scores was roughly equal to the effect size (Deuschl et al., 2006). Over the past 10 years computational models have been used to characterize potential sources of variance in the way DBS is applied (Grill et al., 2004; Johnson and McIntyre, 2008; Dorval et al., 2009, 2010; Santaniello et al., 2011). In general, these studies attempted to characterize how and where stimulation was applied in each patient. With regard to the latter, one critical element for both surgical planning and population research has been co-registration of pre-operative patient MRI to a brain atlas. This is performed prior to surgery to permit indirect targeting of nuclei that have poor contrast on conventional imaging, and it is performed after surgery so that regions of activation for each patient can be expressed in a probabilistic atlas of outcomes (Butson et al., 2011). During this process it has been observed that lead locations often vary within and among surgical sites. This observation has led to questions about errors that could be introduced during atlas registration, and has motivated an evaluation of the accuracy of this registration process. The most important finding from this evaluation was that the observed variability in lead location cannot be attributed to errors introduced during atlas registration. In fact, three different registration algorithms yielded virtually the same results. This information supports the suggestion that the neuromodulation community could benefit from wider adoption and acceptance of open source registration algorithms, several of which have been rigorously developed and tested.

Temporal Pattern of Stimulation as a New Dimension of Therapeutic Innovation

Although DBS is an established therapy for the treatment of movement disorders, debate persists about the mechanisms by which high frequency stimulation reduces symptoms. This probably results in a failure to achieve full optimization of the therapy with maximal benefits and minimal side effects. Thus, an improved understanding of therapeutic mechanisms will be important to enable further innovations in DBS technique and technology.

The cellular effects of DBS on neurons of the central nervous system include simultaneous inhibition of the cell body and activation of the axon (McIntyre et al., 2004). This finding motivated the "informational lesion" hypothesis positing that DBS masks pathological oscillatory activity by normalizing the activity of neurons within the stimulated nucleus. The striking parallel between the frequency-dependent effects of DBS on regularizing the activity of model neurons and the clinical effects on symptoms provides strong correlational evidence for this hypothesis (Grill et al., 2004). The informational lesion hypothesis has been tested in several recent experiments (Zimnik et al., 2015). The changes in representation of kinematic information in the firing patterns of neurons of the globus pallidus and thalamus that occurred during DBS indicate that effective DBS produces at least a partial disruption of neural information (Agnesi et al., 2013).

In contrast, a more recent study concluded that DBS does not disrupt information transmission in the basal ganglia (Zimnik et al., 2015). However, the currents used in this study were orders of magnitude smaller than those required for positive effects on symptoms, and therefore the effects of DBS on neuronal activity were substantially underestimated. Using a highly innovative paradigm to render a temporary direct connection to the brain lead during surgical replacement of the implantable pulse generator (IPG) enabled another test of this hypothesis (Swan et al., 2014). Random patterns of subthalamic nucleus DBS, even when delivered at a high average frequency (130 Hz), were not effective in relieving bradykinesia in patients with Parkinson's disease. These findings reinforced the potential importance of regularization (rather than complete disruption) of neuronal activity for the effectiveness of DBS (Dorval et al., 2010).

The finding that the effects of DBS were dependent on the temporal pattern of stimulation, in addition to the frequency of stimulation, inspired the design and testing of novel temporal patterns of DBS. Patterns were developed that treat the symptoms of Parkinson's disease (PD) more effectively than conventional regularly patterned DBS (Brocker et al., 2013). or alternatively enabled equivalent treatment of symptoms but with a substantial reduction in the required energy. This latter innovation is an important consideration for the size, recharge frequency, and battery life of implanted pulse generators. Collectively, the results demonstrated the utility of an entirely new dimension of neural stimulation parameters—the timing between stimulation pulses—to increase the efficacy and efficiency of stimulation.

Advancements in Lead Design

Emerging DBS device technology will enable controlling of stimulation fields. Three novel lead designs—all with uniquely engineered approaches to achieving this objective—were presented. Two of the presented leads feature electrodes segmented radially about the lead, in contrast with existing leads that are segmented only along the long axis of the lead. The third lead featured an extended span, and brings with it a new kind of current control to DBS. These new leads will allow the stimulating currents to be programmed in order to preferentially stimulate therapeutic targets and avoid stimulating areas prone to side effects. The importance of tuning and directing the stimulating field is based on the observation that electrodes are occasionally sub-optimally placed (Okun et al., 2005) and sometimes quite far from the intended target (Ellis et al., 2008). All three of the lead designs are currently being evaluated in various clinical trials (Contarino et al., 2014; Pollo et al., 2014; Vitek and Starr, 2015). The use of directional electrodes can improve DBS outcomes when electrodes are sub-optimally placed. Preliminary data presented at the Think Tank indicated that targeted stimulation with these approaches is promising, although the long-term benefits of the "directional" leads remain to be demonstrated, particularly in a chronic study. **Figure 3** provides a detailed comparison of these new lead designs.

One lead under investigation (Medtronic-Sapiens) possesses an advanced multiplexer unit that supports a total of 40 electrodes and a span of 7.41 mm. With 10 rows of 4 electrodes per row, and alternating rows offset by 45°, 8 radial electrode directions are possible. Stimulation can be further shaped and aimed radially by choosing various combinations of active electrodes and splitting the current between them; however, details are not yet public regarding how electrodes may be combined and programmed. Additionally, recording of local field potentials (LFPs) is possible from each of the 40 electrodes—potentially yielding spatiotemporal information on pathologic neuronal activity. Preliminary intraoperative testing of this system suggests that it may be possible to utilize intraoperative LFP recordings to assess the effect of stimulation in different electrode combinations and current settings on pathological subthalamic electrical activity (Bour et al., 2015). This field shaping capability can possibly avoid stimulation of unwanted regions and enhance engagement of target areas (Barbe et al., 2014).

Another recently tested lead (Aleva) has a total of eight electrodes (span, 5.5 mm): two are the traditional ring electrodes and the remaining two rings are divided into three segments each, allowing for directional current delivery through each segment (Chase, 2014; Pollo et al., 2014). The electrode corners are rounded so as to avoid "hot spots." Clinical data suggest that this directional lead, when tested in the acute setting in either the subthalamic nucleus (STN) or the ventralis intermedius (VIM) thalamus, can improve the therapeutic index, i.e., enlarge the window between therapeutic effect and adverse effects, and also may possibly use less current to achieve the same therapeutic benefits (Chase, 2014; Pollo et al., 2014).

Another lead (Boston Scientific DB-2201; currently undergoing clinical evaluation in the United States) also possesses eight electrodes (15.5 mm span), current on each of which can be precisely controlled, as the IPG is capable of current steering. The aim of this design, also referred to as Multiple Independent Current Control (MICC), is to achieve more precise targeting of stimulation by enhancing control of the therapeutic electric field. As the IPG associated with this lead is a current control design, it should theoretically enable more stable stimulation. By reducing variability in impedance and permitting the effective use of lower pulse widths, it should also be possible to expand the therapeutic window of effective current amplitudes. Results of a European trial have shown clinical outcomes comparable to existing leads, and during the trial over 70% of programmers utilized the current steering feature (although motivations for this use have not yet been evaluated; Timmermann et al., 2015). The system also has cordless recharging, and the rechargeable IPG utilizes cero volt technology, which helps prevent substantial loss in battery capacity following frequent and/or full discharges. Future capabilities that could be co-deployed with this lead were discussed, such as computer-guided distribution of current across contacts for an optimized or informed programming.

Non-DBS Technology Impacting the Field: Focused Ultrasound

In addition to addressing important improvements in DBS system technology, the Think Tank sought to identify "non-DBS" approaches that could impact the DBS field. In this regard, the use of transcranial high intensity focused ultrasound (HIFU) for treatment of movement disorders was reviewed (Dallapiazza et al., 2014). While effective, stereotactic lesioning of the brain for the treatment of movement disorders has been largely abandoned with the development of DBS (Dallapiazza et al., 2015). However, progress in transcranial MR-guided focused ultrasound technology has renewed an interest in stereotactic lesioning mainly because of the potential for continuous MRI-guidance of an "incisionless" thalamotomy (Wang et al., 2015). Three pilot studies at different institutions have demonstrated significant improvements in hand tremor in patients with severe essential tremor following focused ultrasound thalamotomy (Elias et al., 2013; Wintermark et al., 2014a,b). These studies have suggested functional improvements in activities, disabilities, and quality of life with minimal morbidity. Furthermore, transcranial ultrasound at low intensities can be used to manipulate deep brain circuitry through non-invasive brain mapping prior to lesioning. Clinical trials of HIFU for mapping neural circuitry and treating in essential tremor and PD are currently ongoing.

Proponents of HIFU further highlight that an incision and burr hole are not required to perform the procedure, offering a "lower-cost, less invasive" alternative to DBS that eliminate both the risks of penetrating the brain and the inconvenience and costs imposed by implanted hardware (Lipsman et al., 2013). Dissenters believe this to be an oversimplification. Unlike DBS surgery, HIFU *requires* the head to be completely shaved; patients must remain awake during the procedure and must lie flat within the MRI scanner for a few hours while the target is localized. The MRI environment, while offering the potential for procedural monitoring, can be difficult to work in and some patients cannot tolerate these image-guided procedures. In comparison, DBS targeting scans are obtained in just a few minutes and patients are positioned more comfortably during surgery. Most importantly, HIFU is an ablative and irreversible lesion, and can result in adverse effects especially when used bilaterally.

Direct comparisons of traditional (non-HIFU) thalamotomy and thalamic DBS have already been performed (Tasker, 1998; Schuurman et al., 2000; Pahwa et al., 2001). Three studies conducted at reputable centers in the U.S., Canada, and

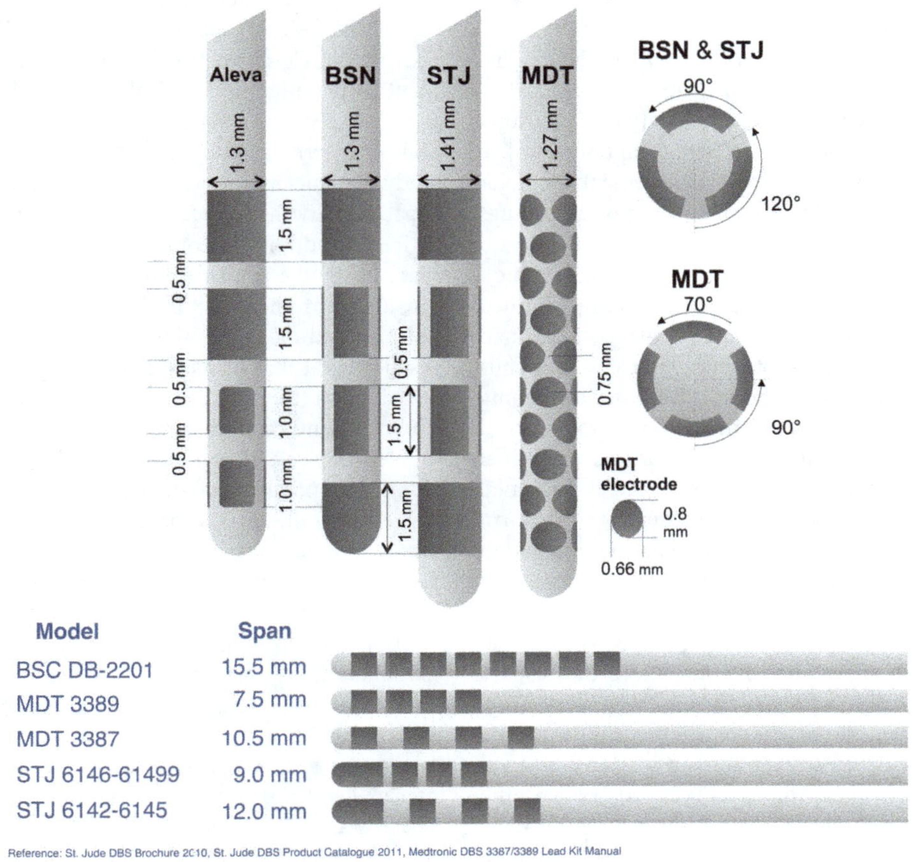

FIGURE 3 | Comparison of emerging DBS electrode lead technology. BSN, Boston Scientific Neuromodulation; STJ, St. Jude Medical; MDT, Medtronic. Reference: St. Jude DBS Brochure 2010, St. Jude DBS Product Catalog 2011, Medtronic DBS 3387/3389 Lead Kit Manual.

Europe have all reached a similar conclusion. While initial tremor control was comparable for the two interventions, thalamic DBS was safer than thalamotomy, causing fewer neurological complications and reducing the need for re-operation in the event of tremor recurrence. Indeed, one member of the University of Virginia HIFU cohort suffered permanent dysesthesia (Elias et al., 2013), and a follow-up study from that group suggests that tremor control may lessen over time as the lesion shrinks in size (Wintermark et al., 2014a). However, it is worth noting that ET can also become refractory to or tolerant of DBS despite increasing currents (Favilla et al., 2012). Clearly, there is a subset of patients who will subjectively prefer HIFU to DBS; however, it remains unknown whether HIFU ablation is objectively better or cheaper than DBS of the thalamus or any other target. Moreover, there are concerns over limitations of this technology including the need for bilateral procedures, the safety profile, and the lack of programmability.

Highlights

1. SEEG-based functional connectivity modeling is helping to predict outcomes of depth electrode placement for epilepsy (Gonzalez-Martinez et al., 2013).
2. Connectivity-based approaches, both functional and structural, suggest that targeting brain networks rather than individual brain sites may improve and personalize DBS.
3. Modifying the temporal pattern of DBS stimulation may offer a new dimension to the therapy.
4. Emerging DBS lead designs incorporating radially segmented electrodes and systems incorporating current steering will enable greater specificity in brain circuit targeting and will improve the benefit/side effect ratio of DBS therapy.
5. Stereotactic ablation with high frequency ultrasound is a less invasive procedure compared to DBS, but carries considerable limitations, including irreversibility and unilaterality.

CLOSING THE LOOP WITH LOCAL FIELD POTENTIALS

Local Field Potentials Provide Insight into Neuropsychiatric Disorders

DBS has shown promise as a therapy for neuropsychiatric disorders; however, advances have been hindered by relatively poor understanding of the neural networks involved in the pathophysiology of these conditions. To address this gap, an ongoing study by researchers at University of California San

Francisco is investigating the mechanisms underlying depression and anxiety in PD patients undergoing awake DBS surgery.

This population of patients is ideal for studying the circuits involved in these depressive and anxious symptoms because they frequently co-occur in varying degrees of severity in Parkinson's disease (Gallagher and Schrag, 2012). These symptoms may be modulated by both DBS and dopamine replacement therapies (Tan, 2012; Storch et al., 2013). High spatial resolution recordings of neuronal activity are performed intraoperatively within brain structures that have been shown to be involved in emotion regulation and cognitive control. Field potentials are recorded from the DBS lead (containing 4 electrode contacts) implanted in the basal ganglia (either the subthalamic nucleus or globus pallidus) and from an additional subdural electrode (containing 28 contacts, spaced 2 mm apart) placed over the prefrontal cortex. Cortical areas targeted include the dorsolateral/medial prefrontal cortex, the orbitofrontal cortex, and the ventrolateral prefrontal cortex. Recordings are performed while patients rest or perform tasks that engage networks involved in emotion regulation and cognitive control. In addition, cortical and subcortical stimulation are used to modulate mood. To identify correlations between neural physiology and symptom severity, depression, mood, and anxiety are characterized both before the surgery using a variety of validated scales, and during the surgery using visual analog mood scales.

Preliminary results of these experiments in the prefrontal cortex suggest that, similar to what has been observed in the motor cortex (Shimamoto et al., 2013; Yang et al., 2014; de Hemptinne et al., 2015), the prefrontal cortex is dominated by beta oscillations that can be coupled to broadband gamma activity (Hammond et al., 2007). It was found that the magnitude of beta rhythm and phase-amplitude coupling varies between patients. In addition, in few patients, it was shown that stimulation delivered to the deepest contact of the DBS lead can induce anxiety, and this effect on mood is associated with a decrease in beta activity and an increase in broadband gamma. Although preliminary, these findings suggest that both the beta oscillations and broadband gamma activity might be relevant to psychiatric symptoms, and that the excessive synchronization observed in cortical-basal ganglia motor networks might also occur in cortical-basal ganglia networks involved in emotion and cognition.

Long-Term Cortical and Subcortical Local Field Potentials (LFPs) in Parkinson's Disease

While DBS is an effective treatment for movement disorders such as PD there are several ways that it might be improved. The current approach is to deliver constant stimulation without adjusting the therapy or controlling for the patient's disease state, medication status, or side effects. A goal of advancing DBS therapy is to implement a "closed-loop" system where electrical signals from the patient's brain are used in real-time as feedback to customize stimulation delivery. Closing the loop can be used to reduce undesired side effects of stimulation and to extend battery life, as well as to improve stimulation effectiveness.

An important step in the development of closed-loop DBS for PD is the characterization of brain signals associated with the disease-relevant network. A recent on-going study aimed at identifying pathophysiological activity related to PD implanted five patients with novel devices capable of both stimulating and long-term recording and storing of LFP data. In this study, patients are implanted with a DBS electrode in the STN capable of both stimulation and sensing/recording electrical activity. In addition, 4-contact electrocorticography (ECoG) strip placed over the primary motor cortex (M1), which is used for sensing/recording only. Each patient is tested multiple times, both on and off medication, and on and off DBS. Preliminary results reveal that in most cases, medication is associated with a reduction in beta (13–30 Hz) power in the STN, while no consistent changes in beta power are recorded from M1. While these results support the importance of beta synchrony throughout basal ganglia-thalamo-cortical loops in PD, they also suggest that there is variability between patients, and that a closed loop signal may need to be optimized on a patient-by-patient basis, and/or that a combination of control signals may be needed.

In addition to identifying markers that are of relevance to hallmark PD symptoms, this study also aimed to assess adverse effects associated with dopaminergic therapy such as the dyskinesias. In two patients experiencing marked contralateral arm dyskinesia, a consistent and reproducible emergence of a narrow-band ~70 Hz increase in cortical power was observed. There was also increased coherence in the same frequency range between STN and M1. Similar patterns of high frequency, narrow-band activity has been previously observed in a rodent model of dyskinesia (Halje et al., 2012), and these may be useful for closed loop approaches.

Long-Term Cortical and Subcortical LFPs in Tourette's Syndrome

Tourette Syndrome (TS) is a paroxysmal neuropsychiatric disorder characterized by involuntary movements and/or vocal outbursts (i.e., - tics) typically preceded by a premonitory urge (Cheung et al., 2007; Kenney et al., 2008). DBS has been used to treat cases of severe and intractable TS (Almeida et al., 2015). It is estimated that ~120 TS patients worldwide have been treated with DBS since 1999, and almost 48 published studies report some degree of motor tic reduction (Schrock et al., 2015). While initial trials have been promising, the mechanisms subserving the effectiveness of DBS in reducing TS signs and symptoms have yet to be identified. Current models of TS hypothesize that thalamocortical-basal ganglia dysfunction is a key network underlying many TS symptoms. Inhibitory input from basal ganglia structures affecting the activity of key thalamic nuclei likely plays a role in patterns of motor behaviors. It may be that inhibition of basal ganglia structures leads to disinhibition of thalamic nuclei, which ultimately evokes initiation of tics (Perlmutter and Mink, 2006). Previous research has demonstrated potential biomarkers of tics (Maling et al., 2012; Bour et al., 2014). Building upon this work, the validity, reliability and relative predictive value of these biomarkers, and the development of an algorithm that can be used in the early detection of tics was presented.

In the presented study, two patients with severe, medication refractory TS were implanted with bilateral DBS devices. Depth leads were placed in the centromedian-parafascicular nucleus of the thalamus (CM-PF) and electrocorticography (ECOG) strips were placed over the precentral gyrus. Experiments consisted of separate interleaved trials in which patients were instructed to (1) tic freely, (2) suppress tics (baseline), and (3) execute volitional movements (shaking hands rapidly, opening and closing hands, raising arms up, and down, talking). Data were recorded intraoperatively and post-operatively. Intraoperative recordings demonstrated that both significantly more low (1–10 Hz) and high (30–100 Hz) frequency CM-PF activity was present during tics but not during volitional movements. A support vector machine (SVM)- based detector (Temko et al., 2011; Wissel et al., 2013) was constructed to investigate the relationship between this activity and tics during each post-operative visit (for a period of 6 months). Three types of tics were recorded including simple, complex, and long complex tics. Long complex tics were shown to be concurrent with a consistently detectable thalamocortical signature. Short complex tics were more difficult to detect than long complex tics, and simple tics were the most difficult to detect. Acute trials of closed loop stimulation using the human tic detector are currently underway.

Local Field Potentials and Depression

A confluence of information prompted exploration of the subcallosal cingulate gyrus (SC) as a DBS target for treatment resistant depression (TRD) (Lozano et al., 2008). Attempts to reduce TRD with SC DBS have shown clinical benefit: a recent study involving 10 patients showed significant response and remission rates following SC DBS (Holtzheimer et al., 2012). However, numerous other targets for TRD, including the nucleus accumbens, dorsolateral prefrontal cortex, and the lateral habenula, have been proposed and subsequently explored in clinical studies, with many of these showing at least some evidence of clinical benefit (Rosa and Lisanby, 2012). The question then arises if and how these targets may be related. The conceptualization of depression as a network disorder suggests that neuromodulation at the purported origin as well as at nodes" of the network can be beneficial (Mayberg, 2009). TAMs of patients who underwent SC DBS for depression demonstrate significant differences between those who responded to therapy and those who did not (Riva-Posse et al., 2014). Specifically, it was shown that responders had greater tract coverage in critical regions.

Recent work has focused on using this information to improve DBS targeting. Prospective work is currently underway to utilize DTI pre-operatively to plan lead placement. This approach has been associated with an increase in the 6-month response rate from 41 to 76%. An important next stage of research will be to identify other markers that can confirm if a lead has been placed in a location that would elicit maximal benefit. Ongoing studies aimed at identifying physiological markers useful in evaluating lead placement and predicting treatment response were presented. These studies focused on intraoperative LFPs from the DBS electrodes in conjunction with intraoperative ECoG and electroencephalograhy (EEG). Previous studies have identified changes in alpha rhythm in depression; the alpha band frequency is increased in the left frontal lobe in depression (Saletu et al., 2010) while alpha is decreased in the right prefrontal cortex (PFC) (Bruder et al., 2001). Preliminary studies of intraoperative LFPs from both ECoG and depth electrodes after stimulation at "effective" contacts (determined by imaging) have demonstrated decreases in the alpha and beta frequencies in the left PFC, as well as a decrease in alpha and beta bands in the subgenual cingulate.

Local Field Potentials and Strides Toward a Closed-Loop DBS

DBS systems currently deployed in the clinic are "open-loop" and do not take into account the potentially intermittent nature of symptoms. By detect the neurophysiologic correlates of symptoms such as tremor, we can determine not only when stimulation may be necessary but also estimate the intensity of stimulation needed. Stimulating only when necessary can increase the battery life of the implanted devices and reduce a patient's exposure to unintended effects.

A novel mobile, wireless platform for investigating closed-loop DBS applications in ambulatory patients was presented (Herron and Chizeck, 2014). The platform consisted of a set of body-worn sensors communicating wirelessly to a host application running on a smartphone or a personal computer. Taking advantage of movement data including inertial measurements, electromyography, and LFPs, these host applications are capable of performing digital signal processing and data fusion in order to make control decisions. These control decisions can include enabling or disabling stimulation or modifying individual stimulation parameters (voltage, pulse width, frequency) in response to changes in neurological symptoms (Herron et al., 2015). These control decisions are then sent wirelessly to an external receiver that then relays packets and control decisions to an implanted neurostimulator. This real-time command link to the implanted device has enabled the implementation of an integrated closed-loop DBS system.

This system confers several important benefits for both research and patient care. Currently, studies are underway to assess clinical performance of the system, and future studies are being planned which utilize the wealth of consistent, chronic data generated from the integrated system to investigate neurological movement disorder, particularly tremor.

Highlights

1. Chronic recording of FPs is permitting greater insight into multiple neuropsychiatric disorders.
2. LFP-based research holds promise for the identification of pathological brain signals that could serve as triggers for responsive stimulation.
3. Closed loop systems are being tested which could use a variety of signals in order to modulate therapy.

INNOVATIVE TARGETS FOR NEW INDICATIONS

Lateral Habenula as a Target for Depression

In 2007, a non-human primate study provided the first electrophysiological evidence that the lateral habenula (LHb) played a role in the brain's reward system. The study demonstrated that reward was associated with suppression of inhibitory input from the LHb and subsequent activation of dopamine neurons, while the reverse was observed for non-rewarding trials (Matsumoto and Hikosaka, 2007). That same year, Alex Sartorius and Fritz Henn advanced the hypothesis of over activation of the habenula in major depressive episodes and argued that DBS of the lateral habenula could be beneficial for TRD (Sartorius and Henn, 2007). More recent studies in humans have corroborated the notion of LHb involvement in the reward system (Salas et al., 2010), and, interestingly, two case reports have since been published (2010, 2013) showing remission of major depression under DBS of the LHb (Sartorius et al., 2010; Kiening and Sartorius, 2013; Schneider et al., 2013). Early results from an on-going open-label trial of six patients undergoing habenular DBS for TRD were presented. The hypothesis that patients who were responsive to electroconvulsive therapy (ECT)—even if for a short duration—could be "better" candidates for habenular DBS was proposed, and is under investigation in the present study. As a DBS target, the LHb poses unique challenges for electrode implantation—among these is the proximity of the target to the third ventricle and the resultant motion artifact observed in imaging studies due to the pulsatile movement of the cerebro-spinal fluid (CSF). Programming-related adverse events observed to date were discussed. Upper extremity paresthesias occurred commonly, although patients mostly habituated to this and the effect was modifiable by gradually increasing the current. Oculomotor abnormalities were also observed which limited current dosing, and it was proposed that current steering could be useful in limiting this side effect.

DBS of the Basolateral Nucleus of the Amygdala for PTSD

Neuromodulation of the amygdala may prove beneficial in disease processes where symptoms arise from the aberrant assignment of an emotion to a specific event or context (Langevin, 2012). In post-traumatic stress disorder (PTSD), patients assign fear to benign situations, which may potentially lead to avoidance behavior. Several neuroimaging studies have demonstrated that the amygdalae of PTSD patients are metabolically overactive during symptomatic episodes (Etkin and Wager, 2007; Hughes and Shin, 2011). The level of activity within the amygdala correlates with the severity of the symptoms as measured by the clinician-administered PTSD scale (CAPS). An important study by Koenigs and colleagues showed that Vietnam veterans who suffered traumatic brain injury to the amygdala never developed PTSD (Koenigs et al., 2008). These results suggest that the amygdala plays a critical role in the production of PTSD symptoms. Focal interference of amygdala activity through DBS may improve PTSD. Although its mechanism is not fully understood, high frequency DBS is thought to functionally inactivate a specific, gray matter target. It was previously shown that DBS of the basolateral nucleus of the amygdala (BLn) reduced the behavior associated with PTSD in a rodent model (Langevin et al., 2010). A subsequent study in the same rodent model demonstrated that BLn DBS was superior to paroxetine—one of the drugs approved by the FDA to treat PTSD (Stidd et al., 2013). These results led to the recent development of a clinical trial to evaluate the feasibility and the safety of this technique in PTSD patients (Koek et al., 2014). An overview of the trial design was presented, as well as an overview of the first surgical subject implanted. In addition, the targeting technique and intra-operative microelectrode recording findings were described. Consideration of the patient's neuroanatomy is critical because of the wide variation in size and shape of the mesiotemporal structures.

DBS for Stroke

The concept of post-stroke neurostimulation does not focus on modulation of the area damaged by ischemia, rather it is intended to (1) augment the perilesional cortex or (2) modulate other areas whose connectivity has been disrupted by the stroke. Direct cortical stimulation as a means of enhancing excitability and plasticity has been investigated (Alonso-Alonso et al., 2007), but has failed to produce the intended benefits in clinical trials. One possible reason for the failure of cortical stimulation was the relationship between cortical axons and the source of stimulation (Manola et al., 2005a,b). In rodent models, axonal arrangement perpendicular to the cathode is predictable. However, in human brains, axonal arrangement is less predictable, and it is possible that axons were inhibited and excited in near equal proportions during cortical stimulation interventions and the net effect washed out. A novel approach to stroke therapy via DBS was discussed; the intention was to stimulate natural fiber pathways to the perilesional cortex in a way that mimics their native function. Preliminary results of this design in a rodent model were presented. Based on motor pathway fiber tracing by Dum and Strick, a cerebellar target (lateral cerebellar nucleus) was selected with the goal of modulating the dentatothalamocortical pathway (Dum and Strick, 2002; Machado and Baker, 2012). Stimulation of this target (particularly at 30 Hz) was shown to evoke cortical excitability. A follow-up study tested the effect of chronic 30 Hz DBS in this target on motor function in a rodent model of stroke (Machado et al., 2013). Animals in the stimulation group showed a significant improvement in motor function compared with post-ischemia baseline performance as well as in comparison with the non-stimulation group (Machado et al., 2013). Moreover, perilesional synaptic density testing showed that animals in the stimulation group had significantly greater numbers of perilesional synapses. Preliminary results of on-going studies of cytoarchitecture in these animals addressing whether these observations reflect neurogenesis in addition to synaptogenesis were also presented. Substantial discussion surrounded the topic of the appropriate level of pre-clinical evidence needed to justify early clinical translation studies.

Highlights

1. Emerging research suggests the viability of DBS as a treatment for new indications, including depression, PTSD, and stroke.
2. Research into novel targets for novel indications requires hypotheses based on animal models (where possible), well-designed clinical trials, and careful attention to potential off-target effects, patient selection, and targeting considerations.

CONCLUSION

These proceedings represent the deliberations of the third Annual Deep Brain Stimulation Think Tank. The group addressed critical issues affecting the progress of the DBS field. These issues span multiple domains, including regulatory and ethical issues as well as study design. There are also important barriers to advance electrophysiology and system engineering. In discussing these challenges, participants in the Think Tank proposed and discussed possible solutions.

Scientific, clinical, and engineering advances that could transform the DBS field in the near future served as a primary focus of the Think Tank. The meeting focused on recent discoveries that may lead to transformative, not just incremental change in DBS therapy. Participants discussed the broad range of potential applications of the new knowledge, techniques, and technologies presented; they also discussed ways in which these advances could be fully exploited to rapidly advance to the next generation of DBS therapy. The future of DBS will depend heavily on building on these advances and on filling knowledge current gaps.

AUTHOR CONTRIBUTIONS

All authors listed, have made substantial, direct and intellectual contribution to the work, and approved it for publication.

REFERENCES

Agnesi, F., Connolly, A. T., Baker, K. B., Vitek, J. L., and Johnson, M. D. (2013). Deep brain stimulation imposes complex informational lesions. *PLoS ONE* 8:e74462. doi: 10.1371/journal.pone.0074462

Almeida, L., Martinez-Ramirez, D., Rossi, P. J., Peng, Z., Gunduz, A., and Okun, M. S. (2015). Chasing tics in the human brain: development of open, scheduled and closed loop responsive approaches to deep brain stimulation for tourette syndrome. *J. Clin. Neurol. Seoul Korea* 11, 122–131. doi: 10.3988/jcn.2015.11.2.122

Alonso-Alonso, M., Fregni, F., and Pascual-Leone, A. (2007). Brain stimulation in poststroke rehabilitation. *Cerebrovasc. Dis. Basel Switz.* 24(suppl. 1), 157–166. doi: 10.1159/000107392

Anderson, J. S., Dhatt, H. S., Ferguson, M. A., Lopez-Larson, M., Schrock, L. E., House, P. A., et al. (2011). Functional connectivity targeting for deep brain stimulation in essential tremor. *AJNR Am. J. Neuroradiol.* 32, 1963–1968. doi: 10.3174/ajnr.A2638

Antony, A. R., Alexopoulos, A. V., González-Martínez, J. A., Mosher, J. C., Jehi, L., Burgess, R. C., et al. (2013). Functional connectivity estimated from intracranial EEG predicts surgical outcome in intractable temporal lobe epilepsy. *PLoS ONE* 8:e77916. doi: 10.1371/journal.pone.0077916

3arbe, M. T., Dembek, T. A., Becker, J., Raethjen, J., Hartinger, M., Meister, I. G., et al. (2014). Individualized current-shaping reduces DBS-induced dysarthria in patients with essential tremor. *Neurology* 82, 614–619. doi: 10.1212/WNL.0000000000000127

3our, L. J., Ackermans, L., Foncke, E. M. J., Cath, D., van der Linden, C., Visser Vandewalle, V., et al. (2014). Tic related local field potentials in the thalamus and the effect of deep brain stimulation in Tourette syndrome: report of three cases. *Clin. Neurophysiol.* 128, 1578–1588. doi: 10.1016/j.clinph.2014.10.217

3our, L. J., Lourens, M. A. J., Verhagen, R., de Bie, R. M. A., van den Munckhof, P., Schuurman, P. R., et al. (2015). Directional recording of subthalamic spectral power densities in parkinson's disease and the effect of steering deep brain stimulation. *Brain Stimulat.* 8, 730–741. doi: 10.1016/j.brs.2015.02.002

rindley, T., and Giordano, D. J. (2014). international standards for intellectual property protection of neuroscience and neurotechnology: neuroethical legal and social (NELS) considerations in light of globalization. *Stanf. J. Law Sci. Policy SJLSP* 7, 33.

rocker, D. T., Swan, B. D., Turner, D. A., Gross, R. E., Tatter, S. B., Koop, M. M., et al. (2013). Improved efficacy of temporally non-regular deep brain stimulation in Parkinson's disease. *Exp. Neurol.* 239, 60–67. doi: 10.1016/j.expneurol.2012.09.008

ruder, G. E., Stewart, J. W., Tenke, C. E., McGrath, P. J., Leite, P., Bhattacharya, N., et al. (2001). Electroencephalographic and perceptual asymmetry differences between responders and nonresponders to an SSRI antidepressant. *Biol. Psychiatry* 49, 416–425. doi: 10.1016/S0006-3223(00)01016-7

Butson, C. R., Cooper, S. E., Henderson, J. M., Wolgamuth, B., and McIntyre, C. C. (2011). Probabilistic analysis of activation volumes generated during deep brain stimulation. *NeuroImage* 54, 2096–2104. doi: 10.1016/j.neuroimage.2010.10.059

Cartreine, J. A., Ahern, D. K., and Locke, S. E. (2010). A roadmap to computer-based psychotherapy in the United States. *Harv. Rev. Psychiatry* 18, 80–95. doi: 10.3109/10673221003707702

Chase, A. (2014). Neurosurgery: directional electrodes widen the therapeutic window for deep brain stimulation in movement disorders. *Nat. Rev. Neurol.* 10, 364. doi: 10.1038/nrneurol.2014.101

Cheung, M.-Y. C., Shahed, J., and Jankovic, J. (2007). Malignant Tourette syndrome. *Mov. Disord.* 22, 1743–1750. doi: 10.1002/mds.21599

Clelland, C. D., Zheng, Z., Kim, W., Bari, A., and Pouratian, N. (2014). Common cerebral networks associated with distinct deep brain stimulation targets for cluster headache. *Cephalalgia Int. J. Headache* 34, 224–230. doi: 10.1177/0333102413509431

Contarino, M. F., Bour, L. J., Verhagen, R., Lourens, M. A. J., de Bie, R. M. A., van den Munckhof, P., et al. (2014). Directional steering: a novel approach to deep brain stimulation. *Neurology* 83, 1163–1169. doi: 10.1212/WNL.0000000000000823

Dallapiazza, R., Khaled, M., Eames, M., Snell, J., Lopes, M. B., Wintermark, M., et al. (2015). Feasibility and safety of MR-guided focused ultrasound lesioning in the setting of deep brain stimulation. *Stereotact. Funct. Neurosurg.* 93, 140–146. doi: 10.1159/000368908

Dallapiazza, R., McKisic, M. S., Shah, B., and Elias, W. J. (2014). Neuromodulation for movement disorders. *Neurosurg. Clin. N. Am.* 25, 47–58. doi: 10.1016/j.nec.2013.08.002

de Hemptinne, C., Swann, N. C., Ostrem, J. L., Ryapolova-Webb, E. S., San Luciano, M., Galifianakis, N. B., et al. (2015). Therapeutic deep brain stimulation reduces cortical phase-amplitude coupling in Parkinson's disease. *Nat. Neurosci.* 18, 779–786. doi: 10.1038/nn.3997

Deuschl, G., Schade-Brittinger, C., Krack, P., Volkmann, J., Schäfer, H., Bötzel, K., et al. (2006). A randomized trial of deep-brain stimulation for Parkinson's disease. *N. Engl. J. Med.* 355, 896–908. doi: 10.1056/NEJMoa060281

Dorval, A. D., Kuncel, A. M., Birdno, M. J., Turner, D. A., and Grill, W. M. (2010). Deep brain stimulation alleviates parkinsonian bradykinesia by regularizing pallidal activity. *J. Neurophysiol.* 104, 911–921. doi: 10.1152/jn.00103.2010

Dorval, A. D., Panjwani, N., Qi, R. Y., and Grill, W. M. (2009). Deep brain stimulation that abolishes Parkinsonian activity in basal ganglia improves thalamic relay fidelity in a computational circuit. *Conf. Proc. IEEE Eng. Med. Biol. Soc.* 2009, 4230–4233. doi: 10.1109/iembs.2009.5333611

Downes, A., and Pouratian, N. (2014). Advanced neuroimaging techniques for central neuromodulation. *Neurosurg. Clin. N. Am.* 25, 173–185. doi: 10.1016/j.nec.2013.08.012

Dum, R. P., and Strick, P. L. (2002). Motor areas in the frontal lobe of the primate. *Physiol. Behav.* 77, 677–682. doi: 10.1016/S0031-9384(02)00929-0

Elias, W. J., Huss, D., Voss, T., Loomba, J., Khaled, M., Zadicario, E., et al. (2013). A pilot study of focused ultrasound thalamotomy for essential tremor. *N. Engl. J. Med.* 369, 640–648. doi: 10.1056/NEJMoa1300962

Ellis, T.-M., Foote, K. D., Fernandez, H. H., Sudhyadhom, A., Rodriguez, R. L., Zeilman, P., et al. (2008). Reoperation for suboptimal outcomes after deep brain stimulation surgery. *Neurosurgery* 63, 754–760. discussion: 760–761. doi: 10.1227/01.neu.0000325492.58799.35

Etkin, A., and Wager, T. D. (2007). Functional neuroimaging of anxiety: a meta-analysis of emotional processing in PTSD, social anxiety disorder, and specific phobia. *Am. J. Psychiatry* 164, 1476–1488. doi: 10.1176/appi.ajp.2007.07030504

Favilla, C. G., Ullman, D., Wagle Shukla, A., Foote, K. D., Jacobson, C. E., and Okun, M. S. (2012). Worsening essential tremor following deep brain stimulation: disease progression versus tolerance. *Brain J. Neurol.* 135, 1455–1462. doi: 10.1093/brain/aws026

Finch, G., Havel, H., Analoui, M., Barton, R. W., Diwan, A. R., Hennessy, M., et al. (2014). Nanomedicine drug development: a scientific symposium entitled "Charting a roadmap to commercialization." *AAPS J.* 16, 698–704. doi: 10.1208/s12248-014-9608-5

Fox, M. D., Buckner, R. L., Liu, H., Chakravarty, M. M., Lozano, A. M., and Pascual-Leone, A. (2014). Resting-state networks link invasive and noninvasive brain stimulation across diverse psychiatric and neurological diseases. *Proc. Natl. Acad. Sci. U.S.A.* 111, E4367–E4375. doi: 10.1073/pnas.1405003111

Fox, M. D., and Raichle, M. E. (2007). Spontaneous fluctuations in brain activity observed with functional magnetic resonance imaging. *Nat. Rev. Neurosci.* 8, 700–711. doi: 10.1038/nrn2201

Gallagher, D. A., and Schrag, A. (2012). Psychosis, apathy, depression and anxiety in Parkinson's disease. *Neurobiol. Dis.* 46, 581–589. doi: 10.1016/j.nbd.2011.12.041

Garcia, M., and Bray, O. (1997). *Fundamentals of Technology Roadmapping.* Albuquerque, NM: Sandia National Laboratories.

Giordano, J. (2012). "Integrative convergence in neuroscience: trajectories, problems, and the need for a progressive neurobioethics," in *Technological Innovations in Sensing and Detection of Chemical, Biological, Radiological, Nuclear Threats and Ecological Terrorism NATO Science for Peace and Security Series A: Chemistry and Biology*, eds A. Vaseashta, E. Braman, and P. Susmann (Springer), 115–130. Available online at: http://link.springer.com/chapter/10.1007/978-94-007-2488-4_10 [Accessed July 2, 2015].

Giordano, J. (2014). "Intersections of 'big data', neuroscience and national security: technical issues and derivative concerns.," in *A New Information Paradigm? From Genes to "Big Data," and Instagrams to Persistent Surveillance: Implications for National Security. Department of Defense*, ed H. Cabayan (Washington, DC: Strategic Multilayer Assessment Group Whitepaper - Joint Staff/J-3/Pentagon Strategic Studies Group), 46–48.

Giordano, J. (2015). A preparatory neuroethical approach to assessing developments in neurotechnology. *Virtual Mentor VM* 17, 56–61. doi: 10.1001/virtualmentor.2015.17.01.msoc1-1501

Gonzalez-Martinez, J., Bulacio, J., Alexopoulos, A., Jehi, L., Bingaman, W., and Najm, I. (2013). Stereoelectroencephalography in the "difficult to localize" refractory focal epilepsy: early experience from a North American epilepsy center. *Epilepsia* 54, 323–330. doi: 10.1111/j.1528-1167.2012.03672.x

Grill, W. M., Snyder, A. N., and Miocinovic, S. (2004). Deep brain stimulation creates an informational lesion of the stimulated nucleus. *Neuroreport* 15, 1137–1140. doi: 10.1097/00001756-200405190-00011

Halje, P., Tamtè, M., Richter, U., Mohammed, M., Cenci, M. A., and Petersson, P. (2012). Levodopa-induced dyskinesia is strongly associated with resonant cortical oscillations. *J. Neurosci.* 32, 16541–16551. doi: 10.1523/JNEUROSCI.3047-12.2012

Hammond, C., Bergman, H., and Brown, P. (2007). Pathological synchronization in Parkinson's disease: networks, models and treatments. *Trends Neurosci.* 30, 357–364. doi: 10.1016/j.tins.2007.05.004

Herron, J., and Chizeck, H. J. (2014). "Prototype closed-loop deep brain stimulation systems inspired by norbert wiener," in *2014 IEEE Conference on*

Herron, J., Denison, T., and Chizeck, H. J. (2015). "Closed-Loop DBS with Movement Intention," in *Neural Engineering (NER), 2015 7th International IEEE/EMBS Conference on* (Montpelier, VT: IEEE).

Holtzheimer, P. E., Kelley, M. E., Gross, R. E., Filkowski, M. M., Garlow, S. J., Barrocas, A., et al. (2012). Subcallosal cingulate deep brain stimulation for treatment-resistant unipolar and bipolar depression. *Arch. Gen. Psychiatry* 69, 150–158. doi: 10.1001/archgenpsychiatry.2011.1456

Hughes, K. C., and Shin, L. M. (2011). Functional neuroimaging studies of post-traumatic stress disorder. *Expert Rev. Neurother.* 11, 275–285. doi: 10.1586/ern.10.198

Johnson, M. D., and McIntyre, C. C. (2008). Quantifying the neural elements activated and inhibited by globus pallidus deep brain stimulation. *J. Neurophysiol.* 100, 2549–2563. doi: 10.1152/jn.90372.2008

Kahan, J., Urner, M., Moran, R., Flandin, G., Marreiros, A., Mancini, L., et al. (2014). Resting state functional MRI in Parkinson's disease: the impact of deep brain stimulation on "effective" connectivity. *Brain J. Neurol.* 137, 1130–1144. doi: 10.1093/brain/awu027

Kelly, M. L., Malone, D., Okun, M. S., Booth, J., and Machado, A. G. (2014). Barriers to investigator-initiated deep brain stimulation and device research. *Neurology* 82, 1465–1473. doi: 10.1212/WNL.0000000000000345

Kenney, C., Kuo, S.-H., and Jimenez-Shahed, J. (2008). Tourette's syndrome. *Am. Fam. Physician* 77, 651–658.

Kiening, K., and Sartorius, A. (2013). A new translational target for deep brain stimulation to treat depression. *EMBO Mol. Med.* 5, 1151–1153. doi: 10.1002/emmm.201302947

Koek, R. J., Langevin, J.-P., Krahl, S. E., Kosoyan, H. J., Schwartz, H. N., Chen, J. W. Y., et al. (2014). Deep brain stimulation of the basolateral amygdala for treatment-refractory combat post-traumatic stress disorder (PTSD): study protocol for a pilot randomized controlled trial with blinded, staggered onset of stimulation. *Trials* 15, 356. doi: 10.1186/1745-6215-15-356

Koenigs, M., Huey, E. D., Raymont, V., Cheon, B., Solomon, J., Wassermann, E. M., et al. (2008). Focal brain damage protects against post-traumatic stress disorder in combat veterans. *Nat. Neurosci.* 11, 232–237. doi: 10.1038/nn2032

Langevin, J.-P. (2012). The amygdala as a target for behavior surgery. *Surg. Neurol. Int.* 3, S40–S46. doi: 10.4103/2152-7806.91609

Langevin, J.-P., De Salles, A. A. F., Kosoyan, H. P., and Krahl, S. E. (2010). Deep brain stimulation of the amygdala alleviates post-traumatic stress disorder symptoms in a rat model. *J. Psychiatr. Res.* 44, 1241–1245. doi: 10.1016/j.jpsychires.2010.04.022

Lipsman, N., Schwartz, M. L., Huang, Y., Lee, L., Sankar, T., Chapman, M., et al. (2013). MR-guided focused ultrasound thalamotomy for essential tremor: a proof-of-concept study. *Lancet Neurol.* 12, 462–468. doi: 10.1016/S1474-4422(13)70048-6

Lozano, A. M., Mayberg, H. S., Giacobbe, P., Hamani, C., Craddock, R. C., and Kennedy, S. H. (2008). Subcallosal cingulate gyrus deep brain stimulation for treatment-resistant depression. *Biol. Psychiatry* 64, 461–467. doi: 10.1016/j.biopsych.2008.05.034

Lujan, J. L., Chaturvedi, A., Choi, K. S., Holtzheimer, P. E., Gross, R. E., Mayberg, H. S., et al. (2013). Tractography-activation models applied to subcallosal cingulate deep brain stimulation. *Brain Stimulat.* 6, 737–739. doi: 10.1016/j.brs.2013.03.008

Machado, A., and Baker, K. B. (2012). Upside down crossed cerebellar diaschisis: proposing chronic stimulation of the dentatothalamocortical pathway for post-stroke motor recovery. *Front. Integr. Neurosci.* 6:20. doi: 10.3389/fnint.2012.00020

Machado, A. G., Cooperrider, J., Furmaga, H. T., Baker, K. B., Park, H. J., Chen, Z., et al. (2013). Chronic 30-Hz deep cerebellar stimulation coupled with training enhances post-ischemia motor recovery and peri-infarct synaptophysin expression in rodents. *Neurosurgery* 73, 344–353. discussion 353. doi: 10.1227/01.neu.0000430766.80102.ac

Maling, N., Hashemiyoon, R., Foote, K. D., Okun, M. S., and Sanchez, J. C. (2012). Increased thalamic gamma band activity correlates with symptom relief following deep brain stimulation in humans with Tourette's syndrome. *PLoS ONE* 7:e44215. doi: 10.1371/journal.pone.0044215

Manola, L., Holsheimer, J., and Veltink, P. (2005a). Technical performance of percutaneous leads for spinal cord stimulation: a modeling study. *Neuromodulation* 8, 88–99. doi: 10.1111/j.1525-1403.2005.00224.x

Manola, L., Roelofsen, B. H., Holsheimer, J., Marani, E., and Geelen, J. (2005b).

potential field, activating functions and responses of simple nerve fibre models. *Med. Biol. Eng. Comput.* 43, 335–343. doi: 10.1007/BF02345810

Matsumoto, M., and Hikosaka, O. (2007). Lateral habenula as a source of negative reward signals in dopamine neurons. *Nature* 447, 1111–1115. doi: 10.1038/nature05860

Mayberg, H. S. (2009). Targeted electrode-based modulation of neural circuits for depression. *J. Clin. Invest.* 119, 717–725. doi: 10.1172/JCI38454

McIntyre, C. C., Grill, W. M., Sherman, D. L., and Thakor, N. V. (2004). Cellular effects of deep brain stimulation: model-based analysis of activation and inhibition. *J. Neurophysiol.* 91, 1457–1469. doi: 10.1152/jn.00989.2003

Okun, M. S., Tagliati, M., Pourfar, M., Fernandez, H. H., Rodriguez, R. L., Alterman, R. L., et al. (2005). Management of referred deep brain stimulation failures: a retrospective analysis from 2 movement disorders centers. *Arch. Neurol.* 62, 1250–1255. doi: 10.1001/archneur.62.8.noc40425

Pahwa, R., Lyons, K. E., Wilkinson, S. B., Tröster, A. I., Overman, J., Kieltyka, J., et al. (2001). Comparison of thalamotomy to deep brain stimulation of the thalamus in essential tremor. *Mov. Disord.* 16, 140–143. doi: 10.1002/1531-8257(200101)16:1<140::AID-MDS1025>3.0.CO;2-T

Perlmutter, J. S., and Mink, J. W. (2006). Deep brain stimulation. *Annu. Rev. Neurosci.* 29, 229–257. doi: 10.1146/annurev.neuro.29.051605.112824

Pollo, C., Kaelin-Lang, A., Oertel, M. F., Stieglitz, L., Taub, E., Fuhr, P., et al. (2014). Directional deep brain stimulation: an intraoperative double-blind pilot study. *Brain J. Neurol.* 137, 2015–2026. doi: 10.1093/brain/awu102

Qattan, M., Demonacos, C., and Krstic-Demonacos, M. (2012). Roadmap to personalized medicine. *Croat. Med. J.* 53, 294–297. doi: 10.3325/cmj.2012.53.294

Rathore, A. S. (2009). Roadmap for implementation of quality by design (QbD) for biotechnology products. *Trends Biotechnol.* 27, 546–553. doi: 10.1016/j.tibtech.2009.06.006

Riva-Posse, P., Choi, K. S., Holtzheimer, P. E., McIntyre, C. C., Gross, R. E., Chaturvedi, A., et al. (2014). Defining critical white matter pathways mediating successful subcallosal cingulate deep brain stimulation for treatment-resistant depression. *Biol. Psychiatry* 76, 963–969. doi: 10.1016/j.biopsych.2014.03.029

Rosa, M. A., and Lisanby, S. H. (2012). Somatic treatments for mood disorders. *Neuropsychopharmacology* 37, 102–116. doi: 10.1038/npp.2011.225

Rossi, P, Machado, A, and Okun, M.S. (2014). Medicare coverage of investigational devices: the troubled path forward for deep brain stimulation. *JAMA Neurol.* 71, 535–536. doi: 10.1001/jamaneurol.2013.6042

Rossi, P. J., Okun, M., and Giordano, J. (2014). Translational imperatives in deep brain stimulation research: addressing neuroethical issues of consequences and continuity of clinical care. *AJOB Neurosci.* 5, 46–48. doi: 10.1080/21507740.2013.863248

Salas, R., Baldwin, P., de Biasi, M., and Montague, P. R. (2010). BOLD responses to negative reward prediction errors in human habenula. *Front. Hum. Neurosci.* 4:36. doi: 10.3389/fnhum.2010.00036

aletu, B., Anderer, P., and Saletu-Zyhlarz, G. M. (2010). EEG topography and tomography (LORETA) in diagnosis and pharmacotherapy of depression. *Clin. EEG Neurosci.* 41, 203–210. doi: 10.1177/155005941004100407

antaniello, S., Fiengo, G., Glielmo, L., and Grill, W. M. (2011). Closed-loop control of deep brain stimulation: a simulation study. *IEEE Trans. Neural Syst. Rehabil. Eng. Publ. IEEE Eng.* 19, 15–24. doi: 10.1109/TNSRE.2010.2081377

artorius, A., and Henn, F. A. (2007). Deep brain stimulation of the lateral habenula in treatment resistant major depression. *Med. Hypotheses* 69, 1305–1308. doi: 10.1016/j.mehy.2007.03.021

artorius, A., Kiening, K. L., Kirsch, P., von Gall, C. C., Haberkorn, U., Unterberg, A. W., et al. (2010). Remission of major depression under deep brain stimulation of the lateral habenula in a therapy-refractory patient. *Biol. Psychiatry* 67, e9–e11. doi: 10.1016/j.biopsych.2009.08.027

challer, R. (2001). "Technological innovation in the semiconductor industry: a case study of the International Technology Roadmap for Semiconductors (ITRS)," in *Portland International Conference on Management of Engineering and Technology, 2001. PICMET'01*, 195, Vol. 1 (Portland, OR).

chneider, T. M., Beynon, C., Sartorius, A., Unterberg, A. W., and Kiening, K. L. (2013). Deep brain stimulation of the lateral habenular complex in treatment-resistant depression: traps and pitfalls of trajectory choice. *Neurosurgery* 72, ons184–ons193. discussion: ons193. doi: 10.1227/neu.0b013e318277a5aa

hrock, L. E., Mink, J. W., Woods, D. W., Porta, M., Servello, D., Visser-Vandewalle, V., et al. (2015). Tourette syndrome deep brain stimulation: a review and updated recommendations. *Mov. Disord.* 30, 448–471. doi: 10.1002/mds.26094

Schuurman, P. R., Bosch, D. A., Bossuyt, P. M., Bonsel, G. J., van Someren, E. J., de Bie, R. M., et al. (2000). A comparison of continuous thalamic stimulation and thalamotomy for suppression of severe tremor. *N. Engl. J. Med.* 342, 461–468. doi: 10.1056/NEJM200002173420703

Shimamoto, S. A., Ryapolova-Webb, E. S., Ostrem, J. L., Galifianakis, N. B., Miller, K. J., and Starr, P. A. (2013). Subthalamic nucleus neurons are synchronized to primary motor cortex local field potentials in Parkinson's disease. *J. Neurosci.* 33, 7220–7233. doi: 10.1523/JNEUROSCI.4676-12.2013

Spencer, W. J., and Seidel, T. E. (1995). "National technology roadmaps: the U.S. semiconductor experience," in *1995 4th International Conference on Solid-State and Integrated Circuit Technology* (Beijing), 211–220.

Stidd, D. A., Vogelsang, K., Krahl, S. E., Langevin, J.-P., and Fellous, J.-M. (2013). Amygdala deep brain stimulation is superior to paroxetine treatment in a rat model of posttraumatic stress disorder. *Brain Stimulat.* 6, 837–844. doi: 10.1016/j.brs.2013.05.008

Storch, A., Schneider, C. B., Wolz, M., Stürwald, Y., Nebe, A., Odin, P., et al. (2013). Nonmotor fluctuations in Parkinson disease: severity and correlation with motor complications. *Neurology* 80, 800–809. doi: 10.1212/WNL.0b013e318285c0ed

Swan, B. D., Grill, W. M., and Turner, D. A. (2014). Investigation of deep brain stimulation mechanisms during implantable pulse generator replacement surgery. *Neuromodulation* 17, 419–424. discussion: 424. doi: 10.1111/ner.12123

Sweet, J. A., Walter, B. L., Gunalan, K., Chaturvedi, A., McIntyre, C. C., and Miller, J. P. (2014). Fiber tractography of the axonal pathways linking the basal ganglia and cerebellum in Parkinson disease: implications for targeting in deep brain stimulation. *J. Neurosurg.* 120, 988–996. doi: 10.3171/2013.12.JNS131537

Tan, L. C. S. (2012). Mood disorders in Parkinson's disease. *Parkinsonism Relat. Disord.* 18(suppl. 1), S74–S76. doi: 10.1016/S1353-8020(11)70024-4

Tasker, R. R. (1998). Deep brain stimulation is preferable to thalamotomy for tremor suppression. *Surg. Neurol.* 49, 145–153. discussion: 153–154. doi: 10.1016/s0090-3019(97)00459-x

Temko, A., Thomas, E., Marnane, W., Lightbody, G., and Boylan, G. (2011). EEG-based neonatal seizure detection with Support Vector Machines. *Clin. Neurophysiol.* 122, 464–473. doi: 10.1016/j.clinph.2010.06.034

Timmermann, L., Jain, R., Chen, L., Maarouf, M., Barbe, M. T., Allert, N., et al. (2015). Multiple-source current steering in subthalamic nucleus deep brain stimulation for Parkinson's disease (the VANTAGE study): a non-randomised, prospective, multicentre, open-label study. *Lancet Neurol.* 14, 693–701. doi: 10.1016/S1474-4422(15)00087-3

Vitek, J. L., and Starr, P. (2015). Deep Brain Stimulation (DBS) for the Treatment of Parkinson's Disease (INTREPID). Available at: https://clinicaltrials.gov/ct2/show/NCT01839396.

Wang, T. R., Dallapiazza, R., and Elias, W. J. (2015). Neurological applications of transcranial high intensity focused ultrasound. *Int. J. Hyperth.* 31, 285–291. doi: 10.3109/02656736.2015.1007398

Wintermark, M., Druzgal, J., Huss, D. S., Khaled, M. A., Monteith, S., Raghavan, P., et al. (2014a). Imaging findings in MR imaging-guided focused ultrasound treatment for patients with essential tremor. *AJNR Am. J. Neuroradiol.* 35, 891–896. doi: 10.3174/ajnr.A3808

Wintermark, M., Huss, D. S., Shah, B. B., Tustison, N., Druzgal, T. J., Kassell, N., et al. (2014b). Thalamic connectivity in patients with essential tremor treated with MR imaging-guided focused ultrasound: *in vivo* fiber tracking by using diffusion-tensor MR imaging. *Radiology* 272, 202–209. doi: 10.1148/radiol.14132112

Wissel, T., Pfeiffer, T., Frysch, R., Knight, R. T., Chang, E. F., Hinrichs, H., et al. (2013). Hidden Markov model and support vector machine based decoding of finger movements using electrocorticography. *J. Neural Eng.* 10:056020. doi: 10.1088/1741-2560/10/5/056020

Yang, A. I., Vanegas, N., Lungu, C., and Zaghloul, K. A. (2014). Beta-coupled high-frequency activity and beta-locked neuronal spiking in the subthalamic nucleus of Parkinson's disease. *J. Neurosci.* 34, 12816–12827. doi: 10.1523/JNEUROSCI.1895-14.2014

Zimnik, A. J., Nora, G. J., Desmurget, M., and Turner, R. S. (2015). Movement-related discharge in the macaque globus pallidus during high-frequency stimulation of the subthalamic nucleus. *J. Neurosci.* 35, 3978–3989. doi: 10.1523/JNEUROSCI.4899-14.2015

12

Proof of Concept of an Online EMG-Based Decoding of Hand Postures and Individual Digit Forces for Prosthetic Hand Control

*Alycia Gailey[1], Panagiotis Artemiadis[2] and Marco Santello[1]**

[1] School of Biological and Health Systems Engineering, Tempe, AZ, USA, [2] School for Engineering of Matter, Transport, and Energy, Arizona State University, Tempe, AZ, USA

Edited by:
Marc Slutzky,
Northwestern University, USA

Reviewed by:
Adenike Adewuyi,
Northwestern University, USA
Matthew R. Williams,
U.S. Department of Veterans Affairs, USA

****Correspondence:***
Marco Santello
marco.santello@asu.edu

Introduction: Options currently available to individuals with upper limb loss range from prosthetic hands that can perform many movements, but require more cognitive effort to control, to simpler terminal devices with limited functional abilities. We attempted to address this issue by designing a myoelectric control system to modulate prosthetic hand posture and digit force distribution.

Methods: We recorded surface electromyographic (EMG) signals from five forearm muscles in eight able-bodied subjects while they modulated hand posture and the flexion force distribution of individual fingers. We used a support vector machine (SVM) and a random forest regression (RFR) to map EMG signal features to hand posture and individual digit forces, respectively. After training, subjects performed grasping tasks and hand gestures while a computer program computed and displayed online feedback of all digit forces, in which digits were flexed, and the magnitude of contact forces. We also used a commercially available prosthetic hand, the i-Limb (Touch Bionics), to provide a practical demonstration of the proposed approach's ability to control hand posture and finger forces.

Results: Subjects could control hand pose and force distribution across the fingers during online testing. Decoding success rates ranged from 60% (index finger pointing) to 83–99% for 2-digit grasp and resting state, respectively. Subjects could also modulate finger force distribution.

Discussion: This work provides a proof of concept for the application of SVM and RFR for online control of hand posture and finger force distribution, respectively. Our approach has potential applications for enabling in-hand manipulation with a prosthetic hand.

Keywords: myoelectric hand, neuroprosthesis, machine learning applied to neuroscience, neurorobotics, brain-machine interface

INTRODUCTION

A significant challenge faced in modern medicine is in replacing a lost hand for upper limb amputees. The human hand performs many complex functions in the activities of daily living. One area of challenge is in the tradeoff between functionality and ease of use. A prosthetic hand that performs more functions will generally require more cognitive effort from the user. In contrast, a prosthetic hand that is simpler to control generally has more limited functionality.

According to an epidemiology study by Dillingham and colleagues (1), from 1988 to 1996 about 134,000 Americans underwent upper limb amputations from trauma and another 29,400 Americans lost their upper limbs to dysvascular disease. Though there are already a number of different upper limb prostheses available, the rate at which individuals with upper limb loss stop using the prostheses is significant. A meta-analysis by Biddiss and Chau (2) showed abandonment rates of 26% in body-powered prosthesis users and 23% in electrically powered prosthesis users. Major reasons for these abandonment rates include heavy weight, lack of functionality and durability, discomfort, poor cosmetic appearance, and finally too much effort required to control the prosthesis.

One of the main remaining challenges for prosthetic hand developers is in allowing the user to reliably control many different hand movements without too much cognitive effort. Body-powered systems are reliable, but their harness system can result in fatigue and strain (2). Furthermore, body-powered prostheses are limited in their functionality. Control systems based on electroencephalographic (EEG) signals can be used to control prosthetic hands for above-elbow amputees and paralyzed individuals (3, 4). However, the implementation of these systems tends to be challenging because EEG signals are associated with many other behaviors besides hand motion, such as proximal musculature involved in hand transport, trunk movement, and so forth. Other methods are being developed to extract signals from within the brain or peripheral nerve tissue, but such methods are invasive and expensive (5).

Myoelectric systems are based on electromyographic (EMG) activity of residual muscles following an amputation and offer several advantages relative to the above-described systems. Specifically, EMG-controlled systems are non-invasive, and they take advantage of signals recorded from residual muscle activity that is specifically involved in the task. Numerous systems have been developed for recording surface EMG signals from the upper limb and extracting features to predict in real-time grasp postures and/or forces, or for individuals with upper limb loss, predicting the user's intended hand movement. Castellini et al. (6) demonstrated the use of EMG in predicting hand postures in healthy able-bodied individuals. Castellini et al. (7) further demonstrated that EMG signals from the residual muscles of amputees can predict five different imagined grasp poses to accuracies around 79–95% and grip force with accuracies between 7 and 17% normalized root mean square error (NRMSE) (7). The grasp poses included open hand, closed fist, 2-digit pinch, tripod (3-digit) grip, and index finger pointing.

In the same year, Yang et al. (8) demonstrated the use of EMG in the forearm to predict one of 18 possible combinations of finger flexion/extension for the thumb, index, and middle finger. It was found that while the classification accuracy was quite high when training and testing on data collected within the same session, training on data in an earlier data collection session and testing on a later session yielded much lower classification accuracies (50–60%). Subsequently, Castellini and Kõiva (9) demonstrated the use of a myoelectric control system that allowed 12 able-bodied subjects to modulate individual finger forces when the hand lay flat on a surface with each finger placed on top of force sensors. Although this system is a good proof of principle of myoelectric control of finger forces, this type of control was not demonstrated in a grasping task when the subject's hand is not laid flat on a surface, but rather is in a fist. In addition, this work does not account for wrist rotation during grasping tasks, although future work should focus on testing the robustness of our decoder across wrist postures that are commonly found in activities of daily living. Later work by Cipriani et al. (10) examined real-time myoelectric control of grasp types by individuals with upper limb loss with nine EMG electrodes placed along either side of the residual forearm muscles. Predicted gestures included open hand, closed fist, thumbs up, index finger pointing with extended thumb, flexed thumb with four extended fingers, and 3-digit grip. Average online control classification accuracy was 79% for transradial amputees and 89% for able-bodied subjects. However, this work did not examine online control of digit forces.

The present work attempts to expand upon the work of Castellini et al. (7) by implementing online control of hand postures—as opposed to offline cross-validation—and online control of individual finger forces, which allow subjects to modulate the distribution of force across the fingers of the prosthetic hand. The system is programed in Matlab, and therefore does not implement true real-time control. However, the delay between a change in EMG signals and a change in desired hand motion is only 0.3 s. For a proof-of-concept demonstration of our approach, we used the commercially available i-limb hand (Touch Bionics) because it has a separate motor for each digit and each digit can exert seven different levels of grip forces, thus allowing for some degree of force modulation by individual digits. We examined several grasping tasks, including lifting the object using a chosen grasp type (2-digit, 3-digit, or whole-hand grasp), alternating between grasp types while holding the object, and modulating the grip force during the object holding phase. Because the i-limb hand has certain limitations (limited speed of motion, limited ability to exert a discrete set of forces per digit), we tested this system mostly by using a computer program to give online feedback of finger forces and grasp type for each loop iteration, while simultaneously instructing the subject to perform different hand poses. The system's performance is demonstrated on able-bodied individuals before future testing on individuals with upper limb loss.

MATERIALS AND METHODS

Subjects

Eight right-handed subjects (age: 23.5 years, SD: ±3.42, five males, three females) participated in the study. We recruited subjects who identified themselves as right handed. Subjects had no history or record of neurological disorders and had never performed tasks involving myoelectric control of an external device. Subjects gave informed written consent to participate in the experiments. The experiments were approved by the Institutional Review Board at Arizona State University and were in accordance with the Declaration of Helsinki. Each experimental session (one session/subject) lasted approximately 1.5–2 h.

Experimental Protocols

We asked subjects to perform two sets of tasks. In the first set of tasks, subjects were asked to perform a series of grasping and finger pointing tasks (*Task 1: hand postures*; **Figure 1A**). In the second set of tasks, subjects were asked to vary the distribution of normal forces among the fingers in a closed fist (*Task 2: digit forces*). For both tasks, we recorded EMG signals from five surface EMG electrodes and extracted features from these signals to train a one-against-one support vector machine (SVM). This SVM was used to distinguish hand poses, and a random forest regression (RFR) was used to predict each of the five digit forces. Subjects performed both tasks in the same experimental session. Below we describe the procedures for both training and testing of our EMG decoder system.

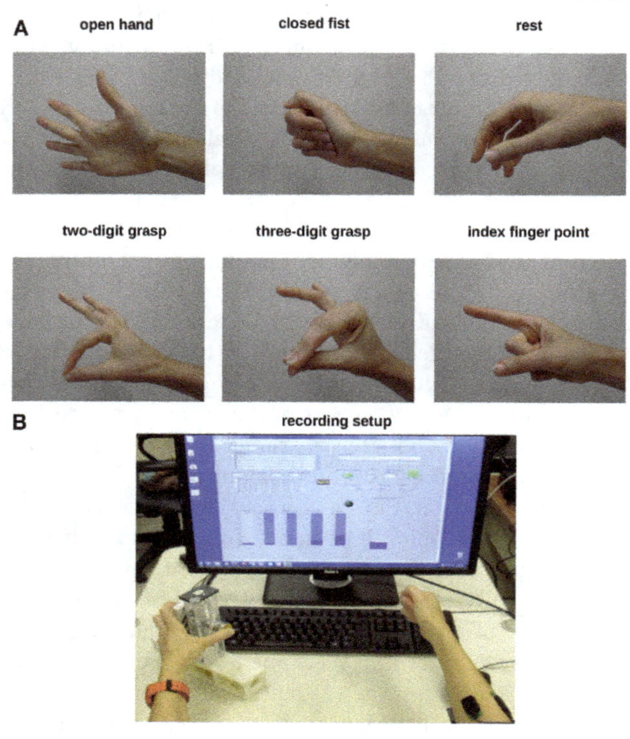

FIGURE 1 | Experimental protocols. (A) For Experiment 1 (Hand postures), subjects were asked to shape their right hand to create six postures (open hand, closed fist, rest, 2-digit grasp, 3-digit grasp, and pointing). **(B)** For Experiment 2 (Digit forces), subjects were asked to change the distribution of finger forces of their right hand while grasping a sensorized object with the left hand. A computer monitor was used to display force data recorded from the sensorized grip device grasped with the left hand. Subjects were given force feedback for each digit in the form of rising bars (one/digit, bottom left display) as well as for all digits (total grip force, bottom right display). For both experiments, we recorded electromyographic activity through surface electrodes placed on the right forearm.

EMG Recording, Signal Processing, and Feature Extraction

We placed five surface EMG electrodes (Delsys) around the circumference of the forearm just below the elbow (**Figure 1B**). The electrodes were roughly equally spaced apart. At least one EMG electrode was placed over the m. extensor digitorum superficialis (finger extensor) on the dorsal surface of the forearm. The other electrodes did not target specific muscles. A reference EMG electrode was placed directly over the lateral epycondyle of the humerus. Prior to EMG electrode placement, the area was cleaned with rubbing alcohol pads. We did not target specific muscles because this approach is not always feasible when using surface EMG from residual muscles in individuals with upper limb loss. Specifically, availability of specific target muscle depends on the extent and state of residual muscle fibers following amputation which, in turn, may affect the EMG signal quality and the extent to which it can be used for hand posture or grasp force decoding. Thus, we aimed at using a muscle-independent EMG decoding approach to resemble a more realistic scenario of extracting features from non-specific forearm muscles.

Our preliminary online and offline testing showed that increasing the number of electrodes did not improve the hand pose classification accuracy. We had also performed preliminary offline testing on a high-resolution electrode array (90 channels) and found that hand pose classification was more difficult due to lower signal quality. Furthermore, work by Castellini et al. (7) showed that five electrodes placed around the circumference of the forearm allowed for prediction of desired hand pose in three amputees. This work, as well as our study, suggested that the quality of the EMG signal might be more important for hand pose and finger force decoding than the number of EMG channels.

All EMG signals during training and testing were analyzed in individual 50-ms non-overlapping time windows for the purpose of enabling online control. Although time windows longer than 50 ms may improve prediction accuracy, we chose a 50-ms time window length based on the need to reduce control delays due to data processing (see below). However, we note that pilot testing revealed that longer time windows would not have significantly improved prediction accuracy. Furthermore Castellini et al. (7) reported that a time window of 50 ms was sufficiently long to make predictions of desired hand motions in amputees. Control was quasi real time as the processing delay was about 0.3 s. For each EMG signal-recording interval, the computed signal average was subtracted to center the signal amplitude about 0. Next, all points in the time interval were normalized to a range spanning −1 to +1 where a value of ±1 represents the EMG magnitude recorded during maximum voluntary contraction (MVC). MVC EMG was recorded by asking subjects to perform six maximum isometric force contractions isometric finger flexion, finger extension, wrist flexion, wrist extension, wrist abduction, and wrist adduction. For each EMG channel, the root mean square (RMS) was computed for each 50-ms time window throughout the entire MVC trial. The maximum RMS value computed for each channel during the MVC recording was used as the EMG magnitude representative of MVC for that channel. All signals collected in that channel in subsequent recordings were centered at 0 and then divided by the MVC magnitude.

Electromyographic signals were amplified in hardware (gain: 1,000; Delsys Bagnoli-8 EMG System) before being digitized and analyzed in software. After subtraction of the mean and normalization of the EMG signal, 60 Hz line noise was filtered by passing the signal through a 60-Hz notch filter with 3-dB cutoff and bandwidth set to 20 Hz. Next, features were extracted from each filtered 50-ms time window. We explored various EMG signal features presented in previous work [e.g., Zecca et al. (11) and Khushaba et al. (12)] including mean absolute value, variance, Willison amplitudes, mean of amplitudes, auto-regressive coefficients, and other novel features presented by Khushaba et al. (12). Of these features, three were found to be most informative for predicting hand posture. The first chosen feature is the RMS, computed according to Eq. 1:

$$\mathrm{RMS} = \sqrt{\frac{1}{N}\sum_{t=t_1}^{t_2} x^2(t)} \tag{1}$$

where the term $x(t)$ denotes the EMG signal value at time t.

The next two features were derived by Khushaba et al. (12). These features were computed by the zero-order moment (same as RMS above), m_0, the second-order moment, m_2, and the fourth-order moment, m_4. These moments were computed according to Eqs 2–4:

$$m_0 = \int_{t-T}^{T} x^2(t)\,dt \tag{2}$$

$$m_2 = \int_{t-T}^{T} \left(\frac{dx}{dt}\right)^2 dt \tag{3}$$

$$m_4 = \int_{t-T}^{T} \left(\frac{d^2x}{dt^2}\right)^2 dt \tag{4}$$

The variable T is the length of time for one time window. After computing the moments, the irregularity factor, IF, and the wavelength variable, WL, were computed according to Eqs 5 and 6:

$$IF = \sqrt{\frac{m_2^2}{m_0 m_4}} \tag{5}$$

$$\mathrm{WL} = \int_{t-T}^{T} \left|\frac{dx}{dt}\right| dt \tag{6}$$

One of the features (f) used was dependent on the zero-order moment or RMS, computed according to Eq. 7:

$$f_2 = \log\left(m_0 / N\right) \tag{7}$$

The variable, N, is the number of samples within each time window. The third feature type was computed according to Eq. 8:

$$f_3 = \log\left(\mathrm{IF} / \mathrm{WL}\right) \tag{8}$$

Each type of feature was computed not only for each individual EMG channel but also for each combination of channel pairs where the feature value of one channel would be subtracted from the feature value of the other channel, thus yielding 15 features of each feature type. To identify non-redundant features, we performed linear correlation between feature pairs. As many features were highly correlated with each other, we did not use all features for hand posture and digit force prediction. Therefore, we chose the 15 features characterized by the weakest correlation with each other. For each pair of features that were highly correlated, we chose the feature that changed the most between grasp types. We found that the features that changed the most between grasp types also were highly correlated with each other, and were therefore redundant. Selecting features least correlated with each other yielded less redundancy, and therefore more information. As such, the same set of features was used in distinguishing all pairs of hand poses.

Force Data Recording and Processing

Normal forces exerted by each digit were measured by five force/torque (F/T) sensors (ATI Industrial Automation) mounted on a grip device grasped by the left hand. Four F/T sensors (Nano-17) were mounted on the finger side of the grip device, and an F/T sensor (Nano-25) was mounted on the thumb side. During recording sessions, the subject grasped the force-sensing device with one digit on each force sensor, and force data were collected synchronously with EMG data to form a mapping between EMG and each digit force.

EMG and Force Data Processing

Electromyographic and force data were acquired at 1 kHz by 12-bit analog-to-digital converter boards (NIDAQ PCI-6225, National Instruments; sampling frequency: 1 kHz). EMG data recording was performed through Matlab (Mathworks), which forces data recording through LabVIEW (version 8.0, National Instruments). EMG data and force data were synchronized by a trigger pulse sent by the LabVIEW program to the NIDAQ board at the start of the recording. This pulse appeared in the EMG recording in Matlab.

Training Data Collection

After recording MVC EMG, the subject was prompted to relax the hand for 1 min while EMG signals were recorded. RMS was computed for each 50-ms time window of the resting period and the resting threshold was computed as 1.5 times the average magnitude of the EMG signal in each channel. When the RMS of all five EMG channels was below their resting threshold, the computer program predicted that the hand was at rest.

The EMG decoder predicts one of six possible hand poses. The hand poses are shown in **Figure 1A**. We chose these poses to capture basic grasp types [2- and 3-digit precision grasps where the thumb contacts the fingertips; closed fist to approximate a "power" grasp (13)], as well as non-prehensile hand postures (rest, open hand, and index finger pointing). To form a mapping between EMG signals and hand pose/digit forces, data were collected from 12 training trials lasting 30 s each. For trials 1 and 2, the subject extended all fingers. About 15 s after the start of the recording, the subject was told to co-contract the hand muscles while keeping fingers extended for about 7–8 s. For trials 3 and 4, the subject shaped the hand into a 2-digit grasping pose where the thumb and index finger pressed against each other at the tips and the other three fingers were extended (**Figure 1A**). Fifteen seconds after the start of the recording, the subject was told to increase the pinch force for about 7–8 s. For trials 5 and 6, the subject did an index finger pointing (**Figure 1A**). Subsequently, the subject was told to increase and then decrease the muscle co-contraction. For trials 7 and 8, the subject did a 3-digit grasp (index finger and middle finger pressing against the tip of the thumb while ring finger and little finger were extended; **Figure 1A**). Fifteen seconds after the start of the recording, the subject was told to increase the pinch force.

For trials 9–12, subjects made a fist with the ipsilateral hand and grasped the force-sensing object with the contralateral hand (**Figure 1B**). The subject was asked to keep flexion forces approximately the same for both hands. For trial 9, the subject began by making a fist using a small grip force, and then the subject shifted most of the force onto the index finger with the ipsilateral hand while still maintaining a closed fist. With the contralateral hand, the subject exerted most or all of the pressure on the force sensors with the thumb and index finger to teach the RFR that most of the force was concentrated on the index finger and thumb. The same procedure was repeated for the middle finger. For trial 10, the process was repeated for the ring finger and little finger. For trials 11 and 12, the subject started the trial with the ipsilateral hand in a relaxed fist and the contralateral hand exerting minimal force on all five force sensors. The subject was then prompted to ramp up the flexion force across all digits on both hands to a moderately high value, maintain the higher grip force for about 5 s, and then ramp the force back down.

The rationale for having subjects make a fist with the right ipsilateral hand during training while grasping the force sensors with the contralateral hand was that this approach is more feasible for training individuals with unilateral (ipsilateral) upper limb loss. Specifically, these individuals can use the intact (contralateral) hand to grasp force-sensing object while sending similar motor commands to the ipsilateral hand to trying to match forces across the two limbs.

One of the goals of the system in the current study is to allow the user to grasp the object with the prosthetic hand by simply making a fist with the real hand, and then pressing the fingers into the palm in order to modulate the distribution of force across the fingers. EMG signals can change depending on the size of the object being grasped. Therefore, if EMG signals are recorded while the subject is grasping a force-sensing object of a certain size, then the subject may need to grasp an object of the same size during online control in order to generate the desired finger forces.

Training the Machine Learning Classifiers and Regressions

Figure 2 shows a block diagram of the training portion and testing portion of our system. 15 The training portion inputs data from the subject to form a mapping between EMG signal and 16 hand pose, and a mapping between EMG signal and finger forces. The testing portion of the 17 system inputs EMG signals and makes online predictions of hand pose and finger forces.

To distinguish among the five hand postures, we used a one-against-one radial basis kernel SVM. Such a system consists of one SVM binary classifier to distinguish each pair of hand poses. When one hand pose is guessed in favor of the other one, the hand pose receives a vote. The hand pose receiving the most votes across the different SVM classifiers gets selected. The hyperparameters were determined by offline testing on preliminary pilot data. Such testing would train on some data and test on the other data. The classification errors were computed for each set of hyperparameters, and the hyperparameters yielding the lowest classification errors were selected. For more information on SVMs and the one-against-one multiclass classification methods, the reader is referred to Hsu and Lin (14). To distinguish each pair of poses, 15 features were selected with the lowest correlation with each other. For digit force predictions, the 15 RMS features were used to train a RFR, which used 50 trees and all 15 features/tree. For a description of RFR algorithm, see Breiman (15). A separate RFR was trained for each digit force.

Online Myoelectric Control: Finger Force Prediction through a Computer Program

Regulation of force is difficult with the i-limb hand because (1) the i-limb hand commands only consist of integer values from −7 to +7, thereby limiting the resolution of force exertion and (2) if force is too high, it is difficult to reduce the force on a given finger by a specific amount unless extensive calibration is employed to determine the duration of the extension command necessary to decrease the force by a specific amount without losing contact. Furthermore, (3) the wireless Bluetooth-based communication required to receive commands tended to be unstable in our setup. Therefore, most of the online testing of the quality of myoelectric control was performed using a custom-made computer program. This program printed to the screen the predicted flexion forces for each digit during each loop iteration (~3 loop iterations/second). The computer program prompted the subject either to perform grasping tasks or to make a fist and vary the force distribution among the fingers.

For simulated grasping tasks using the computer program, 50 ms of EMG data were recorded for each loop/iteration. EMG signal features were extracted and input into the SVM classifiers for hand posture prediction, and RFRs for digit force prediction. Flexion and extension forces for each digit were printed to the screen at the end of the loop iteration. A force value greater or lower than 0 indicated predicted flexion or extension, respectively. A value equal to 0 indicated a predicted resting state. If all printed digit forces were negative, then the predicted hand pose was open hand. If all printed digit forces were positive, then the predicted hand pose was closed fist. If only the top 2-digit forces (index finger and thumb) were positive, then the predicted hand pose was a 2-digit pinch grip. If only the index finger force was negative and all other forces were positive, then the predicted hand pose was an index finger point (which could be performed while grasping an object).

Initially, the subject was given time to familiarize with the computer program used to display predicted finger forces by learning to associate the printed forces on the screen with specific hand poses. If digit force control was not sufficient, then training would be repeated for specific hand poses that were found to be more difficult to predict. To test the quality of myoelectric control, commands were posted on the screen to the subject about what hand posture to adopt and what target force to reach during grasping.

The computer program would summate the normal forces of the digits in contact and print the total grip force in the space below the individual digit forces. When the subject was asked to grasp, a target grasping force was printed to the screen in the area below the predicted total grip force. We chose submaximal target grasping forces (ranging from 6 to 30 N for a 2-digit and power grasp, respectively) as these are typically associated with activities of daily living. An example of force feedback (printed to the screen once per loop iteration) is shown below:

INDEX-THUMB GRASP
Thumb: 5.62
Index finger: 4.32
Middle finger: 0.05
Ring finger: −1
Little finger: −1
9.944 N
Target Force: 6 N

Each grasp task consisted of 100 iterations, at roughly 300 ms/loop iteration. Below is the list of commands given to the subject in chronological order:

- Relax, Open Hand, Index-thumb grasp (target force = 6 N, 12 N), Open Hand, Relax
- Open Hand, Three-digit grasp (target force = 10 N, 20 N), Open Hand, Relax
- Open Hand, Power grasp (target force = 30 N, 25 N, 20 N, 15 N, 10 N), Open Hand
- Relax, Open Hand, Power grasp (target force = 12 N), Index finger point (target force = 12 N), Power grasp, Index finger point, Power grasp, Open hand, Relax
- Open Hand, Power grasp, Index-thumb grasp, Power grasp, Index-thumb grasp, Power grasp, Open Hand, Relax

To factor out response time of subjects to the change in command, the program paused for 4 s whenever there was a change in the command given to the subject.

For the second set of exercises, subjects made a fist the entire force across the digits. For the first 20% of iterations, subjects began with a relaxed fist (minimal flexion forces) and when prompted, made a tight fist. Every 20 iterations, subjects transitioned from tight to relaxed fist, or from relaxed to tight fist. For the second 20% of iterations, subjects were prompted to shift the force to the little finger. For the third 20% of iterations, subjects were prompted to shift the force to the ring finger. For the fourth 20% of iterations, subjects shifted the force to the middle finger. For the fifth 20% of iterations, subjects shifted the force to the index finger. Both sets of trials were performed five times. Subjects alternated between grasping task rounds and force-shifting task rounds, making a total of 10 rounds. We accepted all attempts at achieving the target force. The measure of how close the subject attained the target force was captured the NRMSE, which was computed as the square root of the difference between the target and predicted force divided by the target force.

Testing with the i-Limb Hand

For practical demonstration purposes, the myoelectric control system was tested on a commercially available prosthetic hand, the i-limb (Touch Bionics). For each loop iteration, commands were wirelessly sent to the i-limb hand where the integer value of the flexion command was proportional to the predicted flexion force. The subject was asked to grasp the 5-digit force-sensing object (one force sensor/digit) using a 5-digit grasp, 2-digit pinch grip, and a 3-digit tripod grip. The subject was only required to complete one successful trial for each grasp type. Finally, the subject was prompted to alternate grasp types during object hold. For this trial, the subject used myoelectric control to grasp the object with five digits. Upon command, the subject released the index finger to do an index finger point, and then upon command, the subject returned to the 5-digit grasp. Next, the subject was prompted to release 2 or 3 of the fingers and transition to a 3-digit or 2-digit grasp without losing contact. Finally, the subject released the object. For all grasping tasks with the i-limb hand, a successful trial was defined as a trial during which the subject could hold a grasp for about 5 s without unwanted hand opening, and then release the grasp on verbal command.

To quantify the level of difficulty in completing simple grasping tasks with the i-limb hand, subjects were asked to rate each i-limb task level of difficulty on a scale from 1 to 5. On the scale, 1 = "easy," 2 = "able to do the task," 3 = "able to do the task, but with effort," 4 = "moderately hard," and 5 = "very hard or could not do."

Data Analysis: Predicted Finger Forces and Force Distributions

For trials concerned with grasping tasks, variables of interest included the NRMSE of the grip force across grasp types, and confusion matrix that relates predicted hand posture to desired hand posture. The error of the grip force was computed as the difference between the total predicted grip force and the target force. Total grip force was computed as the summation of normal forces across all digits that were supposed to be flexed. For hand pose predictions, the overall percent accuracy was the predicted hand pose was correct out of the total of 500 loop iterations. Another variable of interest is the number of times that an open hand is predicted when the correct hand pose is a grasp. Such a situation would indicate unwanted loss of contact.

For trials concerned with force distribution across the fingers, the finger forces were summated for each loop/iteration, and then the fraction of the total finger force contributed by each finger was computed. For loop iterations 101–200, the little finger was expected to contribute the highest fraction of total finger force out of all the other fingers. Similarly, for loop iterations 201–300, the ring finger was expected to contribute the highest fraction of total finger force. For loop iterations 301–400, the middle finger was expected to contribute the highest fraction of total finger force. For loop iterations 401–500, the index finger was expected to contribute the highest fraction of total finger force. Data analyses examined the extent to which the force distribution across fingers changed as the subject was prompted to shift the flexion force from one finger to the next. Force distributions were measured as the percent of total finger force that was contributed by each finger during each time epoch. Force distribution index was used as an additional measure of force distribution, with a value of −1 for all force concentrated on the little finger, a value of +1 for all force concentrated on the index finger and a value of 0 for evenly distributed forces.

When force distribution changed across fingers, the myoelectric control system may predict an incorrect grasp type. To investigate this issue, the variable of interest was the percentage of the time that the 5-digit (correct) hand posture was predicted.

Statistical Analysis

The first statistical analysis focused on performance during the in-hand force-shifting task. A repeated-measures analysis of variance (ANOVA) was performed on the force distribution index (range: −1 to 1) with three within-subjects factors: round of trials (*Round*; five levels), time epoch within each round (*Time epoch*; five levels), and first half versus second half of each time epoch (*Sample*; 2 levels). Subjects performed five rounds of the force-shifting tasks. Changes in force distribution across rounds indicate whether there was significant change in performance with practice. Changes in force distribution across time epochs indicate whether there was a significant change in force distribution across the fingers when subjects were prompted to change their force distribution from one finger to the next. The purpose of analyzing the factor *Sample* was to examine if performance was dependent on the length of time that subjects were asked to maintain a force distribution concentrated on one particular finger. Because each loop/iteration lasted approximately 300 ms, each time epoch was about 30 s long.

A second ANOVA was performed on overall hand pose prediction accuracy for the grasping tasks using one within-subject factor (*Round*; five levels). Results of this analysis would indicate whether overall prediction accuracy improved with practice.

RESULTS

The EMG control system design presented here is for demonstrating the use of machine learning techniques to decode five surface EMG signals from the forearm to predict desired hand motion. A machine learning-based mapping was created between EMG signal features and individual finger movements, allowing online control of individual finger movements in a robot hand. The end goal is to allow subjects to open the hand, grasp an object using a chosen grasp type, and execute an index finger pointing for gesturing or typing. When grasping, subjects were told to use the EMG decoder system to modulate

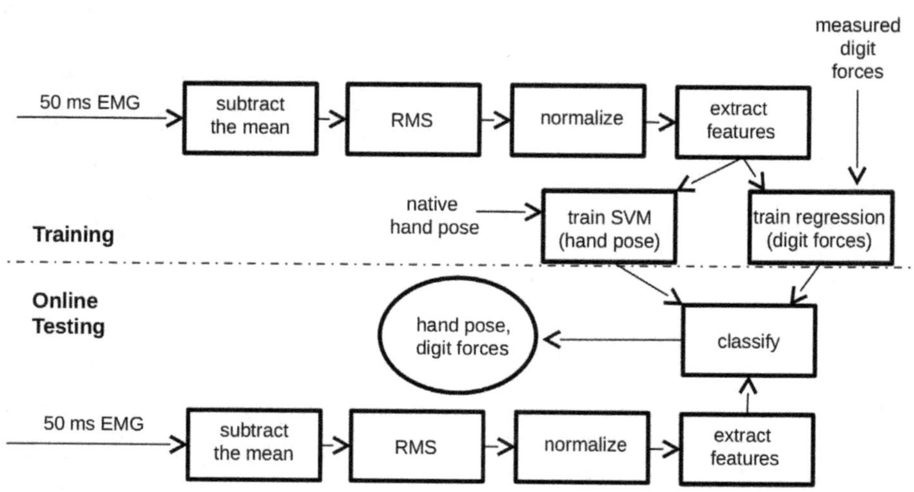

FIGURE 2 | Electromyographic (EMG) decoding system block diagram. For training, the system takes three inputs: EMG signal, force measurements from each digit of the hand, and hand pose. For testing, the system uses only one input, EMG, to predict hand pose and each digit force in real time. Each rectangle in the diagram represents a data processing step. The circle represents the system output. Above the dashed line is the training portion of the system, which forms a mapping between EMG and hand pose as well as a mapping between EMG and each of the five digit forces. Below the dashed line is the portion of the system that inputs EMG, extracts features, and generates a prediction of hand posture and digit forces for online control.

not only the amount of grip force but also the distribution of grip force across the fingers. To test system performance, subjects were prompted to perform grasping tasks and finger pointing tasks with a virtual hand in an *ad hoc* computer program where finger and thumb forces were printed to the computer screen at the end of each loop iteration.

Grasping Task Performance

Figure 3 illustrates task performance during the third round of virtual grasping tasks for a representative subject. Each of the five grasping task rounds consisted of 500 loop iterations, and each grasping task within a round consisted of 100 loop iterations (~300 ms/loop iteration). For the first 100 loop iterations, the subject was prompted to open the hand, do a 2-digit grasp, and then open the hand again. During the next 100 loop iterations, the subject was prompted to repeat with a 3-digit grasp. During loop iterations 200–300, the subject was prompted to perform a 5-digit grasp. During loop iterations 300–400, the subject was prompted to perform a 5-digit grasp, and then transition back and forth between a 5-digit grasp and an index finger point. During loop iterations 400–500, the subject was prompted to perform a 5-digit grasp, and then transition back and forth twice between a 5-digit grasp and a 2-digit grasp. The subjects were instructed to hold each hand pose for a fairly long duration to assess not only subjects' ability to achieve a given hand pose but also to maintain it.

Confusion Matrices

We created confusion matrices to illustrate the performance of the EMG decoder in predicting hand poses (**Table 1**). A confusion matrix not only indicates the overall accuracy of hand pose prediction but also specifies areas of confusion in predicting hand pose. Each entry of the confusion matrices is the median ± SEM across subjects. Entries in each row of the confusion matrix represents the hand pose that the subjects were instructed to adopt. Entries in each column represent the percentage of time that each hand pose was predicted. For example, the confusion matrix for Round 1 shows that when the subject was prompted to open the hand, an open hand was only predicted about 50% of the time (median across subjects). For 14% of the time, a 2-digit grasp was predicted instead. For 1% of the time, a 3-digit grasp was predicted. For 2 ± 6% of the time, a closed fist was predicted. An unclassified hand pose was predicted 5 ± 3% of the time.

For an ideal discrimination of hand postures, a confusion matrix will have a value of 100% along the diagonal and a value of 0% off the diagonal. Non-zero percentages that are off of the diagonal represent areas of confusion between pairs of hand poses. Predictions of an unclassified hand pose occurred when transitioning from one classified hand pose to the next. Some unclassified poses included a closed fist with extension of the little finger, extension of the little finger and index finger, extension of the middle finger and ring finger, and flexion of only the thumb and middle finger. These poses occurred mostly when the subject was attempting an open hand, 2-digit grasp, or 3-digit grasp.

The confusion matrices for each round show an improvement in performance across rounds. However, it should be noted that for some subjects, the EMG decoder was retrained on one of the hand poses only after Round 1, thereby partially explaining the increase in performance from Round 1 to Round 2. From Round 2 to Round 5 however, there was some improvement in the ability to perform a 3-digit grasp and an index finger point that can be attributable only to practice.

Analysis of variance on the overall hand pose prediction accuracy revealed that prediction accuracy varied significantly across grasping tasks (*Time epoch*; $p < 0.05$) with no main effect of *Round* (practice) or interaction between *Round* and *Time epoch*. Although 5- and 2-digit grasping had the highest and lowest prediction accuracy, we found that no significant difference was found between these two grip types. However, we found a main significant effect of experimental session ($p < 0.001$).

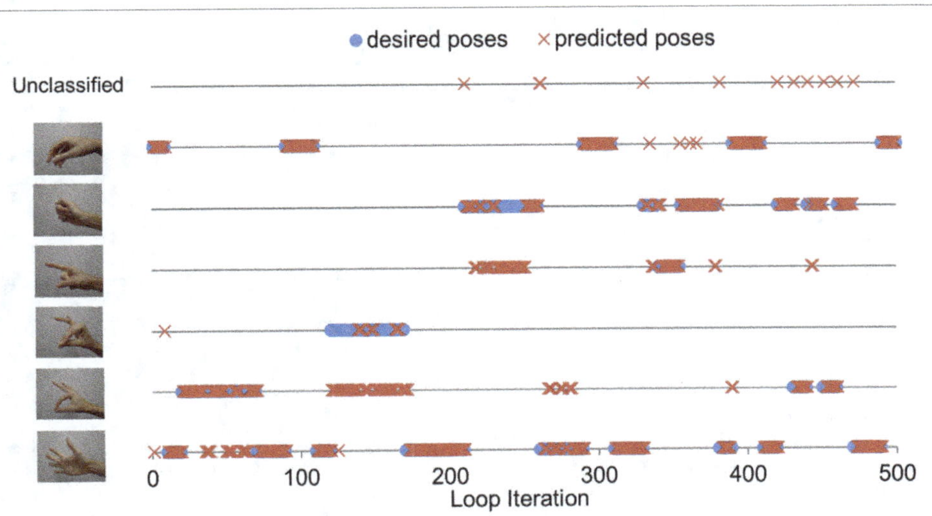

FIGURE 3 | Grasping task performance (third round, one subject). The figure shows the hand pose that the subject was instructed to achieve and maintain (blue circles), and the hand pose that the electromyographic (EMG) decoder predicted (red crosses). Each line corresponds to a specific hand pose. The top line refers to an unclassified hand pose, which happened when the EMG decoder output transitioned from one hand pose to the next.

Achieving Target Forces

During each grasp, subjects were told to reach a target force. The total predicted grip force across the fingers in contact was summated for each loop/iteration. The subject was prompted to attain the predicted total grip force to match the target force as closely as possible. The task was challenging because of the large variation in predicted grip force from one loop iteration to the next. Although the predicted grip force was computed as the average of the previous three loop iterations, there still was significant variability in force predictions across consecutive loop iterations.

Quality of grip force control was measured by the NRMSE. **Table 2** shows the NRMSE for each round of grasping tasks. The first row represents Round 1 and the bottom row represents Round 5 after subjects have undergone practice. The first column is the average NRMSE computed across all grasp types ± SEM. The other columns show the NRMSE for specific grasp types. The NRMSE shows little improvement with practice, but finer control of grip force during the 2-digit grasp. We found a marginally significant effect of number of digits when comparing force production with 2, 3, and 5 digits ($p = 0.057$), with NRMSE being lowest in the 2-digit case. This was most likely due to the fact that the 2-digit grasp only involves control of 2 of the digit flexion forces rather than all 5, leaving less room for variability in total grip force. The overall ANOVA revealed NRMSE from the 2-digit condition to be lower than 3- and 5-digit condition, whereas 3- and 5-digit conditions were not significantly different from each other. We found no interaction or effect of session on NRMSE.

Force Distribution across Fingers

Figure 4 shows how the force distribution across the fingers changes across time epochs. For the first time epoch, subjects were told to make a fist and periodically vary the total force every 20 iterations. For the second time epoch, subjects were told to shift the grip force to the little finger. For the third time epoch, subjects were told to shift the force to the ring finger. For the fourth time epoch, subjects were told to shift the force to the middle finger. For the fifth time epoch, subjects were told to shift the force to the index finger.

TABLE 1 | Confusion matrices, rounds 1 to 5 ± interquartile range.

Performed → Desired ↓	Open hand	2-digit grasp	3-digit grasp	Finger point	Closed fist	Rest	Unclassified
Round 1: 63 ± 39% average success rate							
Open hand	**50 ± 35**	14 ± 12	1 ± 1	0 ± 1	2 ± 22	0 ± 0	5 ± 9
2-digit grasp	6 ± 27	**72 ± 47**	4 ± 9	0 ± 0	4 ± 6	0 ± 0	3 ± 10
3-digit grasp	0 ± 2	11 ± 42	**48 ± 68**	0 ± 0	4 ± 8	0 ± 0	6 ± 24
Finger point	0 ± 0	0 ± 0	0 ± 0	**45 ± 37**	35 ± 37	0 ± 0	0 ± 13
Closed fist	0 ± 17	2 ± 3	0 ± 3	7 ± 15	**77 ± 26**	0 ± 2	5 ± 4
Rest	0 ± 0	3 ± 4	1 ± 1	1 ± 3	4 ± 7	**88 ± 21**	0 ± 4
Round 2: 78 ± 36% average success rate							
Open hand	**81 ± 19**	4 ± 7	1 ± 1	0 ± 1	2 ± 9	0 ± 0	1 ± 7
2-digit grasp	2 ± 19	**86 ± 56**	2 ± 3	0 ± 0	4 ± 6	0 ± 0	3 ± 9
3-digit grasp	0 ± 0	11 ± 36	**57 ± 62**	0 ± 0	2 ± 8	0 ± 0	4 ± 18
Finger pointing	0 ± 0	0 ± 0	0 ± 0	**49 ± 50**	31 ± 22	0 ± 0	0 ± 5
Closed fist	0 ± 2	0 ± 2	0 ± 1	0 ± 8	**93 ± 15**	0 ± 0	1 ± 43
Rest	0 ± 0	0 ± 0	0 ± 0	0 ± 0	0 ± 3	**100 ± 11**	0 ± 0
Round 3: 82 ± 30% average success rate							
Open hand	**78 ± 26**	3 ± 4	1 ± 1	0 ± 1	2 ± 6	0 ± 0	2 ± 3
2-digit grasp	3 ± 19	**85 ± 41**	1 ± 4	0 ± 0	4 ± 4	0 ± 0	3 ± 7
3-digit grasp	0 ± 2	7 ± 24	**74 ± 50**	0 ± 0	2 ± 4	0 ± 0	3 ± 16
Finger pointing	0 ± 0	0 ± 0	0 ± 0	**65 ± 45**	20 ± 7	0 ± 1	0 ± 13
Closed fist	0 ± 1	1 ± 2	0 ± 1	1 ± 3	**90 ± 8**	0 ± 1	2 ± 3
Rest	0 ± 0	0 ± 1	0 ± 0	0 ± 0	1 ± 3	**98 ± 11**	0 ± 0
Round 4: 80 ± 21% average success rate							
Open hand	**83 ± 28**	2 ± 1	1 ± 1	0 ± 1	2 ± 3	0 ± 0	2 ± 3
2-digit grasp	6 ± 11	**86 ± 34**	1 ± 1	0 ± 0	3 ± 4	0 ± 0	2 ± 1
3-digit grasp	0 ± 2	11 ± 24	**64 ± 32**	0 ± 0	1 ± 2	0 ± 0	5 ± 22
Finger pointing	0 ± 0	0 ± 0	0 ± 0	**57 ± 22**	27 ± 22	0 ± 0	0 ± 0
Closed fist	0 ± 1	1 ± 2	0 ± 0	1 ± 3	**93 ± 8**	0 ± 0	3 ± 3
Rest	0 ± 0	0 ± 0	0 ± 0	0 ± 0	1 ± 1	**99 ± 4**	0 ± 0
Round 5: 83 ± 25% average success rate							
Open hand	**86 ± 16**	4 ± 6	1 ± 1	0 ± 1	2 ± 3	0 ± 0	2 ± 2
2-digit grasp	6 ± 19	**83 ± 34**	2 ± 4	0 ± 0	4 ± 4	0 ± 0	3 ± 3
3-digit grasp	0 ± 0	7 ± 38	**73 ± 56**	0 ± 0	1 ± 8	0 ± 0	6 ± 16
Finger pointing	0 ± 0	0 ± 0	0 ± 0	**60 ± 22**	25 ± 20	0 ± 0	0 ± 0
Closed fist	0 ± 2	1 ± 2	0 ± 0	1 ± 3	**94 ± 9**	0 ± 0	1 ± 1
Rest	0 ± 0	0 ± 0	0 ± 0	0 ± 0	1 ± 1	**99 ± 16**	0 ± 0

Numbers in bold represent the percent of the time that each hand pose was 5 correctly predicted.

TABLE 2 | Normalized root mean square error (NRMSE) of grip force control ± SEM.

Experimental round	Average NRMSE (%)	NRMSE 2-digit (%)	NRMSE 3-digit (%)	NRMSE 5-digit (%)
Round 1	26 ± 5	24 ± 5	20 ± 3	26 ± 6
Round 2	23 ± 2	15 ± 2	26 ± 5	24 ± 2
Round 3	22 ± 2	18 ± 2	20 ± 2	23 ± 2
Round 4	22 ± 1	17 ± 2	23 ± 1	23 ± 2
Round 5	25 ± 3	18 ± 2	25 ± 3	25 ± 4

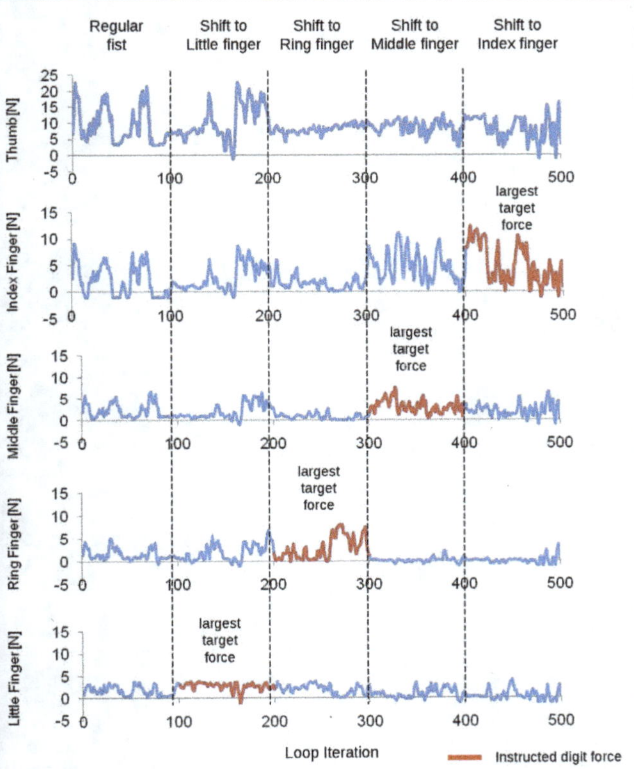

FIGURE 4 | Electromyographic decoder output for each finger flexion force (one subject). The subject was instructed to vary the force distribution across the fingers. The instruction given to the subject is shown on top for each time epoch. Time epochs are separated by vertical dashed lines. Data from each digit are shown on each row. The instructed digit for each task is denoted by a red trace. The little finger is expected to show an increased predicted force during loop iteration 100–200. During loop iteration 200–300, the ring finger is expected to show an increased predicted force. During loop iteration 300–400, the middle finger is expected to show an increased predicted force. During loop iteration 400–500, the index finger is expected to show an increased predicted force.

Figure 5 shows how the percent of total grip force on each inger varied across time epochs (horizontal axis). In time epoch , subjects were told to flex all of the fingers. Naturally, more force vill be on the index finger and middle finger as these fingers can roduce more force than other fingers. In time epoch 2, subjects vere told to shift the force to the little finger. It can be seen that a hift in the force distribution toward the little finger occurred. In ime epoch 3, subjects were told to shift the force to the ring finger. A substantial increase in predicted ring finger force is observed with a drop in predicted little finger force from time epoch 2. In time epoch 4, subjects were told to shift the force to the middle finger. A drop in predicted ring finger force is shown along with an increase in middle finger force and often an increase in index finger force. In time epoch 5, subjects were told to shift the force to the index finger. An increase in predicted index finger force is observed along with a decrease in middle finger force. The upper left plot represents data taken across subjects from Round 1. The lower left plot shows force distribution across time epochs in Round 2 after subjects have benefited from some practice and after retraining was done on one of the subjects for force predictions. The lower right plot represents data taken across subjects from Round 5 after subjects have benefited from more practice without any additional retraining. In Round 5, subjects are better at shifting more force selectively to the pinky and ring finger in time epochs 2 and 3. In both Rounds 1 and 5, subjects can easily shift force to the index finger and less on the little and ring finger.

Another way of illustrating grip force distribution across the fingers is the force distribution index, which is equal to −1 when all force across the fingers is concentrated on the pinky and equal to +1 when all force is concentrated on the index finger. When force is evenly distributed across the fingers, the force distribution index is 0. Force distribution index is computed as follows:

$$F_{dist} = F_{index} * 1 + F_{middle} * 0.5 - F_{ring} * 0.5 - F_{pinky} * 1 \quad (9)$$

When the subject was told to make a fist during the first time epoch, we expected the force distribution index to be greater than 0 because naturally the index finger and middle finger each have a higher grip force than the little finger. **Table 3** shows force distribution indices across time epochs (by row) and subjects (by column). Data from across rounds show more negative values when subjects were told to shift the force to the little finger, and greater positive values are found when subjects were told to shift the force to the index finger. Compared to when subjects were told to make a regular fist, the force distribution index was lower when subjects were told to shift the force to the ring or little finger, and higher when subjects were told to shift the force to the middle or index finger.

We found that subjects were able to shift force distribution across the fingers from one time epoch to the next (significant main effect of *Time epoch*; $p < 0.002$). However, subjects did not improve with practice, and furthermore, we found that the duration of the time epoch did not affect how well subjects could maintain a given force distribution across fingers (no main effect of *Round*, *Sample*, or significant interaction; $p > 0.1$).

Ability to Perform Grasping Tasks without Dropping the Object

A major factor influencing whether a grasping task can be performed successfully with an artificial hand is whether there is an unwanted opening of the hand as this can cause dropping of the object. In the trials involving grasping tasks, an opening of the hand when the hand was not supposed to be open rarely occurred (4.4 ± 1.4% of loop iterations), and there was little change in the incidence of unwanted hand openings across

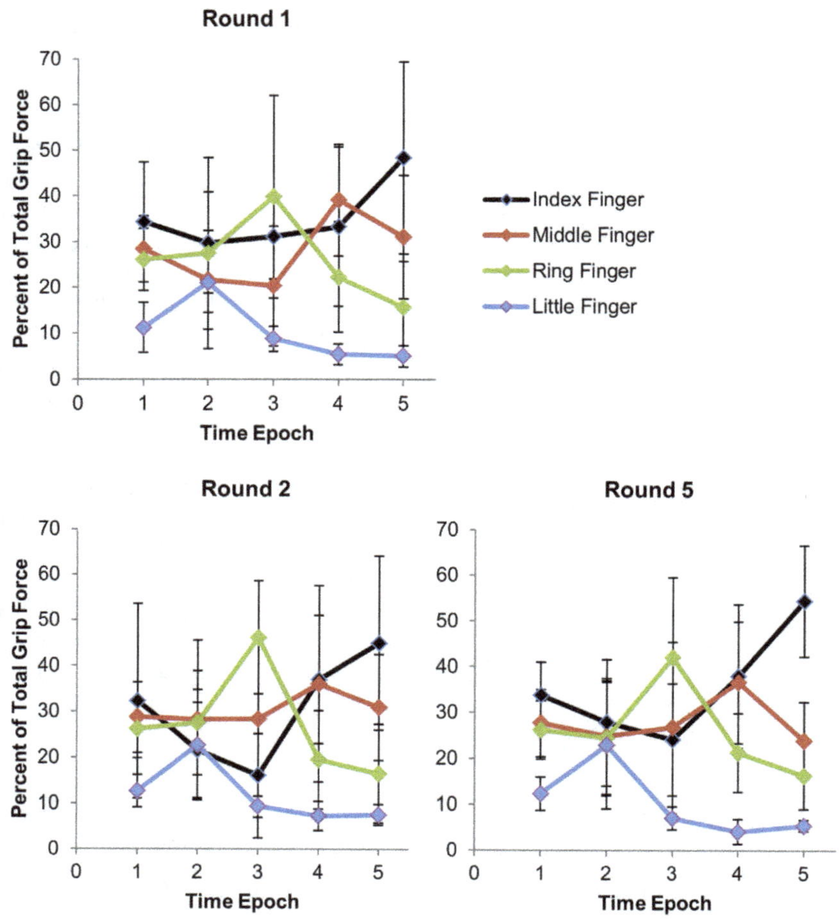

FIGURE 5 | Force distribution across fingers with each time epoch. For epoch = 1, subject made regular closed fist. For epoch = 2, subject shifted force to the pinky. For epoch = 3, subject shifted the force to the ring finger. For epoch = 4, subject shifted the force to the middle finger. For epoch = 5, subject shifted the force to the index finger. Total grip force refers to the sum of the grip forces across the fingers, excluding the thumb. Error bars represent the interquartile range.

rounds. Unwanted hand opening occurred most often for the index-thumb grasp, as illustrated in the confusion matrices (**Table 1**). In trials involving shifts in force distribution across the fingers, unwanted hand opening also occurred very rarely ($2.7 \pm 1.2\%$ of the time).

To further assess the ability to performing grasping tasks, subjects were allowed to myoelectrically control the i-limb hand. For these trials, subjects were instructed to do a few basic grasping tasks. The first task involved simply opening and closing the hand. The second and third tasks involved performing 2- and 3-digit grasps, respectively. The fourth task involved grasping with a 5-digit grasp, transitioning to index finger pointing, transitioning back to a 5-digit grasp, then transitioning to a 2- or 3-digit grasp before opening the hand. All subjects who attempted the opening and closing of the hand succeeded in performing these movements, although some subjects did so more easily than others. All subjects were able to do 2- and 3-digit grasps, but often with difficulty. All but one subject were able to perform the index finger pointing and transition from a 5- to a 3-digit grasp without losing contact. Subject 7 did not attempt the grasping tasks because of insufficient time availability.

Finally, we also asked subjects to report the level of difficulty they experienced while performing online control of each online i-limb task. 1 = "easy," 2 = "able to do the task," 3 = "able to do the task, but with effort," 4 = "moderately hard," and 5 = "very hard or could not do." **Table 4** shows the rating for each subject and task. More than half of the ratings (19/35) were below 3, i.e., subjects found the task to be easy or at least doable. Some of the ratings (9/35) were equal or greater than 3, indicating that subjects found the task moderately or very hard. These tasks were usually the finger pointing or the transition from 5- to 3-digit grasp. Although all subjects were able to transition from a 5- to a 3-digit grasp some had trouble transitioning from a 5- to a 2-digit grasp without accidentally opening the hand. A 2-digit grasp involves flexing of 3 fingers, which could have caused the hand pose to be confused with the open hand pose, which involves flexing of all digits.

DISCUSSION

This work has demonstrated a proof of principle for a system that decodes EMG signals from the upper limb of able-bodied subjects for online prediction of individual digit forces. Subject

TABLE 3 | Force distribution indices for each subject and averages across subjects.

	S1	S2	S3	S4	S5	S6	S7	S8	Average
Round 1									
Regular fist	0.24	0.35	0.20	0.19	0.20	0.08	0.22	0.45	0.24
Shift to pinky	−0.10	0.32	−0.02	0.00	−0.22	0.54	−0.12	0.06	0.06
Shift to ring	0.10	−0.19	0.02	0.45	−0.26	0.73	0.14	0.01	0.12
Shift to middle	0.12	0.07	0.18	0.37	0.47	0.63	0.48	0.58	0.36
Shift to index	0.22	0.51	0.49	0.40	0.73	0.49	0.50	0.74	0.51
Round 2									
Regular fist	−0.02	0.36	0.23	0.14	0.08	0.27	0.30	0.31	0.21
Shift to pinky	−0.13	0.40	0.10	0.13	−0.17	0.21	−0.42	−0.17	−0.01
Shift to ring	−0.02	−0.05	0.11	−0.10	−0.30	0.06	−0.04	0.15	−0.02
Shift to middle	0.39	0.20	0.17	0.19	0.61	0.52	0.38	0.58	0.38
Shift to index	0.38	0.49	0.27	0.23	0.56	0.31	0.60	0.73	0.45
Round 5									
Regular fist	0.21	0.38	0.12	0.16	0.11	0.27	0.19	0.35	0.22
Shift to pinky	0.15	0.39	−0.00	0.20	−0.34	0.06	−0.31	0.25	0.05
Shift to ring	0.09	0.32	−0.07	0.38	−0.27	0.24	0.05	0.00	0.09
Shift to middle	0.62	0.14	0.06	0.51	0.62	0.40	0.46	0.51	0.42
Shift to index	0.32	0.54	0.54	0.42	0.66	0.42	0.70	0.61	0.53

TABLE 4 | Subjective rating of difficulty level of i-limb grasping task.

i-Limb tasks	S1	S2	S3	S4	S5	S6	S7	S8
5-digit grasp	2	2	1	2	2	1	n/a	1
2-digit grasp	3	2	3	2	1	1	n/a	1
3-digit grasp	4	3	2	2	1	1	n/a	4
Finger point	3	4	5	4	4	2	n/a	2
5→3 transition	5	3	4	3	3	1	n/a	3

were able to perform a variety of grasping tasks using an *ad hoc* computer program. The system is to eventually be used on transradial amputees for enabling them to perform grasping tasks and hand gesturing with myoelectric control of a prosthetic hand such as the i-limb hand.

Clearly, predicting individual digit forces alone is insufficient for online prediction of hand motion because the EMG-to-force mapping on a given digit changes depending on which of the other digits is flexed. For example, the EMG-to-force mapping for the middle finger is going to be different for a thumb-middle finger precision grasp versus a closed fist. By incorporating an SVM classifier that distinguishes between hand postures, myoelectric control of hand motion, and individual digit forces for everyday activities becomes more feasible.

As with any myoelectric control system, this system is vulnerable to changes in the EMG signal over time. This issue is particularly relevant for myoelectric control systems that predict multiple hand motions. As the proposed system has not been tested for functionality over time periods of hours or days, future work will examine the sensitivity of our myoelectric control system to prolonged usage. Nevertheless, the impact of changes in EMG signals on myoelectric controllers has been extensively studied and the insight provided by this previous work could potentially be integrated with the proposed approach. Below we discuss previous work on myoelectric prosthesis controller algorithms and the contributions of the present work.

Previous Work on Myoelectric Decoders

Previous work has also explored numerous techniques for using EMG signals to predict desired total grasp force and hand postures. With regard to grasp force prediction, Gijsberts and colleagues (16) demonstrated the use of a supervised non-linear incremental learning method (Incremental Ridge Regression) that makes occasional updates with small batches of training data each time. This approach led to a reduction in normalized mean square error and an increase in the correlation between desired and predicted grip forces.

With regard to hand kinematics, Anam and Al-Jumaily (17) used an online sequential learning method that used small chunks of finger movement data collected online as additional training data. These additional chunks of data were used to update the weights of the trained model without retraining the entire model. The online retraining allowed for a model prediction accuracy to be maintained at 85% day-to-day, whereas the system without online retraining could not. This system could distinguish among 10 movement classes, i.e., 5 individual finger movements and 5 combined finger movements where more than one finger flexed simultaneously. Another group (18) used supervised adaptation-based linear discriminant analysis methods to adapt to drifts in the EMG signal. Offline analysis showed improvements in classification accuracy from 75% without adaptation to 92% with adaptation. For online control, the accuracy increased by 25%. The system distinguished between a mix of hand and wrist movements, which included wrist pronation/supination, wrist flexion/extension, hand open, 2-digit pinch grip, key grip, and no movement. Al-Timemy and colleagues (19) demonstrated classification of up at 15 finger movements with 98% accuracy using only 6 EMG channels in intact subjects and 90% accuracy using 11 EMG electrodes in amputees. Interestingly, the system showed better performance using Orthogonal Fuzzy Neighborhood Discriminant Analysis (OFNDA) for feature selection than principal component analysis (PCA). Unlike PCA, OFNDA takes into account maximum separation of feature values between classes. PCA only takes into consideration maximum variability among feature values in feature space.

Continuous morphing between hand postures has been another attempt at making prosthetic hand movements more natural. Segil and Weir (20) created a mapping between the EMG principal component and joint angle domains for allowing real-time control by able-bodied subjects of 15 joints of a virtual hand displayed on a computer screen. The authors reported accurate control of 13 out of 15 joints in the best-case scenario. In addition, EMG control and joystick control were found to be comparable in controlling joint motions. By using SVMs, Khushaba et al. (21) distinguished 10 classes of individual and combined finger movements, including a hand close movement, with 90.3% accuracy in real-time control experiments on eight able-bodied subjects.

Finally, ultrasound imaging has also been studied as a means to overcome the limitations of surface EMG. Akhlaghi and colleagues (22) implemented a real-time control system that classifies hand motions by sensing mechanical deformations in forearm muscle compartments. Although the results were encouraging, the system is not feasible for eventual integration with hand prosthesis controllers.

Contributions to Previous Work

It should be noted that the above-cited work on myoelectric algorithms has focused mostly on EMG-based prediction of total grasping force. To the best of our knowledge, the use of myoelectric signals to predict individual finger forces has not been investigated. This is a major gap, as successful prediction of flexion force of *individual* fingers from EMG signals could be useful for performing in-hand object manipulation using a prosthetic hand. Another gap in the literature on myoelectric controller algorithms is that there has been no demonstration of smooth transitions between grasp types without losing contact with the object. Although previous work has explored myoelectric control of smooth transitions between hand postures (20), such work did not address how easily such transitions between grasp types could be made without accidental loss of contact with the object.

In the present work, we have demonstrated proof of principle of a unique system that provides online intuitive control of individual finger forces. Subjects simply press their fingers into the palm of their hands, and the force exerted by each finger into the palm is approximately correlated with the flexing force command delivered to the corresponding finger of the robot hand. The training process involves grasping a force-sensing object only with the contralateral hand while pressing with approximately identical finger flexion forces on the ipsilateral hand. In this way, the system could be trained on amputees who have no ipsilateral hand with which to grasp the force-sensing object.

Although the RFR that predicted each finger force was trained only when the subject was making a fist, finger force prediction was transferable to other grasp types such as the 2-digit pinch grip. As long as the subject was given feedback of the digit forces, the subject was able to modulate his/her EMG signals to adjust the total grasping force accordingly. For grasping tasks performed using a computer program to display predicted finger forces, confusion matrices show that most of the improvement in performance across rounds was from Round 1 to Round 2, with smaller improvements shown in subsequent rounds (**Table 1**). In Round 5, our algorithm attained success rates ranging from 60% (index finger pointing) to 94 and 99% for closed fist and resting state, respectively. Some of the improvement from Round 1 to Round 2 was due to retraining on 1–2 hand poses on some of the subjects. Some improvement could thus be attributed to practice and familiarization to the task. Overall, our results show that subjects have voluntary control over the hand pose that the system outputs, although there is room for improvement in the system's prediction accuracy.

Figures 4 and **5** demonstrate the feasibility of EMG control of not only total grip force but also grip force distribution across the fingers during a grasping task. By selectively pressing the fingers into the palm of the hand, subjects can control which fingers have the largest normal force at the system output. This feature of the system allows for more dexterous control of individual finger motions that is intuitive for the user. However, due to high noise in predictions of total grip force, NRMSE is higher than it could have been. Finally, we demonstrate that subjects can use myoelectric control to transition between grasp types without losing contact with the object, as shown in **Figure 3**.

Methodological Considerations

One way of improving the system is incorporation of a Kalman filter for hand posture predictions. A Kalman filter can take into account the degree of uncertainty in each hand posture prediction, and it gives higher weight to predictions with higher levels of certainty. A one-against-one SVM selects the hand posture with the most votes. Therefore, the first possible measure of uncertainty in the SVM is the number of votes in favor of the chosen hand posture relative to the number of votes in favor of the other hand postures. If there are two hand postures that both have the largest number of votes, then there is uncertainty in the hand pose prediction. The second possible measure of uncertainty is in the distance of a data point from the dividing hyperplane in feature space. For distinguishing each pair of hand poses in an SVM, there is a dividing hyperplane in feature space that assigns a specific hand posture to data points on one side of the hyperplane and another hand posture to data points on the other side of the hyperplane. The shorter the distance between a data point and the dividing hyperplane, the larger the degree of uncertainty, and therefore the lower the weight that would be given to that prediction. A third measure of uncertainty would be whether the prediction of hand posture is different from the previous few predictions. When the system has a high enough processing speed to make 20 predictions/second, each prediction can be weighed differently depending on its level of uncertainty.

Even though the trials performed using a computer program to display predicted finger forces were characterized by an unwanted open hand in a small percentage of the trial duration, when using the i-limb it only takes one unwanted hand opening of the hand to classify the grasping task as unsuccessful. As described above, there are several methods that can be implemented for preventing unwanted opening of a prosthetic hand during a real grasping task. One such method is a Kalman filter, which weighs different hand pose predictions depending on their level of uncertainty.

With regard to our delay in hand posture estimation, Farrell and Weir (23) estimated 100–125 ms as optimal delays for fast and slower prehensors, respectively. The optimality of these delays is based on compromising between allowing for sufficient time for EMG decoding and maximizing the responsiveness of the prosthesis. Although our 300-ms delay is more than twice the optimal delay identified by Farrell and Weir (23), it could be significantly improved by at least 10-fold by using a different software platform (i.e., C++ instead of Matlab) to enable a larger number of hand pose predictions to be made per second. Using Kalman filters (see above) would allow for the weighing of different hand pose predictions based on the level of certainty in each prediction.

Potential Applications for Individuals with Bilateral Upper Limb Loss

Some individuals may have both hands amputated, in which case they have no hand with which to grasp a force-sensing device. In such cases, the system can make assumptions about the finger flexion forces at certain time points. For example, when the amputee is asked to concentrate the force on a specific finger, the system can assume an arbitrarily higher flexion force for that finger and a minimal force on the other fingers during that time frame. Amputees also can be prompted to vary the total grip force of a grasp where in some time frames the amputee can be prompted to exert a minimal total grasp force, and in other time frames the amputee can be prompted to exert a high grasping force. For each time frame, the system can make an assumption about the total grasp force and assume how the force would be distributed across the fingers during a grasp such as a regular closed fist depending on previous data from able-bodied individuals. For each case, the opposing thumb force can be assumed to be approximately equal to the summation of the four finger forces. An advantage of this approach is that it requires the same effort across subjects for exerting specific grasping forces because the assumption made of the grasping force for each time frame is independent of the magnitude of EMG signal (because of normalization) and of the overall muscular strength of the subject.

CONCLUSION

We have demonstrated proof of principle in the use of five EMG electrodes for predicting hand pose and individual finger forces using a one-against-one SVM and RFR, respectively. The present system has potential for myoelectric control of dexterous hand prostheses. Future work should explore additional methods of feature selection, signal filtering, machine learning classification, Kalman filtering, and training. New myoelectric control systems should be adjustable with small amounts of new training data without the need to retrain the entire system so that drifts in the EMG signal over time do not decrease classification accuracy.

ETHICS STATEMENT

Subjects gave informed written consent to participate in the experiments. The experiments were approved by the Institutional. Review Board at Arizona State University (Protocol: #1201007252) and were in accordance with the Declaration of Helsinki. Prior the experiment, participants were given time to read a consent form that described the experimental procedure. After reading the form, participants were asked if they had any questions. After any questions were answered, participants were asked to sign and date the consent form. Next, the experimenter signed and dated the consent form. No participants from vulnerable populations were used in this study.

AUTHOR CONTRIBUTIONS

AG designed the prosthetic control system, designed most of the experimental protocol, carried out the experimental protocol, collected data, analyzed data, and made data plots. PA provided expertise in the area of myoelectric control of robotic devices, thereby playing a role in design of the prosthetic control system and experimental protocol design. MS provided expertise in motor control and neuroscience. He contributed to the experimental design and data analysis methods. All authors contributed to manuscript preparation.

ACKNOWLEDGMENTS

The authors thank Dr. Justin Fine for assistance with statistical analysis.

REFERENCES

1. Dillingham TR, Pezzin LE, MacKenzie EJ. Limb amputation and limb deficiency: epidemiology and recent trends in the United States. *South Med J* (2002) 95(8):875–83. doi:10.1097/00007611-200208000-00018
2. Biddiss EA, Chau TT. The roles of predisposing characteristics, established need and enabling resources on upper extremity prosthesis use and abandonment. *Disabil Rehabil Assist Technol* (2007) 2(2):71–84.
3. Hazrati MK, Almajidy RK, Weiss J, Oung S, Hofmann UG. Controlling a simple hand prosthesis using brain signals. *48th Annual Conf of the German Society for Biomedical Engineering*. Hannover (2014).
4. Agashe HA, Paek AY, Zhang Y, Contreras-Vidal JL. Global cortical activity predicts shape of hand during grasping. *Front Neurosci* (2015) 9(121):121. doi:10.3389/fnins.2015.00121
5. Thakor NV. Translating the brain-machine interface. *Sci Transl Med* (2013) 5(210):210ps17. doi:10.1126/scitranslmed.3007303
6. Castellini C, Fiorilla AE, Sandini G. Multi-subject/daily life activity EMG-based control of mechanical hands. *J Neuroeng Rehabil* (2009) 6:41. doi:10.1186/1743-0003-6-41
7. Castellini C, Gruppioni E, Davalli A, Sandini G. Fine detection of grasp force and posture by amputees via surface electromyography. *J Physiol Paris* (2009) 103:255–62. doi:10.1016/j.jphysparis.2009.08.008

8. Yang D, Zhao J, Gu Y, Jiang L, Liu H. EMG pattern recognition and grasping force estimation: improvement to the myocontrol of multi-DOF prosthetic hands. *The 2009 IEEE/RSJ International Conference on Intelligent Robots and Systems*. St Louis, MO (2009). p. 516–21.
9. Castellini C, Kõiva R. Using surface electromyography to predict single finger forces. *The Fourth IEEE RAS/EMBS International Conference on Biomedical Robotics and Biomechatronics*. Roma, Italy (2012). p. 1266–72.
10. Cipriani C, Antfolk C, Controzzi M, Lundborg G, Rosén B, Carrozza MC, et al. Online myoelectric control of a dexterous hand prosthesis by transradial amputees. *IEEE Trans Neural Syst Rehabil Eng* (2011) 19(3):260–70. doi:10.1109/TNSRE.2011.2108667
11. Zecca M, Micera S, Carrozza MC, Dario P. Control of multi-functional prosthetic hands by processing the electromyographic signal. *Crit Rev Biomed Eng* (2002) 30(4–6):459–85. doi:10.1615/CritRevBiomedEng.v30.i456.80
12. Khushaba RN, Takruri M, Miro JV, Kodagoda S. Towards limb position invariant myoelectric pattern recognition using time-dependent spectral features. *Neural Netw* (2014) 55:42–58. doi:10.1016/j.neunet.2014.03.010
13. Cutkosky MR. On grasp choice, grasp models, and the design of hands for manufacturing tasks. *IEEE Trans Robot Auto* (1989) 5(3):269–79. doi:10.1109/70.34763
14. Hsu CW, Lin CJ. A comparison of methods for multi-class support vector machines. *Dept Computer Science and Information Engineering*. National Taiwan University.
15. Breiman L. Random forests. *Mach Learn* (2001) 45:5–32. doi:10.1023/A:1017934522171
16. Gijsberts A, Bohra R, González DS, Werner A, Nowak M, Caputo B, et al. Stable myoelectric control of a hand prosthesis using non-linear incremental learning. *Front Neurorobot* (2014) 8:8. doi:10.3389/fnbot.2014.00008
17. Anam K, Al-Jumaily A. A robust myoelectric pattern recognition using online sequential extreme learning machine for finger movement classification. *Conf Proc IEEE Eng Med Biol Soc* (2015) 2015:7266–9. doi:10.1109/EMBC.2015.7320069
18. Vidovic M, Hwang HJ, Amsuss S, Hahne J, Farina D, Muller KR. Improving the robustness of myoelectric pattern recognition for upper limb prostheses by covariate shift adaptation. *IEEE Trans Neural Syst Rehabil Eng* (2015) 24(9):961–70. doi:10.1109/TNSRE.2015.2492619
19. Al-Timemy AH, Bugmann G, Escudero J, Outram N. Classification of finger movements for the dexterous hand prosthesis control with surface electromyography. *IEEE J Biomed Health Inform* (2013) 17(3):608–18. doi:10.1109/JBHI.2013.2249590
20. Segil JL, Weir RF. Design and validation of a morphing myoelectric hand posture controller based on principal component analysis of human grasping. *IEEE Trans Neural Syst Rehabil Eng* (2013) 22(2):249–57. doi:10.1109/TNSRE.2013.2260172
21. Khushaba RN, Kodagoda S, Takruri M, Dissanayake G. Toward improved control of prosthetic fingers using surface electromyogram (EMG) signals. *Expert Syst Appl* (2012) 39(12):10731–8. doi:10.1016/j.eswa.2012.02.192
22. Akhlaghi N, Baker C, Lahlou M, Zafar H. Real-time classification of hand motions using ultrasound imaging of forearm muscles. *IEEE Trans Biomed Eng* (2015) 63(8):1687–98. doi:10.1109/TBME.2015.2498124
23. Farrell TR, Weir RF. The optimal controller delay for myoelectric prosthesis. *IEEE Trans Neural Syst Rehabil Eng* (2007) 15(1):111–8. doi:10.1109/TNSRE.2007.891391

13

Qualitative-Modeling-Based Silicon Neurons and Their Networks

Takashi Kohno [1], Munehisa Sekikawa [2], Jing Li [3], Takuya Nanami [4] and Kazuyuki Aihara [1]*

[1] *Institute of Industrial Science, University of Tokyo, Tokyo, Japan,* [2] *Department of Mechanical and Intelligent Engineering, Utsunomiya University, Utsunomiya, Japan,* [3] *College of Electronic Engineering, Xi'an Shiyou University, Xi'an, China,* [4] *Department of Electrical Engineering and Information Systems, University of Tokyo, Tokyo, Japan*

Edited by:
Paolo Bonifazi,
Tel Aviv University, Israel

Reviewed by:
Alberto Mazzoni,
Scuola Superiore Sant'Anna, Italy
Maurizio Mattia,
Istituto Superiore di Sanità, Italy

****Correspondence:***
Takashi Kohno
kohno@sat.t.u-tokyo.ac.jp

The ionic conductance models of neuronal cells can finely reproduce a wide variety of complex neuronal activities. However, the complexity of these models has prompted the development of qualitative neuron models. They are described by differential equations with a reduced number of variables and their low-dimensional polynomials, which retain the core mathematical structures. Such simple models form the foundation of a bottom-up approach in computational and theoretical neuroscience. We proposed a qualitative-modeling-based approach for designing silicon neuron circuits, in which the mathematical structures in the polynomial-based qualitative models are reproduced by differential equations with silicon-native expressions. This approach can realize low-power-consuming circuits that can be configured to realize various classes of neuronal cells. In this article, our qualitative-modeling-based silicon neuron circuits for analog and digital implementations are quickly reviewed. One of our CMOS analog silicon neuron circuits can realize a variety of neuronal activities with a power consumption less than 72 nW. The square-wave bursting mode of this circuit is explained. Another circuit can realize Class I and II neuronal activities with about 3 nW. Our digital silicon neuron circuit can also realize these classes. An auto-associative memory realized on an all-to-all connected network of these silicon neurons is also reviewed, in which the neuron class plays important roles in its performance.

Keywords: qualitative modeling, silicon neuron, non-linear dynamics, low-power circuit, neuronal network emulation

1. INTRODUCTION

The nervous system allows individual animals and their populations to survive in severe environments by analyzing a huge amount of information from sensory organs and promptly generating adequate control signals for motor organs. This complex and intelligent information processing ability is autonomously obtained and adaptively maintained on its genetically developed physical basis, the network of neuronal cells. The nervous system consumes a sufficiently low power to allow for operation within the power supply limit of an animals' body; for example, the human brain consumes about 20 W (Clarke and Sokoloff, 1999), which is a lower power than mainstream CPUs. Because it is a network of neuronal cells with a wide variety of complex activities, the mechanisms of its information processing function are still poorly understood. It is attracting increased attention from biological, medical, and engineering fields.

A silicon neuronal network is a network of silicon neurons (SNs) connected via silicon synapses (SSs), which are electronic circuits that reproduce the electrophysiological activity of neuronal cells and synapses, respectively. Unlike neuro-inspired artificial neural networks, it is an approach to neuromimetic systems that realize intelligent, autonomous, robust, and power-efficient information processing via an architecture comparable to the nervous system (Arthur and Boahen, 2011; Brink et al., 2013b; Cassidy et al., 2013; Kohno et al., 2014b; Qiao et al., 2015; Giulioni et al., 2016). Because it is a bottom-up approach with cell-level granularity and reproduces neuronal spiking activities, it is also applicable to biohybrid systems including neuroprosthetic devices that replace damaged nerve tissues (Ambroise et al., 2013). Generally, SN circuits are required to have the capability of reproducing complex neuronal activities, have a low power consumption, and be compact and highly integratable.

In fields where the reproducibility is important, such as the biohybrid systems and high-speed simulators, SN circuits have been designed to solve ionic conductance neuronal models (Simoni and DeWeerth, 2006; Schemmel et al., 2010; Grassia et al., 2011; Saïghi et al., 2011). These models describe the dynamics of ionic currents that generate the dynamical behavior of the membrane potential by charging and discharging the membrane capacitance. They can precisely reproduce neuronal activities, but their equations are described by high-dimensional non-linear differential equations (DEs). It was demonstrated that their circuit implementations (conductance-based SNs) can well reproduce the neuronal activities of their target cells but require a relatively large amount of hardware resources and consume a relatively high power in the range of micro- to milliwatts. The ionic conductance models share a common structure, namely the Hodgkin–Huxley formalism, which allows their circuit implementation to mimic a variety of neuronal cells after fabrication by applying appropriate parameter voltages (Grassia et al., 2011; Saïghi et al., 2011).

In fields where low power consumption and integratability are important, SN circuits that solve integrate-and-fire (I&F) models are widely used. These models describe the neuronal activities with simple DEs by treating a spike as an event and focusing on the timing of spike generation. Their analog and digital circuit implementations (I&F-based SNs) have been developed (Thomas and Luk, 2009; Arthur and Boahen, 2011; Cassidy et al., 2013; Merolla et al., 2014; Mayr et al., 2015; Qiao et al., 2015; Giulioni et al., 2016). Analog I&F-based SNs achieve ultralow power consumption down to several nanowatts and several hundreds of them were integrated on a chip with thousands of SS circuits. Although their digital implementations consume more power, they are more portable, easy-to-operate, and highly integratable. A milestone work is the TrueNorth chip (Merolla et al., 2014) that integrates 1 million SNs and 256 million SSs on an application-specific integrated circuit chip and consumes less than 70 mW. Silicon neuronal networks implemented on field-programmable gate array (FPGA) chips achieve far less integration (about 1000 SNs) and consume higher power, but their low cost and reconfigurability have attracted many researchers. Sophisticated I&F-based models such as the Izhikevich (IZH) (Izhikevich, 2004) and adaptive exponential I&F (Brette and Gerstner, 2005) models incorporate the viewpoint of qualitative neuronal modeling described below, which allows them to reproduce a variety of neuronal activities. In principle, however, they cannot reproduce some neuronal properties related to the variability of spikes, which are reported experimentally and indicated theoretically. For example, it was reported that the amplitude of spikes at an axon terminal in the hippocampus is gradedly dependent on the stimulus intensity (Alle and Geiger, 2006), and a mathematical analysis of neuronal models indicated that a class of neurons, Class II in Hodgkin's classification (Hodgkin, 1948), can generate spikes in the same manner (Rinzel and Ermentrout, 1998). In addition, the parameter setting of the I&F-based models requires careful tuning; for example, we pointed out that the phase response curve (PRC) of the IZH model in the Class II setting is discontinuous at $\theta = 0$, which causes a severe reduction in the retrieval ability of an auto-associative memory in all-to-all connected networks (Osawa and Kohno, 2015). This problem can be solved by increasing the parameter d of the model, which distorts the waveforms of the membrane potential by producing a huge hyperpolarization after each spike. Another example is that the spiking patterns of the IZH model in the intrinsic bursting (IB) setting have different characteristics from IB cells when a strong stimulus is applied (Nanami and Kohno, 2016). These facts suggest the possibility that a network of I&F-based silicon neurons may have limited ability to reproduce particular information processing in the nervous system.

In the field of qualitative neuronal modeling, the mathematical techniques of non-linear dynamics have been effectively applied to ionic-conductance models to produce low-dimensional and simple polynomial equations that qualitatively capture their dynamical properties (Rinzel and Ermentrout, 1998; Izhikevich, 2007). In contrast to the I&F approach, they do not ignore specific phenomena including the spike generation mechanism. The most well-known qualitative model is the FitzHugh–Nagumo (F-N) model (FitzHugh, 1961) that reproduces the dynamical structure in the Hodgkin–Huxley (H-H) model (Hodgkin and Huxley, 1952). The H-H model is described by four-variable non-linear DEs, whereas the F-N model is two-variable and its only non-linear term is cubic. The F-N model is Class II and can produce the graded spike response to a pulse stimulus. The first silicon nerve membrane circuit, the Nagumo circuit (Nagumo et al., 1962), implemented this model using the tunnel diode. Later, several SNs have implemented the F-N and other qualitative models using recent analog and digital circuit technologies (Linares-Barranco et al., 1991; Cosp et al., 2004; Weinstein and Lee, 2006).

In our previous works (Kohno and Aihara, 2005, 2007, 2008a; Sekikawa et al., 2008; Kohno and Aihara, 2010; Li et al., 2012; Kohno and Aihara, 2014a; Kohno et al., 2014b), we proposed a qualitative-modeling-based design approach for SNs. In this approach, a qualitative neuronal model that reproduces the dynamical structure in a target neuronal model is constructed by combining the formulae for the characteristic curves of favorable elemental circuit blocks instead of polynomials. The elemental circuit blocks are selected according to the required features of the SN; for example, subthreshold metal–oxide semiconductor field-effect transistor (MOSFET) circuit blocks may be used for low-power SNs. Such a model is expected to be implemented efficiently in comparison to the direct implementation of polynomial-based qualitative models. In addition, a model that supports the mathematical structures in different classes of neurons can be designed, and one of them is invoked by appropriately selecting the model parameters. We developed a configurable low-power analog SN circuit (Kohno and Aihara, 2008a,b; Sekikawa et al., 2008; Kohno and Aihara, 2010) and a configurable simple digital SN circuit (Kohno and Aihara, 2007; Li et al., 2012, 2013). Our analog SN supports five classes of neuronal activities, Class I and II in the Hodgkin's classification, regular spiking (RS), square-wave bursting, and elliptic bursting (Wang and Rinzel, 2003) by appropriately setting the parameter voltages, and our digital SN supports Class I and II and Class I* (Tadokoro et al., 2011) neuronal activities. Basu and Hasler (2010) developed two ultralow-power analog SNs that consume several nanowatts (Brink et al., 2013b) on the basis of a similar approach; one of them is dedicated to Class I and another to Class II. We are developing an analog SN that supports both classes and consumes a low amount of power that is comparable to their work (Kohno and Aihara, 2014a).

Most silicon neuronal networks incorporate the SS circuits that mimic the signal transmission in chemical synapses. Their three important features are the synaptic efficacy, plasticity, and summation (Destexhe et al., 1998; Song et al., 2000; Dan and Poo, 2004). A large (small) amount of synaptic current is injected into the postsynaptic neuronal cell if the synaptic efficacy is high (low). The synaptic efficacy is modulated on the basis of some factors including the neuronal spikes generated by the pre- and postsynaptic neuronal cells (the synaptic plasticity). It is called the spike-timing-dependent plasticity (STDP) if its rule (a learning rule) is based on the timing of neuronal spikes in the pre- and postsynaptic neuronal cells (Song et al., 2000; Dan and Poo, 2004). The synaptic summation allows a bursting spike input to enhance the effect of synaptic transmission. It was shown that this feature can play a critical role in spike timing recognition (Gütig and Sompolinsky, 2006). Note that the information of an input spike's magnitude can be transmitted via the time period of neurotransmitter release. The compactness and low-power consumption of SS circuits are also an important issue because the number of SSs in a silicon neuronal network is generally larger than that of SNs. In Merolla et al. (2014), the integration of a huge number of digital SSs was realized by limiting the functionality of the SS to the synaptic efficacy. Their synaptic weights have to be calculated by a off-chip system, but this is not a limitation in engineering applications in which "ready-trained" discriminators are required. They reported that this circuit could realize a multiobject detection and classification system. Only the synaptic efficacy was supported also in early FPGA-based silicon neuronal networks (Rice et al., 2009; Thomas and Luk, 2009), but in recent works, the synaptic summation is supported in Ambroise et al. (2013) and all of the three features are supported in Li et al. (2013) and Cassidy et al. (2013). The analog SS circuit in Giulioni et al. (2016, 2015) implements the synaptic efficacy and the plasticity. Their silicon neuronal network chip integrates 128 leaky I&F SNs and 16384 SSs whose synaptic efficacy is stored in a bistable memory and controlled by a Hebbian-type STDP rule (Fusi et al., 2000). They realized an autoassociative visual memory (Giulioni et al., 2015) and motion detectors (Giulioni et al., 2016). The analog SS circuit in Qiao et al. (2015) implements all of the three features of synapses. The synaptic summation is realized by a low-power current-mode integrator circuit called a differential-pair integrator (DPI). To reduce the circuit size, a DPI circuit is shared by multiple synapses by exploiting its linearity. The synaptic efficacy is stored in a bistable memory and controlled by an STDP-based algorithm (Brader et al., 2007). This chip integrates 256 adaptive exponential I&F SNs with more than 128,000 SSs and was applied to image classification tasks. Another full-featured analog SS in Brink et al. (2013b) stores the synaptic efficacy in an analog non-volatile memory based on a floating-gate device and supports an asymmetrical STDP learning rule. This chip integrates 100 Class II SNs with 30000 SSs and realized a winner-take-all network and a rhythm generator (Brink et al., 2013a).

In this article, we briefly review our SN circuits designed by a qualitative-modeling-based approach. The next section summarizes the mathematical methods of qualitative neuronal modeling that are applied to SN design. Section 3 explains our analog and digital SNs and Section 4 concludes this review.

2. QUALITATIVE NEURONAL MODELING

In spiking neuronal cells, fast ionic currents such as the fast sodium and rectifying potassium currents are responsible for spike generation. Slower ionic currents such as the calcium currents and the potassium currents that are controlled by the intracellular calcium concentration modify the dynamics of the spike generation system. Various types of neuronal cells are known and each of them has its own combination of expressed ionic channels, which leads to a variety of neuronal activities. The mechanisms of these dynamical activities have been considerably elucidated from the perspective of non-linear dynamics (Rinzel and Ermentrout, 1998; Wang and Rinzel, 2003; Izhikevich, 2007).

2.1. Spike Generation Systems

It is known that many spike generation systems can be projected onto two-variable systems without critically distorting their dynamics. Typically, the equations of the projected system are in the following form:

$$\frac{dv}{dt} = f_v(v, n) + I_{\text{stim}}, \tag{1}$$

$$\frac{dn}{dt} = f_n(v, n), \tag{2}$$

where v is the membrane potential and n is a variable that abstractly represents the activity of ionic channels. A stimulus current is represented by I_{stim}. **Figures 1A,C** illustrate the phase plane of two typical spike generation systems. The v-nullcline, a set of points on which $\frac{dv}{dt} = 0$, is N-shaped in both systems, which intersects the n-nullcline at three points in (**Figure 1A**) and at one point in (**Figure 1C**). In both cases, $\frac{dv}{dt}$ is negative (positive) above (below) the v-nullcline, and $\frac{dn}{dt}$ is negative (positive) above (below) the n-nullcline.

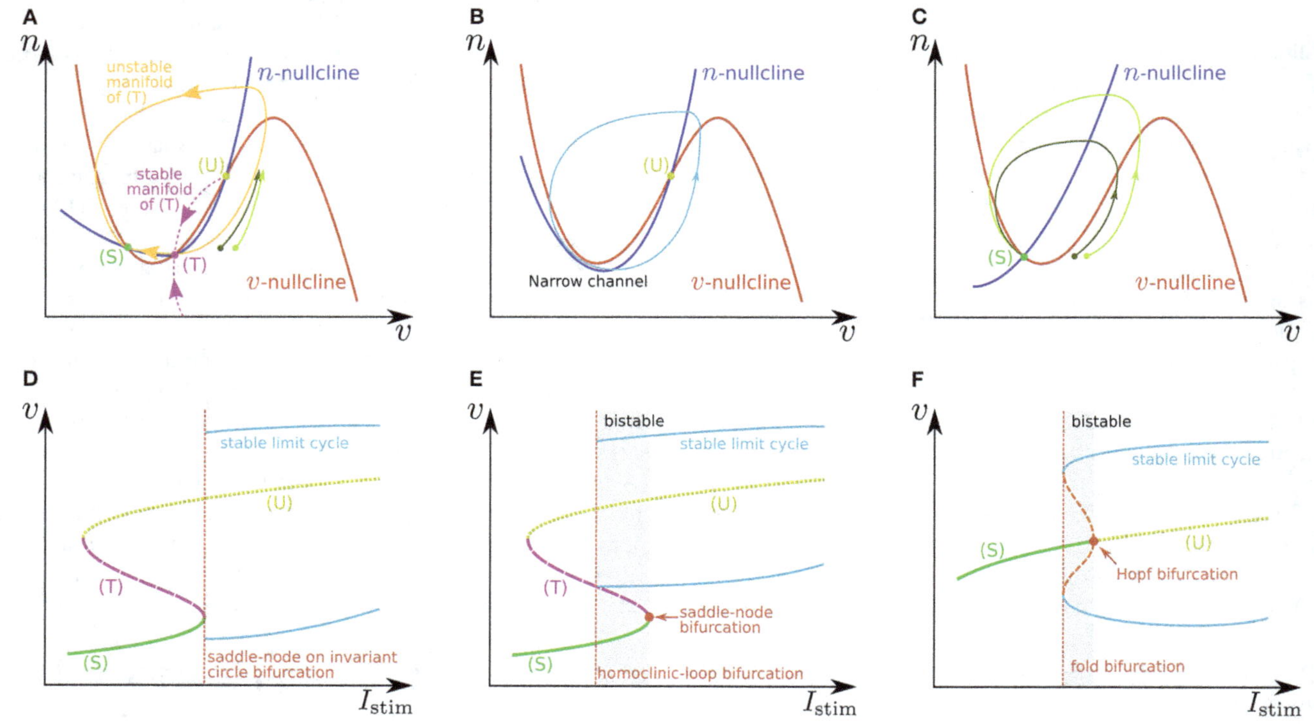

FIGURE 1 | Illustrations of (A–C) phase planes and (D–F) bifurcation diagrams in the fast subsystem. The characteristics of neuronal activities can be adjusted by exploiting their mechanisms explained in the main text. For example in **(A)**, the threshold voltage can be increased while the resting membrane potential is held constant if (T) is displaced rightward while (S) is fixed by tuning the slope of the v- or n-nullcline. The ratio of the time constants of n and v is one of the factors that determine the shape of the stable and unstable manifolds of (T) and the limit cycle.

In **Figure 1A**, the leftmost intersection (equilibrium) (S) is a stable point, the middle (T) is a saddle point, and the rightmost (U) is an unstable point. Without any perturbation, the state point stays at (S), which corresponds to the resting state. If an excitatory instantaneous pulse stimulus is applied to the system, the system state is displaced horizontally rightward because v is the differential voltage of the membrane capacitance to which the stimulus current is directly injected. If the displacement is sufficiently large and the state point crosses the stable manifold of (T), it goes back to (S) along the longer branch of the unstable manifold of (T) by moving upward to the right and then leftward. This temporal increase in v is the mechanism of spike generation. Because the trajectory (the orbit of the state point) is attracted to the unstable manifold of (T), the shape of the spikes is not strongly dependent on the stimulus intensity. The threshold voltage for spike generation is determined by the stable manifold of (T) because if the state point does not cross it, the point goes back to (S) along the shorter branch of the unstable manifold by just moving leftward.

The v-nullcline is displaced upward by the application of an excitatory sustained stimulus I_{stim}. Through this transition, (S) and (T) move toward each other, coalesce, and then disappear, which produces a stable limit cycle from the longer branch of the unstable manifold of (T). While the state point stays on the limit cycle, its v coordinate repeatedly increases and decreases, which is the mechanism of repetitive spiking. This process, the disappearance of two equilibria and the appearance of a limit cycle, is called a saddle-node on invariant circle bifurcation, and the critical value of I_{stim} is a bifurcation point. **Figure 1D** shows a bifurcation diagram illustrating an overview of this transition. The horizontal axis is for I_{stim} (the bifurcation parameter), and the dynamical structure of the phase plane for each value of I_{stim} is projected onto the 1-d space of the vertical axis, v. Here, the limit cycle is represented by its maximum and minimum values of v. As is illustrated in **Figure 1B**, just above the bifurcation point, the limit cycle passes through a region near both of the v- and n-nullclines. Because both $\frac{dv}{dt}$ and $\frac{dn}{dt}$ are small in this region, the state point takes a long time to pass, which extends the period time of the limit cycle. As I_{stim} is closer to the bifurcation point, this effect is stronger. It extends the period time, which diverges to infinity when I_{stim} reaches the bifurcation point. This mechanism accounts for the Class I property in Hodgkin's classification.

If n is sufficiently faster than v, a stable limit cycle is produced via a homoclinic-loop bifurcation before (S) and (T) coalesce (**Figure 1E**). As the system is closer to the homoclinic-loop bifurcation point, the period of the limit cycle is extended to infinity by the extended passing time of a region near (T). Because the limit cycle appears before (S) disappears, the system is bistable in the range of I_{stim} between the homoclinic-loop and saddle-node bifurcation points.

In **Figure 1C**, the unique equilibrium (S) is stable, which corresponds to the resting state. If the state point is displaced beyond the rising part of the v-nullcline by an excitatory instantaneous pulse stimulus, it starts moving rightward because $\frac{dv}{dt} > 0$ below the v-nullcline. It then turns to left when it crosses the v-nullcline again. This is the mechanism of spike generation in this type of system. The magnitude of the spike, which is the maximum value of v on the spike's trajectory, is determined by its intersection with the v-nullcline, which is dependent on the starting point to which the state point is displaced by the stimulus. Thus, the spike shape is dependent on the stimulus intensity, which is referred to as graded response.

When I_{stim} is a positive sustained stimulus, the v-nullcline is displaced upward, by which (S) is transferred upward to the right. At a critical value of I_{stim}, the stability of this point is reversed via a subcritical Hopf bifurcation. In the bifurcation diagram (**Figure 1F**), the appearance of a set of stable and unstable limit cycles via another bifurcation, a fold bifurcation, is seen at a smaller value of I_{stim}. Once (S) loses stability, the state point jumps to the stable limit cycle, and the system starts to spike repetitively. Because there is no dynamical structure that suppresses the velocity of the state point on the stable limit cycle down close to zero, the spiking frequency is always much higher than 0. This accounts for the Class II property in Hodgkin's classification. This system also has bistability composed of the resting state and the stable limit cycle.

2.2. System with Slow Dynamics

Slow hyperpolarizing ionic currents activated by depolarization provide a negative feedback to the spike generation system, which is a most basic mechanism that maintains the spiking behavior "convergent." These currents play a role as inhibitory stimuli to the spike generation system that modify its dynamical structures. In a case that their time constants are similar, they can be projected even onto a single-variable system. It was elucidated that a simple system composed of a two-variable spike generation subsystem and a single-variable slow subsystem can explain the dynamics of several classes of neuronal activities including RS (**Figure 2A**), square-wave bursting (**Figure 2B**), elliptic bursting (**Figure 2C**), and low-threshold spiking (LTS). In this section, the dynamical structures of the first three classes are explained. Here, a slow subsystem is merged into the spike generation system in the previous section as follows:

$$\frac{dv}{dt} = f_v(v, n, q) + I_{\text{stim}}, \tag{3}$$

$$\frac{dn}{dt} = f_n(v, n), \tag{4}$$

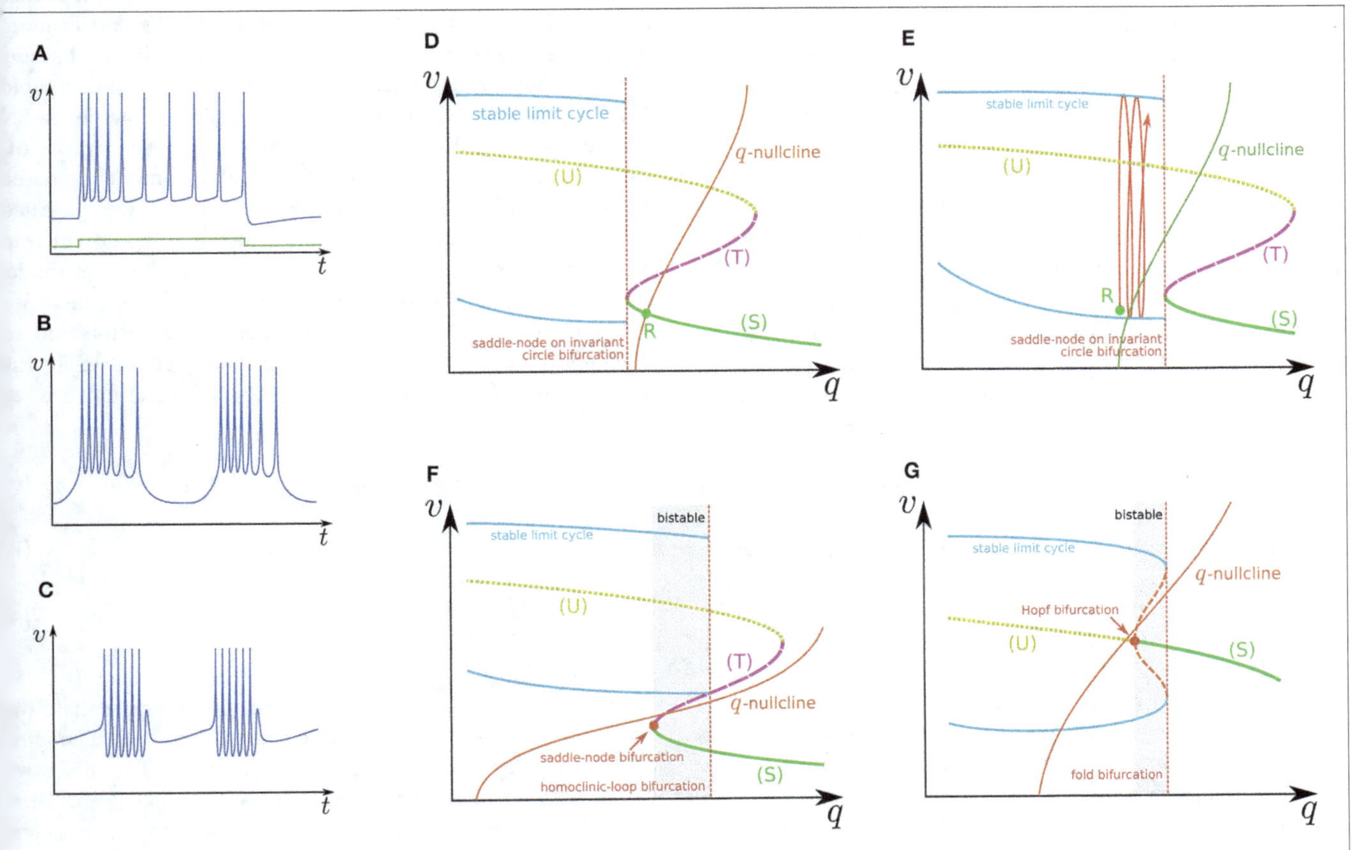

FIGURE 2 | Illustrations of firing patterns and the dynamical structures that account for their mechanism. Waveforms of **(A)** RS, **(B)** square-wave bursting, and **(C)** elliptic bursting. The v–q planes of a simple system that produces the firing patterns of **(D,E)** RS, **(F)** square-wave bursting, and **(G)** elliptic bursting.

$$\frac{dq}{dt} = f_q(v, q). \quad (5)$$

Figure 2D illustrates the q–v plane of a system with a Class I spike generation subsystem. Because q works as an inhibitory stimulus to the spike generation subsystem, the dynamical structure is dependent on q in the opposite manner to I_{stim}. Thus, the dynamical structure drawn in this figure is similar to a horizontal flip of the bifurcation diagram in **Figure 1D**. The q-nullcline illustrates the characteristics of the slow subsystem; above (below) it, $\frac{dq}{dt} < 0$ ($\frac{dq}{dt} > 0$). It has an intersection R with (S), which is a stable equilibrium point and corresponds to the resting state. In response to an appropriate step stimulus, this system produces RS, which is repetitive spiking whose frequency is initially high and then gradually decreases to a lower value (**Figure 2A**). Because the dynamical structure of the spike generation subsystem is displaced rightward by an excitatory sustained stimulus (**Figure 2E**), the state point is released at R at the onset of the step stimulus. It is attracted by the stable limit cycle, which is a repetitive spiking state. The slow variable q slowly increases because most parts of the limit cycle are above the q-nullcline. It converges to a value at which the increase and decrease in the portion of the limit cycle above and below the q-nullcline balance. The spiking frequency decreases as q increases because the spike generation subsystem is Class I, which produces spikes with a lower frequency in response to a stimulus closer to the bifurcation point. Some types of excitatory cells in the neocortex produce this type of activity. In contrast, some types of inhibitory cells generate faster spikes with a weaker frequency adaptation (fast spiking) (Harris and Shepherd, 2015). Such activity can be modeled by the same model with a weaker adaptation of the spike frequency or a Class II spike generation system.

Figure 2F illustrates the q–v plane of a system with the spike generation subsystem in **Figure 1E**. The dynamical structure of the spike generation subsystem is similar to its horizontal flip and the q-nullcline has no intersection with any stable states. If the state point is near (S) at some moment, it is attracted to (S). Because (S) is below the q-nullcline, q slowly decreases, and the state point moves leftward until (S) disappears via the saddle-node bifurcation. The system does not generate any spikes in this phase. The state point is then attracted to the stable limit cycle, which is the only stable state. Because the limit cycle is above the q-nullcline, q slowly increases, and the state point moves rightward until the limit cycle disappears via the saddle-loop bifurcation. Repetitive firing is produced on the limit cycle in this phase. Then the state point is attracted to (S) again. The system repeats the alternation between the tonic firing and silent phases without any stimuli. This is the mechanism of square-wave bursting (**Figure 2B**). This class of neuronal activities is involved in life-supporting rhythm generation networks such as a respiratory rhythm generator and a heartbeat rhythm generator (Hill et al., 2001; Negro et al., 2001).

Figure 2G illustrates the q–v plane of a system with the spike generation subsystem in **Figure 1F**. As in the previous case, the state point is attracted to (S) if the state point is near to it. Because (S) is below the q-nullcline, the state point slowly moves leftward along (S) until it loses stability via the Hopf bifurcation. No spike is generated in this phase. Then the state point is attracted to the stable limit cycle. On the limit cycle, if the increase in q above the q-nullcline exceeds the decrease below, the state point slowly moves rightward, repetitively generating spikes. After the limit cycle disappears by the fold bifurcation, the state point is attracted to (S) again. The repeated alternation between these two phases is the mechanism of elliptic bursting (**Figure 2C**). This class of neuronal activities is observed in sleep spindles (Destexhe et al., 1993), which is a characteristic spiking pattern appearing in the thalamus during non-REM sleep.

3. SILICON NEURON CIRCUITS

The core idea of our qualitative-modeling-based approach is to design an ideal silicon neuronal model that reproduces the dynamical structure of a target neuronal class by combination of "device-native" formulae (Kohno and Aihara, 2008b). For low-power analog circuit implementation, the formulae of the V–I characteristic curves for compact and simple low-power analog circuit blocks can be selected. For digital circuit implementation, polynomials with the lowest order are appropriate because the multiplier is the circuit with the highest cost.

3.1. Low-Power Analog Silicon Neuron

We developed a low-power analog SN circuit that can realize the Class I and II neuronal activities in Hodgkin's classification RS, square-wave bursting, and elliptic bursting. The ideal model of this circuit was designed for implementation by subthreshold MOSFET circuits, which are typically chosen for low-power SN circuits. Because this circuit was intended to be a proof-of-concept for the application of our qualitative-modeling-based approach to integrated circuits, elemental circuits were selected by attaching importance to stability and configurability instead of low-power consumption. The equations of the ideal model are constructed by combining the formulae of the sigmoidal V–I characteristic curves of differential-pair-based circuits and an integration operation with a leak that can be implemented by the Tau-cell circuit (van Schaik and Jin, 2003). The equations are

$$C_v\frac{dv}{dt} = -g(v) + f_m(v) - n - q + I_a + I_{\text{stim}}, \quad (6)$$

$$\frac{dn}{dt} = \frac{f_n(v) - n}{\tau_n}, \quad (7)$$

$$\frac{dq}{dt} = \frac{f_q(v) - q}{\tau_q}, \quad (8)$$

where v, n, and q represent the membrane potential, the abstracted activity of fast ionic channels, and the abstracted activity of slow ionic channels, respectively. The first two variables compose a fast subsystem, namely the spike generation system, and q provides a slow negative feedback to it. Parameters C_v, I_a, τ_n, and τ_q are the membrane capacitance, a constant current, and the time constants of n and q, respectively. Functions $f_x(v)$ ($x = m, n, q$) and $g(v)$ are the formulae of the idealized V–

characteristic curves of the differential pair and transconductance amplifier (**Figures 3A,B**) as follows:

$$f_x(v) = M_x \frac{1}{1 + \exp\left(-\frac{\kappa}{U_T}(v - \delta_x)\right)}, \quad (9)$$

$$g(v) = S \frac{1 - \exp\left(-\frac{\kappa}{U_T}(v - \theta_v)/(1 + 1/\kappa)\right)}{1 + \exp\left(-\frac{\kappa}{U_T}(v - \theta_v)/(1 + 1/\kappa)\right)}, \quad (10)$$

where U_T and κ are the thermal voltage (approximately 26 mV at room temperature) and the capacitive-coupling ratio

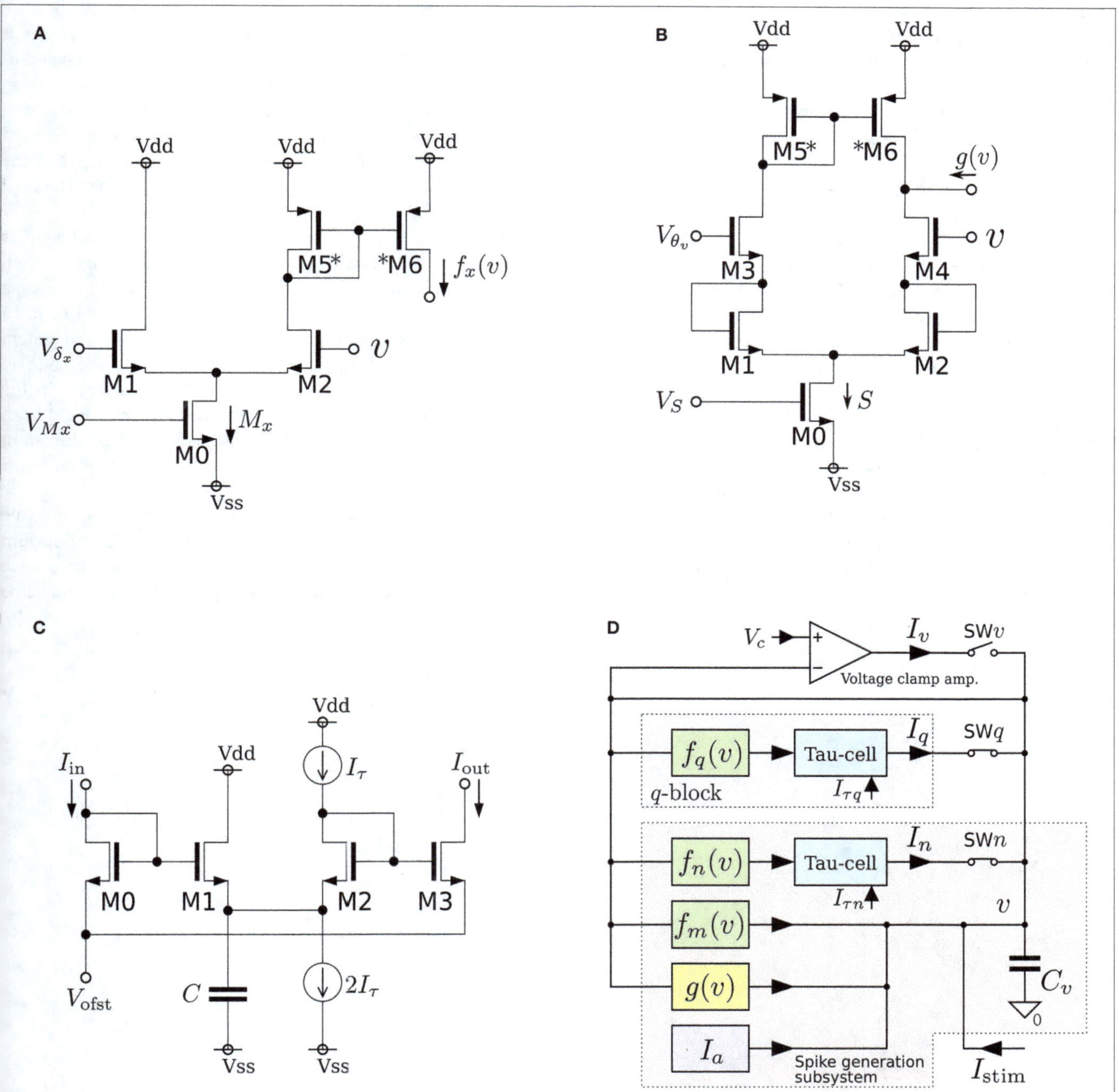

FIGURE 3 | Circuits of our low-power analog silicon neuron. (A–C) Elemental circuits and **(D)** block diagram. The voltage clamp amplifier placed at the top in the block diagram is used to measure the nullclines experimentally. It is a transconductance amplifier that provides a negative feedback loop to the active terminal of C_v. When SW_v is closed, it locks v near V_c, which is an input voltage of the amplifier. If SW_q and SW_n are open, its output current I_v compensates the current generated by the f_m, g_v, and I_a circuits. By scanning V_c in an appropriate range and measuring I_v, I_n, and I_q, the v-, n-, and q-nullclines are measured, respectively. The copied outputs of those currents are available for this purpose. This circuit is exploited to find the appropriate parameter voltages that replicate the dynamical structure in the ideal model, which are altered from their ideal values by fabrication mismatch and the transistors' second effects. Reprinted with modification from Kohno et al. (2014b).

(approximately 0.7 in our environment), respectively. Parameters M_x, δ_x, S, and θ are controlled by the externally applied voltages V_{M_x}, V_{δ_x}, V_S, and V_{θ_v} in the figures. The v-nullcline of this model is given by $n = f_m(v) - g(v) + I_a + I_{\text{stim}}$. Because both $f_m(v)$ and $g(v)$ are sigmoidal curves and the latter is shallower than the former, it can be N-shaped by an appropriate choice of the parameters.

As is drawn in the block diagram of the overall circuit that solves the system equations (**Figure 3D**), Equation (6) is integrated by C_v whose differential voltage corresponds to v and Equations (7) and (8) are solved using the Tau-cell (**Figure 3C**) whose ideal equation is

$$\frac{dI_{\text{out}}}{dt} = \frac{I_{\text{in}} - I_{\text{out}}}{CU_T/I_\tau}, \tag{11}$$

where C is the capacitance in the circuit, and I_τ is a parameter current by which the time constant is arranged. The solutions of Equations (7) and (8) are given by the output current of the Tau-cell circuits (blue boxes in the block diagram) whose input terminals are connected to the outputs of the $f_x(v)$ circuits ($x =$ n, q). The output current of the lower (upper) Tau-cell, I_n (I_q), represents n (q). Parameter currents $I_{\tau x}$ ($x = n$, q) and I_a are generated by integrated V–I converters that are controlled by the externally applied voltages, $V_{\tau n}$, $V_{\tau q}$, and V_a, respectively.

In this review, we focus on the square-wave bursting mode. In this mode, the parameters of the model are selected so that the dynamical structures of the fast subsystem resemble those in **Figure 1A**. **Figure 4A** illustrates an example of the v–n phase plane on which the v- and the n-nullclines are configured for this mode. The reversed N-shape of the v-nullcline is produced by a combination of a rising sigmoidal curve, $f_m(v)$, and a shallower falling sigmoidal curve, $-g(v)$. Thus, M_m is increased to make its rising phase steeper and S is increased to make its falling phases steeper. These factors control the deepness of its U-shaped and reversed U-shaped regions. The threshold voltage for spike generation depends on the former, which controls the distance between (S) and (T). Because the magnitude of the spikes is suppressed by the latter, the former is generally coordinated to be deeper than the latter to obtain sufficiently high spikes in comparison to the threshold, which can be realized by selecting a smaller value for θ_v than δ_m. The spike height is also boosted by increasing the time constant of n, which slightly increases the spike period as well. The actual spike height can be estimated by drawing the unstable manifolds of (T) whose maximum v gives the minimum height. In **Figure 4A**, the spike height is estimated to be at least 20 mV. In this figure, the longer branch of the unstable manifold of (T) is pulled back to (T) because a relatively small value is selected for the time constant of n. In this situation, as described in the previous section, the system undergoes a saddle-loop bifurcation instead of a saddle-node on invariant circle bifurcation in response to the increase in the stimulus current (**Figure 1E**). Because the slow variable q is an inhibitory stimulus current to the v–n subsystem, this bifurcation structure appears on the v–q plane in a horizontally flipped manner (**Figure 4B**).

The appropriate selection of M_q and δ_q places the q-nullcline so that it separates the stable limit cycle and the stable equilibrium (S), which reproduces the dynamical structure in the square-wave bursting illustrated in **Figure 2F**. The position of the q-nullcline

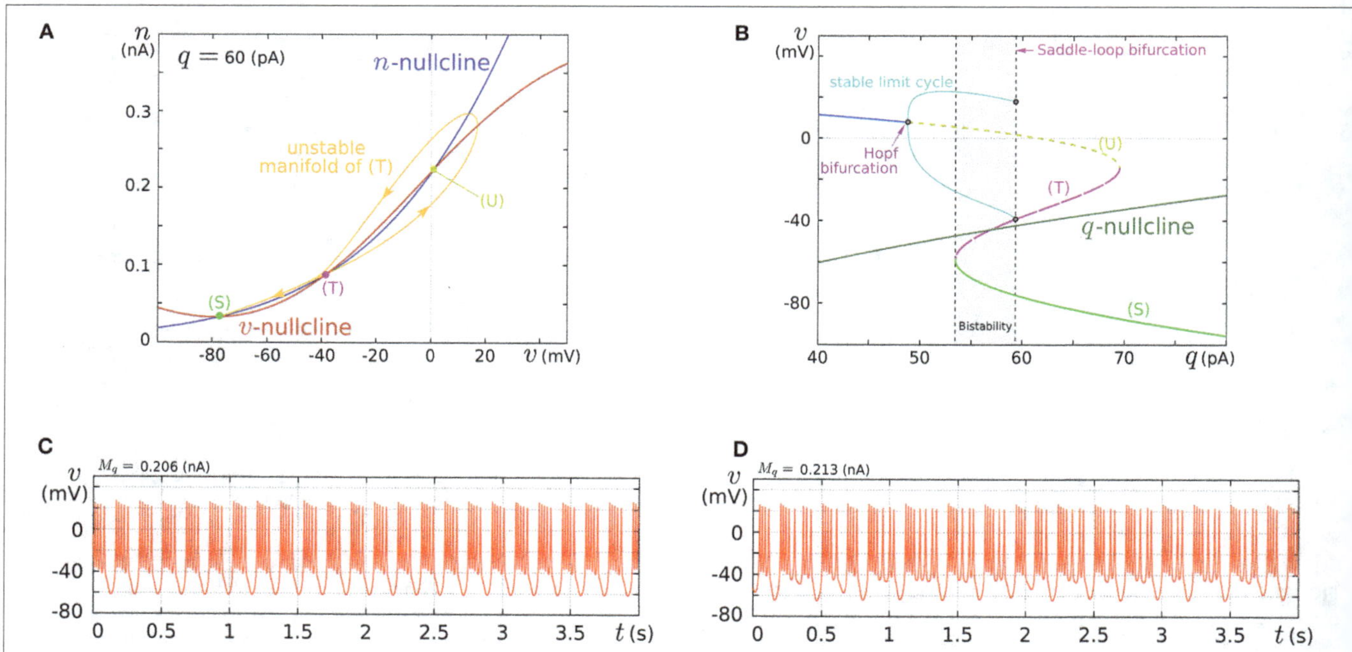

FIGURE 4 | Example of a dynamical structure and the activities of our low-power analog SN model in the square-wave bursting mode. (A) An example of the v–n phase plane of the fast subsystem when q is fixed at 60 pA. **(B)** Bifurcation diagram of the fast subsystem whose bifurcation parameter is q. **(C,D)** Activities of the membrane potential v. Reprinted with modification from Kohno and Aihara (2010) (some parameters are modified).

relative to the stable states of the fast subsystem is a factor that controls the number of spikes in a burst. This dependence was theoretically elucidated in Wang (1993) using the Hindmarsh–Rose model, which is a qualitative square-wave bursting model. When the slow variable's nullcline is close to the limit cycle, tonic spiking is generated. As it departs from the limit cycle, the tonic spiking becomes chaotic via a period doubling bifurcation cascade. Then regular bursting appears and the number of spikes in a burst decreases one by one down to single-spike bursting. At those transitions, chaotic bursting can be observed if the number of spikes is relatively large. This transition was also observed in an ionic-conductance model of the pancreas β cell (Chay and Rinzel, 1985), in which the maximum conductance of a slow current was swept as the bifurcation parameter. The same transition appears in our circuit model when M_q is swept. This parameter abstractly represents the activity of the slow ionic current which corresponds to the bifurcation parameter in Chay and Rinzel (1985). Examples of regular bursting and chaotic bursting are shown in **Figures 4C,D**.

We fabricated this circuit using a Taiwan Semiconductor Manufacturing Company (TSMC) 0.35 μm mixed-signal CMOS process (**Figure 5A**). The parameter voltages were tuned following the procedure explained in the caption for **Figure 5** on the basis of the dynamical structures in **Figure 4**. In **Figure 5C**, a typical bursting activity observed in the circuit experiments is shown. Its activity was always unstable and could not be stabilized by tuning parameters. In Kohno and Aihara (2011, 2013), we pointed out that this fluctuated behavior arises from the intrinsic dynamical structure of square-wave bursting, i.e., the sensitivity to the initial conditions near the saddle-loop bifurcation. By extending the time constant of q (decreasing $I_{\tau q}$), we could obtain a bursting pattern with a longer period that is similar to the activity of autonomous bursting cells in the pre-Bötzinger complex that generate the respiratory rhythm (Negro et al., 2001). In this case, the bursting activity is more stable than that in (c) because the extended time constant of q makes the trajectory of the state point pass closer to the stable equilibrium (S) and its sojourn time near the saddle-loop bifurcation point shorter. In addition to square-wave bursting, we could also realize Class I and II, RS, and elliptic bursting. For any settings, the power consumption of this circuit including the bias-voltage generators for the Tau-cell circuits did not exceed 72 nW.

3.2. Ultralow-Power Analog Silicon Nerve Membrane

The power consumption of the above circuit is one order of magnitude higher than low-power-oriented leading-edge circuits (Basu and Hasler, 2010; Brink et al., 2013b; Qiao et al., 2015). We developed SN circuitry to attain a lower power consumption that is comparable to these works. A two-variable model that supports the Class I and II neuronal activities was designed on the basis of this circuitry to evaluate its practicality (Kohno and Aihara, 2014a). Its ideal model is given by

$$C_v \frac{dv}{dt} = f_v(v) - g_v(v) + I_{av} - r(n) + I_{\mathrm{stim}}, \tag{12}$$

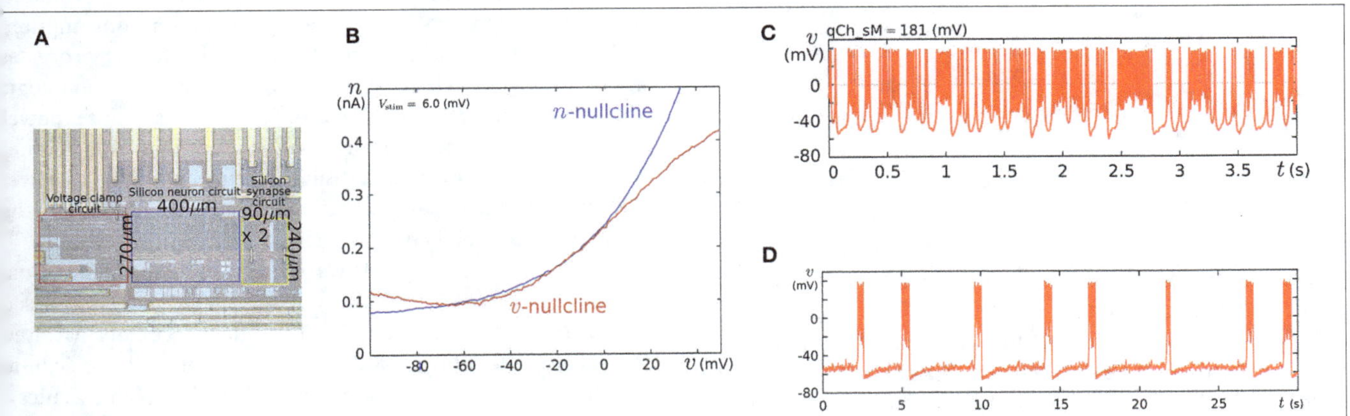

FIGURE 5 | (A) Photograph of the fabricated circuit. **(B)** The nullclines measured using the integrated voltage clamp circuit, which resemble those in **Figure 4A**. Reprinted with modification from Kohno and Aihara (2011). **(C,D)** Square-wave bursting in the circuit. In **(D)**, the time constant of q is extended to mimic the activity of the pre-Bötzinger complex bursting neurons. Reprinted with modification from Kohno et al. (2014b). The appropriate parameter voltages for a fabricated circuit are found by iteration in small modification steps. The starting values are calculated by converting the parameters in the ideal model as follows: $V_{Mx} = \frac{U_T}{\kappa} \ln \frac{M_x}{I_{ON}}$, $V_S = \frac{U_T}{\kappa} \ln \frac{S_V}{I_{ON}}$, $V_{\delta x} = \delta_x$, and $V_{\theta v} = \theta$, where I_{ON} is the current-scaling parameter of the common-sized NMOS transistors M0 in **Figures 3A,B**. In accordance with the characteristics of the V–I converters used to generate I_a, $I_{\tau n}$, and $I_{\tau q}$, the voltages V_a, $V_{\tau n}$, and $V_{\tau q}$ are calculated, whose detailed equations are omitted here. Then, the modification of the parameter voltages is determined so that the shape and position of the v- and n-nullclines measured using the integrated voltage clamp amplifier resemble those in the ideal model. In the iteration of this modification, V_{Mx}, $V_{\delta x}$, V_S, $V_{\theta v}$, and V_a ($x = m, n$) are tuned. After the phase plane structure of the fast subsystem is arranged, $I_{\tau n}$ is modified so that the bifurcation diagram of the fast subsystem in the circuit resembles that in the ideal model. The stable states of the bifurcation diagram can be drawn in circuit experiments by measuring v while slowly scanning $-I_{\mathrm{stim}}$, which is equivalent to q from the fast subsystem's viewpoint. In this measurement, SW$_v$ and SW$_q$ are opened, and SW$_n$ is closed. Because I_{stim} is generated by an integrated V–I converter controlled by the voltage input V_{stim} and equipped with a copied output of I_{stim}, this bifurcation diagram can be translated to the q–v plane. The parameter voltages related to the q-nullcline are selected so that the total q-v plane resembles that of the ideal model. Finally, $V_{\tau q}$ is tuned to obtain bursting activity with the appropriate period.

$$C_n \frac{dn}{dt} = f_n(v) - g_n(v) + I_{an} - r(n), \quad (13)$$

where v and n represent the membrane potential and the abstracted activity of fast ionic channels, respectively. Parameters C_v and C_n are the capacitances that are determined at circuit fabrication, I_{av} and I_{an} are parameter currents, and I_{stim} is the stimulus current. Functions $f_x(v)$, $g_x(v)$, and $r(n)$ ($x = v, n$) are monotonic increasing sigmoidal functions that correspond to the idealized V–I characteristic curves of the elemental circuits shown in **Figures 6A–C**. Their equations are

$$f_x(v) = \frac{M_x}{1 + \exp\left(-\frac{\kappa}{U_T}(v - \delta_x)\right)}, \quad (14)$$

$$g_x(v) = I_{0P}\sqrt{\frac{R_{x20}\exp\left(\frac{\kappa}{U_T}\theta_x\right)}{1 + R_{x21}\exp\left(-\frac{\kappa}{U_T}(v - \theta_x)\right)}}, \quad (15)$$

$$r(n) = I_{0P}\sqrt{\frac{\exp\left(\frac{\kappa}{U_T}\theta_r\right)}{1 + \exp\left(-\frac{\kappa}{U_T}(v - \theta_r)\right)}}. \quad (16)$$

The parameters in these equations are explained in the caption for **Figure 6**. A block diagram of a circuit that solves this model is shown in **Figure 6D**. In this circuit, v and n are coded by the voltage difference between Vdd and the voltage across capacitors C_v and C_n, respectively. Blocks $f_x(v)$ and $g_x(v)$ ($x = v, n$) correspond to the circuits in (a) and (b), respectively. For $g_v(v)$, the transistors in the shadowed region are omitted to simplify the circuit. The two blocks of $r(n)$ correspond to a single circuit of (c).

Equations (12) and (13) are transformed as follows by defining the variable $\tilde{n} \equiv r(n)$:

$$C_v \frac{dv}{dt} = f_v(v) - g_v(v) + I_{av} - \tilde{n} + I_{stim}, \quad (17)$$

$$C_n \frac{d\tilde{n}}{dt} = r'(n)(f_n(v) - g_n(v) + I_{an} - \tilde{n}). \quad (18)$$

By using the two voltage clamp amplifiers, VAV and VAN, in the block diagram, the v- and $\tilde{n}$-nullclines are measured and $r'(n)$ is evaluated (see the caption for **Figure 6**).

The major improvement of this circuitry from the previous SN is a reduction in the static current consumption. In the $f_x(v)$ circuit, M7, M8, M10, and M11 are used to extend the output current range without increasing the tail current I_s. The current consumption of the cascode circuitry in $g_x(v)$ is equal to the output current, whereas the transconductance amplifier in the previous $g_x(v)$ circuit constantly consumes its maximum current. The integration of n is performed by a capacitor instead of the Tau-cell. The Tau-cell is an easy-to-use current-mode integrator with a constant time constant, which supports a wide range of input and output currents. However, it requires additional circuits that generate I_τ, $2I_\tau$, and V_{ofst}. The currents required to drive these circuits are cut off by the direct integration of the currents into a capacitor. In this case, the acceptable range of the variables is limited by the range of $r_n(n)$, on which the time constant of n is dependent. The above nullcline-drawing function helps to find the appropriate parameter values under these limitations; once $r_n(n)$ is specified by the time constant requirement of n, the appropriate dynamical structure for the target neuronal class can be constructed within the acceptable range of the variables by tuning the other parameters utilizing the nullcline drawing function.

By a similar parameter tuning procedure to that for the fast subsystem in the previous SN circuit, we found the parameter values for the Class I and II modes. **Figure 7** shows the simulation results obtained using the Spectre circuit simulator with the TSMC 0.25 μm mixed-signal CMOS process development kit. Capacitances C_v and C_n are implemented by metal–insulator–metal capacitors (MIMCAPs) with capacitances of 1.5 and 2.0 pF, respectively. In the pulse stimulus responses (**Figure 7A**), the height of spike is dependent on the intensity of the stimulus (graded response) in the Class II mode (lower plot), whereas the dependence is weak in the Class I mode (upper plot). In the sustained stimulus response (**Figures 7B,C**), the spike frequency can be reduced close to 0 by applying a sufficiently weak stimulus in the Class I mode [(B)], whereas spike generation is terminated before the spike frequency reaches close to 0 in the Class II mode [(C)]. In both settings, the power consumption increases with the spike frequency and is less than 3.2 nW when the spike frequency is less than 70 Hz.

3.3. A Silicon Neuronal Network by Digital Arithmetic Circuits

Generally, the power consumption of a dynamical digital circuit is higher than that of the subthreshold analog circuits used in the previous sections. However, the continuous evolution of the fabrication process is lowering the power consumption. In Merolla et al. (2014), a combination of ultrafine processes and technologies such as asynchronous and near-threshold logic realized low-power silicon neuronal networks whose power consumption per neuron is only one order of magnitude higher than the lowest-power analog silicon neurons. Reduced power consumption these days is facilitating a fascination with the scalability and stability of digital circuits.

In Li et al. (2012, 2013), we developed a silicon neuronal network in an FPGA based on our qualitative-modeling-based silicon neuronal model for digital arithmetic circuits (Kohno and Aihara, 2007). **Figure 8A** is a block diagram of its basic unit the silicon neuronal network module (SNNM), which executes calculation related to 16 SNs including spike-timing-dependent learning. Larger-scale networks are constructed by connecting more than one of these modules in parallel.

The digital spiking silicon neuron (DSSN) Unit calculates th silicon neuronal model designed with the same principle as abov so that it can be implemented with reduced hardware resource by using the minimum number of multipliers. Its equations ar given by

$$\frac{dv}{dt} = \frac{\phi}{\tau}(f(v) - n + I_0 + I_{stim}), \quad (19)$$

$$\frac{dn}{dt} = \frac{g(v) - n}{\tau}, \quad (20)$$

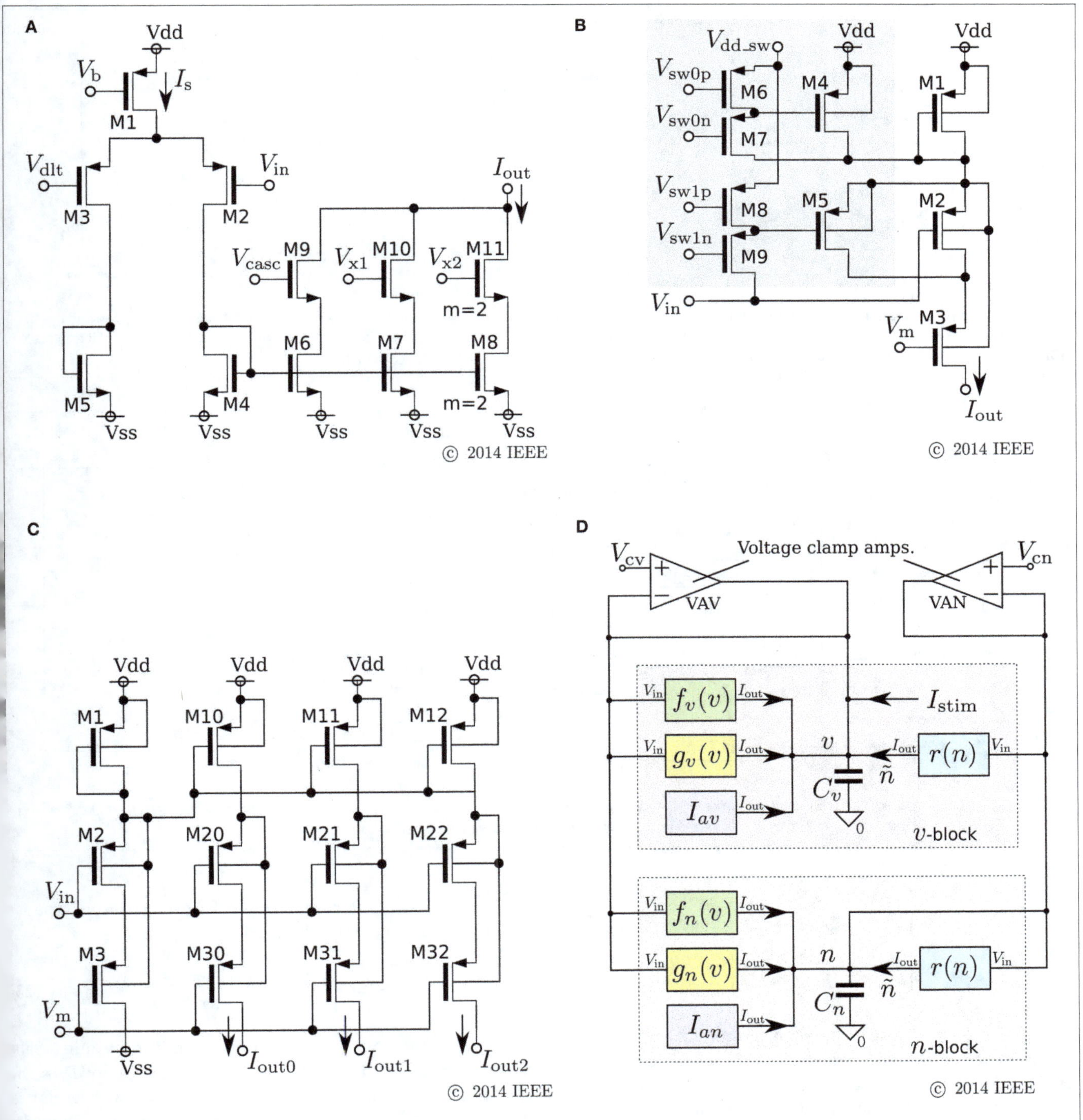

FIGURE 6 | Circuits of our ultralow-power analog silicon neuron. (A–C) Elemental circuits and **(D)** block diagram. In Equations (14)–(16), I_{0P} is the current-scaling parameter of common-sized PMOS transistors [M1 in **(A)**, M1 to M3 in **(B)**, and all of the transistors in **(C)**]. Parameter M_x is the drain current of M1 in **(A)**, which is controlled by V_b. Parameters δ_x ($x = v, n$) and θ_x ($x = v, n, r$) correspond to Vdd - V_{dlt} and Vdd - V_m (Vdd = 1.0 V), respectively. Parameter R_{x20} is 1 (0.5) when M6 is on (off) and M7 is off (on) in panel **(B)**. Parameter R_{x21} is 1 (2) when M8 is on (off) and M9 is off (on). These two parameters are used to shift the curve of $g_x(v)$ horizontally. The two voltage clamp amplifiers, VAV and VAN, in **(D)** are for drawing the v- and $\tilde{n}$-nullclines and evaluating $r'(n)$ in Equations (17) and (18). The output of these transconductance amplifiers is 0 when the two input voltages are the same and positive (negative) when the "+" input voltage is higher (lower) than that of the "−" input. When they are activated and the $r_n(n)$ block is deactivated, their outputs are equal to the sums of $f_x(v)$, $g_x(v)$, and I_{ax} ($x = v, n$). By scanning V_{cv} and maintaining V_{cn} constant, the nullclines are measured. Similarly, when the $r_n(n)$ block is activated and the other blocks are deactivated, the output of VAN is equivalent to $r_n(n)$. By scanning V_{cn}, the dependence of $r_n(n)$ on n is measured, from which $r'(n)$ can be evaluated. Reprinted with modification from Kohno and Aihara (2014a).

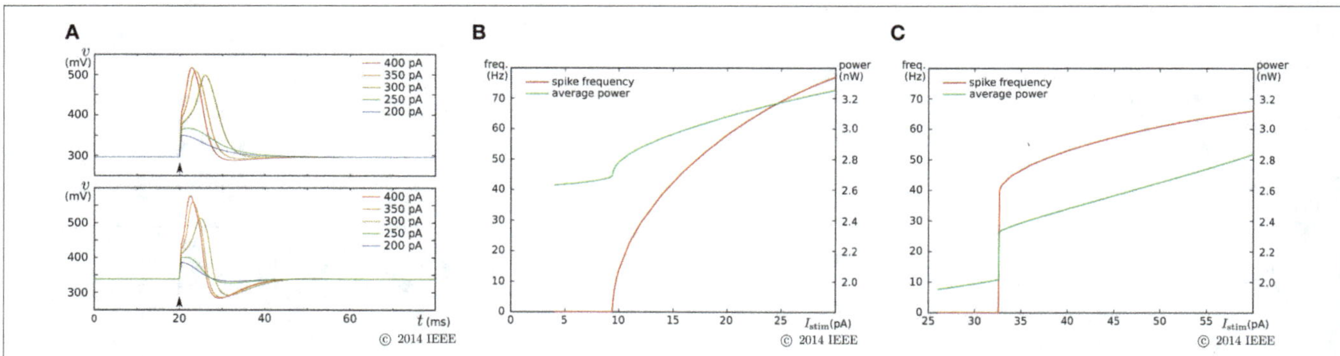

FIGURE 7 | Circuit simulation results of our ultralow-power analog silicon neuron. (A) Responses to a pulse stimulus in the Class I mode (upper) and the Class II mode (lower). **(B,C)** Spiking frequency and power consumption in response to a sustained stimulus. The horizontal axes represent the intensity of the stimulus. **(B)** is for the Class I mode and **(C)** is for the Class II mode. Reprinted with modification from Kohno and Aihara (2014a).

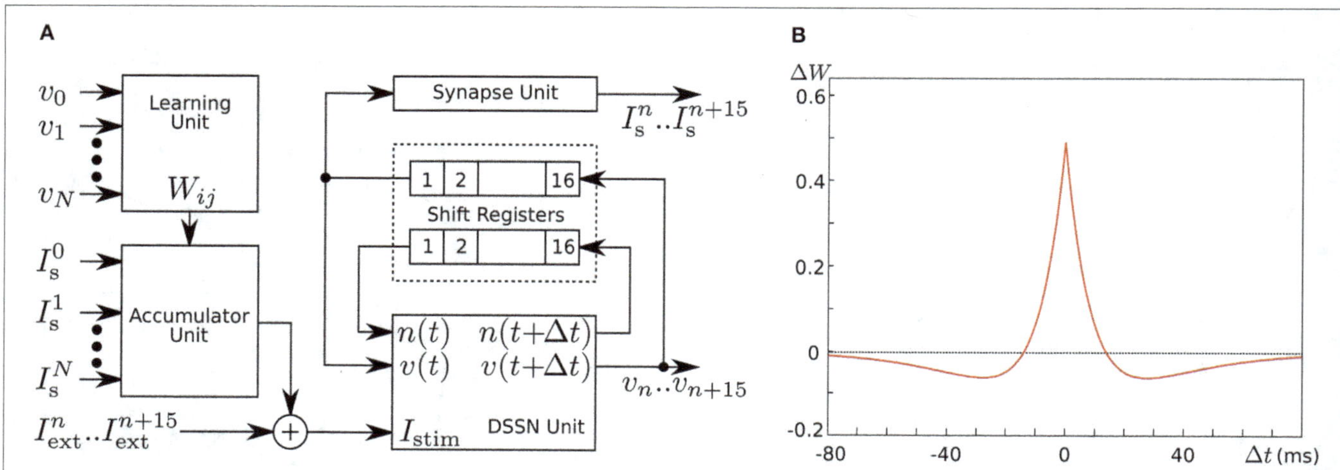

FIGURE 8 | (A) Block diagram of our silicon neuronal network module, which solves the equations for 16 SNs. **(B)** Mexican-hat-type spike-timing-dependent learning curve utilized in the Hebbian-type learning in our digital silicon neuronal network. Reprinted with modification from Li et al. (2013).

$$f(v) = \begin{cases} a_{fn}(v - b_{fn})^2 + c_{fn} \ (v < 0), \\ a_{fp}(v - b_{fp})^2 + c_{fp} \ (v \geq 0), \end{cases} \tag{21}$$

$$g(v) = \begin{cases} a_{gn}(v - b_{gn})^2 + c_{gn} \ (v < r_g), \\ a_{gp}(v - b_{gp})^2 + c_{gp} \ (v \geq r_g), \end{cases} \tag{22}$$

where v and n are variables with no unit that represent the abstracted membrane potential and ionic current activity, respectively. Parameters ϕ and τ configure the time scale of the model's activity. A stimulus input is represented by I_{stim}. The other parameters determine the shape of the nullclines on the v–n phase plane; $n = f(v) + I_0$ for the v-nullcline and $n = g(v)$ for the n-nullcline. The N-shaped v-nullcline is realized by the piecewise quadratic function $f(v)$ instead of a cubic function, which reduces the number of multiplications between variables. Multiplication between a constant and a variable can be implemented by small numbers of shifters and adders if the number of active bits in the constant's binary expression is small. By the parameter tuning procedure similar to our analog SNs, parameter sets that realize the Class I and II activities were found with which this model is solved by Euler's method with fixed-point operations.

The Synapse Unit calculates the following silicon synapse model by Euler's method with fixed-point operations.

$$\frac{dI_{\mathrm{s}}}{dt} = \begin{cases} \alpha(1 - I_{\mathrm{s}}) & \text{when } v \geq 0, \\ -\beta I_{\mathrm{s}} & \text{when } v < 0, \end{cases} \tag{23}$$

where I_{s} is the post-synaptic stimulus received by other SNs. Parameters α and β determine the time constants of I_{s} in the rising and falling phases, respectively. This model was developed on the basis of the kinetic models of chemical synapses (Destexhe et al., 1998) so that it can transmit the analog information of the graded responses in Class II neurons.

The Accumulator Unit calculates the sum of I_{s} given by other SNNMs as follows:

$$I_{\mathrm{ss}}^{j} = c \sum_i W_{ji} I_{\mathrm{s}}^{i}, \tag{24}$$

where c is a scaling parameter, W_{ji} is the synaptic weight from SN i to SN j, and I_{s}^{i} is I_{s} generated by the Synapse Unit for neuron i. The sum of I_{ext}^{j} and I_{ss}^{j} is given to the SN's stimulus input, I_{stim}.

The Learning Unit supports spike-time-dependent learning with exponential-based rules. In Li et al. (2013), we implemented the following Hebbian-type rule:

$$\Delta W_{ji} = A_{+} \exp\left(\frac{-|\Delta t_{ji}|}{\tau_{+}}\right) - A_{-} \exp\left(\frac{-|\Delta t_{ji}|}{\tau_{-}}\right), \qquad (25)$$

where ΔW_{ji} is the modification applied to W_{ji}, and Δt_{ji} is the time between the two nearest spikes of neuron j and neuron i. The time of a spike here is defined as the time when v exceeds 0. Parameters A_{+} and A_{-} configure the amplitude of the learning curve and τ_{+} and τ_{-} specify its time scale. Mexican-hat-type learning curves can be realized by selecting appropriate parameter values (**Figure 8B**).

By implementing 16 SNNMs in an FPGA chip, we constructed an all-to-all connected silicon neuronal network composed of 256 SNs. To verify its functionality, we executed associative memory tasks in which the four patterns shown in **Figure 9A** are stored. A pattern comprises 256 (16 × 16) pixels, each of which has a value of 1 or −1. In the figure, a black (white) pixel has value of 1 (−1). Firstly, these patterns were stored by correlation learning without using the Learning Unit as follows:

$$W_{ij} = \begin{cases} \frac{1}{4} \sum_{u=1}^{4} x_i^u x_j^u & \text{when } i \neq j, \\ 0 & \text{when } i = j, \end{cases} \qquad (26)$$

where x_i^u represents the value of the ith pixel in pattern u. In the retrieval process, all SNs are repetitively spiking owing to the application of an appropriate sustained stimulus I^i_{ext} for all i. Their initial spiking phases are arranged by a short positive external input applied before the sustained stimulus only to the SNs that correspond to the pixel with a value of 1 in the input pattern. The input patterns were generated by flipping the values of randomly selected pixels in a stored pattern. **Figure 9B** plots examples of observed retrieval processes, in which the time step for numerical integration is 375 μs. In the left column, M_u, an index that reflects the correlation between the current spiking pattern and the uth pattern, is plotted. This value is 0 when the spiking pattern has no relation with the uth pattern and approaches 1 as the pattern matches to it. In the right column, the phase synchronization index (PSI) that reflects the degree of synchronization is plotted. It is 0 when the SNs are spiking fully asynchronously and approaches 1 as their spike timing is synchronized. In the upper row, 10% of the pixels in pattern (1) are flipped and applied as inputs. In this case, M_1 quickly increases and remains near 1, which indicates the successful retrieval of pattern (1). In the lower row, 40% of the pixels are flipped. Then, none of the values of M_u remain close to 1, which indicates that no pattern was retrieved. The PSI plotted in the right column stayed near 1 when a correct pattern was retrieved but not when no pattern was retrieved. We executed 100 retrieval processes: 10 different levels of flipped (error) pixels from 5 to 50% in 5% increments and 10 patterns for each error level. The red and blue plots in **Figure 9C** show the rate of successful retrieval when the SNs are in the Class I and II modes, respectively. The network could retrieve a correct pattern from a

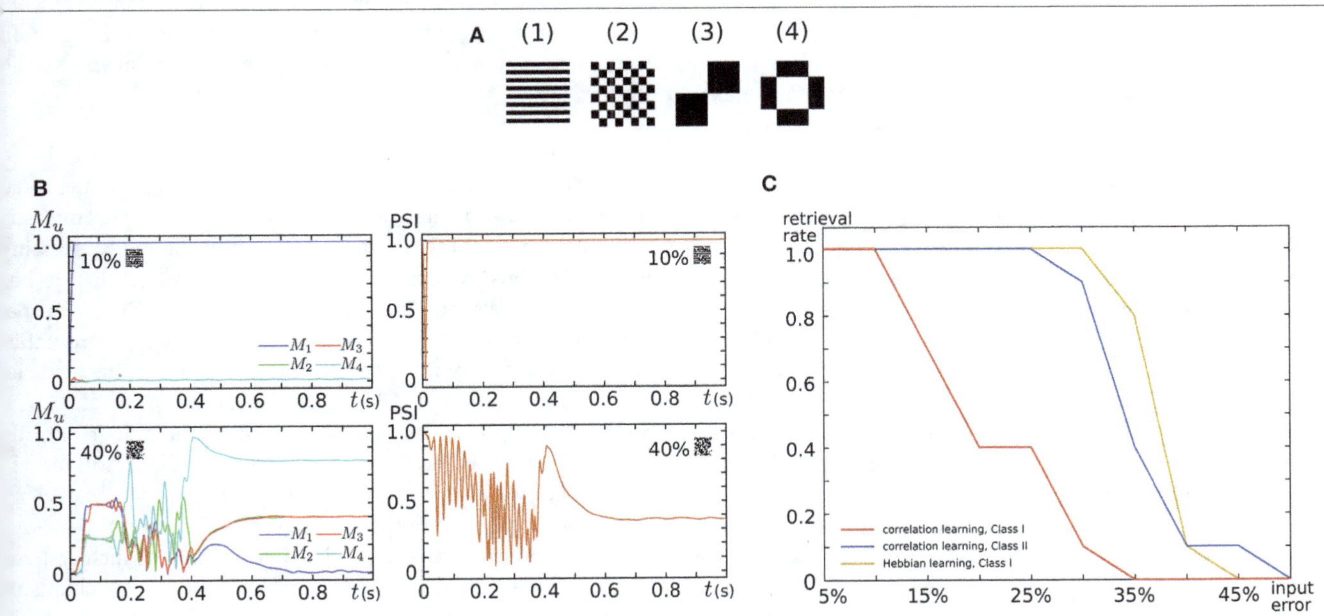

FIGURE 9 | Auto-associative memory tasks executed in our all-to-all digital silicon neuronal networks. (A) Stored patterns. Each pattern is composed of 256 (16 × 16) pixels with a value of 1 or −1. Black (white) pixels have a value of 1 (−1). Reprinted with modification from Li et al. (2012). **(B)** Examples of the transition of M_U and PSI when the input pattern has 10 and 40% flipped pixels. Reprinted with modification from Li et al. (2012). **(C)** Error recovery performance when the patterns are stored by correlation learning and the SNs are in the Class I mode (red) and in the Class II mode (blue). The yellow plot is for the case where the patterns are stored by Hebbian-type spike-timing-dependent learning and the SNs are in the Class I mode. The horizontal axis is the ratio of the flipped pixels to the total number of pixels (the error level). The vertical axis represents the rate of successful retrieval rate. For each error level, 10 trials were executed. Reprinted with modification from Li et al. (2013).

larger number of errors when the SNs are in the Class II mode than when they are in the Class I mode. This indicates that the spiking dynamics may play important roles in auto-associative memory tasks.

Second, the four patterns were stored by activating the Learning Unit as follows. The stored patterns were applied to the network in the sequence of (1), $\overline{(1)}$, (1), $\overline{(1)}$, .. (2), $\overline{(2)}$, .. (3), $\overline{(3)}$, .. (4), $\overline{(4)}$, .. (1), $\overline{(1)}$, .., where $\overline{(n)}$ means the reversed pattern of (n). A couple of a stored pattern and its reversed pattern was repeated eight times in a block. This sequence was applied until one of the values of W_{ij} reached 1 or -1 by the modification in Equation (26). In the retrieval process, the Learning Unit was deactivated and input patterns with errors were applied in the same way as above. The yellow plot in **Figure 9C** shows the rate of successful retrieval when the SNs are in the Class I mode. The error recovery performance exceeded both results with correlation learning. In our preliminary results with SNs in the Class II mode, this performance was further boosted (not shown in the figure). The spiking dynamics may also be important in auto-associative memory with spike-timing-dependent learning rules.

4. DISCUSSION

As reviewed above, our silicon neuron circuits can realize different classes of neuronal activities by selecting appropriate parameter values and their characteristics can be modified by finely tuning the parameters as shown in **Figure 5D**. This high configurability is advantageous not only for bio-silico hybrid systems but also for constructing " field-programmable" silicon neuronal networks in which each SN can be reconfigured after fabrication or each SN autonomously obtains appropriate dynamical properties on the basis of the history of stimulus inputs as in the brain. This high configurability arises from the fact that the activity of many neuronal classes can be explained using common dynamical structures that are reproduced in our models by a combination of implementation-efficient formulae. In contrast, the circuitry is simplified by supporting only one neuronal class in the non-I&F-based SN circuits developed by a similar approach (Basu and Hasler, 2010; Brink et al., 2013b). These circuits realize ultralow power consumption down to several nanowatts at the expense of configurability. In their SN network systems, the configurability is supplemented by accommodating a sufficiently large SN circuit pool, in which the appropriate SNs for a desired network are activated. Our circuit in Section 3.2 supports both Class I and II neuronal activities and consumes a similar power; however, it has the drawback of high configurability. The circuit has to be configured appropriately by tuning a number of parameter values, and additional circuits are required for storing parameter values. The complexity of the configuration process is solved by parameter tuning procedures that utilize the nullcline drawing circuits as explained in detail in Section 3.1. This procedure is still not straightforward, but all of the students who worked on our circuit learned to be able to finish the tuning procedure within several tens of minutes. For a large-scale silicon neuronal network, this procedure has to be automated. It may be done by metaheuristic approaches similar to those utilized in Grassia et al. (2011). The power consumption and area occupied by additional circuits for storing parameter values may be reduced by evolving non-volatile memory technologies such as memristors.

In digital silicon neuronal networks, the accumulation of synaptic inputs consumes a considerably larger amount of hardware resources than SN circuits. Thus, the compactness of the SN circuit is not a major issue. The advantage of our circuit is that its model is non-I&F-based and thus can mimic the spike-generation-related properties in neuronal activities more finely than I&F-based circuits. One of these properties is the graded response in Class II neurons. Because the graded response is found in the brain, as mentioned in the introduction, there is possibility that it plays some roles in information processing in the brain. Our silicon neuronal network model intends to provide a platform in which a wide variety of neuronal activities including the dynamics of spike generation is qualitatively reproduced without a major increase in hardware resource consumption. For this goal, our SN model is being expanded so that it can realize more classes of neurons including RS, LTS, and IB as well as autonomous bursting supported by our analog SN. It has four variables (two original and two additional slow variables) but still can be solved by one multiplication per a numerical integration step. The details of this model is explained in Nanami and Kohno (2016).

A goal of our analog silicon neuronal circuits is to establish an ultralow-power general-purpose silicon neuronal network platform that will be applicable to neuromimetic computing when the mechanism of information processing in the nervous system is elucidated. We expect that it has an advantage also in the application to large-scale neuronal network simulators (Schemmel et al., 2010; Stromatia et al., 2013) and brain-prosthetic devices such as an artificial hippocampus (Berger et al., 2012; Hampson et al., 2013; Song et al., 2015), an artificial cerebellum (Hogri et al., 2015), and an artificial prefrontal cortex (Hampson et al., 2012) because our circuits meet their requirements of low power consumption and the ability to mimic various complex neuronal activities finely. Construction of such systems may contribute to the elucidation of the brain's mechanism by the "analysis by synthesis" approach. Our digital silicon neuronal network platform is also applicable to neuromimetic computing and large-scale neural network simulation. It consumes more power than analog circuits but has advantage in scalability.

AUTHOR CONTRIBUTIONS

MS performed circuit experiments on analog silicon neurons. JL implemented, simulated, and performed experiments on digital silicon neuronal networks. TN expanded the digital silicon neuron model. KA checked the mathematical correctness of the research. TK did all other things.

ACKNOWLEDGMENTS

The works reviewed in this article were supported by the VLSI Design and Education Center (VDEC), The University of Tokyo with the collaboration with Cadence Design Systems, Inc. and Mentor Graphics, Inc.

REFERENCES

Alle, H., and Geiger, J. R. P. (2006). Combined analog and action potential coding in hippocampal mossy fibers. *Science* 311, 1290–1293. doi: 10.1126/science.1119055

Ambroise, M., Levi, T., Joucla, S., Yvert, B., and Saïghi, S. (2013). Real-time biomimetic central pattern generators in an fpga for hybrid experiments. *Front. Neurosci.* 7:215. doi: 10.3389/fnins.2013.00215

Arthur, J. V., and Boahen, K. A. (2011). Silicon-neuron design: a dynamical systems approach. *IEEE Trans. Circ. Syst. I* 58, 1034–1043. doi: 10.1109/TCSI.2010.2089556

Basu, A., and Hasler, P. E. (2010). Nullcline-based design of a silicon neuron. *IEEE Trans. Circ. Syst. I* 57, 2938–2947. doi: 10.1109/TCSI.2010.2048772

Berger, T. W., Song, D., Chan, R. H. M., Marmarelis, V. Z., LaCoss, J., Wills, J., et al. (2012). A hippocampal cognitive prosthesis: multi-input, multi-output nonlinear modeling and VLSI implementation. *IEEE Trans. Neural Syst. Rehabil. Eng.* 20, 198–211. doi: 10.1109/TNSRE.2012.2189133

Brader, J. M., Senn, W., and Fusi, S. (2007). Learning real-world stimuli in a neural network with spike-driven synaptic dynamics. *Neural Comput.* 19, 2881–2912. doi: 10.1162/neco.2007.19.11.2881

Brette, R., and Gerstner, W. (2005). Adaptive exponential integrate-and-fire model as an effective description of neuronal activity. *J. Neurophysiol.* 94, 3637–3642. doi: 10.1152/jn.00686.2005

Brink, S., Nease, S., and Hasler, P. (2013a). Computing with networks of spiking neurons on a biophysically motivated floating-gate based neuromorphic integrated circuit. *Neural Netw.* 45, 39–49. doi: 10.1016/j.neunet.2013.02.011

Brink, S., Nease, S., Hasler, P., Ramakrishnan, S., Wunderlich, R., Basu, A., et al. (2013b). A learning-enabled neuron array ic based upon transistor channel models of biological phenomena. *IEEE Trans. Biomed. Circ. Syst.* 7, 71–81. doi: 10.1109/TBCAS.2012.2197858

Cassidy, A., Georgiou, J., and Andreou, A. G. (2013). Design of silicon brains in the nano-cmos era: spiking neurons, learning synapses and neural architecture optimization. *Neural Netw.* 45, 4–26. doi: 10.1016/j.neunet.2013.05.011

Chay, T. R., and Rinzel, J. (1985). Bursting, beating, and chaos in an excitable membrane model. *Biophys. J.* 47, 357–366. doi: 10.1016/S0006-3495(85)83926-6

Clarke, D. D., and Sokoloff, L. (1999). "Circulation and energy metabolism of the brain," in *Basic Neurochemistry: Molecular, Cellular and Medical Aspects*, 6th *Edn.*, eds G. J. Siegel, B. W. Agranoff, R. W. Albers, S. K. Fisher, and M. D. Uhler (Philadelphia: Lippincott Williams and Wilkins), 637–669.

Cosp, J., Madrenas, J., Alarcó, E., Vidal, E., and Villar, G. (2004). Synchronization of nonlinear electronic oscillators for neural computation. *IEEE Trans. Neural Netw.* 15, 1315–1327. doi: 10.1109/TNN.2004.832808

Dan, Y., and Poo, M.-M., (2004). Spike timing-dependent plasticity of neural circuits. *Neuron* 44, 23–30. doi: 10.1016/j.neuron.2004.09.007

Destexhe, A., Mainen, Z. F., and Sejnowski, T. J. (1998). "Kinetic models of synaptic transmission," in *Methods in Neural Modeling, 2nd Edn.*, eds C. Koch and I. Segev (Cambridge, MA: MIT Press), 1–25.

Destexhe, A., Mccormick, D. A., and Sejnowski, T. J. (1993). A model for 8–10hz spindling in interconnected thalamic relay and reticularis neurons. *Biophys. J.* 65, 2473–2477. doi: 10.1016/S0006-3495(93)81297-9

FitzHugh, R. (1961). Impulses and physiologcal states in theoretical models of nerve membrane. *Biophys. J.* 1, 445–466. doi: 10.1016/S0006-3495(61)86902-6

Fusi, S., Annunziato, M., Badoni, D., Salamon, A., and Amit, D. J. (2000). Spike-driven synaptic plasticity: Theory, simulation, VLSI implementation. *Neural Comput.* 12, 2227–2258. doi: 10.1162/089976600300014917

Giulioni, M., Corradi, F., Dante, V., and del Giudice, P. (2015). Real time unsupervised learning of visual stimuli in neuromorphic VLSI systems. *Sci. Rep.* 5, 1–10. doi: 10.1038/srep14730

Giulioni, M., Lagorce, X., Galluppi, F., and Benosman, R. B. (2016). Event-based computation of motion flow on a neuromorphic analog neural platform. *Front. Neurosci.* 10:35. doi: 10.3389/fnins.2016.00035

Grassia, F., Buhry, L., Levi, T., Tomas, J., Destexhe, A., and Saïghi, S. (2011). Tunable neuromimetic integrated system for emulating cortical neuron models. *Front. Neuroscience* 5:134. doi: 10.3389/fnins.2011.00134

Gütig, R., and Sompolinsky, H. (2006). The tempotron: a neuron that learns spike timing-based decisions. *Nat. Neurosci.* 9, 420–428. doi: 10.1038/nn1643

Hampson, R. E., Gerhardt, G. A., Marmarelis, V., Song, D., Opris, I., Santos, L., et al. (2012). Facilitation and restoration of cognitive function in primate prefrontal cortex by a neuroprosthesis that utilizes minicolumn-specific neural firing. *J. Neural Eng.* 9:056012. doi: 10.1088/1741-2560/9/5/056012

Hampson, R. E., Song, D., Opris, I., Santos, L. M., Shin, D. C., Gerhardt, G. A., et al. (2013). Facilitation of memory encoding in primate hippocampus by a neuroprosthesis that promotes task specific neural firing. *J. Neural Eng.* 10:066013. doi: 10.1088/1741-2560/10/6/066013

Harris, K. D., and Shepherd, G. M. G. (2015). The neocortical circuit: themes and variations. *Nat. Neurosci.* 18, 170–181. doi: 10.1038/nn.3917

Hill, A. A. V., Lu, J., Masino, M. A., and Calabrese, R. L. (2001). A model of a segmental oscillator in the Leech heartbeat neuronal network. *J. Comput. Neurosci.* 10, 281–302. doi: 10.1023/A:1011216131638

Hodgkin, A. L. (1948). The local electric changes associated with repetitive action in a non-medullated axon. *J. Physiol.* 107, 165–181. doi: 10.1113/jphysiol.1948.sp004260

Hodgkin, A. L., and Huxley, A. F. (1952). A quantitative description of membrane current and its application to conduction and excitation in nerve. *J. Physiol.* 117, 500–544. doi: 10.1113/jphysiol.1952.sp004764

Hogri, R., Bamford, S. A., Taub, A. H., Magal, A., Del Giudice, P., and Mintz, M. (2015). A neuro-inspired model-based closed-loop neuroprosthesis for the substitution of a cerebellar learning function in anesthetized rats. *Sci. Rep.* 5, 1–8. doi: 10.1038/srep08451

Izhikevich, E. M. (2004). Which model to use for cortical spiking neurons ? *IEEE Trans. Neural Netw.* 15, 1063–1070. doi: 10.1109/TNN.2004.832719

Izhikevich, E. M. (2007). *Dynamical Systems in Neuroscience.* Cambridge, MA: The MIT Press.

Kohno, T., and Aihara, K. (2005). A MOSFET-based model of a class 2 nerve membrane. *IEEE Trans. Neural Netw.* 16, 754–773. doi: 10.1109/TNN.2005.844855

Kohno, T., and Aihara, K. (2007). "Digital spiking silicon neuron: concept and behaviors in gj-coupled network," in *Proceedings of International Symposium on Artificial Life and Robotics 2007* (Beppu), OS3–OS6.

Kohno, T., and Aihara, K. (2008a). A design method for analog and digital silicon neurons -mathematical-model-based method-. *AIP Conf. Proc.* 1028, 113–128. doi: 10.1063/1.2965080

Kohno, T., and Aihara, K. (2008b). Mathematical-model-based design method of silicon burst neurons. *Neurocomputing* 71, 1619–1628. doi: 10.1016/j.neucom.2007.04.003

Kohno, T., and Aihara, K. (2010). "A mathematical-structure-based aVLSI silicon neuron model," in *Proceedings of the 2010 International Symposium on Nonlinear Theory and its Applications* (Krakow), 261–264.

Kohno, T., and Aihara, K. (2011). "Reducing a fluctuation in burst firing of a square-wave burster silicon neuron model," in *Proceedings of Physcon 2011*, IPACS Electronic Library, Available online at: http://lib.physcon.ru/doc?id=8b4e8b1b12f1

Kohno, T., and Aihara, K. (2013). Improving noise resistance of intrinsic rhythms in a square-wave burster model. *BioSystems* 112, 276–283. doi: 10.1016/j.biosystems.2013.03.016

Kohno, T., and Aihara, K. (2014a). "A qualitative-modeling-based low-power silicon nerve membrane," in *Proceedings of 21st IEEE International Conference on Electronics Circuits and Systems* (Marseille), 199–202. doi: 10.1109/icecs.2014.7049956

Kohno, T., Li, J., and Aihara, K. (2014b). Silicon neuronal networks towards brain-morphic computers. *Nonlin. Theory Appl. IEICE* 5, 379–390. doi: 10.1587/nolta.5.379

Li, J., Katori, Y., and Kohno, T. (2012). An fpga-based silicon neuronal network with selectable excitability silicon neurons. *Front. Neurosci.* 6:183. doi: 10.3389/fnins.2012.00183

Li, J., Katori, Y., and Kohno, T. (2013). "Hebbian learning in fpga silicon neuronal network," in *Proceedings of The 1st IEEE/IIAE International Conference on Intelligent Systems and Image Processing 2013* (Kitakyushu), 83–90. doi: 10.12792/icisip2013.020

Linares-Barranco, B., Sénchez-Sinencio, E., Rodríguez-Vázquez, A., and Huertas, J. L. (1991). A cmos implementation of fitzhugh-nagumo neuron model. *IEEE J. Solid-State Circ.* 26, 956–965. doi: 10.1109/4.92015

Mayr, C., Partzsch, J., Noack, M., Hänzsche, S., Scholze, S., Höppner, S., et al. (2015). A biological-realtime neuromorphic system in 28 nm cmos using low-leakage switched capacitor circuits. *IEEE Trans. Biomed. Circ. Syst.* 10, 243–254. doi: 10.1109/TBCAS.2014.2379294

Merolla, P. A., Arthur, J. V., Alvarez-Icaza, R., Cassidy, A. S., Sawada, J., Akopyan, F., et al. (2014). A million spiking-neuron integrated circuit with a scalable communication network and interface. *Science* 345, 668–673. doi: 10.1126/science.1254642

Nagumo, J., Arimoto, S., and Yoshizawa, S. (1962). An active pulse transmission line simulating nerve axon. *Proc. IRE* 50, 2061–2070. doi: 10.1109/JRPROC.1962.288235

Nanami, T., and Kohno, T. (2016). Simple cortical and thalamic neuron models for digital arithmetic circuit implementation. *Front. Neurosci.* 10:181. doi: 10.3389/fnins.2016.00181

Negro, C. A. D., Johnson, S. M., Butera, R. J., and Smith, J. C. (2001). Models of respiratory rhythm generation in the pre-Bötzinger complex. iii. experimental tests of model predictions. *J. Neurophysiol.* 86, 59–74.

Osawa, Y., and Kohno, T. (2015). Associative memory with class i and ii izhikevich model. *J. Robot. Netw. Artif. Life* 1, 312–315. doi: 10.2991/jrnal.2015.1.4.12

Qiao, N., Mostafa, H., Corradi, F., Osswald, M., Stefanini, F., Sumislawska, D., et al. (2015). A reconfigurable on-line learning spiking neuromorphic processor comprising 256 neurons and 128k synapses. *Front. Neurosci.* 9:141. doi: 10.3389/fnins.2015.00141

Rice, K. L., Bhuiyan, M. A., Taha, T. M., and Vutsinas, C. N. (2009). "Fpga implementation of izhikevich spiking neural networks for character recognition," in *Proceedings of 2009 International Conference on Reconfigurable Computing and FPGAs* (Cancún), 451–456. doi: 10.1109/ReConFig.2009.77

Rinzel, J., and Ermentrout, G. B. (1998). "Analysis of neural excitability and oscillations," in *Methods in Neural Modeling, 2nd Edn.*, eds C. Koch, and I. Segev (Cambridge, MA: MIT Press), 251–291.

Saïghi, S., Bornat, Y., Tomas, J., Le Masson, G., and Renaud, S. (2011). A library of analog operators based on the hodgkin-huxley formalism for the design of tunable, real-time, silicon neurons. *IEEE Trans. Biomed. Circ. Syst.* 5, 3–19. doi: 10.1109/TBCAS.2010.2078816

Schemmel, J., Brüderle, D., Grübl, A., Hock, M., Meier, K., and Millner, S. (2010). "A wafer-scale neuromorphic hardware system for large-scale neural modeling," in *Proceedings of 2010 IEEE International Symposium on Circuits and Systems* (Paris), 1947–1950. doi: 10.1109/ISCAS.2010.5536970

Sekikawa, M., Kohno, T., and Aihara, K. (2008). An integrated circuit design of a silicon neuron and its measurement results. *J. Artif. Life Robot.* 13, 116–119. doi: 10.1007/s10015-008-0530-8

Simoni, M. F., and DeWeerth, S. P. (2006). Two-dimensional variation of bursting properties in a silicon-neuron half-center oscillator. *IEEE Trans. Neural Syst. Rehabil. Eng.* 14, 281–289. doi: 10.1109/TNSRE.2006.881537

Song, D., Hampson, R. E., Robinson, B. S., Opris, I., Marmarelis, V. Z., Deadwyler, S. A., et al. (2015). "Nonlinear dynamical modeling of human hippocampal ca3-ca1 functional connectivity for memory prostheses," in *Proceedings of 7th Annual International IEEE EMBS Conference on Neural Engineering* (Montpellier), 316–319. doi: 10.1109/ner.2015.7146623

Song, S., Miller, K. D., and Abbott, L. F. (2000). Competitive hebbian learning through spike-timing-dependent synaptic plasticity. *Nat. Neurosci.* 3, 919–926. doi: 10.1038/78829

Stromatias, E., Galluppi, F., Patterson, C., and Furber, S. (2013). "Power analysis of large-scale, real-time neural networks on spinnaker," in *Proceedings of the 2013 International Join Conference on Neural Networks* (Dallas, TX), 1–8. doi: 10.1109/IJCNN.2013.6706927

Tadokoro, S., Yamaguti, Y., Fujii, H., and Tsuda, I. (2011). Transitory behaviors in diffusively coupled nonlinear oscillators. *Cogn. Neurodyn.* 5, 1–12. doi: 10.1007/s11571-010-9130-0

Thomas, D. B., and Luk, W. (2009). "Fpga accelerated simulation of biologically plausible spiking neural networks," in *Proceedings of the 17th IEEE Field Programmable Custom Computing Machines* (Napa, CA), 45–52. doi: 10.1109/fccm.2009.46

van Schaik, A., and Jin, C. (2003). "The tau-cell: a new method for the implementation of arbitrary differential equations," in *Proceedings of IEEE International Symposium on Circuits and Systems 2003* (Bangkok), 569–572. doi: 10.1109/iscas.2003.1205627

Wang, X.-J. (1993). Genesis of bursting oscillations in the Hindmarsh-Rose model and homoclinicity to a chaotic saddle. *Phys. D* 62, 263–274. doi: 10.1016/0167-2789(93)90286-A

Wang, X.-J., and Rinzel, J. (2003). "Oscillatory and bursting properties of neurons," in *The Handbook of Brain Theory and Neural Networks, 2nd Edn.*, ed M. A. Arbib (Cambridge, MA: MIT Press), 835–840.

Weinstein, R. K., and Lee, R. H. (2006). Architectures for high-performance fpga implementations of neural models. *J. Neural Eng.* 3, 21–34. doi: 10.1088/1741-2560/3/1/003

14

A Bidirectional Brain-Machine Interface Featuring a Neuromorphic Hardware Decoder

Fabio Boi [1†], Timoleon Moraitis [2†], Vito De Feo [1†], Francesco Diotalevi [3], Chiara Bartolozzi [4], Giacomo Indiveri [2] and Alessandro Vato [1]*

[1] Neural Computation Laboratory, Istituto Italiano di Tecnologia, Rovereto, Italy, [2] Institute of Neuroinformatics, University of Zurich and ETH Zurich, Zurich, Switzerland, [3] Robotics, Brain and Cognitive Sciences, Istituto Italiano di Tecnologia, Genova, Italy, [4] iCub Facility, Istituto Italiano di Tecnologia, Genova, Italy

Edited by:
Timothée Levi,
University of Bordeaux 1, France

Reviewed by:
Christoph Richter,
Technische Universität München, Germany
Mikhail Lebedev,
Duke University, USA

***Correspondence:**
Fabio Boi
fabio.boi@iit.it

† These authors have contributed equally to this work.

Bidirectional brain-machine interfaces (BMIs) establish a two-way direct communication link between the brain and the external world. A decoder translates recorded neural activity into motor commands and an encoder delivers sensory information collected from the environment directly to the brain creating a closed-loop system. These two modules are typically integrated in bulky external devices. However, the clinical support of patients with severe motor and sensory deficits requires compact, low-power, and fully implantable systems that can decode neural signals to control external devices. As a first step toward this goal, we developed a modular bidirectional BMI setup that uses a compact neuromorphic processor as a decoder. On this chip we implemented a network of spiking neurons built using its ultra-low-power mixed-signal analog/digital circuits. On-chip on-line spike-timing-dependent plasticity synapse circuits enabled the network to learn to decode neural signals recorded from the brain into motor outputs controlling the movements of an external device. The modularity of the BMI allowed us to tune the individual components of the setup without modifying the whole system. In this paper, we present the features of this modular BMI and describe how we configured the network of spiking neuron circuits to implement the decoder and to coordinate it with the encoder in an experimental BMI paradigm that connects bidirectionally the brain of an anesthetized rat with an external object. We show that the chip learned the decoding task correctly, allowing the interfaced brain to control the object's trajectories robustly. Based on our demonstration, we propose that neuromorphic technology is mature enough for the development of BMI modules that are sufficiently low-power and compact, while being highly computationally powerful and adaptive.

Keywords: bidirectional BMI, neuromorphic decoder, on-line learning, modular system, spiking neural network

1. INTRODUCTION

The possibility of controlling a prosthetic device through a direct interface with the central nervous system represents a promising solution for restoring sensory-motor functionalities in patients with limb amputations or peripheral and neurological deficits due to spinal cord injury, amyotrophic lateral sclerosis, or stroke. In the last two decades, a fast-growing worldwide scientific community has developed several brain-machine or brain-computer interfaces (respectively, BMIs or BCIs) toward the clinical application of these devices. Such interfaces offer also a powerful tool for exploring the sensory-motor mechanisms of control, adaptation, and learning that are employed by the central nervous system. This research has been assisted both by progress in our understanding of the underlying neural processes that take place in the brain, and by technological advances that have dramatically improved the quality of the signals recorded from the brain and the possibility of managing and processing large amount of data in real-time (Wolpaw et al., 2000; Lebedev and Nicolelis, 2006; Wander and Rao, 2014). Encouraging results have been recently obtained in controlling a robotic arm by using motor neural activity in tetraplegic patients (Hochberg et al., 2012) and by restoring cortical control of movement in humans with quadriplegia (Bouton et al., 2016) but these setups still have limitations that prevent their clinical use on a large scale (Baranauskas, 2014).

The development of a BMI system aiming for large clinical application requires crucial improvements of the hardware and software components. The hardware components need to be (a) fully implantable for long term use and therefore miniaturizable; (b) able to reliably process neural signals with a limited power budget; (c) powerful enough to implement non-trivial computational tasks involved in a BMI system. Additionally, the decoding algorithms need to be (d) sufficiently flexible to be implemented with different types of hardware components, and (e) able to dynamically adapt to changes in the neural activity due to the interaction with the artificial device (Dangi et al., 2011; Orsborn et al., 2014).

Neuromorphic devices comprise compact, energy-efficient, and adaptive circuits that have been demonstrated to be optimal for tasks that involve learning from real-world observations in an on-line fashion (Chicca et al., 2014). They achieve this by employing silicon emulations of biological neurons and synapses that can be physically configured to implement algorithms inspired by the asynchronous massively parallel computations performed in biological neural networks. Additionally, input to and output from neuromorphic chips is provided with asynchronous digital pulses that encode information in their analog timing, similarly to action potentials of biological neurons. Because of these features, neuromorphic processing chips are very promising candidates for implementing reliable and energy-efficient decoding of neural activity, that could ultimately be evolved to be portable, implantable, and directly interfaced with neural tissue.

For this reason we directed our efforts toward the development of a fully implantable BMI by prototyping a neuromorphic processor chip (Qiao et al., 2015) integrated in a bidirectional brain-machine interface, trained to decode neural signals recorded on-line, and to provide suitable outputs useful for controlling actuators and end effectors. In order to assess the performance of this system, we took the following steps: first we developed suitable spike-based decoding methods that could be implemented by the neuromorphic processor chip, then we configured the chip to implement these methods in real-time and adapted the bidirectional BMI designed and tested in our lab (Vato et al., 2012) to include in the processing chain this neuromorphic component. Finally, we tested this neuromorphic bidirectional BMI in a closed-loop real-time experimental setup that involved the control of the motion of an external device by the decoded neural signals recorded from the brain of an anesthetized rat. Here, we describe in detail the properties of the neuromorphic processor, and the network of spiking neurons that was implemented by the chip to carry out the decoding task. We present the main hardware and software modules that we developed to interface the chip with the other components of the BMI, and describe the experimental paradigm that we used to test the system.

Our approach differs from those of currently-developed BMIs, which are *ad hoc* ensembles of hardware and software elements designed to perform specific tasks, and which are difficult to replicate, generalize, or modify for use in other tasks or different environments (Leuthardt et al., 2006). As these are limitations that hinder collaborations between laboratories we chose to emphasize a modular approach in designing our BMI by developing a system that is compatible with a wide range of different hardware and software standards, and which is composed of a main control core module and multiple possible recording, stimulating, decoding, and encoding modules. We argue that the combination of this modular bidirectional BMI setup with the use of neuromorphic hardware modules can give a crucial contribution to the development of the next generation of brain-machine interfaces for large-scale clinical applications.

2. MATERIALS AND METHODS

We begin by describing the general scheme of this novel bidirectional BMI in Section 2.1 and the experimental procedure used to test the performance of the neuromorphic decoder in Section 2.2. In Section 2.3, we describe in details the main modules comprising the system and finally we present the hardware and the software implementation of the neuromorphic chip, respectively, in Sections 2.4 and 2.5.

2.1. General Scheme of the Modular Bidirectional BMI

We extended the Dynamic Neural Interface described in Szymanski et al. (2011) and Vato et al. (2012, 2014) with the inclusion of a neuromorphic decoder module. This system uses the neural signals collected from a rat's brain to control the movement of an external object by means of a sensory and motor interface. In designing it we took inspiration from earlier studies in frogs (Bizzi et al., 1991), rats (Tresch and Bizzi, 1999) and cats (Lemay and Grill, 2004) by emulating the functioning of the spinal cord that combines sensory information with brain instructions and organizes the movement of the limb along dynamically stable trajectories. We set up a decoding and an encoding interface which generate a dynamic control policy in the form of a force field and robustly drive the movement of the controlled object. The neural signals are recorded from the motor cortex of the anesthetized rat by means of a recording multielectrode array. These signals are transformed by the decoder into a force vector to be applied to a device that can control the motion of the object. After receiving this external input, the device moves the object, according to its dynamics, for a predefined amount of time. An encoder maps each position of the object in the workspace to a pattern of intracortical microstimulation (ICMS) delivered to the somatosensory cortex of the rat. This is achieved by means of a stimulating multielectrode array which provides the brain with information about the position of the controlled object. A calibration procedure of the interface establishes a control policy based on an approximation of a radial force field with the aim of driving the controlled object toward a target location defined by the central equilibrium point of the field. In the implementation described here we use four different patterns of intracortical stimulation and, consequently, the workspace is divided into four different contiguous sensory regions. The four stimulation patterns differ from each other only in the combination of the electrodes chosen to deliver the stimulation. Each stimulation pattern consists of a train of 10 biphasic pulses (100 μA, 100 μs/phase, cathodic first) delivered at 333 Hz (Butovas and Schwarz, 2007; Semprini et al., 2012). After each stimulation, the decoder considers the first 256 ms of the evoked motor neural signal to produce the driving force for the external device. In **Figure 1**, we report the post-stimulus time course of the time-dependent firing rate (mean $\pm$ sem over 50 trials) of the evoked neural activity recorded from all the electrodes of the array. The raster plots represent the time occurrences of at least one spike recorded from all the electrodes of the multielectrode array.

The calibration force corresponding to each region was defined by a vector pointing from the region's centroid to the target (colored thick arrows depicted in **Figure 8**). The task of the decoder consists in extracting from each evoked neural response a resulting force, calculated as a weighted sum of the four calibration forces defining the force field. In particular, the decoder needs to extract the four coefficients corresponding to the contribution of each of the four calibration forces to the decoded force.

2.2. Experimental Procedure

Neural data were collected from male Long-Evans rats (300–400 g) anesthetized for the entire duration of the experimental sessions by means of Xylazine (5 mg/kg) and a mixture of Tiletamine and Zolazepam (30 mg/kg). Two craniotomies were

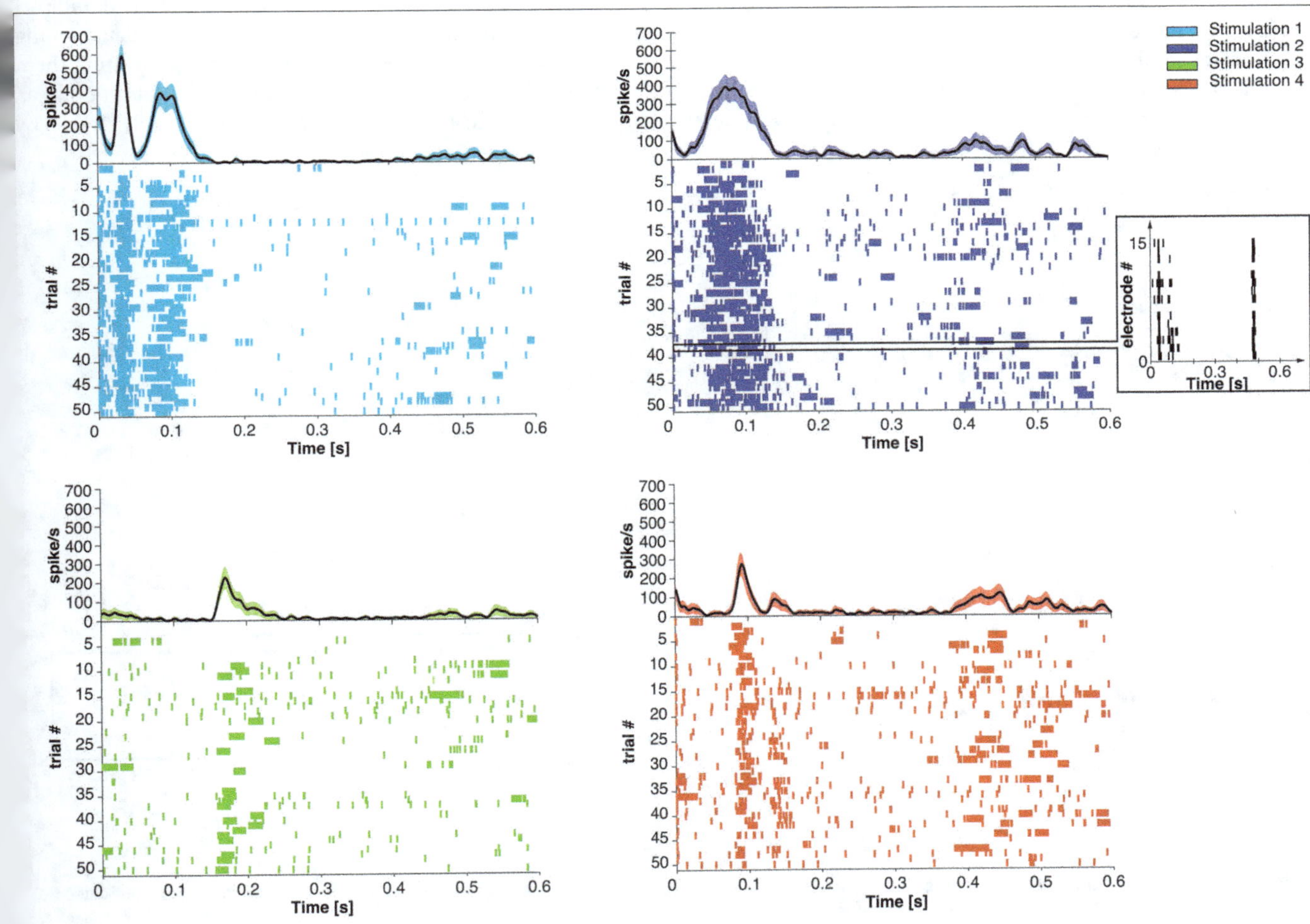

FIGURE 1 | Post-stimulus time course of the time-dependent firing rate (mean ± SEM across trials) and raster plot of the recorded neural activity evoked by four different stimulation patterns. Each short vertical line in the raster plots represents the occurrence of at least one spike recorded from all the electrodes on the recording array in a 1 ms time bin. In the inset, we report the neural activity recorded from each electrode of the microwire array during a single trial.

performed above the somatosensory (S1) and the motor (M1) cortex representing the whiskers on the same hemisphere. The stimulation microwire array (Tucker Davis Technologies—TDT) was lowered perpendicular to the somatosensory cortex 300–500 μm under the surface (AP -3.5 mm, LM $+4$ mm with respect to the most posterior medial electrode of the array). The recording array was placed at depth 900–1100 μm below the pia (AP -1.5 mm, LM $+0.5$ mm with respect to the most posterior medial electrode of the array) using a hydraulic microdrive. These locations have been chosen for the presence of several cortico-cortical connections between the two regions(Mao et al., 2011). Both arrays are composed of 16 microelecrodes (2 rows of 8 electrodes, 50 μm diameter) each one separated from the neighboring ones by 250 and 375 μm along and across the rows, respectively. All the experiments have been performed in accordance with DL116/92 of the Italian legal code and approved by the institutional review board of the University of Ferrara and by the Italian Ministry of Health (73/2008-B).

2.3. Main Modules of the BMI System

The modular bidirectional BMI was designed around a core unit named Managing Unit (MU) that can be connected to satellite modules, each dedicated to specific tasks as decoding the neural signal, controlling the movement of an external device, and encoding the information collected from the external environment to provide sensory feedback. The MU does not require any information about the specific implementation of each module, which can be a software running on general purpose processing units, a dedicated programmable hardware such as Field Programmable Gate Arrays (FPGA) or a neuromorphic chip. This modularity ensures a fast and flexible prototyping phase required during research and development, whereby different software modules can allow testing the algorithms to be implemented on custom low-power, miniaturized implantable hardware.

In this implementation, we connected five different satellite modules to the MU realizing the functionalities required by a bidirectional BMI: Acquisition Unit, Stimulation Unit, Decoder, Encoder and Dynamical System, as shown in **Figure 2** that have been described in details in Boi et al. (2015a). The Dynamical System (see Boi et al., 2015b) consists of a small mobile cart connected to a water/pellet dispenser mounted on a vertical wall in a custom-made behavioral box for rodents and controlled by two servomotors spanning an area of 38 $\times$ 38 cm. The cart is protected by a transparent acrylic glass sheet with a slot that allows the rat to grab the food if the cart is positioned in the desired position. The Dynamical System was designed, developed, and tested in this way to be used in future experimental sessions with behaving subjects.

The main algorithm running on the MU named *mbBMI algorithm* is in charge of reading the spiking neural data coming from the Acquisition System module and communicating them to the decoder. Once the decoder generates an output signal, the algorithm transforms it into motor commands usable by

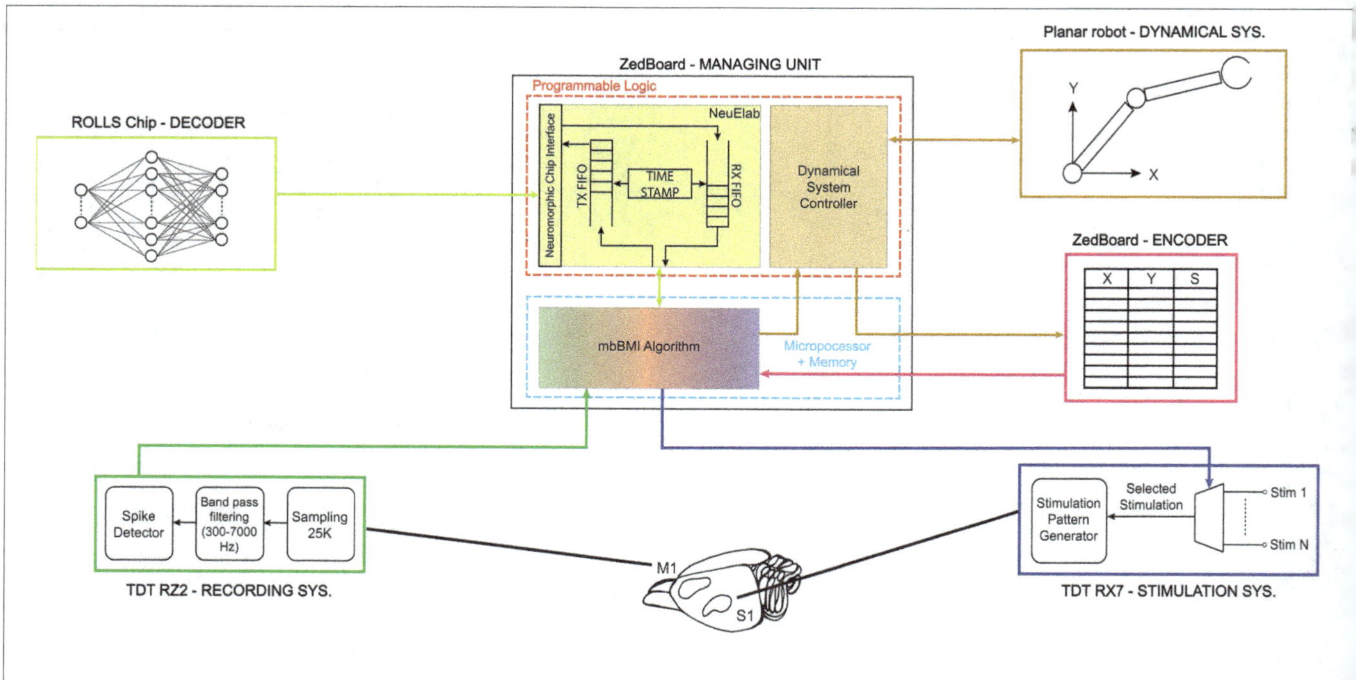

FIGURE 2 | Real implementation of a modular bidirectional BMI. The Managing Unit is implemented on a ZedBoard development board that communicates via User Datagram Protocol (UDP) with a *TDT RZ2 BioAmp Processor*—Tucker-Davis Technologies—(acquisition system) and a *TDT RX7 Stimulator Base* (stimulation system). The ZedBoard is connected to the ROLLS neuromorphic processor (decoder) that implements a neural network that is able to learn to decode the neural signal coming from the rat's motor cortex. The decoder's output is translated by the Managing Unit into a two-dimensional force which is converted into digital signals to drive the motors installed on the 2° of freedom robotic device (dynamical system). The dynamical system communicates to the encoder its final state which is transformed into a stimulation pattern that is subsequently delivered by the TDT RX7 into the somatosensory cortex of the subject and closes the loop.

the Dynamical System. To close the loop on the brain, the algorithm acquires the current position reached from the external device and communicates it to the encoder that returns the next stimulus to be communicated to the Stimulation System module.

2.3.1. Managing Unit

We implemented the Managing Unit by using the development board ZedBoard™ equipped with a Xilinx Zynq®-7000 All Programmable System On Chip (SoC). The Zynq®-7000 family integrates a feature-rich dual-core ARM Cortex™-A9 based processing system (PS) and 28 nm Xilinx programmable logic (PL) in a single device. In our implementation, the PL runs a custom module that can interface with neuromorphic chips and implements two software modules named NeuElab and Dynamical System Controller. The NeuElab module acquires the pre-processed brain signals from the *mbBMI algorithm* and routes them to the decoder and vice versa, via its hardware interface (Zynq2Neuro described in Section 2.3.1).

The MU stores the temporal offset of each recorded action potential with respect to the last delivered stimulation, as a list of time-stamps associated with the identity (or address) of the emitting electrode. At the end of each recording period, spike trains are generated from the recorded spike time-stamps according to the decoder's requirements (Section 2.5 and **Figure 5**) and then forwarded to the neuromorphic chip. The MU communicates with the decoder using the native neuromorphic asynchronous communication protocol, known as Address Event Representation (AER) protocol (Mortara, 1998), where the information is encoded in the implicit timing between digital pulses (or spikes) and in the identity (or address) of the neuron that has emitted the pulse. The decoder's output AER spikes are acquired by the MU and forwarded to its Dynamical System Controller part.

When acquired on the MU clocked system, the implicit temporal information in the AER spike sequence is explicitly paired with the address of the spike by the TimeStamp block of the NeuElab part of the MU. NeuElab is composed of two different FIFOs that drive the data flow from/to the neuromorphic chip. The TX FIFO is filled with the address of the neuron that shall receive the spike and the time relative to the other spikes, by associating a delay time value by the TimeStamp block. NeuElab reads the TX FIFO and sends a spike to the neuromorphic chip at the time specified by the delay, the address associated to the spike allows the receiving chip to rout the spike to the corresponding neuron. The RX FIFO is filled with the spikes from the neurons of the neuromorphic chip. The received pairs of address and relative time-stamp are then sent to the BMI algorithm that translates the recorded neural activity into commands for the Dynamical System.

Besides managing the AER communication with the neuromorphic chip, the NeuElab interface is critical for the chip's configuration, through digital configuration bits and a number of tunable analog voltages or currents (biases) that set the operating point of the analog circuits. NeuElab can be used, in principle, for interfacing the BMI with any neuromorphic chip that uses the AER communication protocol. In this implementation, the output spiking activity of the neuromorphic chip is translated into a bidimensional force applied to the Dynamical System by means of a pair of Pulse Width Modulated (PWM) analog signals generated by the ZedBoard that drive the external object.

2.4. Hardware Aspects of the Neuromorphic Decoder

The decoder that transforms the recorded brain activity into motor commands is implemented on a neuromorphic chip. In the following, we describe the chip and the printed circuit board (PCB) that we developed to connect the chip with the rest of the system.

2.4.1. The ROLLS Neuromorphic Processor

The Reconfigurable On-line Learning Spiking (ROLLS) Neuromorphic Processor is a general-purpose spiking neural network chip (Qiao et al., 2015). **Figure 3** shows the chip micrograph. It was fabricated using a standard 6-metal 180 nm CMOS process, occupies an area of 51.4 mm^2 and has approximately 12.2 million transistors. It comprises 256 adaptive exponential integrate-and-fire neurons implemented in a mixed signal analog/digital circuit design.

There are 128 K synapses, of which 64 K that can implement a Hebbian plasticity rule (Brader et al., 2007; Mitra et al., 2009) [Long-Term Plasticity (LTP) synapses] (Mostafa et al., 2014). The rest 64 K synapses can exhibit short term depression and short-term facilitation dynamics [Short-Term Plasticity (STP) synapses], and have two possible programmable weights resolution, in addition to the possibility to configure them as either excitatory or inhibitory. These two synaptic matrices (LTP and STP) allow arbitrary on-chip connectivity thanks to a crossbar structure. In principle all-to-all connections are possible through the programmable logic state of the synapses. Additional circuits next to the neurons' array represent the calcium concentration at the post-synaptic side, needed to implement the spike-based LTP weight update algorithm (Brader et al., 2007). We refer the reader to Qiao et al. (2015) for a detailed description of the circuits.

Both the neural network architecture and the parameters of the neuromorphic core are fully programmable via a high-level Python framework (Stefanini et al., 2014). The combination of reconfigurable hardware with the Python-based configuration framework supports the exploration of a wide range of spiking neural network architectures, and their real-time emulation in closed-loop setups. Here, these enabled us to configure a hardware implementation of a spiking neural network that learns on-line to decode patterns of recorded spike sequences.

2.4.2. The Zynq2Neuro (Z2N)

With the aim to manage, program, and interface neuromorphic chips with the Managing Unit, we designed and developed the Zynq2Neuro (Z2N) PCB that can host up to two daughterboards (DTB) that mount neuromorphic chips. The Z2N connects the neuromorphic chips to the FNC connector of the ZedBoard, supplies power to the chips and supports the AER communication and the chip configuration signals. Analog biases that configure the parameters of the silicon neural and synaptic models on the neuromorphic chip can be set either

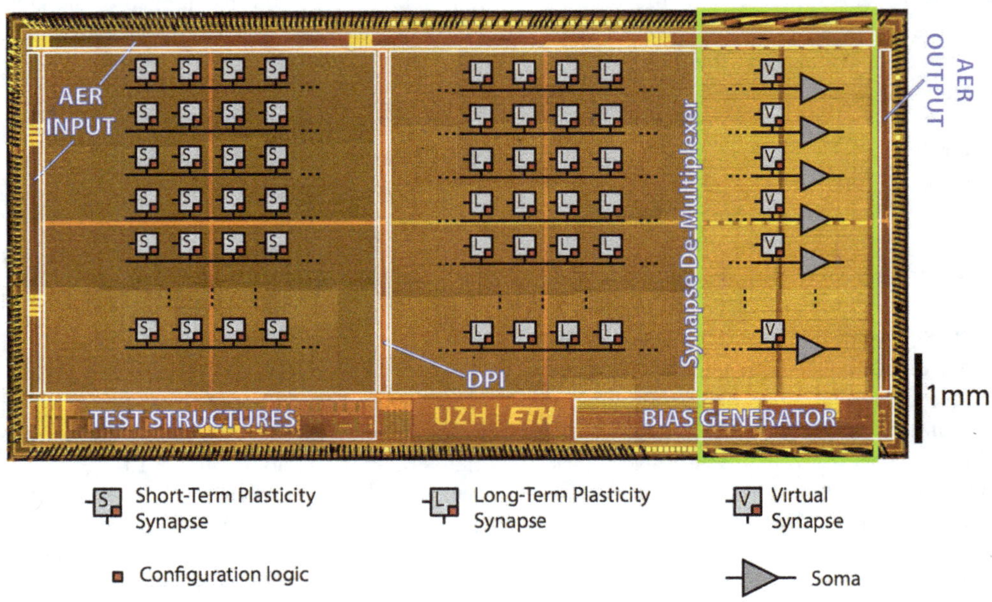

FIGURE 3 | ROLLS Neuromorphic Processor: micrograph of a neuromorphic processor chip that allocates most of its area to non-linear synapse circuits for memory storage and distributed massively parallel computing. The test structures in the lower left part of the chip contain extra low power neural amplifier circuits and spike-based neural signal Analog-to-Digital conversion circuits that have not been used in this work.

by means of external digital to analog converters (DAC), or by on-chip programmable bias generators (BG) (Delbruck and Lichtsteiner, 2006). NeuElab, together with the Zynq2Neuro board, can drive both systems, the Zynq2Neuro board hosts 64 DACs that can be programmed through an SPI interface and also hosts the necessary signals for programming different types of BGs, managed by NeuElab, hence supporting a large library of neuromorphic chips. The Z2N board is already configured to support future chip functionalities by means of I/O expanders and I^2C protocol. The AER addressing space can be expanded up to 30 bits (configurable as inputs or outputs). The Z2N (**Figure 4**) can support logic levels, power supply and biases from Digital to Analog Converters of 3.3 or 1.8 V, as selected from the first DTB. This means that the two DTBs need to host chips that are homogeneous for the logical levels. In general, the Z2N can support chips fabricated on the 350 nm (3.3 V) and 180 nm process of the latest generation (1.8 V and mixed 1.8/3.3 V). To optimize the design, AER address lines, some bits of the Bias Generator programming, I^2C and I/O expander are shared among the two DTBs. The sharing of the AER address lines is based on the assumption that they are in tri-state when the chip is not sending or receiving an event. This is guaranteed by the SCX protocol (Mortara, 1998), but can be supported also for the P2P protocol (Boahen, 2000), by adding buffers on the DTB driven by the handshake signals (ACK) from the ZedBoard. The correct addressing of the event to/from the chip is guaranteed by the reserved handshake signals (REQ/ACK and Bias LATCH) that target only one of the two chips. The Z2N specifically targets compatibility with neuromorphic chips such as the ROLLS (Qiao et al., 2015), but is a more general tool for most of existing neuromorphic chips based on parallel (or word-serial Boahen, 2004) AER protocols, on Bias Generators externally configurable by means of SPI-like serial interfaces, or on external voltage tuning. Some examples of supported chips are the Dynamic Vision Sensor (Lichtsteiner et al., 2008), the AER EAR (Chan et al., 2007), the Selective Attention Chip (Bartolozzi and Indiveri, 2009), the spiking Winner-Take-All chip (Chicca et al., 2014), and the Asynchronous Time-Based Image Sensor (Posch et al., 2010).

2.5. Algorithmic Aspects of the Neuromorphic Decoder

We approached the neuromorphic decoding task by combinin the constraints of a multi-class classification task with thos of spiking neural networks with limited resolution synapti weights, and with the BMI-specific requirements related to th simultaneous contribution of all four classes to each decode force (see Section 2.1).

2.5.1. The Silicon Spiking Neural Network

We configured the ROLLS chip to implement a feed-forwar spiking neural network that exploits the spike-timing depende plasticity of the chip's LTP synapses to learn how to extract th pattern of four calibration forces that should result in the ne desired force, from the recorded neural activity. Each of th output neurons of the network was trained to act as a binar classifier by re-weighting the features of its input that wer distributed across its synapses, so as to ultimately yield, via it activation function, a higher output spike rate for one, positiv class of input compared to the other three, negative classe Neurons were grouped into four ensembles, each correspondin to one of the four stimuli. The spike counts output by th

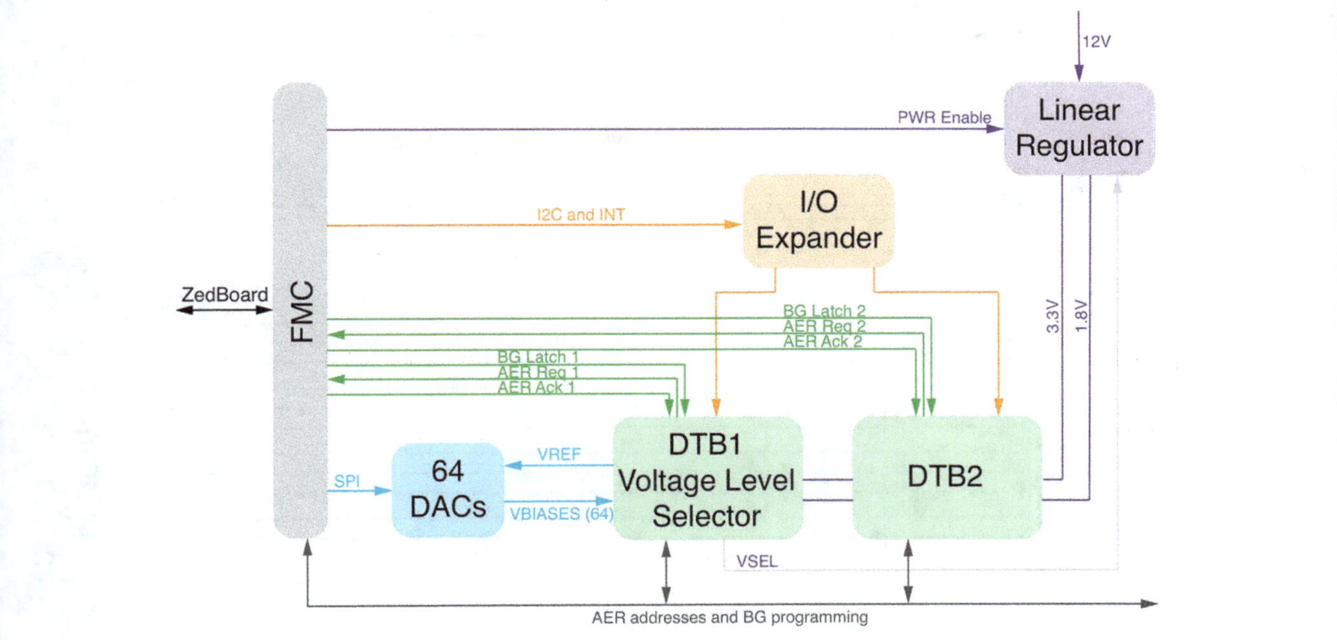

FIGURE 4 | Zynq2Neuro schematic: block diagram of the board allowing the use of neuromorphic chips in the bmBMI. It hosts DTBs with neuromorphic chips and connects them to the ZedBoard through the FMC connector. Chip configuration is supported by Digital to Analog Converters or Bias Generator programming and by IO expander for digital configuration. AER input/output communication supports P2P and SCX protocols.

four ensembles during the presentation of the recordings to the network were directly used as the coefficients that weight the contributions of the four component forces acting on the BMI's end effector.

2.5.2. Mapping the Neural Recordings to the ROLLS Neuromorphic Processor

The spike-based learning algorithm implemented on the chip is based on the model proposed in Brader et al. (2007). Using this model, feed-forward neural networks can learn to classify patterns based on their mean rates. However, in the neural data we recorded, the principal feature that distinguishes one class from the others is the precise timing of the recorded spikes, aligned to the offset of the sensory micro-stimulation (**Figure 1**). Therefore a transformation of the input spike sequence into an array of firing rates is required before it reaches the output layer. Furthermore, the number of non-redundant features in the data needs to be sufficiently high to support robust discrimination across all classes, but the recorded activity was very similar across all recording channels (see **Figure 1**, inset). Therefore it is likely impossible to find a single-layer feed-forward network configuration that can classify the recordings based on features corresponding directly to the recording channels.

To reconcile the characteristics of the data with the network requirements we mapped uncorrelated sub-samples of the spike sequence to different synapses of the classifier neuron, using a mean-rate encoding. Specifically, we binned the recorded spike trains in time bins of 1 ms (**Figure 5B**) and associated each bin with one input synapse of each neuron of the network (**Figure 5C**). We provided a 400 ms high mean-rate (100 Hz) Poisson spike train to the learning synapses for time bins that contained recorded spikes, and no input to the rest of the synapses (**Figure 5C**).

Under the constraint of a finite number (256) of available synapses per neuron, there was a trade-off among the number of recording channels, the duration of the recording patterns, and the temporal precision desired. The first 200–300 ms of each recorded pattern included significant differences across the four different classes (**Figure 1**), that would potentially be sufficient for the classifier to discriminate between them. Based on this, together with the observation that the distributions of spike timings were very similar across different recording channels, we merged the 15 recording channels into a single spike train, and we used the first 256 ms of the recordings, thus acquiring a temporal precision of one ms per time bin. Longer recording duration with a two-millisecond or lower precision was found to diminish decoding performance.

2.5.3. The Neural Network's Task

The aim of the BMI is to best approximate the desired force field over the duration of the experimental session, through weighting the four force components. To achieve this aim, there are two criteria based on which the decoder has to simultaneously optimize its learning. Firstly, it needs to learn to classify the patterns, i.e., to correctly output the single class to which each presented recording truly belongs, as expressed by the "winning" (i.e., the most firing) ensemble of output neurons. Secondly, the decoder also needs to prevent the other three "losing" ensembles from biasing the force field toward particular directions on average over the trajectory of the end effector. That is, it

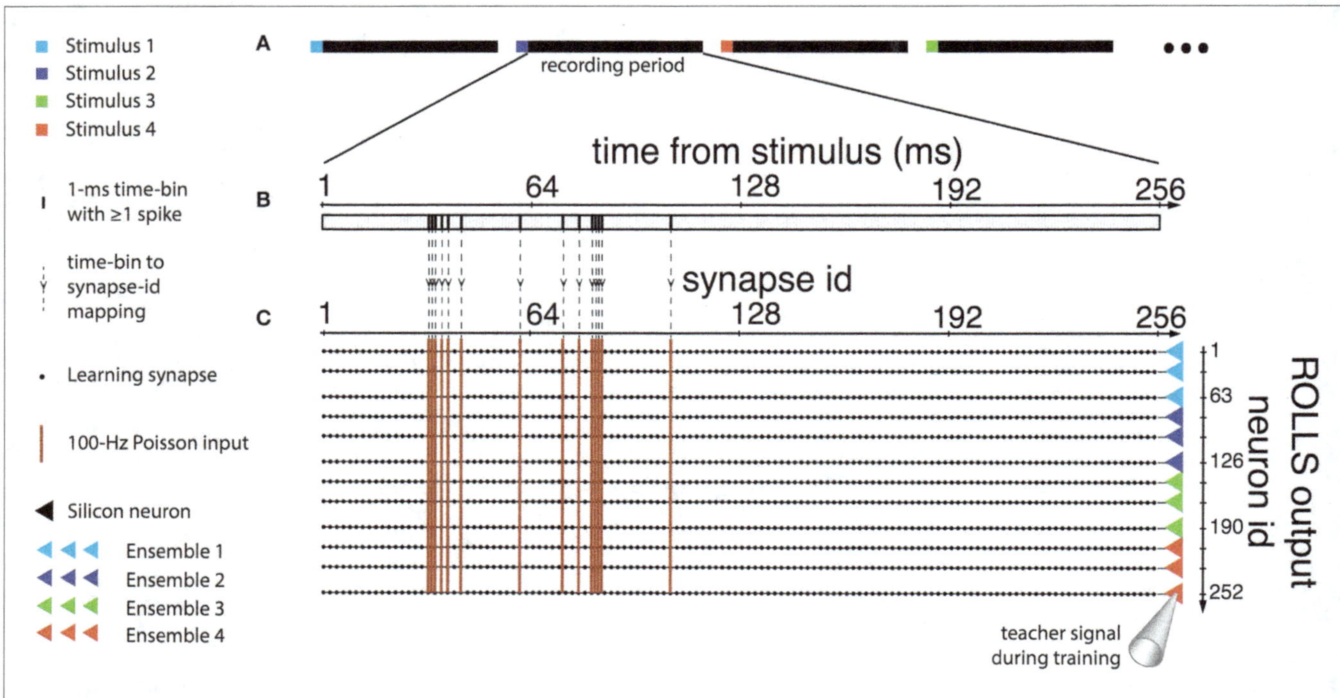

FIGURE 5 | Input, training, and use of the neuromorphic decoder. (A) To train the decoder, four different stimuli were provided to the rat's sensory cortex. Stimuli were provided in random order, 40 times each, and the activity in the motor cortex was recorded during the session. **(B)** The activity in the first 256 ms *after* the end of each stimulus was used with the decoder. The recording was binned in 1 ms time bins, and bins where at least one action potential was detected across any of the recording channels were marked. **(C)** Each time bin was mapped to a column of 252 learning synapses on the ROLLS, whereby each synapse belonged to a different post-synaptic neuron on the chip. Synapses corresponding to time bins in the recording that included detected spikes received a Poisson spike train with a mean rate of 100 Hz. Synapses corresponding to empty time bins received no input. In addition, the silicon neurons were stimulated by a teacher signal, as follows. The 252 post-synaptic neurons were separated in four ensembles of 63, and we associated each ensemble with one of the four stimuli provided to the rat's sensory cortex. During the presentation of each recording to the chip, the ensemble corresponding to the preceding cortical stimulus was stimulated by a Poisson spike train of 75 Hz as a teacher signal, while the other three neuronal ensembles received a teacher signal of 25 Hz. After training, the ROLLS received no teacher signal, and each recording was decoded into a force applied to the end effector, by weighting four force components by the number of spikes output by each of the four ensembles.

needs to classify the recordings under the constraint of learning to equalize the average outputs of "losing" ensembles. Thus, despite the similarities to a classifier, classification of individual recordings is only partly the decoder's task.

2.5.4. Biased Similarities and Differences between Classes of Recordings: Addressing Them with Heterosynaptic Competition

The decoder had to address certain additional characteristics of the recordings to achieve its goal of approximating the desired force field over the experiment's course. Specifically, different classes of recordings differed in number of recorded spikes on average, and this difference in the input energy could be reflected as a bias in the chip's output and consequently in the direction of the decoded force in each trial. Moreover, even though spike timing was the principal difference between recordings of different classes, some spike timings were common between classes. This increased the difficulty in distinguishing between different classes. That is, the different classes had a certain level of overlap between their features, which could increase classification errors. Additionally, this overlap was not of the same extent for all pairs of classes, i.e., some classes were more similar to some than to others in terms of common spike timings (**Figure 1**). This asymmetry could result in additional biases in the weighting of the force components by the decoder, thus misshaping the resulting force field in certain parts of the working space.

To address these points, we used the "stop learning" feature of the ROLLS chip learning circuits (see Brader et al., 2007) which prohibits potentiation of synapses when the post-synaptic firing rate exceeds a threshold. When a certain number of synapses that correspond to a neuron's positive class are potentiated, the increased excitation from the input causes the neuron to stop learning. This introduces heterosynaptic competition (Royer and Paré, 2003) to the chip's output neurons, which serves (a) to normalize the network's output in response to different classes, (b) to make potentiated synapses a scarce resource hence biasing potentiation toward non-overlapping features, and (c) to equalize the output of "losing" ensembles. In addition, combined with device mismatch on the neuromorphic circuits, it biases different members of each ensemble to learn a slightly different decision boundary. This is similar to boosting techniques employed in machine learning and improves the classification performance by allowing for non-linear decision boundaries for the ensemble through the aggregation of the multiple linear boundaries defined by the ensemble's member neurons.

2.5.5. Training the Neuromorphic Decoder

To train the neuromorphic decoder, we used an experimental session composed of 40 repetitions of each stimulation pattern (i.e., 160 evoked recordings). During the training procedure were randomly interleaved (**Figure 5A**) and presented to the ROLLS processor the 160 training trials, according to the method described in Section 2.5.2 (**Figures 5B,C**), along with a teacher signal representing the label of the presented example, i.e., the type of sensory microstimulation that produced the recorded neural response. Sixty-three output neurons were assigned to each class (**Figure 5C**, right). The teacher signal biased each neuron to be tuned to one class, by causing it to fire with a rate that maximized the probability that the neurons synapses got potentiated when an example of that class was presented, and depressed when an example of the other classes was presented. The mean rate of the Poisson spike train that would act as a teacher signal with these properties, as well as the analog parameters of the silicon neurons and synapses of the ROLLS processor were configured to match the characteristics of the input data with the requirements of the learning and of the decoding task.

2.6. Assessing the BMI's Performance

Once the decoding and encoding interfaces were properly calibrated, in order to test the system we ran the BMI by decoding from each neural trial a bidimensional force and by encoding each position of the controlled object through an ICMS pattern. We used a test dataset of neural recordings acquired by 10 repetitions of each of the four stimulation patterns (i.e., 40 evoked recordings), which were unseen by the BMI during its training. We selected eight different equispaced and equidistant positions as starting points in which the dynamical system was initialized and we ran the BMI 100 times starting from each initial position by obtaining 800 trajectories. We tested the system under two conditions: under normal operation (encoder-ON condition), each test recording was selected according to the dynamical system's current position. An alternate condition (encoder-OFF) was used to test the bidirectionality of the BMI and the learned coordination between the encoder and decoder modules. In the encoder-OFF condition, each test trial was randomly selected among all 40 test recordings.

To assess the repeatability, the speed and the optimality of the generated trajectories we measured the number of steps required to converge to the target and the mean *within-trajectory variance* (abbreviated to *wtv*). In particular, each trajectory's *wtv* is defined as $\sqrt{C_x^2 + C_y^2}$, where C_x and C_y is the covariance of the distribution of the per-step displacement along the x and the y axis, respectively. We obtained the mean *wtv* by averaging the *wtv* computed for each set of trajectories that started from one initial position.

3. RESULTS

3.1. Decoding Performance

To assess the decoder we used test datasets, which were previously unseen by the decoder, as described in Section 2.6. For each decoded pattern, the output spikes produced by each neuronal ensemble (**Figure 6A**) were counted. Given a stimulus, the average spike count of the ensemble of silicon neurons corresponding to that stimulus was higher than the other three (**Figure 6B**).

In addition, as a result of the introduction of "stop learning" to the silicon neurons average spike counts were relatively uniform across the other three ensembles despite the biases in pairwise similarities between input classes (see Section 2.5.4). The chip learned to suppress this bias, and, consequently, decoded resultant forces for each stimulus were, as originally intended, most similar to one of the four forces used during the calibration phase (colored thick arrows shown in **Figure 8B**).

While the task of the decoder was not a pure classification task and it was not optimized to perform as a classifier, we also evaluated its performance in correctly classifying the recordings, as expressed by the maximally firing ensemble of neurons. For 20 different random splits between the training and the test sets, the classification performance on the test set ranged between 50 and 70% correct, with the chance performance level being at 25%.

3.2. BMI Performance

In order to assess the BMI performance, we performed two different testing sessions: during the first session we set the maximum number of steps to 100 as stopping rule for the obtained trajectories (**Figure 7**). The BMI moved the object freely according to the sequence of forces that the closed-loop set-up applied and we placed the target as the origin of the axes. In each trial, the controlled object was initialized at one of eight starting positions and the BMI generated one trajectory of 100 encoding + decoding steps. We marked and plotted in the figure the point that was closest to the origin of the axes considered as the target point (**Figure 7A**). For each starting position we repeated the experiment 100 times, yielding 800 points in each of the two conditions (blue points for "Encoder ON" and red points for "Encoder OFF"). In condition ON, when a stimulus was provided to the sensory cortex, it was according to the current position of the object. In condition OFF, the stimulus was selected randomly among the four possible stimuli, thus not encoding the current position of the object. The distributions of the two sets of points (**Figure 7B**) are statistically different (independent samples t-test, $p < 0.001$) showing a decrease of 99% in the distance from the target and demonstrating that closing the loop in the proposed BMI is crucial in order to correctly drive the dynamical system toward a target.

In the second testing session, we simulated a real experiment in order to generate motor commands that drive a mobile cart from predefined initial positions toward a target position represented by a slot in the glass that allows the rat to get the reward (Boi et al., 2015b). In this session to distinguish between convergent and non-convergent trajectories, we defined the target as a circular region with radius set to 3.6 cm placed in the center of the workspace. A trial was considered successful as soon as the generated trajectory reached the borders of this area. When this happened the BMI was disconnected and the cart was automatically positioned in the center of the slot to allow the subject to receive the reward.

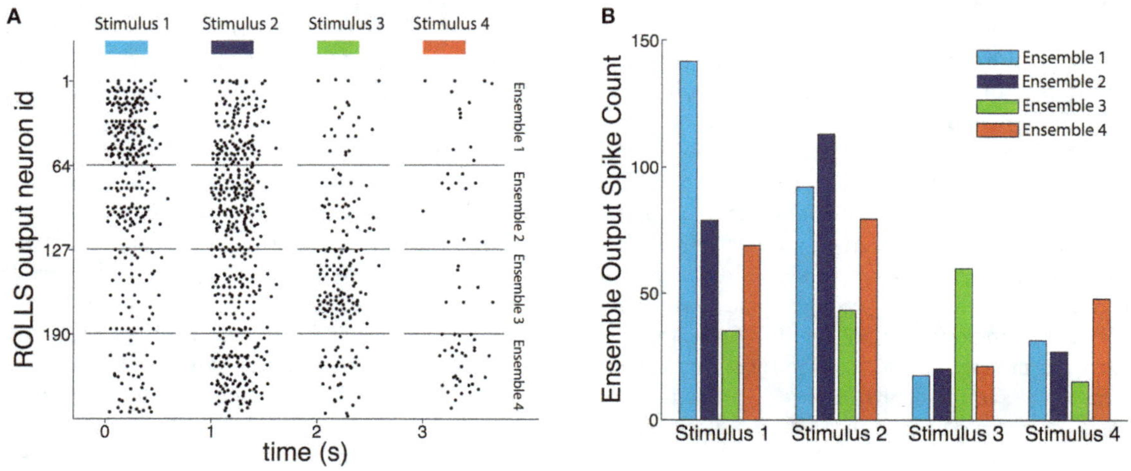

FIGURE 6 | Output of the trained decoder. (A) Raster plot of the output spikes of the trained ROLLS chip during presentation of four example test recordings each resulting from a different type of stimulus. The length of the bars on top shows the 400 ms long presentation of the input. During presentation of the four examples, the most active ensemble of output neurons corresponds to the true stimulus that caused the input recording. The spike count of the output each of the four neuronal ensembles was directly used to weight each of the four components of the force field to result in the motor command, i.e., force, that acted on the controlled object. The chip's neurons maintained some activity till shortly after the input stopped, mainly due to excitatory current leaking between the firing neuronal electronic circuits. **(B)** Average output spike count for each ensemble of neurons, for each type of stimulus that caused the decoded recording. For each stimulus, its corresponding ensemble fires on average more than the other three, demonstrating the classification aspect of the decoder's task. In addition, the decoder learned for each stimulus to partially equalize the response amplitudes of the three non-corresponding ensembles, compared to the extent of the differences between input classes (cf. **Figure 1** and see Section 3.1).

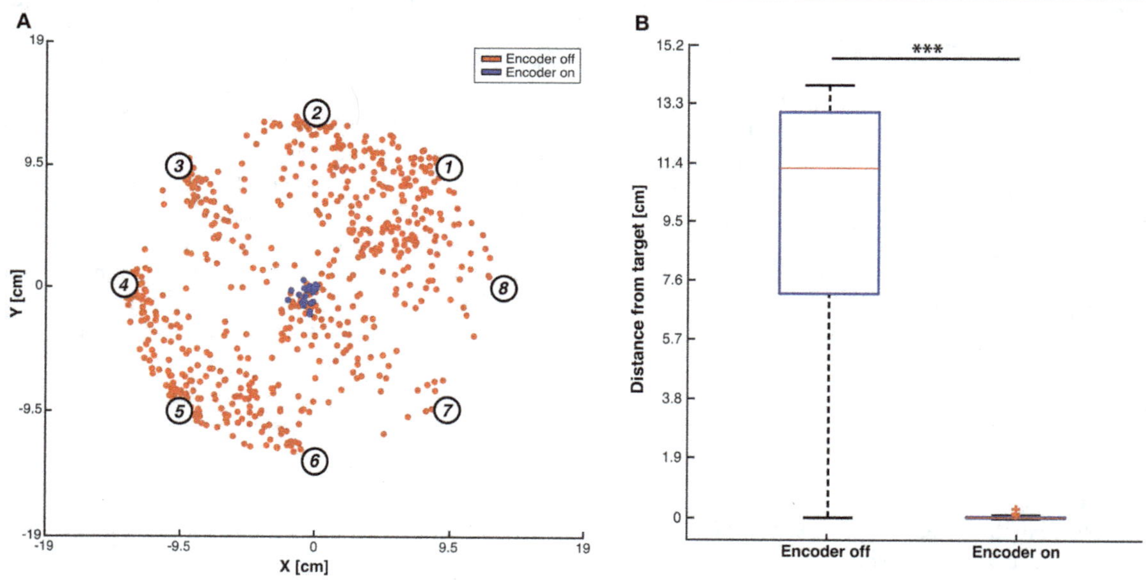

FIGURE 7 | Testing of BMI performance with 100-steps stopping rule. (A) Trajectories closest points to target. Red dots indicate, for each trajectory, the closest points to the workspace axis origin with the encoder switched OFF while blue dots represent the same points for the trajectories generated with the encoder ON. Data were collected by running the BMI 100 times for each of the eight predefined initial positions (i.e., numbered circles) both with the encoder turned ON and OFF. **(B)** Box plots of the trajectories closest points distributions with the encoder ON and OFF. Two-sample *t*-test, $^{***}p < 0.001$.

Figure 8A shows the mean trajectories (blue lines) and the covariance (light blue area) generated during this experimental session with the encoder turned ON. Two distinct behaviors are distinguishable (see Figure S1C): if the pathway from the starting position to the target region lies inside the same sensory region, we obtained an almost straight trajectory. On the other hand, when the controlled device crosses the border of one region, the systems oscillates along the border of the two adjacent region

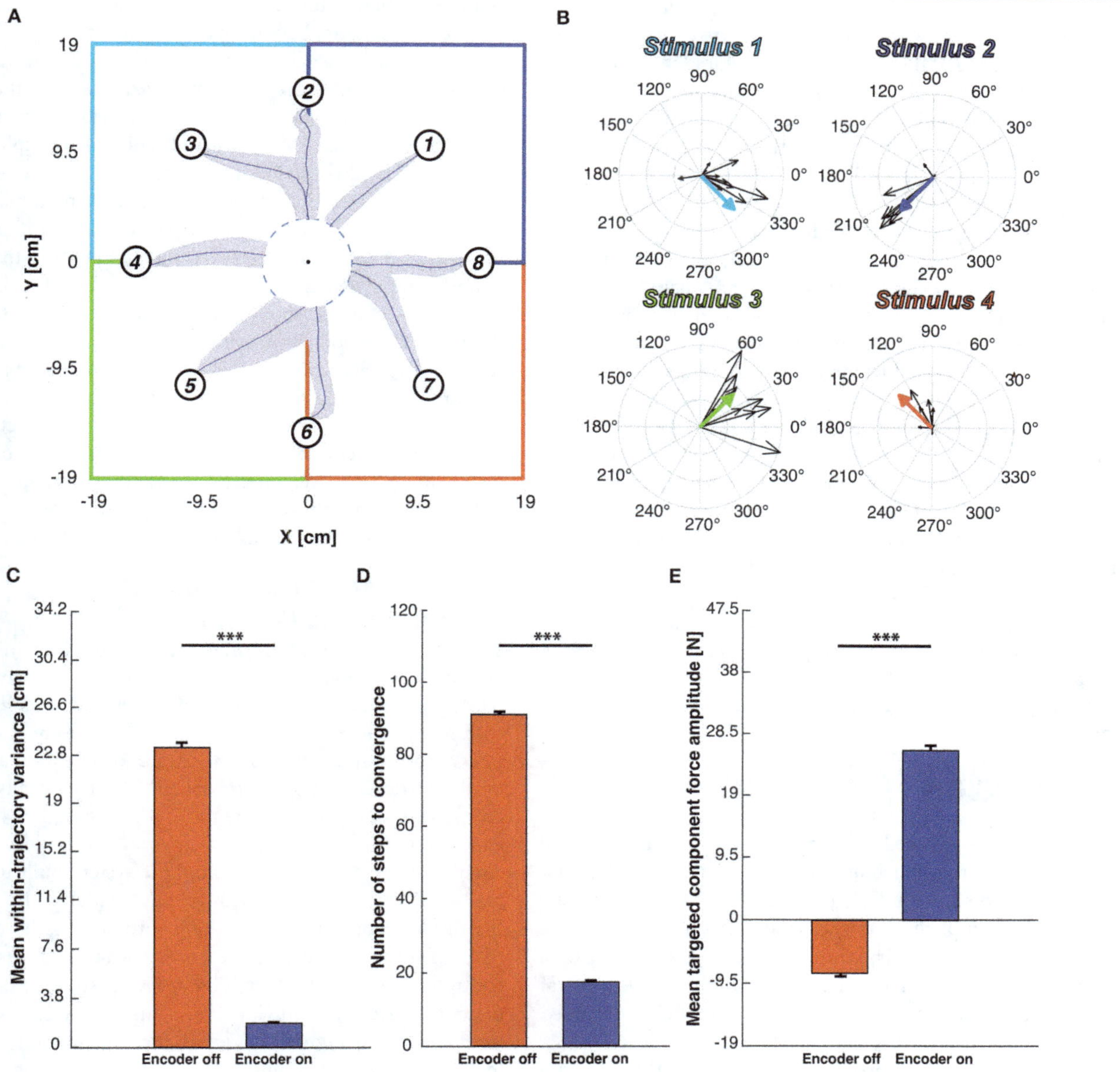

FIGURE 8 | Testing of BMI performance with target-region stopping rule. (A) Mean trajectories plot. Starting from each starting point depicted with a numbered circle, the blue lines represents the mean trajectories and light blue areas represent the covariance of the trajectories along 100 trials. The workspace is subdivided into four sensory regions, one per each stimulation, highlighted by four different colors. We defined a target region centered in the origin of the axes and whenever the mobile cart reaches its edge the BMI considers the task accomplished. **(B)** Black arrows represent the decoded forces computed during the BMI test phase. Colored thick arrows represent the four calibration forces associated to the sensory regions. Forces were grouped on the basis of the stimulus that generates them. **(C)** Mean *within-trajectory variance (wtv)* ± SEM of all the 800 trajectories recorded both with the encoder turned ON (blue bar) and OFF (red bar). **(D)** Mean number of steps to convergence ± SEM. The red bar, obtained with the encoder turned OFF, is quite close to the maximum step allowed (100 steps) while when the encoder is active the steps number necessary to reach the target region is significantly lower. **(E)** Mean *DT* component magnitude ± SEM. Each decoded force has been split into *Directed to the target - DT* (magnitude of the force that points toward the target) and *Orthogonal to the target - OT* one (part of the force perpendicular to the directive component). The mean magnitude of the DT component obtained from forces generated with the encoder turned off (red bar)is much higher than when the encoder activated (blue bar). Two sample *t*-test, $^{***}p < 0.001$.

'his particular behavior does not represent a decoding error ut rather reflects the limitation of having only four different timulation patterns encoding the information about the region 1 which the device is, disregarding the precise position inside : (Tehovnik, 1996; Romo et al., 1998). The BMI converges to 1e target region with a 100% success, and it does so in a very stable and straight path because the decoded forces obtained in response to the same stimulation pattern are very similar to each other, both in terms of direction and magnitude. This is demonstrated in the compass plots in **Figure 8B** showing that the forces decoded from the neural activity evoked from each stimulation pattern and used during the testing phase (i.e., black arrows) are almost overlapping. In order to further assess the neuromorphic decoding capabilities we also report the forces used to calibrate the BMI motor interface (colored thick arrows in **Figure 8B**) that, especially in terms of direction, are almost equal to most of the related forces decoded during the BMI run. In the encoder-ON case the mean *wtv* and the steps needed to reach the target region significantly decrease (respectively, 92 and 80%) with respect to the encoder-OFF case (**Figures 8C,D**).

Finally, for each force produced by the decoding process, we measured the magnitude of two components: the component of the force that points toward the target point, named *Directed to the target—DT*, and the component orthogonal to it, named *Orthogonal to the target—OT*. The mean of the DT-component is strongly positive (directed to the target) in the case of encoder-ON and slightly negative (divergent from the target) when the encoder is turned OFF (**Figure 8E** shows an increase of 69%). In both conditions (ON and OFF), the mean OT-components are almost null compared to the mean *DT* obtained with the encoder-ON (respectively, 90 and 97% less). In the OFF condition, this can be attributed to the randomness of the motion. In the ON condition, combined with the increased DT force, this is an indication of successful decoding.

Figures S1A,B show the complete set of trajectories collected without using the target-region stopping rule, respectively, with the encoder switched ON and OFF. Figures S1C,D shows the set of trajectories used to build the different panels of **Figure 8**.

4. DISCUSSION

In this paper, we showed the applicability of neuromorphic hardware in a brain-machine interface system, in the first demonstration of this kind. In particular, the decoder module of the BMI was implemented by a spiking neural network on a mixed-signal analog/digital neuromorphic processor, the ROLLS, that learned to perform on-line the decoding of the neural recordings into commands that addressed the brain-controlled device.

The analog neuromorphic circuits of the ROLLS neuromorphic processor emulate functions of biological neurons and synapses by replacing biophysical properties with analogous properties of the sub-threshold physics of transistors. The resulting spiking neural networks operate on a power-efficient and compact system for applications of pattern recognition such as a BMI decoder's task. On the other hand, because of these underlying principles of operation, analog neuromorphic circuits like the ones found on the ROLLS are imprecise and variable, similar to biological neural elements, in sharp contrast to simulations of spiking neurons and synapses on digital neuromorphic or general-purpose processors. The neuromorphic decoding task was further complicated by the variability in the recorded data, and by the overlap in spike-timings between the to-be-discriminated classes.

Further difficulty arose by the fact that the decoder's task was not a standard classification task, as the BMI required the decoder to output a contribution of all potential classes of recorded activity simultaneously, while preventing the average chip output from being biased toward any pair of classes, even though the pair-wise similarities between classes were biased.

Despite these particularities, the spiking network we designed successfully learned the decoding task, enabling the BMI to perform at similar levels of a previous non-neuromorphic version of the bidirectional BMI. This was achieved by exploiting two key characteristics of the ROLLS chip: variability between silicon synapses and neurons deployed into an ensemble learning technique that aggregated multiple weak classifiers into a powerful one, and the heterosynaptic competition through the "stop-learning" feature of synapses on the ROLLS chip, which enabled the network to focus on the discriminative features of the input, thus both improving classification performance and reducing the reflection of biased similarities in the input onto the output of the trained network. A key feature of the decoder is that the spiking output of the neuromorphic chip is directly used to compute the force controlling the end-effector. The components of the force were weighted by the spike counts of the chip's output, an important step toward using neuromorphic hardware not only as a decoder, but also as prosthetic controller.

4.1. Features of the Proposed Neuromorphic Decoder

The set-up we propose has been designed as an initial proof of concept prototype to evaluate the potential of neuromorphic hardware computing in BMIs, and to determine its limitations; within this context, this work shows that, even at this level, integration of neuromorphic hardware in set-ups characterized by the intricacy of a bidirectional BMI is technically possible. Our results show that, despite the low precision, low resolution, and noisy (but compact and low-power) analog electronic circuits in the neuromorphic chip, the system built in this way can recognize multi-dimensional input patterns. In particular, the results demonstrate how this neuromorphic hardware can be configured to produce the correct average forces over the controlled object's trajectory (**Figure 8A**), despite the fact that the forces decoded from individual recordings could strongly deviate from the target (**Figure 8B**) due to the contributions of all four force components combined with unbalanced inputs (**Figure 1**). A unique aspect of the specific neuromorphic hardware used is represented by its ability to learn these computationally demanding tasks, with on-chip real-time spike-based plasticity circuits, as opposed to learning the network parameters off-line and configuring them at run-time. The flexibility provided by the digital event-based communication infrastructure, and the digital registers embedded in the chip, next to the subthreshold analog neuromorphic circuits, allow this system to be used in a variety of tasks that require real-time decoding or classification of sensory inputs, or real-time encoding of desired outputs. Although, the analog circuits have time constants of the order of millisecond (in order to provide biological realism, and importantly, to minimize power consumption), the real-time response properties of the chip at network level have latencies that are extremely small (e.g., below tens of microseconds). This allows the chip to decode the neural activity on line in the BMI's loop, within one time step of the dynamical system's operation, whose bottleneck is determined not by the decoder, but by the inter-stimulus interval

The average power consumption of the chip, which has been measured to be approximately 4 mW, is competitive with state-of-the-art DSPs and much lower of general purpose low-power computing units that could be used to run the pattern recognition software. It is worth noting however, that since in the current set-up the neuromorphic chip is interfaced to additional devices mainly used for prototyping and debugging, the overall system requires additional relatively high power and area.

4.2. Limitations of the System and Proposed Future Additions

The simplicity of the single-layer feed-forward network of only 252 neurons that was employed for this particular application demonstrates the limitations and computational power of physical instantiations of spiking neural networks and suggests that further development of analog neuromorphic hardware and spike-based algorithms may yield a computationally powerful, yet low-power consuming alternative to software and conventional processors for a broad spectrum of tasks. With respect to the neuromorphic BMI decoder in particular, further work could enable two specific improvements and additions.

Firstly, the present implementation addresses the complex temporal dynamics of the recordings with a processing step introduced between the neural recording and the output layer of the neural network, and performed off-chip, which transforms the temporal dynamics of the recordings to a spatial pattern input to the chip. While the method proposed is suitable for the presented system, we have been investigating alternative algorithms and spiking neural network architectures that can potentially decode and recognize these types of spatio-temporal patterns entirely on the chip. In this way, the chip could directly receive the recorded spike train, and operate on it with no need for an intermediate off-chip storage step. This would be possible because of the ROLLS' real-time operation, with time constants that match those of real neurons. To this direction, Corradi and Indiveri (2015) perform a binary classification task on spatio-temporal recordings from the zebra finch, using reservoir computing on the ROLLS' silicon neurons, which demonstrates that future development of these types of methods can permit their application on a BMI.

On a separate but related note, here the BMI operated in discrete time steps. This permitted us to insert the processing step that inputs the recorded spike timings as rate-coded patterns into the ROLLS chip, without loss the system's continuity. Nonetheless, this will be a crucial obstacle for the decoding module's integration in future continuously operating BMIs. On the other hand, the limitation does not originate in the ROLLS chip itself. The chip does not have an internal clock that must be synchronized with the chosen time points. It rather recognizes inputs in which time represents itself in the spike train's statistics. This implies that removing any off-chip transformation that intermediates the input would also enable the on-line use of the chip in continuous-time BMI set-ups.

As a further future improvement, the fact that the network learns on line could be used to allow the decoder to adapt to changes in the neural responses with time. Specifically, in the current implementation, the decoder updates itself incrementally after the presentation of each training pattern. Training inputs are combined with a teacher signal that biases different neurons to strengthen or weaken their connections to different features of the input, through imposing different levels of output firing during the presentation of different input classes. After training, we use the chip to decode new recordings of brain activity. The on-line learning feature is not crucial for demonstrating the performance of the BMI in its current instantiation, but can become useful in future chronically implanted setups, that have to adapt to continuous slow changes in the nature of the signals being recorded. In such a future implementation, learning could continue during the chip's use as a trained decoder. As the trained silicon neurons respond with high firing rates to their corresponding input classes, and with lower rates to the other classes, the neurons could bias themselves to continue correctly adapting their synapses to the input patterns in the absence of an externally provided teacher signal. This would be made possible after tuning the parameters of STDP synaptic dynamics of the ROLLS to enable potentiation and depression in the ranges of firing rate that the trained neurons output when decoding the input.

4.3. BMI Modularity

As technological and scientific progress accelerates, it brings new opportunities for improving the quality of life of millions of people. The interdisciplinary field of brain-machine interfaces largely relies on the rapid evolution in the diverse fields that are involved (Nicolas-Alonso and Gomez-Gil, 2012). Nevertheless, the complexity of BMI systems, the interdependence of their components cause them to be very difficult to manage, test, modify, and upgrade. Our work suggests a possible solution to this issue by proposing a new modular implementation that allows to modify or update each module without changing the entire system.

The modularity allows to develop different parts of the BMI in different labs and assemble the complete system by plugging in these parts as modules. This structure makes easier and more reliable both the implementation of the single module and its integration in the complete system. Parallel development of components could also accelerate the ultimate realization of a device compact and powerful enough to be used as clinical tool able to transfer data between the brain and external devices wirelessly through an implanted interface (Azin et al., 2011; Fan et al., 2011; Borton et al., 2013; Angotzi et al., 2014). In this work, we also demonstrated that the modular architecture does not affect BMI performances, showing results comparable with the ones achieved in Vato et al. (2012); this result suggests that BMI systems developed in other labs could also be re-implemented in a modular manner. To help the interested scientist in doing this, most of the material used in this project is freely available on Si-Code website : http://www.sicode.eu/results/software.

5. CONCLUSIONS

The relevance of neuromorphic technology in the design of brain-machine interfaces is demonstrated by the flourishing work in this domain (see Dethier et al., 2013; Barsakcioglu et al., 2014; Hogri et al., 2015, as non-exhaustive examples). The main features of neuromorphic implementations are low power consumption, real-time operation, adaptability, and compactness. Simulations show that hardware Spiking Neural Networks can successfully decode the activity of neurons for closed-loop cortical implants (Dethier et al., 2013) and an ad-hoc working prototype is able to substitute a cerebellar learning function in the rat (Hogri et al., 2015). Our work extends this approach in proposing a modular and reconfigurable scheme whereby the neuromorphic chip can be exploited for implementing different algorithms and BMI functions; in particular, we demonstrated this approach by using the chip as neural decoder. We also explored the impact of using a neuromorphic decoder in such a closed-loop system by comparing its performance with the one previously developed in our lab.

As in Vato et al. (2012), we closed the loop with the brain by decoding the neural activity evoked by different patterns of intracortical micro-stimulation selected by the encoder. Even if we are not decoding from the anesthetized subjects any volitional input, this system, establishing a bidirectional interaction between the brain and an external device, needs to be considered the first necessary step toward the design of future experiments involving behaving subjects controlling the movements of a small mobile cart connected to a water or food dispenser (Boi et al., 2015b). The unique characteristics of the neuromorphic decoder will allow our modular bidirectional BMI to integrate the volitional component of brain activity in the decoding scheme and to explore the integration of the volitional input with the automatic brain response in controlling the movement of the external device.

AUTHOR CONTRIBUTIONS

FB, VD, FD, and CB designed, built, and debugged the hardware and software infrastructure for the mbBMI. TM and GI implemented the spike-based learning and decoding algorithm on the ROLLS neuromorphic processor. FB and AV performed the experiments and collected the neural data. FB, VD, and TM performed all the analysis presented in the paper. All the authors contributed in writing and editing the manuscript.

ACKNOWLEDGMENTS

Research supported by the EU Future & Emerging Technologies (FET) program under Grant "SI-CODE" (284553), the EU ERC Grant neuroP (257219), and the Samsung Advanced Institute of Technology (SAIT)s Global Research Outreach (GRO) Program.

REFERENCES

Angotzi, G. N., Boi, F., Zordan, S., Bonfanti, A., and Vato, A. (2014). A programmable closed-loop recording and stimulating wireless system for behaving small laboratory animals. *Sci. Rep.* 4:5963. doi: 10.1038/srep05963

Azin, M., Guggenmos, D. J., Barbay, S., Nudo, R. J., and Mohseni, P. (2011). A battery-powered activity-dependent intracortical microstimulation ic for brain-machine-brain interface. *IEEE J. Solid State Circ.* 46, 731–745. doi: 10.1109/JSSC.2011.2108770

Baranauskas, G. (2014). What limits the performance of current invasive brain machine interfaces? *Front. Syst. Neurosci.* 8:68. doi: 10.3389/fnsys.2014.00068

Barsakcioglu, D. Y., Liu, Y., Bhunjun, P., Navajas, J., Eftekhar, A., Jackson, A., et al. (2014). An analogue front-end model for developing neural spike sorting systems. *IEEE Trans. Biomed. Circ. Syst.* 8, 216–227. doi: 10.1109/TBCAS.2014.2313087

Bartolozzi, C., and Indiveri, G. (2009). Selective attention in multi-chip address-event systems. *Sensors* 9, 5076–5098. doi: 10.3390/s90705076

Bizzi, E., Mussa-Ivaldi, F. A., and Giszter, S. (1991). Computations underlying the execution of movement: a biological perspective. *Science* 253, 287–291.

Boahen, K. A. (2000). Point-to-point connectivity between neuromorphic chips using address events. *IEEE Trans. Circ. Syst. II Analog Digit. Signal Process.* 47, 416–434. doi: 10.1109/82.842110

Boahen, K. A. (2004). A burst-mode word-serial address-event link-i: transmitter design. *IEEE Trans. Circ. Syst. Regular Pap.* 51, 1269–1280. doi: 10.1109/TCSI.2004.830703

Boi, F., Diotalevi, F., Stefanini, F., Indiveri, G., Bartolozzi, C., and Vato, A. (2015a). "A modular configurable system for closed-loop bidirectional brain-machine interfaces," in *7th International IEEE/EMBS Conference on Neural Engineering (NER)* (Montpellier: IEEE), 198–201.

Boi, F., Semprini, M., Ivaldi, F. A. M., Panzeri, S., and Vato, A. (2015b). "A bidirectional brain-machine interface connecting alert rodents to a dynamical system," in *37th Annual International Conference of the IEEE Engineering in Medicine and Biology Society (EMBC)* (Milan: IEEE), 51–54.

Borton, D. A., Yin, M., Aceros, J., and Nurmikko, A. (2013). An implantable wireless neural interface for recording cortical circuit dynamics in moving primates. *J. Neural Eng.* 10:026010. doi: 10.1088/1741-2560/10/2/026010

Bouton, C. E., Shaikhouni, A., Annetta, N. V., Bockbrader, M. A., Friedenberg, D. A., Nielson, D. M., et al. (2016). Restoring cortical control of functional movement in a human with quadriplegia. *Nature* 533, 247–250. doi: 10.1038/nature17435

Brader, J. M., Senn, W., and Fusi, S. (2007). Learning real-world stimuli in a neural network with spike-driven synaptic dynamics. *Neural Comput.* 19, 2881–2912. doi: 10.1162/neco.2007.19.11.2881

Butovas, S., and Schwarz, C. (2007). Detection psychophysics of intracortical microstimulation in rat primary somatosensory cortex. *Eur. J. Neurosci.* 25, 2161–2169. doi: 10.1111/j.1460-9568.2007.05449.x

Chan, V., Liu, S.-C., and van Schaik, A. (2007). Aer ear: a matched silicon cochle pair with address event representation interface. *IEEE Trans. Circ. Syst. Regular Pap.* 54, 48–59. doi: 10.1109/TCSI.2006.887979

Chicca, E., Stefanini, F., Bartolozzi, C., and Indiveri, G. (2014). Neuromorphic electronic circuits for building autonomous cognitive systems. *Proc. IEEE* 10[illegible], 1367–1388. doi: 10.1109/JPROC.2014.2313954

Corradi, F., and Indiveri, G. (2015). A neuromorphic event-based neural recording system for smart brain-machine-interfaces. *IEEE Trans. Biomed. Circ. Syst.* [illegible], 699–709. doi: 10.1109/TBCAS.2015.2479256

Dangi, S., Gowda, S., Héliot, R., and Carmena, J. M. (2011). "Adaptive kalman filtering for closed-loop brain-machine interface systems," in *5th International IEEE/EMBS Conference on Neural Engineering (NER)* (Cancun: IEEE), 609–612.

Delbruck, T., and Lichtsteiner, P. (2006). "Fully programmable bias current generator with 24 bit resolution per bias," in *2006 IEEE International Symposium on Circuits and Systems* (Kos: IEEE), 4.

Dethier, J., Nuyujukian, P., Ryu, S. I., Shenoy, K. V., and Boahen, K. (2013). Design and validation of a real-time spiking-neural-network decoder for brain–machine interfaces. *J. Neural Eng.* 10:036008. doi: 10.1088/1741-2560/10/3/036008

Fan, D., Rich, D., Holtzman, T., Ruther, P., Dalley, J. W., Lopez, A., et al. (2011). A wireless multi-channel recording system for freely behaving mice and rats. *PLoS ONE* 6:e22033. doi: 10.1371/journal.pone.0022033

Hochberg, L. R., Bacher, D., Jarosiewicz, B., Masse, N. Y., Simeral, J. D., Vogel, J., et al. (2012). Reach and grasp by people with tetraplegia using a neurally controlled robotic arm. *Nature* 485, 372–375. doi: 10.1038/nature11076

Hogri, R., Bamford, S. A., Taub, A. H., Magal, A., Del Giudice, P., and Mintz, M. (2015). A neuro-inspired model-based closed-loop neuroprosthesis for the substitution of a cerebellar learning function in anesthetized rats. *Sci. Rep.* 5:8451. doi: 10.1038/srep08451

Lebedev, M. A., and Nicolelis, M. A. (2006). Brain–machine interfaces: past, present and future. *Trends Neurosci.* 29, 536–546. doi: 10.1016/j.tins.2006.07.004

Lemay, M. A., and Grill, W. M. (2004). Modularity of motor output evoked by intraspinal microstimulation in cats. *J. Neurophysiol.* 91, 502–514. doi: 10.1152/jn.00235.2003

Leuthardt, E. C., Schalk, G., Moran, D., and Ojemann, J. G. (2006). The emerging world of motor neuroprosthetics: a neurosurgical perspective. *Neurosurgery* 59, 1–14. doi: 10.1227/01.NEU.0000221506.06947.AC

Lichtsteiner, P., Posch, C., and Delbruck, T. (2008). A 128× 128 120 db 15 μs latency asynchronous temporal contrast vision sensor. *IEEE J. Solid State Circ.* 43, 566–576. doi: 10.1109/JSSC.2007.914337

Mao, T., Kusefoglu, D., Hooks, B. M., Huber, D., Petreanu, L., and Svoboda, K. (2011). Long-range neuronal circuits underlying the interaction between sensory and motor cortex. *Neuron* 72, 111–123. doi: 10.1016/j.neuron.2011.07.029

Mitra, S., Fusi, S., and Indiveri, G. (2009). Real-time classification of complex patterns using spike-based learning in neuromorphic VLSI. *IEEE Trans. Biomed. Circ. Syst.* 3, 32–42. doi: 10.1109/TBCAS.2008.2005781

Mortara, A. (1998). "A pulsed communication/computation framework for analog VLSI perceptive systems," in *Neuromorphic Systems Engineering*, ed T. S. Lande (Boston, MA: Kluwer Academic Publishers), 201–215.

Mostafa, H., Corradi, F., Stefanini, F., and Indiveri, G. (2014). "A hybrid analog/digital spike-timing dependent plasticity learning circuit for neuromorphic VLSI multi-neuron architectures," in *IEEE International Symposium on Circuits and Systems (ISCAS)* (Melbourne: IEEE), 854–857.

Nicolas-Alonso, L. F., and Gomez-Gil, J. (2012). Brain computer interfaces, a review. *Sensors* 12, 1211–1279. doi: 10.3390/s120201211

Orsborn, A. L., Moorman, H. G., Overduin, S. A., Shanechi, M. M., Dimitrov, D. F., and Carmena, J. M. (2014). Closed-loop decoder adaptation shapes neural plasticity for skillful neuroprosthetic control. *Neuron* 82, 1380–1393. doi: 10.1016/j.neuron.2014.04.048

Posch, C., Matolin, D., and Wohlgenannt, R. (2010). "A QVGA 143db dynamic range asynchronous address-event pwm dynamic image sensor with lossless pixel-level video compression," in *IEEE International Solid-State Circuits Conference-(ISSCC)* (San Francisco, CA: IEEE), 400–401.

Qiao, N., Mostafa, H., Corradi, F., Osswald, M., Stefanini, F., Sumislawska, D., et al. (2015). A reconfigurable on-line learning spiking neuromorphic processor comprising 256 neurons and 128k synapses. *Front. Neurosci.* 9:141. doi: 10.3389/fnins.2015.00141

Romo, R., Hernández, A., Zainos, A., and Salinas, E. (1998). Somatosensory discrimination based on cortical microstimulation. *Nature* 392, 387–390.

Royer, S. and Paré, D. (2003). Conservation of total synaptic weight through balanced synaptic depression and potentiation. *Nature* 422, 518–522. doi: 10.1038/nature01530

Semprini, M., Bennicelli, L., and Vato, A. (2012). "A parametric study of intracortical microstimulation in behaving rats for the development of artificial sensory channels," in *2012 Annual International Conference of the IEEE Engineering in Medicine and Biology Society* (San Diego, CA), 799–802.

Stefanini, F., Neftci, E. O., Sheik, S., and Indiveri, G. (2014). Pyncs: a microkernel for high-level definition and configuration of neuromorphic electronic systems. *Front. Neuroinform.* 8:73. doi: 10.3389/fninf.2014.00073

Szymanski, F. D., Semprini, M., Mussa-Ivaldi, F. A., Fadiga, L., Panzeri, S., and Vato, A. (2011). "Dynamic brain-machine interface: a novel paradigm for bidirectional interaction between brains and dynamical systems," in *2011 Annual International Conference of the IEEE Engineering in Medicine and Biology Society* (Boston, MA: IEEE), 4592–4595.

Tehovnik, E. J. (1996). Electrical stimulation of neural tissue to evoke behavioral responses. *J. Neurosci. Methods* 65, 1–17.

Tresch, M. C., and Bizzi, E. (1999). Responses to spinal microstimulation in the chronically spinalized rat and their relationship to spinal systems activated by low threshold cutaneous stimulation. *Exp. Brain Res.* 129, 401–416.

Vato, A., Semprini, M., Maggiolini, E., Szymanski, F. D., Fadiga, L., Panzeri, S., et al. (2012). Shaping the dynamics of a bidirectional neural interface. *PLoS Comput. Biol.* 8:e1002578. doi: 10.1371/journal.pcbi.1002578

Vato, A., Szymanski, F. D., Semprini, M., Mussa-Ivaldi, F. A., and Panzeri, S. (2014). A bidirectional brain-machine interface algorithm that approximates arbitrary force-fields. *PLoS ONE* 9:e91677. doi: 10.1371/journal.pone.0091677

Wander, J. D., and Rao, R. P. (2014). Brain–computer interfaces: a powerful tool for scientific inquiry. *Curr. Opin. Neurobiol.* 25, 70–75. doi: 10.1016/j.conb.2013.11.013

Wolpaw, J. R., Birbaumer, N., Heetderks, W. J., McFarland, D. J., Peckham, P. H., Schalk, G., et al. (2000). Brain-computer interface technology: a review of the first international meeting. *IEEE Trans. Rehab. Eng.* 8, 164–173. doi: 10.1109/TRE.2000.847807

15

A Personalized Multi-Channel FES Controller Based on Muscle Synergies to Support Gait Rehabilitation after Stroke

Simona Ferrante [1*†], *Noelia Chia Bejarano* [1†], *Emilia Ambrosini* [1,2], *Antonio Nardone* [3,4], *Anna M. Turcato* [3,4], *Marco Monticone* [2,5], *Giancarlo Ferrigno* [1] and *Alessandra Pedrocchi* [1]

[1] Neuroengineering and Medical Robotics Laboratory, Department of Electronics, Information and Bioengineering, Politecnico di Milano, Milan, Italy, [2] Physical Medicine and Rehabilitation Unit, Scientific Institute of Lissone, Fondazione Salvatore Maugeri (IRCCS), Lissone, Monza Brianza, Italy, [3] Posture and Movement Laboratory, Division of Physical Medicine and Rehabilitation, Scientific Institute of Veruno, Fondazione Salvatore Maugeri (IRCCS), Veruno, Novara, Italy, [4] Department of Translational Medicine, University of Eastern Piedmont, Novara, Italy, [5] Department of Public Health, Clinical and Molecular Medicine, University of Cagliari, Cagliari, Italy

Edited by:
Paolo Massobrio, University of Genoa, Italy

Reviewed by:
Erika G. Spaich, Aalborg University, Denmark
Marco Knaflitz, Polytechnic University of Turin, Italy

***Correspondence:**
Simona Ferrante
simona.ferrante@polimi.it

†*Co-first authors.*

It has been largely suggested in neuroscience literature that to generate a vast variety of movements, the Central Nervous System (CNS) recruits a reduced set of coordinated patterns of muscle activities, defined as muscle synergies. Recent neurophysiological studies have recommended the analysis of muscle synergies to finely assess the patient's impairment, to design personalized interventions based on the specific nature of the impairment, and to evaluate the treatment outcomes. In this scope, the aim of this study was to design a personalized multi-channel functional electrical stimulation (FES) controller for gait training, integrating three novel aspects: (1) the FES strategy was based on healthy muscle synergies in order to mimic the neural solutions adopted by the CNS to generate locomotion; (2) the FES strategy was personalized according to an initial locomotion assessment of the patient and was designed to specifically activate the impaired biomechanical functions; (3) the FES strategy was mapped accurately on the altered gait kinematics providing a maximal synchronization between patient's volitional gait and stimulation patterns. The novel intervention was tested on two chronic stroke patients. They underwent a 4-week intervention consisting of 30-min sessions of FES-supported treadmill walking three times per week. The two patients were characterized by a mild gait disability (walking speed > 0.8 m/s) at baseline. However, before treatment both patients presented only three independent muscle synergies during locomotion resembling two different gait abnormalities. After treatment, the number of extracted synergies became four and they increased their resemblance with the physiological muscle synergies, which indicated a general improvement in muscle coordination. The originally merged synergies seemed to regain their distinct role in locomotion control. The treatment benefits were more evident for one patient, who achieved a clinically important change in dynamic balance (Mini-Best Test increased from 17 to 22) coupled with a very positive perceived treatment effect (GRC = 4). The treatment had started the neuro-motor relearning process also on the second subject, but twelve sessions were not enough to achieve clinically relevant improvements. This attempt to apply the novel theories of neuroscience research in stroke rehabilitation has provided promising results, and deserves to be further investigated in a larger clinical study.

Keywords: functional electrical stimulation, stroke rehabilitation, locomotion, treadmill, muscle synergies

INTRODUCTION

The rehabilitation of neurological patients strongly benefits of task-oriented, immersive, repetitive exercises when the patient experiences an enriched, augmented sensorial feedback. Indeed, such interventions stimulate the activity-dependent plasticity of the Central Nervous System (CNS) thus facilitating motor relearning (Ting et al., 2015). Activity-dependent plasticity is further enhanced when Functional Electrical Stimulation (FES) is synchronized with task-oriented volitional exercises (Sheffler and Chae, 2007; Chae et al., 2008; Gandolla et al., 2014, 2016; Kafri and Laufer, 2015), such as cycling (Ferrante et al., 2008; Ambrosini et al., 2011, 2012) and walking (Kesar et al., 2009; Embrey et al., 2010; Sabut et al., 2010, 2011; Daly et al., 2011; Kim et al., 2012). Indeed, the increased afferent feedback provided by FES modulates motor cortex function and excitability to facilitate recovery (Ridding et al., 2000; Gandolla et al., 2014, 2016).

The first FES-based gait systems were designed for the treatment of foot drop, combining single-channel stimulation of the peroneal nerve with a pressure sensor to detect the initial contact of the foot with the ground (Melo et al., 2015). Since then, multi-channel FES strategies have been proposed and tested in stroke patients (Kesar et al., 2009; Ambrosini et al., 2010; Embrey et al., 2010; Sabut et al., 2010, 2011; Daly et al., 2011; Kim et al., 2012). However, in all FES-based gait systems, only the two main gait phases (i.e., the stance and swing phase) were detected and used to trigger the stimulation of the different muscles involved in the movement. The stimulation waveforms were mainly trapezoidal (Melo et al., 2015). These waveforms use a ramp up of stimulation amplitude at a constant pulse width to avoid sudden and jerky muscle responses both in the agonist and antagonist muscles, and a ramp down to avoid a sudden and unpleasant slap of the foot on the ground. Biomimetic stimulation controllers, which modulate the stimulation amplitude based on physiological EMG activations, were proposed for a single-channel drop-foot stimulator and were tested on a single patient, resulting to be more efficient than trapezoidal profiles (O'Keeffe et al., 2003). Biomimetic multi-channel FES systems have shown promising therapeutic benefits when applied in stroke patients during cycling (Ferrante et al., 2008; Ambrosini et al., 2011, 2012). However, to the authors' knowledge, a biomimetic multi-channel FES system has not yet been proposed and tested during gait.

To design a biomimetic FES controller, it is essential to mimic the neural solutions adopted by the CNS to generate movements. It has been largely suggested in neuroscience literature that in order to generate a vast variety of movements, the CNS recruits a reduced set of coordinated patterns of muscle activities, defined as muscle synergies or motor modules (d'Avella et al., 2003; d'Avella and Bizzi, 2005). Further, a study on spinalized rats has provided experimental evidence that the CNS simplifies the complexity and high dimensionality of neural commands and mechanical outputs by means of a modular organization at the neuromuscular level (Mussa-Ivaldi and Bizzi, 2000).

The concept of muscle synergy has been formalized with a mathematical model based on factorization algorithms that decompose the EMG signals into the product of two components. The weighting component reveals the muscle composition of each synergy and the relative level of activation of each muscle, whereas the temporal component reflects the activation timing of each synergy throughout the execution of the movement. Each muscle synergy contributes to the mechanical output needed to generate task-specific biomechanical functions, also called biomechanical correlates (Lacquaniti et al., 2012). Many studies on physiological gait have agreed in the definition of four synergies as responsible of the main biomechanical correlates on healthy subjects (Clark et al., 2010; Barroso et al., 2014; Routson et al., 2014):

Synergy 1 (weight acceptance): activation of the hip and knee extensors during early stance that is associated with weight acceptance;

Synergy 2 (push off): activation of the ankle plantar-flexors in late stance that is associated with forward propulsion;

Synergy 3 (foot clearance): activation of the rectus femoris and the tibialis anterior during early stance and early swing, which provides foot dorsi-flexion immediately after heel strike and ground clearance of the foot, respectively;

Synergy 4 (leg deceleration): activation of the hamstrings during late swing and early stance to decelerate the leg and propel the body.

An additional synergy can be found when the trunk muscles are also recorded (Ivanenko et al., 2005). Simulation studies have confirmed the validity of the biomechanical correlates of the muscle synergies (Neptune et al., 2009; Allen and Neptune, 2012).

Muscle synergies have been shown to be "fixed" because they are consistent across different subjects despite variability and noise in the neuro-musculo-skeletal system, but also "flexible" so that they can adapt to slight changes in the environment or be affected by pathologies and then modulated with rehabilitation training (Santello and Lang, 2014). For instance, during locomotion post-stroke individuals exhibit a reduced number of synergies in their paretic side due to the merging of motor modules that imply a non-functional muscle co-contraction reflecting walking dysfunctions (Bowden et al., 2010; Clark et al., 2010; Ting et al., 2015). It is likely that this reduction is caused by a lack of independence of the corticospinal drive to the spinal cord, which ultimately causes a poor muscle control.

Muscle-synergy analysis is currently considered a useful methodology to assess sensorimotor individual deficits (Safavynia et al., 2011). Further, it could be a potential ground upon which novel therapies aimed at enhancing motor relearning could be designed (Ting et al., 2015). In this scope, a FES training based on healthy muscle synergies has been recently proposed for a balance control task. However, the experimental apparatus was rather complex, discouraging its translation to the clinical practice (Galeano et al., 2014).

Our study merges the potentialities of FES-based gait treatments with the strength of muscle-synergy training approach. Indeed, this study was aimed at designing a personalized, biomimetic, multi-channel stimulation controller to support gait rehabilitation after stroke, integrating the following novel aspects:

1) the FES strategy is based on the physiological muscle synergies obtained during overground locomotion.
2) the FES strategy is personalized according to an initial locomotion assessment of the patient, and is used to properly activate impaired biomechanical correlates.
3) the FES strategy is mapped accurately on the altered gait kinematics taking advantage of a segmentation algorithm able to discriminate in real time between 6 gait phases (Chia Bejarano et al., 2015b), allowing a maximal synchronization between the subject's volitional gait and the stimulation patterns.

Preliminary results obtained from two chronic stroke patients with the proposed FES gait controller will be presented in order to show the potentiality of this novel intervention.

MATERIALS AND METHODS

The Stimulation Controller Architecture

The FES-controller architecture includes the subject that can walk overground or on a treadmill, a PC running Linux RTAI, which hosts the whole control system, and a current-controlled stimulator (Rehastim®, Hasomed GmbH) delivering biphasic pulses to surface electrodes (Pals®, Axelgaard Manufacturing Co., Ltd.) placed on up to 8 muscles of the paretic leg. The subjects wear two inertial sensors (Mtx®, Xsens Technology), on both shanks, which provide a real-time kinematic measure used to accurately synchronize the stimulation to the gait cycle. The control system comprises a graphical user interface (GUI) implemented in Qt™software and two real-time applications. The GUI allows the therapist to customize the treatment on the single patient, to start, pause, and stop the treatment, to save data, and to access the stored data. The first real-time application of the control system is the *gait segmentation block* (see **Figure 1**), which receives the signals from the inertial sensors and estimates the Initial Contact (IC), the End Contact (EC), and the Mid-Swing (MS) gait events for each leg. This algorithm was adapted from Chia Bejarano et al. (2015b), in order to be used robustly also in a magnetically disturbed environment, and was validated on healthy subjects using the force-sensitive resistors as a gold standard (Chia Bejarano et al., 2015a). The algorithm demonstrated an excellent accuracy in detecting the IC and EC events (F1-score of 0.98 for the IC and 0.96 for the EC), and allows the detection of the following 6 gait phases: paretic double support, non-paretic initial swing, non-paretic terminal swing, non-paretic double support, paretic initial swing, paretic terminal swing (**Figure 1**).

The second real-time application is the *multi-channel synergy-based stimulation controller* that is personalized on each patient following the steps reported in **Figure 2** and detailed below.

Healthy Muscle Synergies

The starting point of the stimulation controller is the definition of a set of representative healthy muscle synergies. Thirteen healthy subjects (7 men and 6 women; age: 24.8 ± 1.3 years; height: 1.73 ± 0.11 m, weight: 60.8 ± 11.4 kg) volunteered to participate in this study. They were asked to walk overground and on a treadmill at their self-selected speed. The EMG was measured on the following muscles of the dominant leg: gluteus maximus (GM), rectus femoris (RF), vastus medialis (VM), hamstring medialis (HM), hamstring lateralis (HL), gastrocnemius medialis (MG), and tibialis anterior (TA). Kinematics data were acquired at 50 Hz by means of 2 inertial and magnetic sensors (MTx, Xsens) worn on both shanks (Chia Bejarano et al., 2015b).

The EMG signals were acquired at 1024 Hz, band-pass filtered (3rd-order Butterworth filter, cut-off frequencies of 40 and 400 Hz), rectified, and low-pass filtered (3rd-order Butterworth filter, cut-off frequency of 5 Hz) to obtain the EMG envelopes. Afterwards, the envelopes were segmented into single strides using the first contacts of the ipsilateral foot with the pavement (IC events). Then, each stride was normalized in time by interpolating the signals into 100 points, and in amplitude by dividing the EMG signals of each muscle by the median maximum value obtained across strides for each walking condition (treadmill and overground). After removing the initial acceleration and the final deceleration phases from each acquisition, 20 representative strides for each subject and condition were extracted as suggested by Oliveira et al. (2014). The non-negative matrix factorization (NMF) algorithm was applied separately to the 20 envelopes obtained for each subject and walking condition, in order to extract their muscle synergies (Lee and Seung, 1999). The quality of the factorization was measured by computing the variability accounted for (VAF) and the number of muscle synergies was chosen as the smallest number that allowed the reconstruction with a total VAF higher than 90%, or that did not improve the single-muscle VAF more than 5% when adding a new synergy (Clark et al., 2010). The individual muscle synergies of each walking condition were extracted using the most representative number of synergies obtained according to the chosen VAF criterion. Then, the weights of each individual muscle synergy were normalized to have a unitary norm, applying the corresponding transformation to their respective activations profiles, to maintain constant their product. For each walking condition, the average set of muscle synergies across subjects was calculated. To compare the healthy muscle synergies obtained during overground and treadmill walking, the mean and standard deviation of the following metrics were computed: (1) the similarity, i.e., the normalized scalar product between the weights (W) extracted in the two walking conditions; (2) the circular cross correlation between the activation profiles (H) extracted in the two conditions; (3) the

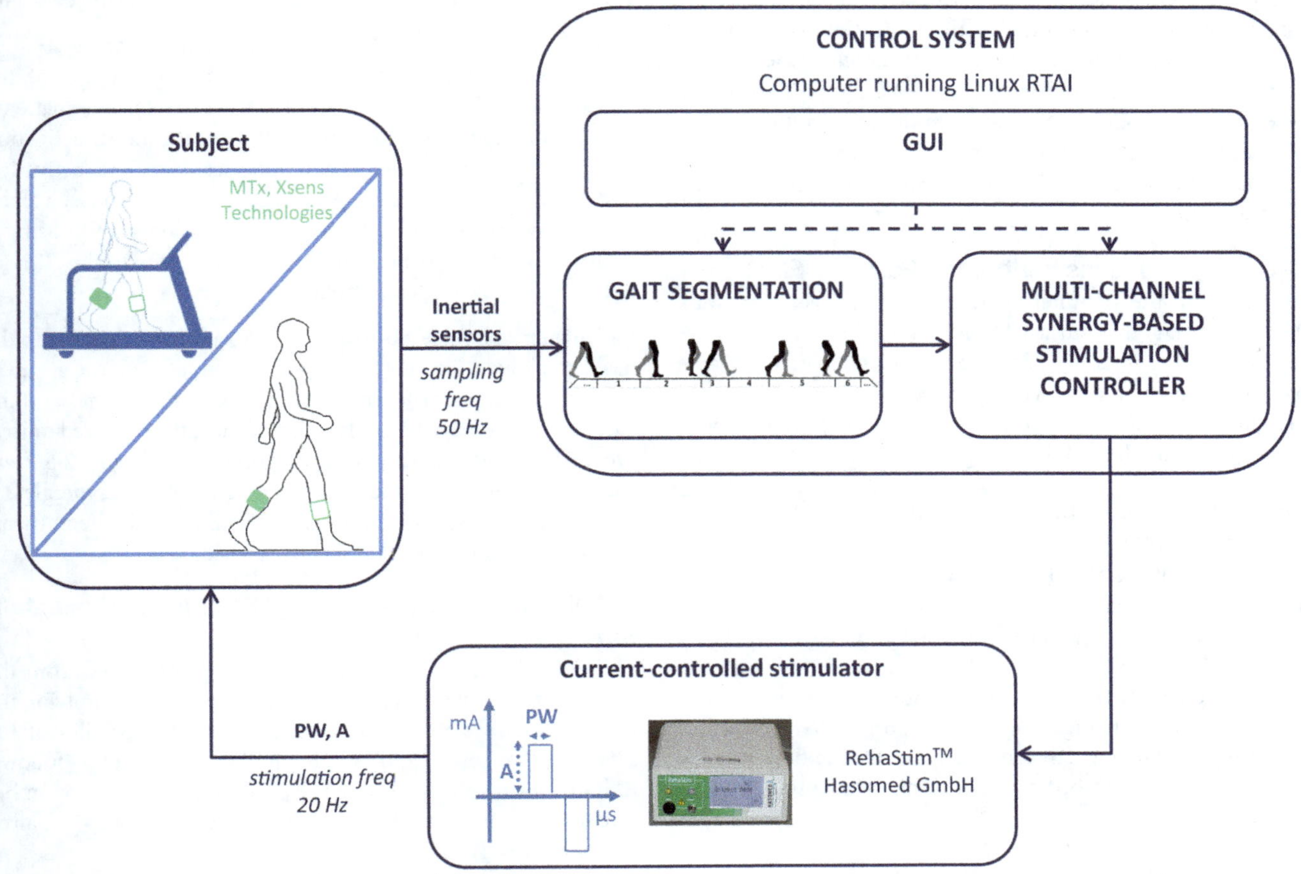

FIGURE 1 | The stimulation controller architecture. In the control system block, real-time signals and non-real-time signals are indicated with solid and dashed arrows respectively. GUI, graphical user interface; freq, frequency; PW, pulse width; A, amplitude.

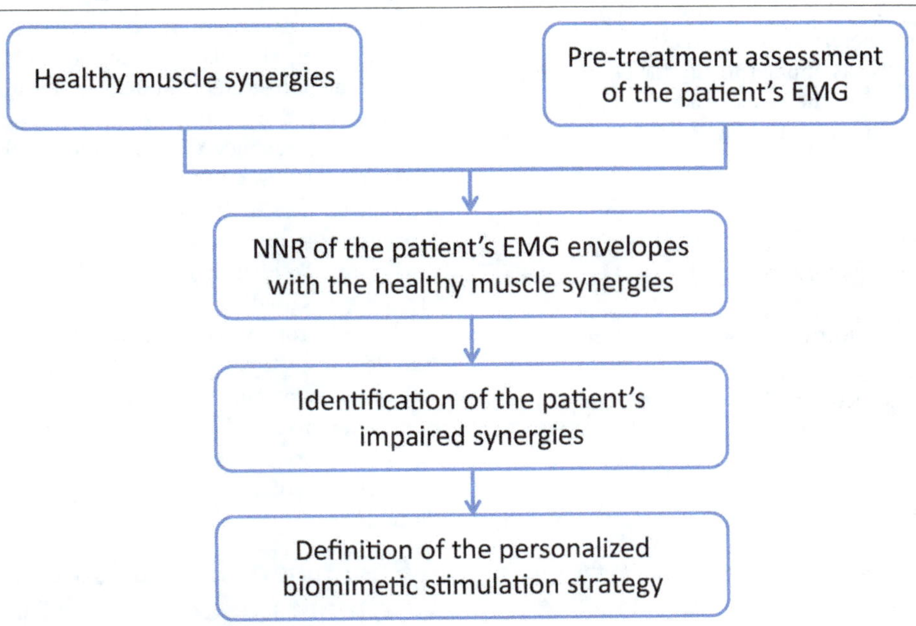

FIGURE 2 | The methodology used to define the personalized biomimetic stimulation strategy. NNR, Non-Negative Matrix Reconstruction.

lag in percentage of gait cycle in which the maximal circular cross correlation was obtained. If the two walking conditions were comparable in terms of muscle synergies, the healthy synergies extracted from the overground walking condition could be used both as a reference to evaluate the overground waking coordination of patients before and after treatment, and to build the biomimetic stimulation strategy to be applied during treadmill training.

Pre-treatment Assessment of the Patient's EMG

Before starting the treatment, the patient was asked to walk overground and the surface EMG activation signals were measured on eight muscles of the paretic leg following the same protocol described in the previous paragraph for healthy subjects. Analogously, the signal processing procedure described above was used to obtain the EMG envelopes.

NNR of the Patient's EMG Envelopes with the Healthy Muscle Synergies

The mean set of weights ($W_{HEALTHY}$) and activation profiles ($H_{HEALTHY}$) obtained during overground walking in healthy subjects were used to perform the two Non-Negative Matrix Reconstructions (NNR) of the EMG envelopes obtained on the paretic side during the patient's pre-treatment assessment. The NNR was applied by fixing the synergy vectors as $W_{HEALTHY}$ and letting only the synergy activation coefficients H update at every algorithm iteration, according to the following multiplicative update rule:

$$H \leftarrow H \frac{\left(W_{HEALTHY}^{T} \cdot M\right)}{\left(W_{HEALTHY}^{T} \cdot W_{HEALTHY} \cdot H\right)}$$

where M is the matrix of the EMG envelopes measured on the 8 muscles during 20 gait cycles. Each vector of $W_{HEALTHY}$ was normalized to unit norm before applying NNR.

Afterwards, the NNR was applied to the EMG envelopes of the specific patient by fixing the synergy activation coefficients $H_{HEALTHY}$ and deriving the patient's weights, using the following update rule:

$$W \leftarrow W \frac{\left(M \cdot H_{HEALTHY}^{T}\right)}{\left(W \cdot H_{HEALTHY} \cdot H_{HEALTHY}^{T}\right)}$$

Identification of the Patient's Impaired Muscle Synergies

Each of the four reconstructed patient's muscle synergies were compared to the mean healthy synergies by computing the following metrics:

- the similarity between the patient's reconstructed weights and $W_{HEALTHY}$.
- the circular cross correlation computed between the patient's reconstructed activation profiles and $H_{HEALTHY}$.
- the time lag computed as: $Tlag = 1 - \left|\frac{lag}{100}\right|$, where lag is the percentage of gait cycle (lag value can vary between −50 and 50) in which the maximal correlation between the reconstructed activation profile and $H_{HEALTHY}$ was obtained.
- the activation duration was defined as: $Act = 1 - \frac{\left|Act_{Hp} - Act_{H_{healthy}}\right|}{100}$, where Act_{Hp} and $Act_{H_{healthy}}$ are the durations, in percentage of the gait cycle, of the activation phases. These were computed on the patient's reconstructed activation profile and on the mean activation profile of the healthy group, respectively. The activation duration was defined based on the onset and offset values, which were determined from the activation profile using a threshold fixed at the minimum of each profile plus 20% of the cycle peak-to-peak amplitude.

For all metrics a value close to 1 indicates a behavior similar to the healthy subjects. The metrics were first computed on the group of healthy subjects in order to obtain the normality ranges and the specific thresholds to be used to discriminate the impaired muscle synergies. For each metric, a cut-off point of the mean $-2{\cdot}SD$ was chosen to define a threshold common to all muscle synergies. A patient's muscle synergy was defined as impaired when at least one of the metrics resulted under threshold.

Definition of the Personalized Biomimetic Stimulation Strategy

The individual muscle activations were reconstructed from the representative physiological muscle synergies by multiplying the mean muscle weights and the mean activation profiles of the synergies that resulted to be impaired in the patient as follows: $EMG_{N\times 100} = W_{healthy\ N\times J} * H_{healthy J\times 100}$ where N is number of considered muscles ($N = 8$) and J the number of impaired synergies ($J \leq 4$).

To avoid excessive fatigue due to FES, the stimulation of each muscle was set to zero when the profile was lower than a threshold defined as the value of the baseline plus the 20% of the peak-to-peak amplitude. Finally, when muscles were characterized by very similar activation profiles, if possible, they were grouped to be activated by a single stimulation channel using stimulation electrodes covering both muscles. The stimulation strategy modulated the stimulation pulse width between 0 and a predefined maximum value of 400 μs. The stimulation frequency was common to all muscles and was set to 20 Hz, whereas the stimulation amplitude was identified individually for each muscle, during an initial calibration procedure, in order to produce a visible contraction without discomfort. To identify the stimulation amplitude a pulse width of 400 μs was used.

The control system adapted the predefined biomimetic stimulation strategy to changes in walking speed within session. Indeed, when a subject entered a new gait phase, the average of its duration over the last five strides was computed. This estimate was used to stretch or expand the corresponding part of the stimulation profile in order to fully adapt to the subject's gait timing.

A Preliminary Evaluation of the FES Treatment Effect on Two Chronic Stroke Patients

Two patients with chronic hemiparesis due to ischemic strok[e] (**Table 1**) were asked to undergo a 4-week intervention consistin[g] of 30-min sessions of FES-supported treadmill walking thre

TABLE 1 | Patient details.

	Age (years)	Gender	Time from stroke	Hemiparetic side
S1	67	Man	11 years	Left
S2	64	Man	9 months	Right

times per week. Each session consisted of 5 min of warming up without FES, 20 min of gait supported by the multi-channel personalized FES controller, and 5 min of cooling down without FES. The patient was asked to select his preferred walking velocity during the warming up phase. Before and after the end of the intervention, two clinical scales were assessed: the motor sub-scale of the Functional Independence Measure (FIM) which evaluates the patient's motor disability during daily life activities and ranges from 13 to 91 (independent), (Kidd et al., 1995) and the Mini Best test (MBT) which evaluated the dynamic balance and ranges from 0 to 28 (normal balance; Franchignoni et al., 2010). To evaluate specific improvements in terms of walking ability, the same test used to identify the patient's impaired muscle synergies was repeated at the end of the intervention. Both kinematics and EMG data were collected. The mean cadence was computed from the kinematics data. EMG envelopes were computed and the NMF algorithm was applied to extract the muscle synergies as previously described for healthy subjects. At the end of the intervention, the patients were also asked to rate the global perceived effect of the treatment using the global rating change (GRC), which is an 11-point scale (-5 = made things worse; 0 = not changed; 5 = completely recovered; Kamper et al., 2009).

The protocol was approved by the Central Ethics Committee of the Fondazione Salvatore Maugeri (IRCCS) and both patients provided their written informed consent before participation.

RESULTS

Functioning of Multi-Channel Synergy-Based Stimulation Controler

Healthy Muscle Synergies

The $W_{HEALTHY}$ and $H_{HEALTHY}$ during overground walking are reported in **Figure 3**. All healthy subjects were characterized by four muscle synergies corresponding to the four gait sub-functions identified in literature: Weight Acceptance (WA), Push Off (PO), Foot Clearance (FC) and Leg Deceleration (LD). The same modular organization, both in terms of spatial composition and temporal recruitment, was obtained during treadmill walking. Indeed, comparing the extracted muscle synergies in the two walking conditions and averaging across subjects, a mean (Standard Deviation, SD) similarity of 0.89 (0.11), a circular cross correlation of 0.94 (0.06), and a time lag of 2 (1) in percentage of the gait cycle were found. This confirms that the two walking conditions share the same muscle coordination and thus it is possible to define both a treadmill and an overground treatment based on the same set of physiological muscle synergies.

The synergies extracted from the overground walking condition were used to perform the two NNR of the EMG envelopes obtained on the paretic side during the patient's pre-treatment assessment.

NNR of the Patient's EMG Envelopes with the Healthy Synergies

Figure 4 shows the NNR results obtained for both patients. The obtained VAF values were 0.85 and 0.77 for S1, and 0.90 and 0.84 for S2 when the NNR was applied fixing $W_{HEALTHY}$ and $H_{HEALTHY}$, respectively.

Identification of the Patient's Impaired Muscle Synergies

Table 2 reports for each metric and each muscle synergy, the thresholds computed on the healthy subjects group (last column) and the values obtained by the two patients during the pre-treatment assessment.

The metrics confirmed what was visually observed by the reconstructed synergies: S1 had an impaired spatial composition in the WA synergy (similarity was under threshold for WA), a wider activation timing of PO and LD synergies, and a delayed recruitment of the FC synergy. Concerning S2, a low cross correlation was found for FC and LD synergies. Thus, all four synergies were defined as impaired for S1 and only FC and LD were considered impaired synergies for S2.

Definition of the Personalized Stimulation Strategy

The final FES strategy obtained and used for both patients is shown in **Figure 5**. The medial and lateral hamstrings and the medial gastrocnemius and soleus showed similar activation profiles and therefore the FES strategy coupled into one stimulation channel both hamstrings, and the calf muscles into another. Thus, a total of six muscle groups were stimulated.

S1 had a FES strategy based on all four healthy synergies, whereas for S2 only the FC and LD synergies was used to obtain the muscle stimulation profiles. When a reduced number of synergies was used to create the stimulation strategy, a subset of the six muscle groups was stimulated. In particular, the calf muscles, which were not recruited by the FC and LD healthy synergies, were not stimulated for S2.

Figure 5 also shows the different kinematic patterns of the two patients. Indeed, both patients were characterized by a prolonged double support, but S1 extended the paretic double support phase (gait phase 1) whereas S2 extended the non-paretic double support phase (gait phase 4). In both cases, the FES strategy was able to adapt to these changes in gait pattern, mapping the stimulation profiles accordingly.

For both patients the first (upper panels) and last (lower panels) sessions of the intervention are shown to highlight the differences in gait speed together with slight differences in the kinematic pattern. In the first session of FES-supported gait, S1 presented an impaired kinematic pattern characterized by a double support phase of the paretic leg (phase 1) lasting the 48% of the gait cycle and a very short paretic single support (21% of the gait cycle). In the last treatment session, this kinematic pattern changed: the duration of the paretic double support was the 25% of the gait cycle and the duration of the paretic single support was 29%. These improvements in the kinematic pattern

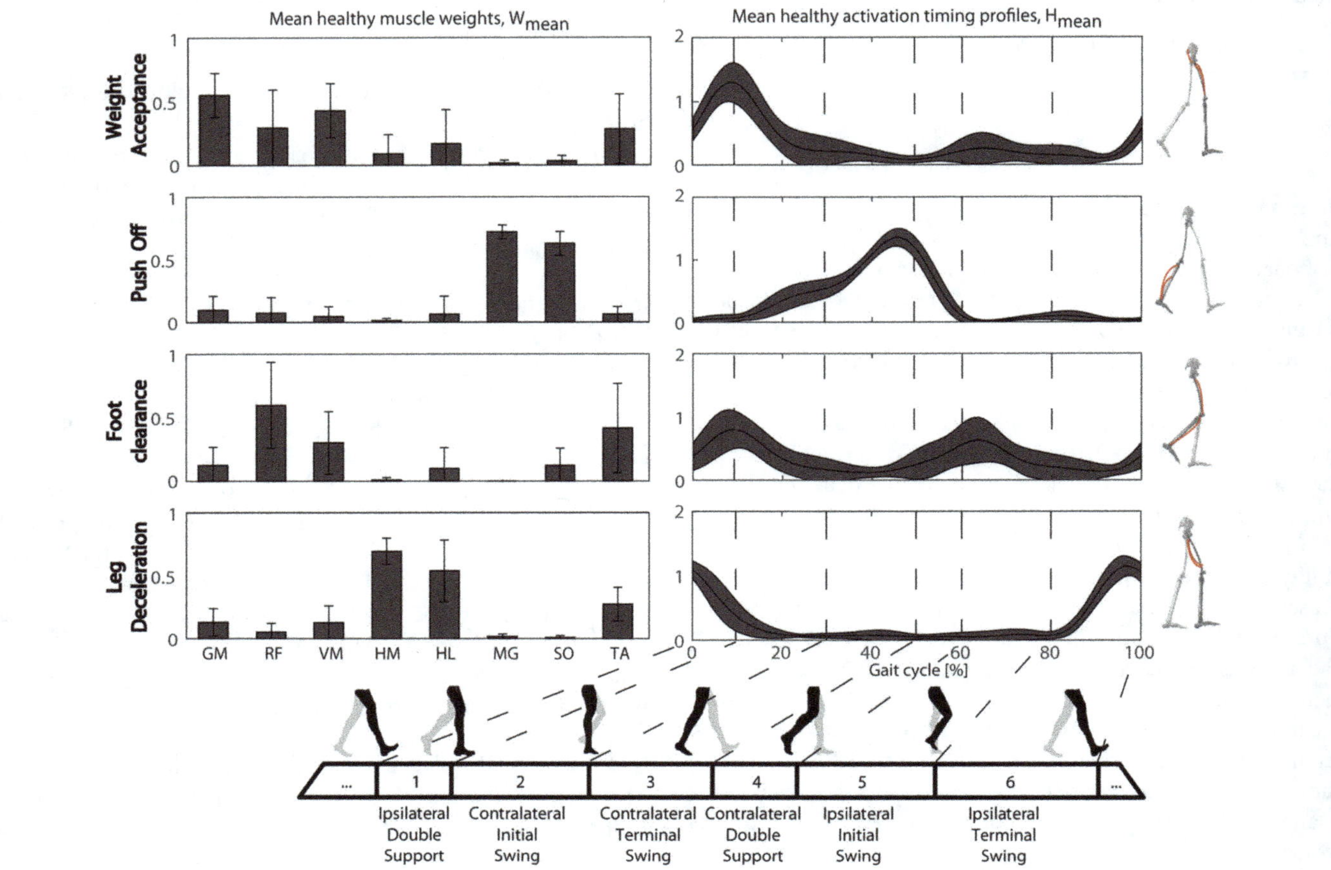

FIGURE 3 | The physiological muscle synergies: muscle weights (Left panel) and temporal activation profiles (Right panel) obtained during overground walking. Mean values and standard deviation are reported in both panels. GM, gluteus maximus; RF, rectus femoris; VM, vastus medialis; HM, hamstring medialis; HL, hamstring lateralis; MG, gastrocnemius medialis; TA, tibialis anterior.

corresponded to a walking speed that in the last session doubled its value with respect to the first session. Concerning S2, the kinematics pattern in the first session was characterized by a reduced paretic swing phase that was augmented by 52% in the last session, achieving a final duration equal to the 38% of the gait cycle.

The FES Treatment Effect on the Two Chronic Stroke Patients

Both patients completed the treatment without difficulties and reported a positive global perceived effect of the treatment (GRC was +4 (improved a lot) and +2 (improved) for S1 and S2, respectively). The treadmill speed used in the first and last day of treatment increased from 0.43 to 0.83 m/s, and from 0.38 to 0.68 m/s for S1 and S2, respectively.

The extracted muscle synergies before and after the treatment during the overground walking tests are shown in **Figures 6**, **7** for S1 and S2, respectively. The treatment induced an increase of the number of extracted synergies in both patients from 3 to 4 indicating a general improvement in muscle coordination. The VAF was 0.87 before and 0.88 after treatment, and 0.90 before and 0.93 after treatment for S1 and S2, respectively. The visual comparison between the extracted synergies obtained before intervention for S1 and the healthy synergies (**Figure 6**) suggests that the first extracted synergy (S1-1) resembles the FC synergy except for the GM activation, the second extracted synergy (S1-2) mostly recruits the MG and SO muscles as it is in the PO synergy with an anticipatory activation profile, and the third synergy (S1-3) merges the WA and LD synergies. After treatment, fou[r] muscle synergies were found, generally resembling the spatia[l] composition of the healthy muscle synergies in **Figure 3**. A[n] early recruitment of the plantar-flexors is still present in the PC synergy.

Concerning S2 (**Figure 7**), before treatment the first synerg[y] (S2-1) can be associated to the WA synergy, the second (S2-2) seems to be the merging of the FC and LD synergies, and th[e] third (S2-3) seems to be the PO synergy with a slight contributio[n] of the hamstring muscles. After treatment, four synergies wer[e] obtained displaying a behavior more similar to healthy subjects however, an early activation of the plantar-flexors is still visible i[n] PO synergy.

The clinical evaluation of the two patients is reported i[n] **Table 3**. Both patients had a mild motor disability at baseline. I[n] both cases the improvement gained in muscle coordination wa[s] not yet enough to be transferred into a significant difference i[n] general motor disability.

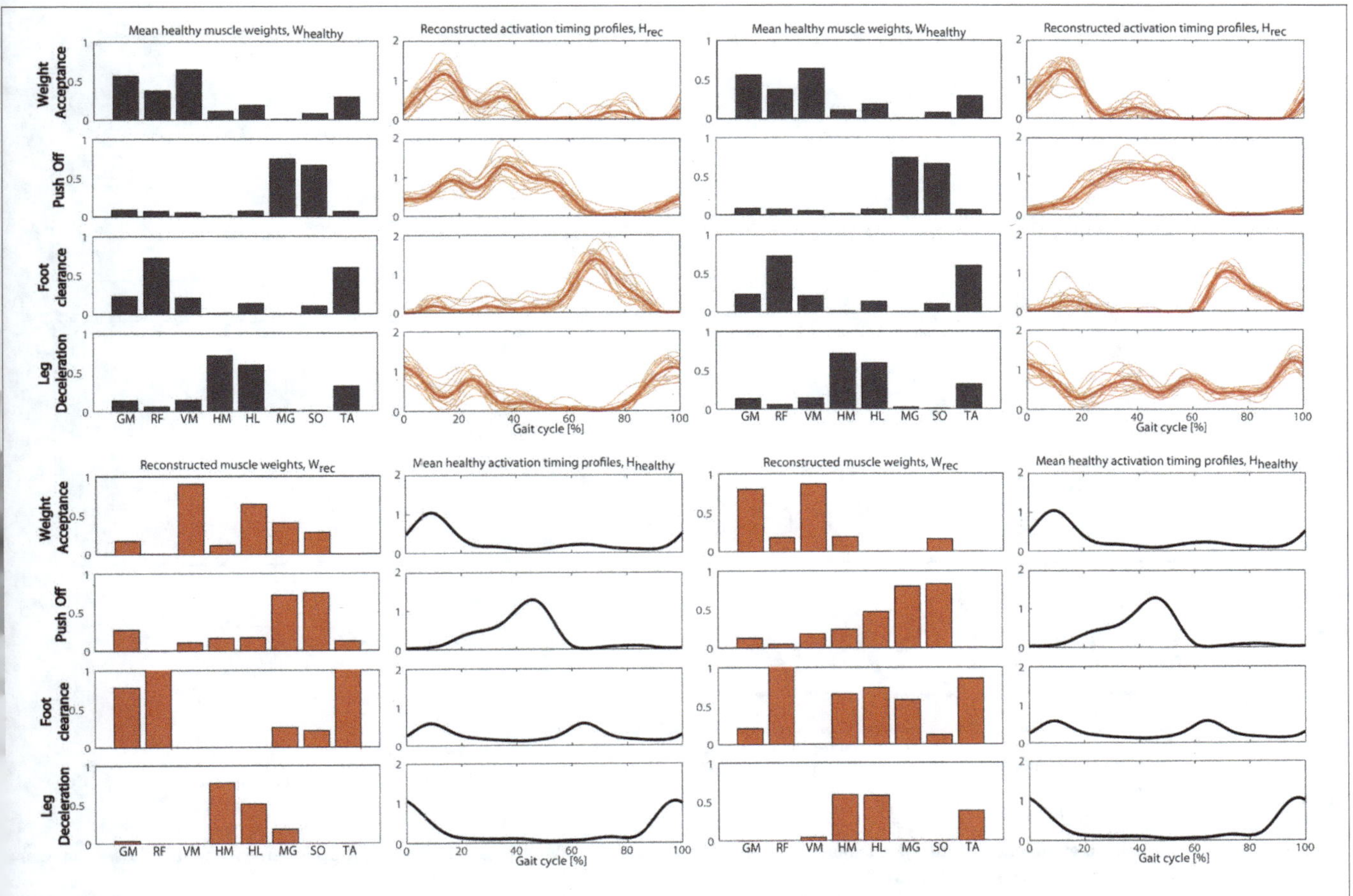

FIGURE 4 | The reconstructed muscle synergies obtained for S1 (Left panels) and S2 (Right panels) using $W_{HEALTHY}$ (Upper panels) of $H_{HEALTHY}$ (Lower panels). In both NNR results, the fixed component is shown in black and the reconstructed one in red. When the activation profiles are reconstructed, both the single-stride profile (thinner lines) and the mean profile (thicker line) are reported.

TABLE 2 | Metrics computed on the reconstructed muscle synergies of S1 and S2 for each muscle synergy.

	WA	PO	FC	LD	Thresholds
S1					
Similarity	**0.67**	0.97	0.95	0.91	0.79
Correlation	0.95	**0.89**	**0.77**	0.92	0.90
-Lag	0.94	0.96	**0.61**	0.99	0.96
Activation	0.85	**0.71**	**0.65**	**0.77**	0.82
S2					
Similarity	0.90	0.93	0.80	0.98	0.79
Correlation	0.96	0.93	**0.79**	**0.85**	0.90
-Lag	0.96	0.98	0.99	0.99	0.96
Activation	0.99	0.83	0.97	0.99	0.82

The last column indicates the thresholds obtained in the group of healthy subjects. The values below the predefined threshold are highlighted in bold.

DISCUSSION

The high heterogeneity of stroke patients and the high variability in their response to treatments demand for novel personalized assessment methodologies able to unveil the specific impaired sub-functions to be recovered and for novel training procedures adapted to single subject's disability. Most of the outcome measures used to assess the patients' condition are focused on the overall motor function (such as the walking speed) and do not have the power to discriminate specific impairments that underlie the general functional deficit (Ting et al., 2015). Recent neurophysiological studies recommended the analysis of muscle synergies to finely assess the impairment of the subject, to design rehabilitation treatments personalized on the specific nature of the individual impairment, and to assess the eventual treatment outcome (Clark et al., 2010; Ting et al., 2015). In this scope, we developed a multi-channel FES controller to support gait training based on physiological muscle synergies and we personalized it to the individual impairment obtained by means of a baseline assessment of gait muscle synergies. The proposed treatment is goal-oriented, task-specific, and challenging, since the subjects are asked to walk for 30 min at a comfortable speed. FES patterns have been accurately aligned in time with the gait phases of the subject so to assure the maximal synchronization between the FES input and the volitional activity. Thus, it should harness activity-dependent neuro-plasticity (Lamontagne and Fung, 2004; Gandolla et al., 2014).

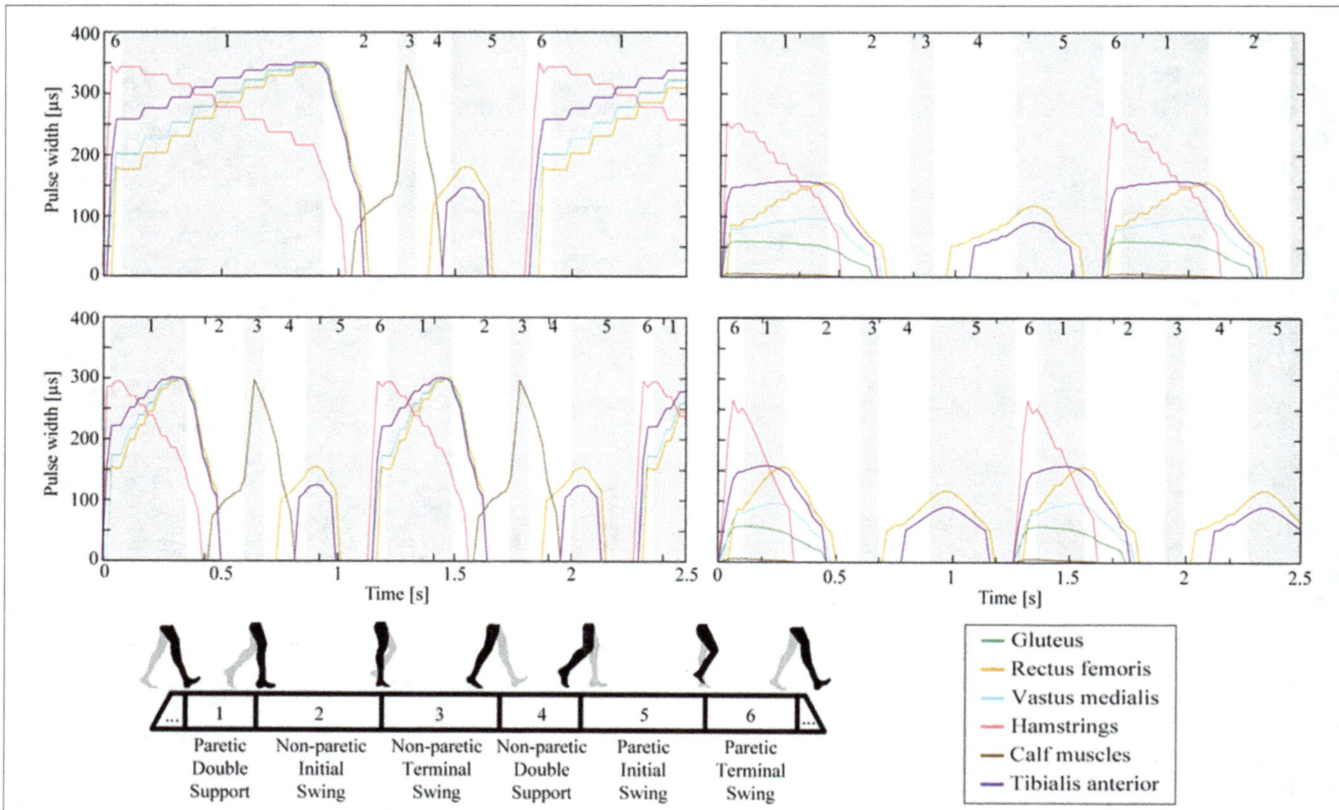

FIGURE 5 | The personalized stimulation strategy obtained for S1 (Left panels) and S2 (Right panels) in the first (Upper panels) and last (Lower panels) sessions of the intervention. Same labels as in **Figure 3**.

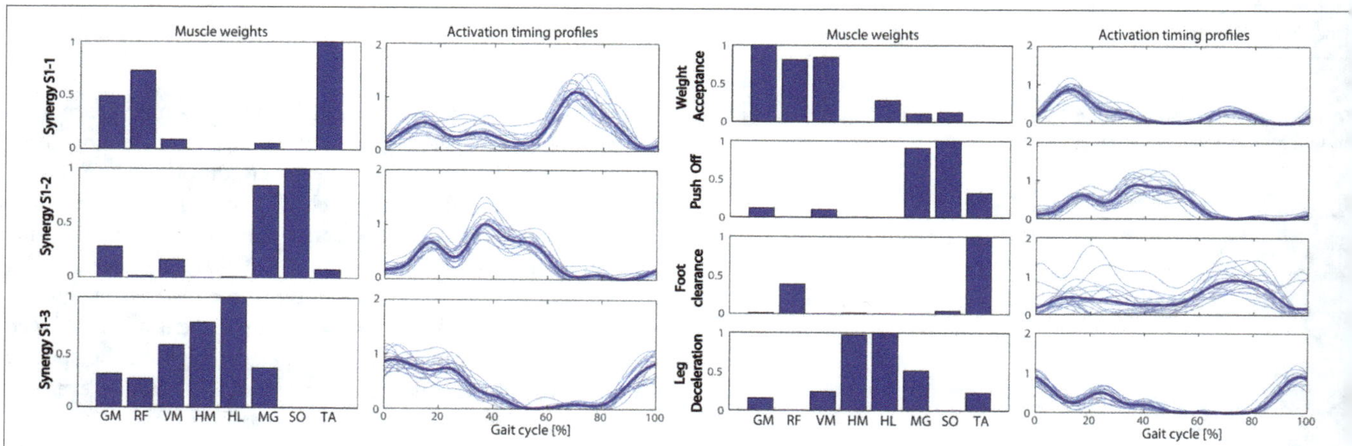

FIGURE 6 | The extracted muscle synergies obtained for S1 before (Left panel) and after (Right panel) treatment. Same labels as in **Figure 3**.

In literature, FES controllers have been based on very simple segmentation algorithms able to discriminate between the stance and swing phases and the FES strategy has been linearly mapped through the gait stride adopting sub-optimal time rules in order to automatically deactivate stimulation (Daly et al., 2011). The novelty of our proposed control system lies in the capability to accurately map the subject's gait timing based on the real-time detection of six gait phases. This mapping is able to stretch or extend the stimulation profiles according to the actual duration of all six phases. For instance, if a patient's gait pattern is characterized by an extended double support phase the stimulation profile of the muscles supporting this phase are extended accordingly in order to follow the correct muscle timing and coordination involved in this phase (see **Figure 5**). This choice avoids the unwanted activation of antagonist muscles in the extended kinematic phase that could increase the instabilit

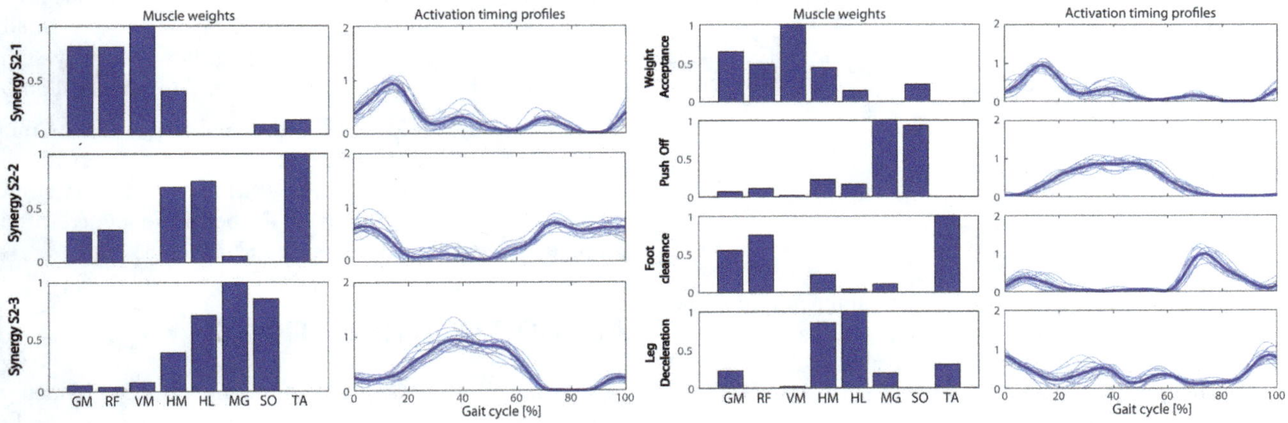

FIGURE 7 | The extracted muscle synergies obtained for S2 before (Left panel) and after (Right panel) treatment. Same labels as in **Figure 3**.

of the gait instead of fostering the relearning process. This novel modality to map the individual kinematics is an important personalization factor, since the duration of each gait phase is highly dependent on the patient's level of impairment (Olney and Richards, 1996).

The starting point to design the proposed biomimetic multi-channel FES controller was the identification of the physiological set of synergies during walking. Results obtained in healthy subjects confirmed that a common motor-control strategy based on four muscles synergies, was shared across walking conditions (overground and treadmill). The identified muscle synergies corresponded well to the four biomechanical functions proposed in the literature (Clark et al., 2010) and confirmed the equivalence in motor coordination between the two walking conditions (Kautz et al., 2011). The physiological muscle synergies used to design the stimulation strategy were extracted from a group of healthy subjects, which were younger than the average stroke patient; nevertheless, it has been shown that synergies are invariant with aging (Monaco et al., 2010).

The two patients included in the pilot study were quite independent in daily-life activities before treatment and were characterized by a mild gait disability (gait speed higher than 0.8 m/s; Tilson et al., 2010). However, a more specific analysis based on muscle synergies during overground gait highlighted an altered motor coordination characterized by only 2 independently recruited muscle synergies for both patients. The underlying gait abnormality was different for the two patients. S1 merged the control of the proximal extensors with the hamstrings (i.e., the WA and LD synergies) and showed an early activation of the plantar-flexors, which is a typical behavior of stroke patients (Clark et al., 2010). S2 merged the FC and LD synergies and also showed an early recruitment of the plantar-flexors presumably connected to an increased excitability of the monosynaptic stretch reflex (Crenna and Frigo, 1987). These two different impairments in terms of muscle coordination produced a proper personalized treatment that resulted in a FES strategy based on all 4 or just 2 muscle synergies for S1 and S2, respectively. Comparing the first and last session of treatment (**Figure 5**), a different kinematic pattern is noticeable. The first patient was able to reduce by half the duration of his paretic double support phase. This represents a big improvement although it was still higher than the physiological duration, which is about 10% of the gait cycle (Perry and Burnfield, 1992). Analogously, the paretic single support increased by 38% becoming closer to the physiological value (Perry and Burnfield, 1992). The second subject improved the duration of his paretic swing phase. For both subjects the improvements across treatment sessions in gait timing were coupled with a faster speed in the training execution.

The assessment after the end of the intervention showed that both patients improved their muscle coordination; indeed, four muscle synergies were extracted for both of them. The originally merged synergies seemed to regain their distinct role in locomotion control, even if the PO synergy maintained an anticipated recruitment and a prolonged timing in both patients. The benefits of the treatment were more evident for S1 and this was confirmed by the patient's perceived effect; indeed, S1 stated that, thanks to the treatment, he was able to achieve a very good walking improvement (GRC = 4). The improvement in motor coordination was also coupled with a clinically important improvement in the dynamic balance. Indeed, the pre-post change of the Mini Best Test overcame 4 points (**Table 3**) that is the minimal clinical important difference for patients with balance disorders (Godi et al., 2013). Concerning S2, the treatment was able to induce a beginning of neuro-motor relearning, but probably the 12 treatment sessions were not enough to translate the motor-coordination progress into relevant clinical improvements, in line with the lower benefit perceived by the patient (GRC = 2).

The duration of the donning and setting up of the FES controller was performed by the physiotherapists and, excluding the first day of training, it lasted an average of 5–10 min, which was compatible with a clinical use.

This study has two main limitations. First, the treatment was tested only with two chronic stroke patients and the results obtained, even if encouraging, should be considered as

TABLE 3 | Comparison of the outcome measures before and after training.

	S1		S2	
	T0	T1	T0	T1
Mini Best Test (0–28)	17	22	21	23
FIM motor subscale (13–91)	78	78	85	85
Cadence (strides/s) (SD)	0.98 (0.03)	1.01 (0.03)	0.81 (0.03)	0.80 (0.02)

preliminary. Second, the speed used during training was too slow. For instance, the second subject never reached his self-selected speed overground during training. Recent studies demonstrated that combining a 2-channel FES with fast treadmill walking yielded larger improvements in gait mechanics than when FES was combined with self-selected speed treadmill walking (Kesar et al., 2011; Awad et al., 2016). Thus, future studies using this personalized biomimetic FES controller should consider the use of fast speed during training.

CONCLUSION

In this study we have developed and tested a personalized multi-channel FES controller to support gait rehabilitation after stroke. The treatment was personalized to the specific gait abnormality of each patient. Indeed, once the impaired biomechanical functions were revealed by an assessment based on muscular synergies analysis, the exercise was shaped in order to train only the muscle coordination associated with those biomechanical functions. The muscle-synergy analysis was also exploited to assess the effects of treatment and confirmed to be very effective in identifying improvements in motor coordination. The results presented in this pilot case study were encouraging; however, they should be confirmed by a wider statistical study (e.g., a randomized controlled study). Additionally, the application of this multi-channel FES controller could be extended to people with post-acute stroke, whose lack of a well-learnt compensatory strategy by the CNS could help improving the benefits obtained with the proposed treatment in case of chronic patients.

AUTHOR CONTRIBUTIONS

SF designed the work, drafted the manuscript, refined the data analysis, interpreted the results, revised and approved the manuscript. NC designed the work, collected the data, carried out the data analysis, interpreted the results and revised and approved the manuscript. EA designed the work, interpreted the results, revised and approved the manuscript. AN designed the work, recruited the patients, supervised the intervention, revised and approved the manuscript. AT performed the clinical scale assessment, carried out the intervention, revised and approved the manuscript. MM revised and approved the manuscript. GF designed the work, revised and approved the manuscript. AP designed the work, revised and approved the manuscript.

ACKNOWLEDGMENTS

The authors would like to acknowledge Axelgaard Manufacturing Ltd. for donating the stimulation electrodes.

REFERENCES

Allen, J. L., and Neptune, R. R. (2012). Three-dimensional modular control of human walking. *J. Biomech.* 45, 2157–2163. doi: 10.1016/j.jbiomech.2012.05.037

Ambrosini, E., Ferrante, S., Pedrocchi, A., Ferrigno, G., and Molteni, F. (2011). Cycling induced by electrical stimulation improves motor recovery in postacute hemiparetic patients: a randomized controlled trial. *Stroke* 42, 1068–1073. doi: 10.1161/STROKEAHA.110.599068

Ambrosini, E., Ferrante, S., Ferrigno, G., Molteni, F., and Pedrocchi, A. (2012). Cycling induced by electrical stimulation improves muscle activation and symmetry during pedaling in hemiparetic patients. *IEEE Trans. Neural Syst. Rehabil. Eng.* 20, 320–330. doi: 10.1109/TNSRE.2012.2191574

Ambrosini, E., Ferrante, S., Schauer, T., Ferrigno, G., Molteni, F., and Pedrocchi, A. (2010). Design of a symmetry controller for cycling induced by electrical stimulation: preliminary results on post-acute stroke patients. *Artif. Organs* 34, 663–667. doi: 10.1111/j.1525-1594.2009.00941.x

Awad, L. N., Reisman, D. S., Pohlig, R. T., and Binder-Macleod, S. A. (2016). Reducing the cost of transport and increasing walking distance after stroke: a randomized controlled trial on fast locomotor training combined with functional electrical stimulation. *Neurorehabil. Neural Repair* 30, 661–670. doi: 10.1177/1545968315619696

Barroso, F., Torricelli, D., Moreno, J. C., Taylor, J., Gomez-Soriano, J., Esteban, E. B., et al. (2014). Shared muscle synergies in human walking and cycling. *J. Neurophysiol.* 112, 1984–1998. doi: 10.1152/jn.00220.2014

Bowden, M. G., Clark, D. J., and Kautz, S. A. (2010). Evaluation of abnorma synergy patterns poststroke: relationship of the fugl-meyer assessment t hemiparetic locomotion. *Neurorehabil. Neural Repair* 24, 328–337. do 10.1177/1545968309343215

Chae, J., Sheffler, L., and Knutson, J. (2008). Neuromuscular electrical stimulatio for motor restoration in hemiplegia. *Top. Stroke Rehabil.* 15, 412–426. do 10.1310/tsr1505-412

Chia Bejarano, N., Ambrosini, E., Baccinelli, W., Nardone, A., Monticone, M Ferrigno, G., et al. (2015a). A multi-channel biomimetic neuroprosthesis t support treadmill gait training in stroke patients. *Conf. Proc. IEEE Eng. Mec Biol. Soc.* 2015, 7159–7162. doi: 10.1109/EMBC.2015.7320043

Chia Bejarano, N., Ambrosini, E., Pedrocchi, A., Ferrigno, G., Monticone, M., an Ferrante, S. (2015b). A novel adaptive, real-time algorithm to detect gait even from wearable sensors. *IEEE Trans. Neural Syst. Rehabil. Eng.* 23, 413–422. do 10.1109/TNSRE.2014.2337914

Clark, D. J., Ting, L. H., Zajac, F. E., Neptune, R. R., and Kautz, S. A. (2010 Merging of healthy motor modules predicts reduced locomotor performanc and muscle coordination complexity post-stroke. *J. Neurophysiol.* 103, 844–85 doi: 10.1152/jn.00825.2009

Crenna, P., and Frigo, C. (1987). Excitability of the soleus H-reflex a during walking and stepping in man. *Exp. Brain Res.* 66, 49–60. dc 10.1007/BF00236201

Daly, J. J., Zimbelman, J., Roenigk, K. L., McCabe, J. P., Rogers, J. M., Butler, K et al. (2011). Recovery of coordinated gait: randomized controlled stroke trial Functional Electrical Stimulation (FES) versus No, FES, with weight-supporte treadmill and over-ground training. *Neurorehabil. Neural Repair* 25, 588–596. doi: 10.1177/1545968311400092

d'Avella, A., and Bizzi, E. (2005). Shared and specific muscle synergies in natural motor behaviors. *Proc. Natl. Acad. Sci. U.S.A.* 102, 3076–3081. doi: 10.1073/pnas.0500199102

d'Avella, A., Saltiel, P., and Bizzi, E. (2003). Combinations of muscle synergies in the construction of a natural motor behavior. *Nat. Neurosci.* 6, 300–308. doi: 10.1038/nn1010

Embrey, D. G., Holtz, S. L., Alon, G., Brandsma, B. A., and McCoy, S. W. (2010). Functional electrical stimulation to dorsiflexors and plantar flexors during gait to improve walking in adults with chronic hemiplegia. *Arch. Phys. Med. Rehabil.* 91, 687–696. doi: 10.1016/j.apmr.2009.12.024

Ferrante, S., Pedrocchi, A., Ferrigno, G., and Molteni, F. (2008). Cycling induced by functional electrical stimulation improves the muscular strength and the motor control of individuals with post-acute stroke. Europa Medicophysica-SIMFER 2007 Award Winner. *Eur. J. Phys. Rehabil. Med.* 44, 159–167.

Franchignoni, F., Horak, F., Godi, M., Nardone, A., and Giordano, A. (2010). Using psychometric techniques to improve the balance evaluation systems test: The Mini-BESTest. *J. Rehabil. Med.* 42, 323–331. doi: 10.2340/16501977-0537

Galeano, D., Brunetti, F., Torricelli, D., Piazza, S., and Pons, J. L. (2014). A tool for balance control training using muscle synergies and multimodal interfaces. *BioMed. Res. Int.* 2014:565370. doi: 10.1155/2014/565370

Gandolla, M., Ferrante, S., Molteni, F., Guanziroli, E., Frattini, T., Martegani, A., et al. (2014). Re-thinking the role of motor cortex: context-sensitive motor outputs? *NeuroImage* 91, 366–374. doi: 10.1016/j.neuroimage.2014.01.011

Gandolla, M., Ward, N. S., Molteni, F., Guanziroli, E., Ferrigno, G., and Pedrocchi, A. (2016). The neural correlates of long-term carryover following functional electrical stimulation for stroke. *Neural Plast.* 2016:4192718. doi: 10.1155/2016/4192718

Godi, M., Franchignoni, F., Caligari, M., Giordano, A., Turcato, A. M., and Nardone, A. (2013). Comparison of reliability, validity, and responsiveness of the mini-bestest and berg balance scale in patients with balance disorders. *Phys. Ther.* 93, 158–167. doi: 10.2522/ptj.20120171

Ivanenko, Y. P., Cappellini, G., Dominici, N., Poppele, R. E., and Lacquaniti, F. (2005). Coordination of locomotion with voluntary movements in humans. *J. Neurosci.* 25, 7238–7253. doi: 10.1523/JNEUROSCI.1327-05.2005

Kafri, M., and Laufer, Y. (2015). Therapeutic effects of functional electrical stimulation on gait in individuals post-stroke. *Ann. Biomed. Eng.* 43, 451–466. doi: 10.1007/s10439-014-1148-8

Kamper, S. J., Maher, C. G., and Mackay, G. (2009). Global rating of change scales: a review of strengths and weaknesses and considerations for design. *J. Man. Manip. Ther.* 17, 163–170. doi: 10.1179/jmt.2009.17.3.163

Kautz, S. A., Bowden, M. G., Clark, D. J., and Neptune, R. R. (2011). Comparison of motor control deficits during treadmill and overground walking poststroke. *Neurorehabil. Neural Repair* 25, 756–765. doi: 10.1177/1545968311407515

Kesar, T. M., Perumal, R., Reisman, D. S., Jancosko, A., Rudolph, C. S., Higginson, J. S., et al. (2009). Functional electrical stimulation of ankle plantarflexor and dorsiflexor muscles: effects on poststroke gait. *Stroke* 40, 3821–3827. doi: 10.1161/STROKEAHA.109.560375

Kesar, T. M., Reisman, D. S., Perumal, R., and Jancosko, A. M. (2011). Combined effects of fast treadmill walking and functional electrical stimulation on post-stroke gait. *Gait Posture* 33, 309–313. doi: 10.1016/j.gaitpost.2010.11.019

Kidd, D., Stewart, G., Baldry, J., Johnson, J., Rossiter, D., Petruckevitch, A., et al. (1995). The functional independence measure: a comparative validity and reliability study. *Disabil. Rehabil.* 17, 10–14. doi: 10.3109/09638289509166622

Kim, J. H., Chung, Y., Kim, Y., and Hwang, S. (2012). Functional electrical stimulation applied to gluteus medius and tibialis anterior corresponding gait cycle for stroke. *Gait Posture* 36, 65–67. doi: 10.1016/j.gaitpost.2012.01.006

acquaniti, F., Ivanenko, Y. P., and Zago, M. (2012). Patterned control of human locomotion. *J. Physiol.* 590 (Pt 10), 2189–2199. doi: 10.1113/jphysiol.2011.215137

amontagne, A., and Fung, J. (2004). Faster is better: implications for speed-intensive gait training after stroke. *Stroke* 35, 2543–2548. doi: 10.1161/01.STR.0000144685.88760.d7

ee, D. D., and Seung, H. S. (1999). Learning the parts of objects by non-negative matrix factorization. *Nature* 401, 788–791. doi: 10.1038/44565

Melo, P. L., Silva, M. T., Martins, J. M., and Newman, D. J. (2015). Technical developments of functional electrical stimulation to correct drop foot: sensing, actuation and control strategies. *Clin. Biomech.* 30, 101–113. doi: 10.1016/j.clinbiomech.2014.11.007

Monaco, V., Ghionzoli, A., and Micera, S. (2010). Age-related modifications of muscle synergies and spinal cord activity during locomotion. *J. Neurophysiol.* 104, 2092–2102. doi: 10.1152/jn.00525.2009

Mussa-Ivaldi, F. A., and Bizzi, E. (2000). Motor learning through the combination of primitives. *Philos. Trans. R. Soc. Lond. B Biol. Sci.* 355, 1755–1769. doi: 10.1098/rstb.2000.0733

Neptune, R. R., Clark, J., and Kautz, S. A. (2009). Modular control of human walking: a simulation study. *J. Biomech.* 42, 1282–1287. doi: 10.1016/j.jbiomech.2009.03.009

O'Keeffe, D. T., Donnelly, A. E., and Lyons, G. M. (2003). The development of a potential optimized stimulation intensity envelope for drop foot applications. *IEEE Trans. Neural Syst. Rehabil. Eng.* 11, 249–256. doi: 10.1109/TNSRE.2003.817678

Oliveira, A. S., Gizzi, L., Farina, D., and Kersting, U. G. (2014). motor modules of human locomotion: influence of EMG averaging, concatenation, and number of step cycles. *Front. Human Neurosci.* 8:335. doi: 10.3389/fnhum.2014.00335

Olney, S. J., and Richards, C. (1996). Hemiparetic gait following stroke. Part I: characteristics. *Gait Posture* 4, 136–148. doi: 10.1016/0966-6362(96)01063-6

Perry, J., and Burnfield, J. M. (1992). *Gait Analysis: Normal and Pathological Function. 2nd Edn.* Thorofare, NJ: Slack Incorporated.

Ridding, M. C., Brouwer, B., Miles, T., S., Pitcher, J., B., and Thompson, P. D. (2000). Changes in muscle responses to stimulation of the motor cortex induced by peripheral nerve stimulation in human subjects. *Exp. Brain Res.* 131, 135–143. doi: 10.1007/s002219900269

Routson, R. L., Kautz, S. A., and Neptune, R. R. (2014). Modular organization across changing task demands in healthy and poststroke gait. *Physiol. Rep.* 2:e12055. doi: 10.14814/phy2.12055

Sabut, S. K., Sikdar, C., Kumar, R., and Mahadevappa, M. (2011). Functional electrical stimulation of dorsiflexor muscle: effects on dorsiflexor strength, plantarflexor spasticity, and motor recovery in stroke patients. *Neurorehabilitation* 29, 393–400. doi: 10.3233/NRE-2011-0717

Sabut, S. K., Sikdar, C., Mondal, R., Kumar, R., and Mahadevappa, M. (2010). Restoration of gait and motor recovery by functional electrical stimulation therapy in persons with stroke. *Disabil. Rehabil.* 32, 1594–1603. doi: 10.3109/09638281003599596

Safavynia, S. A., Torres-Oviedo, G., and Ting, L. H. (2011). Muscle synergies: implications for clinical evaluation and rehabilitation of movement. *Top. Spinal Cord Inj. Rehabil.* 17, 16–24. doi: 10.1310/sci1701-16

Santello, M., and Lang, C. E. (2014). Are movement disorders and sensorimotor injuries pathologic synergies? when normal multi-joint movement synergies become pathologic. *Front. Human Neurosci.* 8:1050. doi: 10.3389/fnhum.2014.01050

Sheffler, L. R., and Chae, J. (2007). Neuromuscular electrical stimulation in neurorehabilitation. *Muscle Nerve* 35, 562–590. doi: 10.1002/mus.20758

Tilson, J. K., Sullivan, K. J., Cen, S. Y., Rose, D. K., Koradia, C. H., Azen, S. P., et al. (2010). Meaningful gait speed improvement during the first 60 days poststroke: minimal clinically important difference. *Phys. Ther.* 90, 196–208. doi: 10.2522/ptj.20090079

Ting, L. H., Chiel, H. J., Trumbower, R. D., Allen, J. L., McKay, J. L., Hackney, M. E., et al. (2015). Neuromechanical principles underlying movement modularity and their implications for rehabilitation. *Neuron* 86, 38–54. doi: 10.1016/j.neuron.2015.02.042

16

Evoked Electromyographically Controlled Electrical Stimulation

Mitsuhiro Hayashibe *

Institut National de Recherche en Informatique et en Automatique (INRIA), University of Montpellier, Montpellier, France

Edited by:
Timothée Levi,
University of Bordeaux, France

Reviewed by:
Ping Zhou,
University of Texas Health Science Center at Houston, USA
Thierry Keller,
Tecnalia Research & Innovation, Spain

***Correspondence:**
Mitsuhiro Hayashibe
mitsuhiro.hayashibe@inria.fr

Time-variant muscle responses under electrical stimulation (ES) are often problematic for all the applications of neuroprosthetic muscle control. This situation limits the range of ES usage in relevant areas, mainly due to muscle fatigue and also to changes in stimulation electrode contact conditions, especially in transcutaneous ES. Surface electrodes are still the most widely used in noninvasive applications. Electrical field variations caused by changes in the stimulation contact condition markedly affect the resulting total muscle activation levels. Fatigue phenomena under functional electrical stimulation (FES) are also well known source of time-varying characteristics coming from muscle response under ES. Therefore, it is essential to monitor the actual muscle state and assess the expected muscle response by ES so as to improve the current ES system in favor of adaptive muscle-response-aware FES control. To deal with this issue, we have been studying a novel control technique using evoked electromyography (eEMG) signals to compensate for these muscle time-variances under ES for stable neuroprosthetic muscle control. In this perspective article, I overview the background of this topic and highlight important points to be aware of when using ES to induce the desired muscle activation regardless of the time-variance. I also demonstrate how to deal with the common critical problem of ES to move toward robust neuroprosthetic muscle control with the Evoked Electromyographically Controlled Electrical Stimulation paradigm.

Keywords: electrical stimulation, evoked electromyography, personalized stimulation, muscle activation control electrode effect cancelation

1. CHALLENGES IN TRANSCUTANEOUS (SURFACE) ELECTRICAL STIMULATION -AN INTRODUCTION

Electrical stimulation of the nervous system is a technique which is frequently used in physical therapy as it offers clinical diagnosis on neuromuscular activation, physiological investigation, and functional control of paralyzed extremities (Merletti et al., 1992). In diagnostic applications, it is used to ascertain the integrity of neuromuscular junctions and reflex loops, as well as the excitability of motor neuron pools, nerves, and muscle fibers (Merletti et al., 1992; DeLuca and Erim, 1994). In therapeutic treatments, continuous usage of electrical stimulation can help to maintain muscle volume and enhance blood circulation following lesions of the nervous system. It can prevent muscle atrophy due to non-use, which can readily occur in spinal cord injured patients, and also in stroke patients during the immobilization period. In orthotic treatments, electrical stimulation can be used to provide functional control of paralyzed muscles, which is called functional electrical stimulation (FES).

FES and neuroprosthetic muscle control have been used to compensate motor functions or produce movements in patients with complete spinal cord injury (SCI; Kobetic et al., 1997), as well as in stroke patients with other sensory-motor deficiencies such as drop foot syndrome (Liberson et al., 1961). In the late 1990s, progress in microprocessor technology provided the means for computer-controlled FES systems (Donaldson et al., 1997; Kobetic et al., 1997; Guiraud et al., 2006). Electrical stimulation strategies are wide-ranging, from implanted stimulation (Triolo et al., 1996; Johnston et al., 2003; Guiraud et al., 2006), spinal stimulation (North, 2008) to transcutaneous surface stimulation (Mangold et al., 2005). In real-world applications, transcutaneous surface stimulation (TES) is the most frequently applied technique for muscle and nerve activation despite the significant efforts made for implantable technology developments (Keller and Kuhn, 2008), simply because TES is an easier solution in practice. Electrodes are placed on the skin at locations where the underlying tissue is intended to be activated. Electrical current is injected through a pair of bipolar electrodes and generates a potential gradient over the targeted area. This artificially generated gradient depolarizes excitable tissue beneath the electrodes that serve as cathodes, thus activating the underlying muscles.

TES has already been popularly utilized for muscular massage purpose. Portable electrical stimulators for home use are widely commercially available. Impulses are generated by a device and delivered through electrodes on the skin in direct proximity to the muscles to be stimulated. TES has also been receiving increasing attention in the last few years because of its potential to serve as a muscle strength training tool for healthy subjects and athletes and as a preventive tool for partially immobilized patients (Maffiuletti et al., 2011). Strength training promotes neural and muscular adaptations that are complementary to the well-known effects of voluntary resistance training. These types of TES devices for muscular massage and strength training are technically equivalent to TES systems which are applied by clinical specialists for therapeutic and functional purposes.

Following the wide availability of TES, many people now have experience on testing transcutaneous surface electrodes for stimulation in massage or training settings. If one has experienced to use surface stimulation electrodes, he would likely have noticed that the muscle status under TES is sometimes suddenly changed by the electrode contact condition to the skin. This is indeed a universal problem in all TES applications. A slight contact condition change can markedly affect the real muscle activation status, even if the same stimulation input is constantly applied. This is related to the correct electrode placement issue, which can cause reduced muscle contraction, especially in dynamic muscle contractions (Keller and Kuhn, 2008). There have been many FES studies of TES applications, it ranges from foot drop correction (O'Keeffe et al., 2003; Azevedo Coste et al., 2014) to upper limb muscle control (Chan et al., 2009). However, in these TES papers, variations in actual muscle activation due to the electrode condition is normally ignored in real applications, as it is hard to deal with the time-variant muscle response issue. As many FES researchers/users frequently encounter muscle activation changes due to electrode effects in TES, it is not negligible level of effect in terms of muscle activation changes. This intra-subject variability in muscle activation under TES is due to electrode dependency. There is also inter-subject variability coming from the muscle strength differences between different subjects. An able-bodied subject's muscle response could be more substantial than the weak muscle response in motor-impaired subjects. This factor also limits the controllability of muscles by ES, a problem that should be addressed via personalized modeling for FES. In this perspective article, I introduce a way to capture muscle activation changes through the concept of Evoked Electromyographically Controlled Electrical Stimulation, which was previously developed to compensate for muscle fatigue variations under FES. I address these issues below by outlining the research studies that have been carried out so far:

1. Personalized Electrical Stimulation through Evoked Electromyography (EMG).
2. Muscle fatigue prediction and compensation in FES.
3. Muscle activation predictive control and cancelation of the stimulation electrode effect.

2. PERSONALIZED ELECTRICAL STIMULATION THROUGH EVOKED EMG

The challenge in implementing the present FES system arises with the problem of how to process the high nonlinearity and complexity of the neuro-muscular system (Durfee, 1993; Riener, 1999). Another challenge concerns time-varying muscle dynamics due to physiological and biochemical factors (such as fatigue, reflexes), as these need to be compensated in order to augment FES applications. Subject-specific modeling and time-variance compensation are essential to improve the performance of motor neuroprosthetics beyond the current limited use. A use of a mathematical model can improve the development of neuroprosthetics by optimizing their functionality for individual patients (Riener, 1999).

To achieve a reliable stimulation pattern and compensate muscle property changes during FES, in Ferrarin et al. (2001) the authors suggested using model-based approaches involving a feedforward controller to improve the control performance. In Jezernik et al. (2004), a sliding model closed-loop control method was proposed to control shank movement. In another work (Ajoudani and Erfanian, 2009), classic sliding model control and a neural network were combined to control FES to track the desired knee joint trajectory. A Feedback Error Learning controller for FES was developed by applying an antireset windup scheme (Watanabe and Fukushima, 2010). In a recent work (Freeman, 2014), iterative learning control was applied to control joint angles via stimulation of an arbitrary set of muscles with a Hammerstein-type muscle-activation recruitment relation.

Most closed-loop FES systems addressed in previous works were established between the electrical stimulus and joint angle since it is more convenient to measure and process the joint angle than joint torque or muscle force. However, in order to take the immediate effect of muscle activity induced by FES control into account, introducing biofeedback into closed-loops should be considered for further FES development (Bruns et al., 2013; Hayashibe et al., 2015), thus contributing to individualized modeling and control to manage different muscle responses from each different subject.

As muscle contraction is induced by artificial stimulation in FES, the drawback of closed-loop control of joint motion is that the resultant motion may not only derive from stimulation but also from external forces (such as environmental contact and gravity). The motion is the result of both external forces and the muscle contractions activated by the stimulation. The motion itself may not be directly related to the stimulation inputs. A stimulation pattern based only on motion signals is likely to be unsafe and unreliable in this case. In addition, it should be kept in mind that the muscle is a very slow actuator in terms of motion control. Error feedback by position information thus can not be instantly compensated, contrary to electromagnetic motor control in robotics. The muscle response to the same stimulation input is also not very consistent due to the physiological time-variant muscle response. Thus, considering the usage of biosignal feedback such as EMG from the muscle itself is a natural way for taking those potential physiological changes into account. By taking advantage of EMG signals, an EMG-triggered FES control system was presented through a pattern recognition (Dutta et al., 2008). This addresses mainly the FES start timing issue by using remained voluntary contractions rather than adapting the stimulation pattern itself. Then it does not handle time-variant muscle responses under FES.

Evoked EMG (eEMG) offers a way to study the myoelectric features of neuromuscular activation associated with electrical stimulation. Motor units activated by electrical stimulation have synchronous activity, with the so-called M-wave present in the EMG signal. When processing FES-evoked EMG signals, stimulation artifacts that appear at the onset of each stimulation impulse, and which are much larger than Mwaves, must be dealt with. In order to retrieve the signal of interest, i.e., M-waves, suitable techniques such as the blanking window method should be implemented to remove stimulation artifacts. The eEMG signal was found to be highly correlated with FES-induced muscular torque under various stimulation situations (Chesler and Durfee, 1997), and a similar phenomenon was also found in an implanted FES SCI subject (Hayashibe et al., 2011b). Moreover, M-waves extracted from the eEMG can be an effective detector for tracking potential muscle fatigue (Heasman et al., 2000). A pioneer work (Erfanian et al., 1998) proposed a predictive model of muscle force production under an isometric percutaneous continuous FES system. After comparing the performance of force prediction from stimulation and from EMG, the authors suggested using measured EMG signals instead of stimulation signals to predict muscle torque. This study was mainly carried out to predict joint torque as a kind of muscle force sensor in FES, and it has not yet been really used to achieve systematic FES closed-loop control based on evoked EMG. In our team, a new control strategy, i.e., EMG-Feedback Predictive Control (EFPC; Zhang et al., 2013), was proposed to adaptively control stimulation patterns to compensate time-varying muscle state changes. This facilitates the prediction of the muscle response and then the system can respond to time-variant muscle state changes toward muscle-response-aware FES control. It was further implemented combined with a wireless portable stimulator (Toussaint et al., 2010) to achieve real-time FES control (Li et al., 2015).

3. MUSCLE FATIGUE PREDICTION AND COMPENSATION IN FES

Muscle fatigue has been defined as a failure to maintain the required or expected force from a repeatedly activated muscle (Edwards, 1981). In voluntary contraction, a variety of biological and motivational factors contribute to muscle fatigue (Gandevia et al., 1995), such as reduced motor drive by the CNS, failure of peripheral electrical transmission, and failure of the muscular contractile mechanism. The rate of muscle fatigue during FES is much greater than that which occurs during natural contractions (Binder-Macleod and Snyder-Mackler, 1993). This fast fatigue phenomenon is complex and is not yet fully understood. Currently, it is understood as follows: (1) the inverse size principle, according to which artificial stimulation recruits the motor neurons from the largest to the smallest (Hamada et al., 2004), and the larger the motor neuron, the more fatigable the muscle fiber; (2) motor units are activated in a synchronized manner with artificial stimulation, which is different from asynchronous activation during natural contraction. This situation requires a much higher stimulation frequency in synchronous stimulation to achieve quasi-tetanic contraction. The high stimulation frequency causes fatigue; and (3) the constant order of recruitment, with fast fatigable motor units activated first, then slow fatigue-resistant motor units. Another factor related to fast fatigue with FES is that the fatigue resistance of paralyzed muscles decreases after injury (Pelletier and Hicks, 2011). Systematic fatigue monitoring is especially important in paraplegic patients suffering from a lack of sensory feedback from their paralyzed muscles, because it can be used to adjust stimulation to prevent failure. Second, force prediction is essential if the muscle force has to be used as feedback in closed-loop stimulation.

Various fatigue models have been drawn up, based on physiological and mathematical interpretation or fitting from experimental measurements. A biomechanical model was developed to predict the shank motion induced by FES (Riener et al., 1996). A five-element musculotendon model was developed to predict the force generation capacity of activated muscles and a fatigue recovery function based on the metabolic profile was introduced (Mizrahi et al., 1997). In Cai et al. (2010) a Wiener-Hammerstein model was proposed to predict FES induced muscle force in unfatigued and fatigued muscle, and the model was verified by stimulating Soleus in SCI patients.

Some researchers have attempted to predict force/torque variations with fatigue based on eEMG. An exponential function was proposed to predict the force of FES-activated quadriceps muscles from eEMG Peak-to-Peak (PTP; Mizrahi et al., 1994). PTP was suggested as a fatigue index at a constant cycling speed in (Chen and Yu, 1997). A close correlation between the EMG mean absolute value (MAV) and knee torque was found under continuous stimulation in paraplegic subjects (Erfanian et al., 1996). In their following work (Erfanian et al., 1998), they proposed a predictive model of muscle force production under an isometric percutaneous continuous FES system. A metabolic model was presented to predict force decline and recovery from EMG signals under intermittent condition (Levin and Mizrahi, 1999). In Ziai and Menon (2011), re-training the model was suggested to regain the high estimation quality lost as a result of degraded estimation accuracy over time. Therefore, the online estimation method proposed in this study is preferable to characterize muscle contraction dynamics for real-time FES control. However, the fatigue properties vary with different fatigue levels and recovery processes, which complicates the identification of the fatigue model. A fatigue model cannot work when the desired stimulation pattern is unknown in advance.

As in **Figure 1**, an online model estimation method is proposed for FES-induced torque prediction and muscle fatigue tracking through Kalman filter update (Zhang et al., 2011a,b). Muscle contraction dynamics modeled by a polynomial Hammerstein model (PHM) to represent joint torque from muscle activity based on evoked EMG, is updated systematically through Kalman filter with forgetting factor to correspond to the time-variant muscle contraction dynamics. This is further extended toward robust estimation with a nonlinear autoregressive with external input (NARX) model-based recurrent neural network (RNN) to predict torque with evoked EMG (Li et al., 2014b). The computational efficacy also makes it feasible for real-time implementation (Li et al., 2014a, 2016).

On the basis of the good predictive performance of the proposed estimation method, a new control strategy, i.e., EMG-Feedback Predictive Control, is proposed to explicitly control joint torque under FES (Hayashibe et al., 2011a; Zhang et al., 2013). Both muscle excitation and contraction dynamics are modeled by PHM. The eEMG signal is used for a dual-purpose: to correlate stimulation with the muscle electrical behavior in the muscle excitation process and to correlate the muscle electrical behavior with the muscle mechanical behavior in the muscle contraction process. Evoked EMG signal was used to feedback actual muscle states to track desired joint torque while considering the time-variant muscle dynamics. The EFPC control problem was resolved as a solution of two Nonlinear Predictive Control problems in series corresponding to activation and stimulation controller, respectively, as shown in **Figure 1**. The personalized models for excitation and contraction processes are developed for each subject for the model predictive controller to compute the inversed solutions. The activation controller solves the necessary muscle activation pattern to track the desired mechanical output reference. The stimulation controller solves the necessary stimulation sequence to achieve the necessary muscle activations. Once the torque deviates from the desired trajectory due to the effects of variations in muscle states such as fatigue, the controller adaptively generates the appropriate stimulation pattern in a systematic way to achieve the desired torque as long as it does not conflict with the stimulation constraints. This control framework provides satisfactory control accuracy and notable robustness in terms of joint torque control in FES (Zhang et al., 2013). This control strategy has a capacity to perform muscle fatigue compensation benefited from evoked EMG feedback.

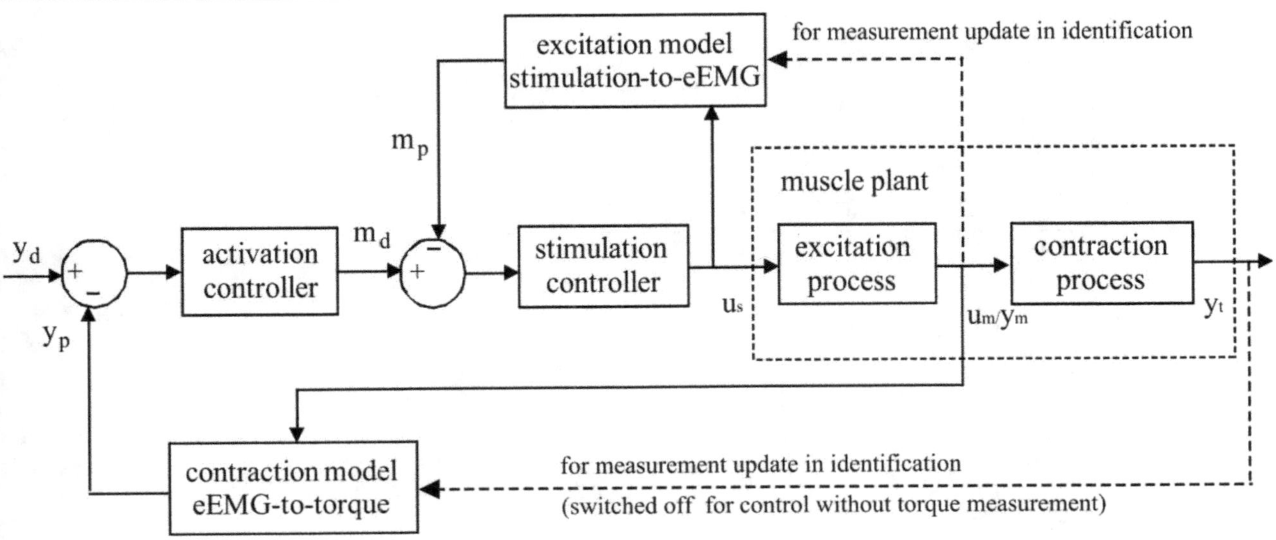

FIGURE 1 | Schematic representation of Evoked Electromyographically Controlled Electrical Stimulation. Muscle activation is explicitly modeled as an intermediate variable between the stimulation input and the mechanical torque output. Muscle activation is obtained through evoked Electromyography under FES. Personalized modeling is performed for one block of muscular excitation process between stimulation and eEMG, and also for the other block of contraction process between eEMG and joint torque. Through the established models, the inversed solutions of stimulation input sequence could be systematically generated with model-predictive controllers to follow the desired mechanical output reference.

4. MUSCLE ACTIVATION PREDICTIVE CONTROL AND CANCELATION OF THE STIMULATION ELECTRODE EFFECT

This section presents muscle activation closed-loop FES control through evoked EMG. It can be regarded as a simple version of EFPC regarding stimulation and muscle activation only.

This muscle activation control can present an advantage of Evoked Electromyographically Controlled Electrical Stimulation. In conventional FES, we normally specify the stimulation pattern and there is no way to check if the muscle is really responding as needed. As the electromagnetic motor is normally observed through the encoder, it is advantageous to monitor the reaction of muscles to electrical stimulation. Since evoked EMG can always be observable through the acquisition system, eEMG could be used for updating the stimulus-to-eEMG model. This could improve the modeling precision of the plant and guarantee the accuracy of the predictive model controller.

A real-time implementation of the predictive model controller for online control of muscle activation is as follows (Li et al., 2015):

1. The reference muscle activation trajectory is prepared before beginning estimation and control;
2. Trapezoidal shape pulse width stimulation at different amplitude levels is tested while recording the eEMG to personalize the model regarding the relationship between the pulse width and MAV of eEMG via Kalman filter;
3. After the identification phase ends, the FES system goes into control mode. The stimulator is driven by a predictive controller to modulate the pulse width to track the desired muscle activation trajectory while the stimulation-to-eEMG model is being updated to correspond to the time-variant properties.

In this way, muscle activation can be fully specified in the framework of Evoked Electromyographically Controlled Electrical Stimulation, instead of specifying the stimulation parameters. This can be useful to compensate for time-variant processes in FES. **Figure 2** shows an example of cancelation of the stimulation electrode effect. At the time 65 s, part of the electrode is suddenly detached without informing it to the system, as indicated by the circle. Muscle activation can be easily influenced by this situation. However, as the change is observed with evoked EMG signal from the targeted muscle (tibialis anterior), the controller systematically modifies the stimulation input to be increased so as to track the desired reference pattern of muscle activation. It is pulse width control then it may not fully cancel

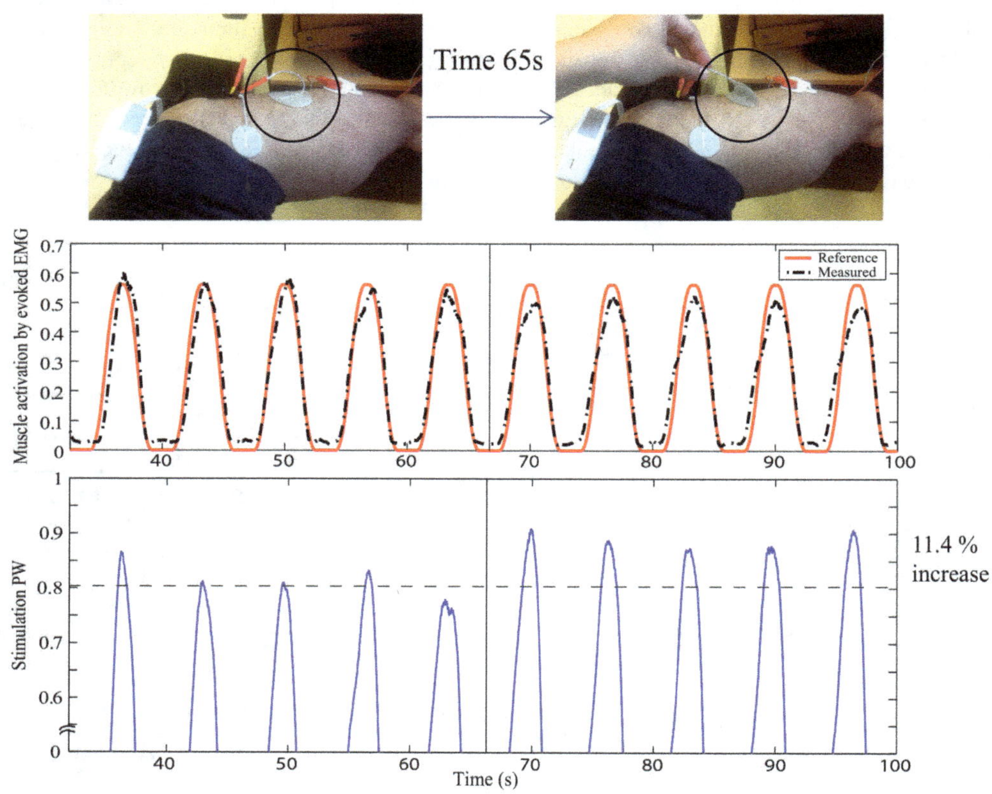

FIGURE 2 | Stimulation electrode effect cancelation in FES: The upper figure represents the experimental setup with typical foot drop correction montage for the stimulation electrode to stimulate the peroneal nerve for the dorsi flexion of the ankle. EMG is measured for the tibialis anterior muscle. At time 65 s, one electrode is detached, as indicated by the circle. The first plot shows the muscle activation obtained by evoked EMG. The second plot shows the stimulation pulse width. Y-axes are in normalized scale. Note that the stimulation is systematically modified to compensate for the effect of the electrode detachment. Muscle activation could thus still be maintained to minimize the effect of the stimulation field variation.

the effect but it could minimize the effect of sudden muscle activation changes by the detachment or the contact condition changes of the electrode. The stimulation electrodes are with typical montage for foot drop correction by FES.

5. CONCLUSION

Transcutaneous electrical stimulation (TES) is the technique most frequently applied for muscle and nerve activation. It is known that it has high sensitivity to the electrode contact condition for electrical stimulation. To compensate the intersubject (muscle strength) and intrasubject variability (stimulation electrode contact change, muscle fatigue), it is essential to monitor the real muscle responses under FES. Evoked Electromyographically Controlled Electrical Stimulation could be one solution to deal with this important issue. This framework contributes to augmenting the FES system in several aspects. First, an appropriate personalized muscle response model under FES (stim-emg, emg-torque) could be quickly established. Prediction of joint torque affected by muscle fatigue could be performed based on evoked EMG. This allows us to systematically compute and control electrical stimulation so as to achieve the desired muscle activation even under time-variant disturbances such as muscle fatigue and contact changes of stimulation electrode. An example of stimulation electrode effect cancelation was demonstrated to show the promising performance of Evoked Electromyographically Controlled Electrical Stimulation, which enables us to induce stable muscle activation in TES.

AUTHOR CONTRIBUTIONS

MH wrote the perspective article along with previous research activities he has performed as a PI of this work.

ACKNOWLEDGMENTS

The author thanks Dr. Qin Zhang (Huazhong University of Science and Technology, China) and Dr. Zhan Li (University of Electronic Science and Technology of China, China) for their contributions during the PhD studies at our team, and Dr. David Guiraud (INRIA, France) for helpful discussions.

REFERENCES

Ajoudani, A., and Erfanian, A. (2009). A neuro-sliding-mode control With adaptive modeling of uncertainty for control of movement in paralyzed limbs using functional electrical stimulation. *IEEE Trans. Biomed. Eng.* 56, 1771–1780. doi: 10.1109/TBME.2009.2017030

Azevedo Coste, C., Jovic, J., Pissard-Gibollet, R., and Froger, J. (2014). Continuous gait cycle index estimation for electrical stimulation assisted foot drop correction. *J. Neuroeng. Rehabil.* 11:118. doi: 10.1186/1743-0003-11-118

Binder-Macleod, S., and Snyder-Mackler, L. (1993). Muscle fatigue: clinical implications for fatigue assessment and neuromuscular electrical stimulation. *Phys. Ther.* 73, 902–910.

Bruns, T. M., Wagenaar, J. B., Bauman, M. J., Gaunt, R. A., and Weber, D. J. (2013). Real-time control of hind limb functional electrical stimulation using feedback from dorsal root ganglia recordings. *J. Neural Eng.* 10:026020. doi: 10.1088/1741-2560/10/2/026020

Cai, Z. J., Bai, E.-W., and Shields, R. K. (2010). Fatigue and non-fatigue mathematical muscle models during functional electrical stimulation of paralyzed muscle. *Biomed. Signal Process. Control* 5, 87–93. doi: 10.1016/j.bspc.2009.12.001

Chan, M. K.-L., Tong, R. K.-Y., and Chung, K. Y.-K. (2009). Bilateral upper limb training with functional electric stimulation in patients with chronic stroke. *Neurorehabil. Neural Repair* 23, 357–365. doi: 10.1177/1545968308326428

Chen, J. J., and Yu, N. Y. (1997). The validity of stimulus-evoked EMG for studying muscle fatigue characteristics of paraplegic subjects during dynamic cycling movement. *IEEE Trans. Rehabil. Eng.* 5, 170–178. doi: 10.1109/86.593288

Chesler, N. C., and Durfee, W. K. (1997). Surface EMG as a fatigue indicator during FES-induced isometric muscle contractions. *J. Electromyogr. Kinesiol.* 7, 27–37. doi: 10.1016/S1050-6411(96)00016-8

DeLuca, C. J., and Erim, Z. (1994). Common drive of motor units in regulation of muscle force. *Trends Neurosci.* 17, 299–305. doi: 10.1016/0166-2236(94)90064-7

Donaldson, N. D., Perkins, T. A., and Worley, A. C. (1997). Lumbar root stimulation for restoring leg function: stimulator and measurement of muscle actions. *Artif. Organs* 21, 247–249. doi: 10.1111/j.1525-1594.1997.tb04660.x

Durfee, W. K. (1993). Control of standing and gait using electrical stimulation: influence of muscle model complexity on control strategy. *Prog. Brain Res.* 97, 369–381. doi: 10.1016/S0079-6123(08)62296-7

Dutta, A., Kobetic, R., and Triolo, R. J. (2008). Ambulation after incomplete spinal cord injury with EMG-triggered functional electrical stimulation. *IEEE Trans. Biomed. Eng.* 55, 791–794. doi: 10.1109/TBME.2007.902225

Edwards, R. H. (1981). Human muscle function and fatigue. *Ciba Found. Symp.* 82, 1–18.

Erfanian, A., Chizeck, H. J., and Hashemi, R. M. (1996). "Excitation-contraction fatigue during sustained electrical stimulation of paralyzed muscle," in *Proceedings of the 18th Annual International Conference of the IEEE Engineering in Medicine and Biology Society (EMBC96)*, Vol. 4 (Amsterdam), 1460–1461.

Erfanian, A., Chizeck, H. J., and Hashemi, R. M. (1998). Using evoked EMG as a synthetic force sensor of isometric electrically stimulated muscle. *IEEE Trans. Biomed. Eng.* 45, 188–202.

Ferrarin, M., Palazzo, F., Riener, R., and Quintern, J. (2001). Model-based control of FES induced single joint movements. *IEEE Trans. Neural Syst. Rehabil. Eng.* 9, 245–257. doi: 10.1109/7333.948452

Freeman, C. (2014). Newton-method based iterative learning control for robot-assisted rehabilitation using FES. *Mechatronics* 24, 934–943. doi: 10.1016/j.mechatronics.2014.04.001

Gandevia, S., Enoka, R. M., McComas, A. J., Stuart, D. G., and Thomas, C. K., (eds.). (1995). *Fatigue: Neural and Muscular Mechanisms*. New York, NY: Plenum Press.

Guiraud, D., Stieglitz, T., Koch, K. P., Divoux, J.-L., and Rabischong, P. (2006). An implantable neuroprosthesis for standing and walking in paraplegia: 5-year patient follow-up. *J. Neural. Eng.* 3, 268–275. doi: 10.1088/1741-2560/3/4/003

Hamada, T., Kimura T., and Moritani, T. (2004). Selective fatigue of fast motor units after electrically elicited muscle contractions. *J. Electromyogr. Kinesiol.* 14, 531–538. doi: 10.1016/j.jelekin.2004.03.008

Hayashibe, M., Guiraud, D., Pons, J. L., and Farina, D. (2015). Editorial: biosignal processing and computational methods to enhance sensory motor neuroprosthetics. *Front. Neurosci.* 9:434. doi: 10.3389/fnins.2015.00434

Hayashibe, M., Zhang, Q., and Azevedo-Coste, C. (2011a). "Dual predictive control of electrically stimulated muscle using biofeedback for drop foot correcti," in *Proceeding in IEEE/RSJ International Conference on Intelligent Robots and Systems* (San Francisco), 1731–1736.

Hayashibe, M., Zhang, Q., Guiraud, D., and Fattal, C. (2011b). Evoked EMG based torque prediction under muscle fatigue in implanted neural stimulation. *J. Neural Eng.* 8, 6. doi: 10.1088/1741-2560/8/6/064001

Heasman, J. M., Scott, T. R. D., Vare, V. A., Flynn, R. Y., Gschwind, C. R., Middleton, J. W., et al. (2000). Detection of fatigue in the isometric electrical activation of paralyzed hand muscles of persons with tetraplegia. *IEEE Trans. Neural Syst. Rehabil. Eng.* 8, 286–296. doi: 10.1109/86.867870

Jezernik, S., Wassink, G. V., and Keller, T. (2004). Sliding mode closed-loop control of FES: controlling the Shank movement. *IEEE Trans. Biomed. Eng.* 51, 263–272. doi: 10.1109/TBME.2003.820393

Johnston, T. E., Betz, R. R., Smith, B. T., and Mulcahey, M. J. (2003). Implanted functional electrical stimulation: an alternative for standing and walking in pediatric spinal cord injury. *Spinal Cord* 41, 144–152. doi: 10.1038/sj.sc.3101392

Keller, T., and Kuhn, A. (2008). Electrodes for transcutaneous (surface) electrical stimulation. *J. Automatic Control* 18, 35–45. doi: 10.2298/JAC0802035K

Kobetic, R., Triolo, R. J., and Marsolais, E. B. (1997). Muscle selection and walking performance of multichannel FES systems for ambulation in paraplegia. *IEEE Trans. Rehabil. Eng.* 5, 23–29. doi: 10.1109/86.559346

Levin, O., and Mizrahi, J. (1999). EMG and metabolite-based prediction of force in paralyzed quadriceps muscle under interrupted stimulation. *IEEE Trans. Rehabil. Eng.* 7, 301–314.

Li, Z., Guiraud, D., Andreu, D., Benoussaad, M., Fattal, C., and Hayashibe, M. (2016). Real-time estimation of FES-induced joint torque with evoked EMG-application to spinal cord injured patients. *J. Neuroeng. Rehabil.* 13:60. doi: 10.1186/s12984-016-0169-y

Li, Z., Hayashibe, M., Andreu, D., and Guiraud, D. (2014a). "A system for real-time estimation of joint torque with evoked EMG under electrical stimulation," in *Replace, Repair, Restore, Relieve Bridging Clinical and Engineering Solutions in Neurorehabilitation SE - 76*, volume 7 of *Biosystems & Biorobotics*, eds W. Jensen, O. K. Andersen, and M. Akay (Springer International Publishing), 513–520.

Li, Z., Hayashibe, M., Andreu, D., and Guiraud, D. (2015). "Real-time closed-loop FES control of muscle activation with evoked EMG feedback," in *7th International IEEE/EMBS Conference on Neural Engineering (NER), 2015* (Montpellier), 623–626.

Li, Z., Hayashibe, M., Fattal, C., and Guiraud, D. (2014b). Muscle fatigue tracking with evoked EMG via recurrent neural network: toward personalized neuroprosthetics. *IEEE Comput. Intell. Mag.* 9, 38–46. doi: 10.1109/MCI.2014.2307224

Liberson, W., Holmquest, H., and Scott, M. (1961). Functional electrotherapy: stimulation of the common peroneal nerve synchronised with the swing phase of gait of hemiplegic subjects. *Arch. Phys. Med. Rehabil.* 42, 202–205.

Maffiuletti, N. A., Minetto, M. A., Farina, D., and Bottinelli, R. (2011). Electrical stimulation for neuromuscular testing and training: state-of-the art and unresolved issues. *Eur. J. Appl. Physiol.* 111, 2391–2397. doi: 10.1007/s00421-011-2133-7

Mangold, S., Keller, T., Curt, A., and Dietz, V. (2005). Transcutaneous functional electrical stimulation for grasping in subjects with cervical spinal cord injury. *Spinal Cord* 43, 1–13. doi: 10.1038/sj.sc.3101644

Merletti, R., Knaflitz, M., and DeLuca, C. J. (1992). Electrically evoked myoelectric signals. *Crit. Rev. Biomed. Eng.* 19, 293–340.

Mizrahi, J., Levy, M., Ring, H., Isakov, E., and Liberson, A. (1994). EMG as an indicator of fatigue in isometrically FES-activated paralyzed muscles. *IEEE Trans. Neural Syst. Rehabil.* 2, 57–65. doi: 10.1109/86.313147

Mizrahi, J., Seelenfreund, D., Isakov, E., and Susak, Z. (1997). Predicted and measured muscle forces after recoveries of differing durations following fatigue in functional electrical stimulation. *Artif. Organs* 21, 236–239.

North, R. (2008). Neural interface devices: spinal cord stimulation technology. *Proc. IEEE* 96, 1108–1119. doi: 10.1109/JPROC.2008.922558

O'Keeffe, D. T., Donnelly, A. E., and Lyons, G. M. (2003). The development of a potential optimized stimulation intensity envelope for drop foot applications. *IEEE Trans. Neural Syst. Rehabil. Eng.* 11, 249–256. doi: 10.1109/TNSRE.2003.817678

Pelletier, C., and Hicks, A. L. (2011). Muscle fatigue characteristics in paralyzed muscle after spinal cord injury. *Spinal Cord* 49, 125–130. doi: 10.1038/sc.2010.62

Riener, R. (1999). Model-based development of neuroprosthesis for paraplegic patients. *Philos. Trans. R. Soc. Lond. Series B Biol. Sci.* 354, 877–894. doi: 10.1098/rstb.1999.0440

Riener, R., Quintern, J., and Schmidt, G. (1996). Biomechanical model of the human knee evaluated by neuromuscular stimulation. *J. Biomech.* 29, 1157–1167. doi: 10.1016/0021-9290(96)00012-7

Toussaint, M., Andreu, D., Fraisse, P., and Guiraud, D. (2010). "Wireless distributed architecture for therapeutic functional electrical Stimulation: a technology to design network-based muscle control," in *Engineering in Medicine and Biology Society (EMBC), 2010 Annual International Conference of the IEEE* (Buenos Aires: IEEE), 6218–6221.

Triolo, R., Bieri, C., Uhlir, J., Kobetic, R., Scheiner, A., and Marsolais, E. (1996). Implanted functional neuromuscular stimulation systems for individuals with cervical spinal cord injuries: clinical case reports. *Arch. Phys. Med. Rehabil.* 77, 1119–1128. doi: 10.1016/S0003-9993(96)90133-1

Watanabe, T., and Fukushima, K. (2010). An approach to applying feedback error learning for functional electrical stimulation controller: computer simulation tests of wrist joint control. *Adv. Artif. Neural Syst.* 2010, 1–8. doi: 10.1155/2010/814702

Zhang, Q., Hayashibe, M., and Azevedo-Coste, C. (2013). Evoked electromyography-based closed-loop torque control in functional electrical stimulation. *IEEE Trans. Biomed. Eng.* 60, 2299–2307. doi: 10.1109/TBME.2013.2253777

Zhang, Q., Hayashibe, M., Fraisse, P., and Guiraud, D. (2011a). FES-induced torque prediction with evoked EMG sensing for muscle fatigue tracking. *IEEE/ASME Trans. Mechatron.* 16, 816–826. doi: 10.1109/TMECH.2011.2160809

Zhang, Q., Hayashibe, M., and Guiraud, D. (2011b). "Muscle fatigue tracking based on stimulus evoked EMG and adaptive torque prediction," in *Proceeding of IEEE International Conference on Robotics and Automation (ICRA 2011)* (Shanghai), 1433–1438.

Ziai, A., and Menon, C. (2011). Comparison of regression models for estimation of isometric wrist joint torques using surface electromyography. *J. Neuroeng. Rehabil.* 8:56. doi: 10.1186/1743-0003-8-56

17

A Review of Control Strategies in Closed-Loop Neuroprosthetic Systems

James Wright[1]*, *Vaughan G. Macefield*[1,2,3], *André van Schaik*[1] *and Jonathan C. Tapson*[1]

[1] *Biomedical Engineering and Neuroscience, The MARCS Institute, University of Western Sydney, Sydney, NSW, Australia,* [2] *School of Medicine, University of Western Sydney, Sydney, NSW, Australia,* [3] *Neuroscience Research Australia, Sydney, NSW, Australia*

Edited by:
Michela Chiappalone,
Istituto Italiano di Tecnologia, Italy

Reviewed by:
Paolo Del Giudice,
Italian National Institute of Health, Italy
Dennis J. McFarland,
Wadsworth Center for Laboratories and Research, USA

***Correspondence:**
James Wright
james.wright@uws.edu.au

It has been widely recognized that closed-loop neuroprosthetic systems achieve more favorable outcomes for users then equivalent open-loop devices. Improved performance of tasks, better usability, and greater embodiment have all been reported in systems utilizing some form of feedback. However, the interdisciplinary work on neuroprosthetic systems can lead to miscommunication due to similarities in well-established nomenclature in different fields. Here we present a review of control strategies in existing experimental, investigational and clinical neuroprosthetic systems in order to establish a baseline and promote a common understanding of different feedback modes and closed-loop controllers. The first section provides a brief discussion of feedback control and control theory. The second section reviews the control strategies of recent Brain Machine Interfaces, neuromodulatory implants, neuroprosthetic systems, and assistive neurorobotic devices. The final section examines the different approaches to feedback in current neuroprosthetic and neurorobotic systems.

Keywords: neuroprosthetics, control theory, closed-loop, brain-machine interface, feedback

INTRODUCTION

A neuroprosthetic is a device or system that has an interface with the nervous system and supplements or substitutes functionality in the patient's body. For the purpose of this review we have included neuromodulatory systems and brain computer interfaces under the general description of neuroprosthetics, as well as rehabilitation systems such as exoskeletons. The key identifying characteristic of the neuroprosthetic is that it has an interface with the subject's nervous system, as distinct from an implantable devices such as an pacemaker or an insulin pump. Consequently there are a broad range of devices that we consider neuroprosthetics. To date there have been a number of reviews of neuroprosthetic systems. There is significant literature on classification algorithms and detection strategies (Schwartz, 2004; Lotte et al., 2007; Green and Kalaska, 2011; Borton et al., 2014; Morimoto and Kawato, 2015), including comparison and evaluation of the relative strengths of different approaches. However, there are fewer examinations the authors are aware of that investigate the different control approaches that have been implemented in neuroprosthetic settings. Performing such a review is made more difficult due to the small number of studies that have compared different control approaches within the same experiment, and the fact that many neuroprosthetic studies have by necessity been conducted with very small sample sizes, sometimes involving a single subject. Additionally many of the devices examined in this review are experimental or investigational, and are not yet in use in clinical or therapeutic settings (Sun and Morrell, 2014).

When considering these devices in the context of control and feedback it can be helpful to place them along a number of axes (**Figure 1**) to partition the large variety of systems and approaches. The first axis we have considered is the location of the interface with the nervous system, with the Central Nervous System (CNS) subdivided into the brain and the spinal cord, and then the Peripheral Nervous System (PNS), consisting of afferent and efferent pathways. Along this axis and additional distinction can be drawn between single channel systems that use a single electrode as the interface to the subject's nervous system, and multichannel systems which utilize many parallel channels for interface. Finally the channel can be unidirectional for simplex communication, or bidirectional for half-duplex, or full duplex communication.

Another axis to consider is the invasiveness of the interface. At one end we place noninvasive interfaces such as Electroencephlogram (EEG), Magnetic Resonance Imaging (MRI), and Electromyography (EMG). These interfaces are hampered by a variety of issues, including low spatial resolution and low signal to noise ratios. The advantage they enjoy is that they can be deployed with little risk, which has meant they are a popular platform for neuroprosthetic development. Next are minimally invasive interfaces such as microwire EMG and microneurographic recordings from the PNS. With a more invasive interface there are better quality signals, but still minimal intervention with the subject's body, reducing risk of complications. These interfaces are susceptible to movement, leading to changes in the quality of the recorded signal. The most invasive interfaces require surgical implantation, and come with risks associated with surgery as well as risk of damage to the part of the nervous system. Within this category a distinction can be drawn between the less invasive, such as cuff electrodes around PNS sites and Electrocorticogram (ECog)—these interfaces do not disrupt the blood brain barrier; and the more invasive Multi Electrode Arrays (MEA) in PNS nerves, motor or somatosensory cortex, Deep Brain Stimulators (DBS) to treat Parkinson's Disease with electrodes in the Globus Pallidus, Sub Thalamic Nucleus, or the Pedunculopontine Nucleus. These multichannel interfaces offer high resolution, but comparatively small spatial coverage (Krook-Magnuson et al., 2015). These electrodes come with risks that are still not fully understood. These primarily involve the physical trauma due to the insertion of the electrode, with effects occurring over different timescales. Shortly after insertion there is bleeding and swelling, as well as physical damage to neurons (Fernandez et al., 2014). Over longer timescales the presence of the recording device compromises the blood-brain barrier, allowing ingress of cellular and molecular components from elsewhere in the body (Schwartz, 2004). Additionally the long term stability of the recording site is often compromised, due to immune and mechanical actions on the microelectrodes (Krook-Magnuson et al., 2015). At the furthest extent of this axis are the interfaces that reconfigure the subject's nervous system. Targeted Muscle Reinnervation (TMR) surgically rewires an amputee subject's PNS, by deinnervating muscles that have no biomechanical role after the amputation and redirecting the preserved nerves from the amputated limb to the deinnervated muscles (Kuiken et al., 2009), allowing for high quality EMG recordings as control inputs to a prosthetic. Optogenetic techniques offer a non-electrical interface to neurons, by using light to activate special ion-channels. This technique enables individual neurons to be targeted, which is extremely difficult with cortical microelectrodes, as well as the

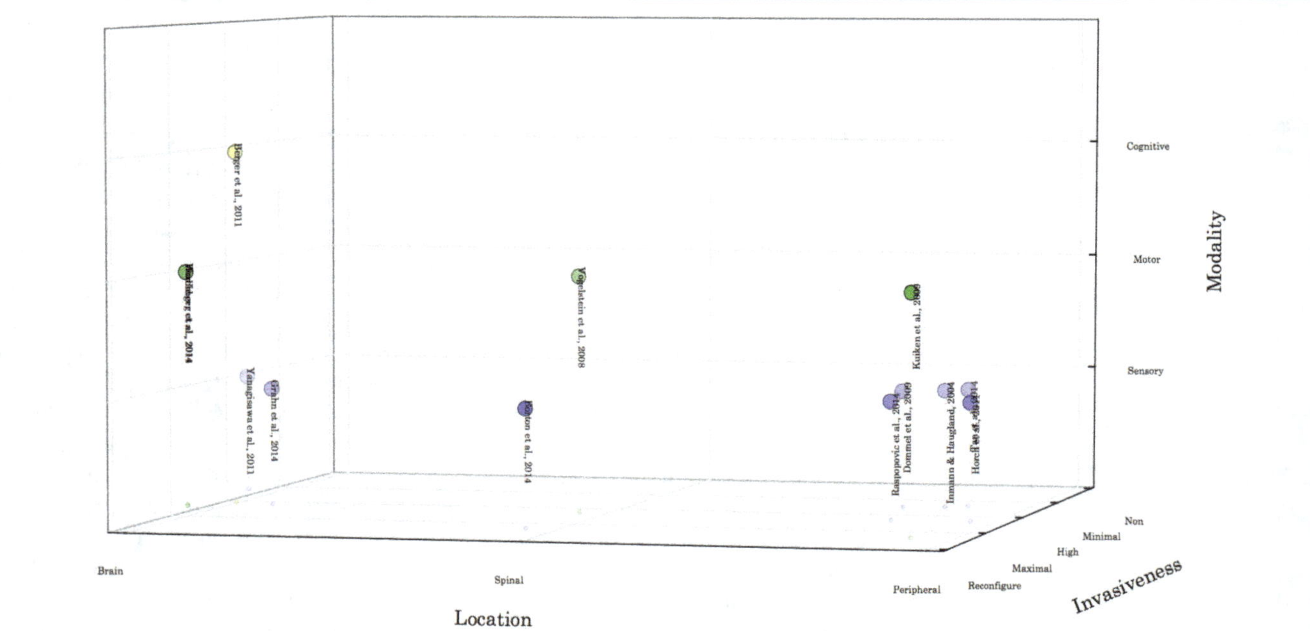

FIGURE 1 | Neuroprosthetic Systems. An illustration of the conceptual space of neuroprosthetic devices. Devices can be classified as similar if they provide assistance in the same Modality, have an equivalent level of Invasiveness, or interface with the user's nervous system in the same Location.

possibility of selectively activating a class of neurons such as excitatory neurons instead of inhibitory (Krook-Magnuson et al., 2015). However, optogentic approaches require the introduction of genes that encode for light activated ion-channels (Deisseroth, 2011), and the issues associated with this may preclude this technique in humans.

The final axis is the modality of the prosthesis. Sensory neuroprosthetics offer input from artificial sensors, as in a cochlear implant or bionic eye, or modulate sensory input as is the case in neurostimulators for treating chronic pain. Systems to treat motor impairment are frequently referred to as Brain Machine Interfaces (BMI) or Brain Computer Interfaces (BCI) and infer motor intent from the subject in order to control a virtual or physical effector. Cognitive devices modulate the activity of the CNS and include devices such as DBS stimulators for Parkinson's Disease, depression, and hippocampal stimulators for memory.

NEUROPROSTHETICS

The following examples are representative, but not exhaustive, and are placed in **Figure 1** to illustrate the wide variety of devices that can be described as having a neuroprosthetic interface. Many of these devices are experimental demonstrations, and not clinically approved interventions. Adjacent to the choice of controller, there are choices about the location and method for acquiring a suitable input signal (Grill et al., 2009; Andersen et al., 2010), and questions about the consequences of long term use of these and similar devices that have not yet been answered.

Peripheral nervous system interfaces are attractive as they are less invasive than the central nervous system alternatives, while still offering a rich source of information for neuroprosthetic control. Inmann and Haugland (2004) used a cuff electrode around the median nerve to record nerve activation due to touch and that input was used to modulate the Functional Electrical Stimulation of the subjects muscles. Horch et al. (2011) demonstrated that human subjects who were provided with intrafascicular electrical stimulation of the median and ulnar nerves derived from sensors on a myoelectric prosthetic limb were able to use the feedback to perform object recognition tasks by digital manipulation. Tan et al. (2014) used non-penetrating cuff electrodes on the median, ulnar and radial nerves of human subjects to provide natural sensations of touch while operating a myoelectric prosthetic allowing for improved performance of manual tasks. Raspopovic et al. (2014) showed that a bidirectional interface with the median and ulnar nerves could be used to provide artificial sensory feedback related to the forces exerted on a sensorized prosthetic limb, and that the artificial sensations allowed the subject to improve their ability to sense characteristics of the objects being manipulated. Targeted Muscle Reinnervation generates a rich high density signal for surface Electromyography (EMG) that enables simultaneous operation of multiple degrees of freedom in a myoelectric prosthetic limb (Kuiken et al., 2009). The tissue serves as a bioamplifier for the nerve signal, allowing a large array of surface electrodes to be deployed on the subject. The array provides a rich signal suitable for pattern recognition, and combined with a high performance prosthetic limb gives the subject an improved experience. As a sensory modality prosthetic, (Dommel et al., 2009) are testing a vision prosthesis for electrical stimulation of the retina. Spinal cord stimulation may be able to generate gait patterns suitable for locomotion in paralyzed patients. Vogelstein et al. (2008) describes the design of a system that is capable of generating primitive locomotion in anesthetized felines. Borton et al. (2014) developed an electrochemical spinal neuroprosthesis to reactivate the circuits in a damaged spinal cord, allowing hindlimb movement sufficient to enable walking in paralyzed rats.

Yanagisawa et al. (2011) used ECog electrodes placed over the sensorimotor cortex of a stroke patient in order to control a supernumerary robotic hand that was able to mimic the hand posture of the subject. Berger et al. (2011) implanted microwire electrodes in the hippocampus of rats and recorded the activity while the animals were trained to complete a memory task. Subsequent stimulation of the electrodes according to the trained model improved the performance of the rats at the cognitive task. Neuromodulators for Deep Brain Stimulation have been used to treat the symptoms of Parkinson's disease and depression (Grahn et al., 2014). Multi Electrode Arrays implanted in motor cortex have been successfully used to acquire signals for the multi degree of freedom control of robotic limbs (Hochberg et al., 2012; Wodlinger et al., 2015). Guggenmos et al. (2013) describe a Brain Machine Brain Interface in rats that utilizes microwire recordings from a premotor area to detect spiking activity leading to stimulation of the somatosensory area. The Activity Dependant Stimulation via the neuroprosthetic prototype enabled rats with injury to the motor area to recover reach and grasp behavior.

This list of devices is not exhaustive, and serves only to illustrate the different axes of Modality, Invasiveness and Location when considering neuroprosthetic designs. For a more thorough description of the available neuroprosthetic devices and interface technologies, the reader is directed to the following excellent reviews (Navarro et al., 2005; Grill et al., 2009; Micera et al., 2010; Ortiz-Catalan et al., 2012). These reviews focus on the interface techniques with the nervous system, and provide a detailed discussion of the limits of current interfaces.

INTRODUCTION TO CONTROL

The design of a neuroprosthetic varies significantly between different modalities. Because it is a multidisciplinary field often the language used to describe the system can vary between devices. The terms "closed-loop," "feedback," and "online" may take on different meanings. Identifying and acquiring a suitable input signal is a non-trivial task (Krook-Magnuson et al., 2015). This makes the fabrication of a substitute system in the case of impairment a complex endeavor. Developing a suitable simplified model for embodiment as an open-loop system is often a first step. But it is not always straightforward; take motor control as example—many models of muscles exist. Highly biophysical models (such as cross-bridge models) of muscles become large systems of non-linear differential equations when describing whole muscles or limbs (Ionescu and De Keyser, 2006). Similarly modeling the individual neurons that act as part of the Basal Ganglia, in a complex network of interconnections across the CNS (Broccard et al., 2014), rapidly becomes an intractable problem when developing an open-loop model for DBS to treat Parkinson's Disease. As a consequence the Basal Ganglia has often been modeled internally by a neurologist (Hosain et al., 2014), rather than explicitly within the DBS device, with stimulation parameters adjusted by the clinician observing the patient's symptoms instead of in response to a model. It is also possible that the control problem for a given neuroprosthetic has more than a single loop that needs to be considered, possibly due to the interaction of different physiological systems and different timescales (Houk, 1988). In this case control may best be achieved by a hierarchy of controllers, or a series of adaptive controllers that can be tuned at different stages of design (McFarland et al., 2006).

Nervous System Control

All parts of the human body have evolved to operate by extremely complex closed-loop control. Different subsystems, such as the cardiovascular system or the immune system operate under closed-loop control, with sensors and effectors operating at micro (LeDuc et al., 2011) and macroscopic scales (Houk, 1988). Sensory organs can be directly connected to the nervous system, such as stretch receptors, or they can be indirectly coupled by messenger systems such as hormone signaling. Command of these systems can be voluntary, or have a voluntary component, but they may also be completely automatic. Substituting or supplementing the performance of an element of the body is the aim of a neuroprosthetic device. Achieving this involves the fabrication of an effector, such as a prosthetic limb, that can replicate at least a subset of the body's functionality. But there is no function without control, so it is also necessary to model, and potentially integrate with, the different control loops within the human body. There has been some good success with simpler systems, possibly due to the high level state abstraction of the control within the nervous system (Holinski et al., 2013), as in the control of the hand. By examining the joint angles for fingers during different hand postures (grasping different objects) using principal component analysis it has been shown that the first 3 principal components can account for 90% of the variability. However, the grasp posture data describes the hand only in the final state, it does not describe the trajectory the fingers took to achieve the position around the object. When joint angle data was recorded continuously from subjects performing natural hand movements, 8–9 principal components were needed to describe 90% of the variance (Danziger, 2014). Thus, classifying hand states, and transitioning between fixed postures in a prosthetic is a more straightforward task than attempting the dexterous control of individual fingers (Aggarwal et al., 2011). Although we can treat a robotic effector as part of the body and nervous system of the operator, all current techniques for recording neural activity involve the projection of the high dimensional space of hundreds to thousands of neurons down through the recording electrode array to the much lower dimensionality of the end point of the effector (Carmena, 2013).

Feedforward Control

Feedforward or open-loop control generates a command for the plant that is expected to produce the correct output. However, there is no measurement of the output from the plant, and hence no measurement of error, so the controller has no mechanism to modulate a command (Houk, 1988). A block diagram of open-loop control is shown as **Figure 2**. Implicit within open-loop control is the assumption of a perfectly described system that can be used to generate a control. Leaving aside the difficulties in creating a perfect model of any system, open-loop approaches do not take noise or measurement error into account.

Feedback Control

Feedback, or closed-loop control requires the inclusion of sensors in the system under control. The feedback controller generates a command for the plant, and the sensors measure the output of the plant in response to the command. If a measurement, such as the angle of a joint differs from the expected output, then the error signal can be used by the feedback controller to modify the generated commands. There are many mathematical approaches that can be used to modify feedback controller output (Crago et al., 1996).

Adaptive Control

Adaptive control can be applied to both feedforward and feedback controllers. By using sensors to measure the input and output of the system adaptive control strategies seek to adjust the controller in response to perturbations in the environment or the controlled system (Crago et al., 1996). Adaptive controllers enable the development of a control strategy without requiring complete knowledge of the system being controlled, however, as a consequence adaptive controllers are rarely optimal.

Internal Model Control

Internal Model Control (IMC) is an approach to feedback controller design that incorporates a model of the system that

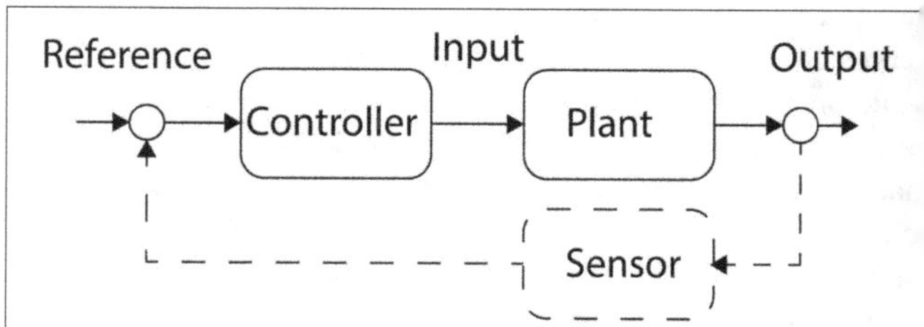

FIGURE 2 | Feedforward and Feedback Control. Feedforward or open-loop control is shown here in the solid line. The controller generates a command that is applied to the system, or Plant. In response to the command the system performs an action at the Output. Closed-loop or feedback control is achieved by the inclusion of the Sensor component, shown here as the dashed line. The Sensor measures the Output enabling the Controller to assess the error and adjust the next Input to the Plant.

is being controlled (García et al., 1989). The model can be developed based only on the relationship between the inputs and outputs of the system, or alternatively a partial model or complete model of the system can be utilized (LeDuc et al., 2011). At each time step the internal model is evaluated forward to a horizon, offering a prediction of the system behavior in response to the controller's input, and the control inputs are evaluated against a cost function to find the optimum command to be executed at the next time step (Pan et al., 2015). A block diagram illustrates IMC as **Figure 3**.

Classification

A Classifier breaks a system into discrete states, and maps a relationship between an input and a system state (Schwartz, 2004). Classifiers can be supervised or unsupervised. Supervised systems are trained on an input-output relationship in a data set, and attempt to generalize the relationship to new data, while unsupervised systems attempt to partition or cluster the dataset.

Actor-Critic

The Actor-Critic architecture separates the control policy from the evaluation of the action. The Actor component of the systems choses a policy, which affects the state of the system. The Critic component assesses the state of the system in accordance with a cost function, and provides the evaluation to the Actor (Mahmoudi and Sanchez, 2011). The goal based evaluation differs from the error signal of other control approaches, and does not require that the Actor has a model of the system's behavior (Mahmoudi et al., 2013).

CONTROL ALGORITHMS

Table 1 summarizes the Control Algorithms.

Control policies can be implemented by classification, model independent, or model based approaches (Kameneva et al., 2015).

Control Policies with Independent Models

Consider the system state to be independent at each time step.

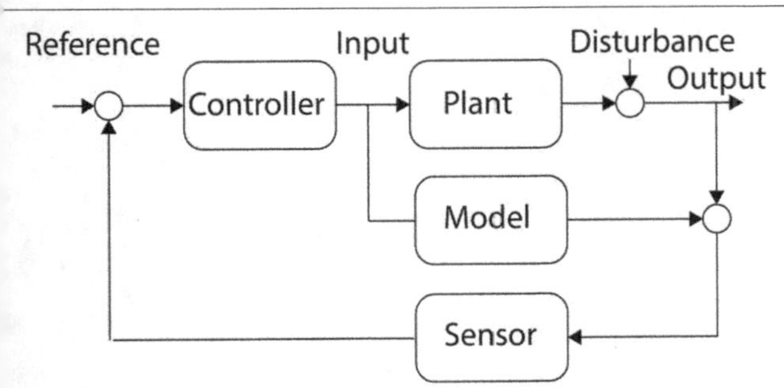

FIGURE 3 | Internal Model Control. The inclusion of a model of the Plant allows for the Controller to incorporate some of the dynamics of the system into the control policy.

Bang-Bang Control

Also referred to as On-Off control, in this scheme when a threshold for a measured variable is crossed a program is activated. Although simple this control scheme has been used successfully to automate tasks that have previously required human intervention, such as the delivery of cortical electrical stimulation after ECog seizure detection (Peters et al., 2001), or the mapping of stimulus thresholds in high electrode count implanted neurostimulators (Wilder et al., 2009).

Finite State Machine

A State Machine is a model of a system. It can be considered a more complex implementation of Bang-Bang control. The measurement of a system value, combined with the modeled system's current state triggers an action and a state transition (Markovic et al., 2014). If the modeled system is periodic, such as gait during walking, then it can be possible to have transitions due to timing (Holinski et al., 2013), in which case the neuroprosthetic enables state transitions in response to deviants from the periodic behavior, such as starting or stopping the gait.

Population Vector Algorithm

The biomechanics of the arm make motor control a difficult problem. Additionally the mechanisim of control within the motor cortex remains an open question. Is the cortical representation in an area such as the activity recorded from M1 encoding the lengthening or shortening of individual muscles (Schwartz, 2004), or is it representing the kinematics of movement (Ajemian et al., 2008)? In either case there is evidence for a forward and inverse model representation of motor control existing within the brain (Andersen et al., 2010; Green and Kalaska, 2011). The Population Vector Algorithm (PVA) is a popular method to decode neural activity recorded from cortical MEA in the motor cortex for the control of a robotic effector, or cursor in a 2D or 3D space. This control algorithm rests on the observation that different neurons have directional preferences—they have higher spike rates for movements in some directions (Shpigelman et al., 2009). Individual neurons do not offer enough specificity to be useful, but a large enough population of neurons, recorded from simultaneously, can be used to determine the intended direction and movement velocity by linear regression. Neuroprosthetic control can then be performed by relying on a "targeting" strategy of decoding the end point trajectory apparent in each cell's activity.

In Helms Tillery et al. (2003) a non-human primate's BMI was extracting an X, Y, and Z signal for the end effector on the robotic arm and the other degrees of freedom of the arm were under the control of the robotic device. In Hatsopoulos et al. (2005) a human participant with 128 electrode array implanted in the precentral gyrus was able to achieve 2D cursor control on a laptop.

Initial implementations of PVA utilized cortical recordings made while the participant watched cursor movement, or the movement of a limb. However, although a PVA decoder created in this way may show good performance in offline testing, the closed-loop performance will not be better, and may be worse (Chase et al., 2009).

TABLE 1 | Summary of Control Strategies.

	Bang-Bang	FSM	PVA	Kalman Filter	PPF	R-L	Feedback Control	LDA	ANN	SVM	LSHDI
FES		Holinski et al., 2013					Ionescu and De Keyser, 2006				
Prosthetic limb		Armiger et al., 2013; Markovic et al., 2014									
DBS	Herron and Chizeck, 2014								Grahn et al., 2014		
Motor BMI			Helms Tillery et al., 2003; Hatsopoulos et al., 2005; Chase et al., 2009	Kim et al., 2008; Li et al., 2009; Dangi et al., 2011, 2014; Gowda et al., 2012; Orsborn et al., 2012, 2014; Corbett et al., 2013, 2014; Jarosiewicz et al., 2013; Marathe and Taylor, 2013; Golub et al., 2014; Matlack et al., 2014; So et al., 2014; Yeom et al., 2014	Shanechi and Carmena, 2013; Shanechi et al., 2014	Mahmoudi et al., 2008, 2013; DiGiovanna et al., 2009; Mahmoudi and Sanchez, 2011	Pan et al., 2015	Zhang et al., 2012; Williams et al., 2013; McCreadie et al., 2014; Iturrate et al., 2015; Xu et al., 2015	Aggarwal et al., 2008; Chang et al., 2009; Shpigelman et al., 2009	Hu et al., 2003; Olson et al., 2005; Olson and Si, 2010	Dethier et al., 2011, 2013
Exo	Cisotto et al., 2013						Nagasako et al., 2015	Xu et al., 2014			
Vision								Peters et al., 2001; Wilder et al., 2009			
Other	Peters et al., 2001; Wilder et al., 2009	Mendez et al., 2013		Marzullo et al., 2010			Shanechi et al., 2013; Iolov et al., 2014	Agashe and Contreras-Vidal, 2011			

Control Policies with Dynamic Models

There are methods that rely on having a model of the dynamic system describing the parameter the neuroprosthetic is controlling. This might be a model of the spiking behavior of a region of the CNS that is to be modulated by a DBS, or a model of the kinematics of the trajectory of a cursor in a motor BMI, or the kinematics of the gait of an exoskeleton. Models can be linear or non-linear. Using the model, and an error signal, and modeling feedback the next state can be predicted using a variety of methods described below. These approaches are iterative, and work well as part of a closed-loop as they represent the process of the subject modifying the input control signal in response to the feedback signal.

A simple linear state model for velocity can be represented as:

$$x_t = Ax_{t-1} + w_{t-1}$$
$$y_t = Cx_{t-1} + q_{t-1}$$

where $\boldsymbol{x}_t$ is the velocity as a 3 dimensional vector at time step $\boldsymbol{t}$, $\boldsymbol{A}$ is a matrix of parameters describing the trajectory and $\boldsymbol{w}_{t-1}$ is a noise term. The second equation describes the measurement model of the neural activity, $\boldsymbol{y}_t$. $\boldsymbol{C}$ is a matrix of parameters that relate velocity to the neural activity and $\boldsymbol{q}_t$ is a noise term. This model can be expanded with the inclusion of an additional term to model the input of the control signal on the system state as follows:

$$x_t = Ax_{t-1} + Bu_{t-1} + w_{t-1}$$

where $\boldsymbol{u}_t$ is the control signal at time step $\boldsymbol{t}$, and $\boldsymbol{B}$ is a matrix of parameters describing the trajectory. The task of the following algorithms is to predicte the state in order to generate an error, the difference between the predicted and observed state, which can be used to adjust the control signal.

There are a number of assumptions within the model, including that the sensory feedback to the subject of the current state $\boldsymbol{x}_t$ is error free and instantaneous (Shanechi and Carmena, 2013). The matrix $\boldsymbol{B}$ is tightly coupled to a particular task, making it difficult for the subject to use the control input $\boldsymbol{u}_t$ to drive the neuroprosthetic if the task order changes during use (Matlack et al., 2014). Williams et al. (2013) points to the utility in including both a "hold" state and a "rest" state in the design of tasks for motor BMI decoders, and which is often not included as part of the model state. Finally, Hogri et al. (2015) illustrate a clear box modeling approach (LeDuc et al., 2011) where a simplified cerebellar microcircuit is implemented as a VLSI chip and interfaced to anesthetized rats.

Kalman Filter

The Kalman Filter (KF) is a recursive optimal estimator and is good at extracting signal from noisy measurements. It has been widely deployed in industrial automation and control systems engineering for over half a century. In its original form the state and measurement models needed to be linear. The extended Kalman Filter (EKF) models non-linear processes where a linearization has been performed, and implementations such as the Unscented Kalman Filter (Li et al., 2009) can utilize non-linear models. A number of variants have been proposed for neuroprosthetic closed-loop control, including SmoothBatch (Orsborn et al., 2012) and ReFIT (Gilja et al., 2012) which capture elements of the neuroprosthetic task in the model and updates the decoder parameters during the operation of the system. Updating the decoder in this manner is referred to as closed-loop decoder adaption (CLDA). In Dangi et al. (2014) Recursive Maximum Likelihood is used as part of CLDA to continuously adjust the KF. This is probably useful because the recording of the neural signal may be non-stationary due to factors (electrode drift, movement artifacts, external noise) as well as the fact that the subject may have changes in attention during the operation of the device, and the learning process may change the parameters for error and modeling (Chase et al., 2009). When examining various parameters that can be tuned in the decoder, (Cunningham et al., 2011) determined that bin width has a large impact on the performance of the KF, and should be optimized. Potentially due to the subjects ability to interact with the closed-loop system, shorter bin widths of 25–50 ms provide improved performance over longer bin widths.

Point Process Filters

The activity of individual neurons in the ensemble can be modeled as point processes with each spike being an event, which enables the filter to respond much more rapidly then methods that rely on binned spike counts or estimates of instantaneous firing rates (Li et al., 2009).

Reinforcement-Learning

In Actor-Critic architectures two coupled systems work together with complimentary models of the task. The two systems adapt using a Reinforcement Learning approach (DiGiovanna et al., 2009). The user of the system supplies a signal indicating success or failure to the Critic, which supplies a training signal to the Actor to allow adaption (Mahmoudi et al., 2008). By trial and error the Actor interacts with the environment, and the Critic's feedback rewards successful actions. The Actor-Critic approach may also be well-suited to neuroprosthetic control in a real world usage scenario where the task and associated trajectory varies from moment to moment, and achieving the goal may be the only reinforcement signal available (DiGiovanna et al., 2009). Mahmoudi et al. (2008) describes a neuroprosthetic for a Sprague Dawley rat with 32 electrodes implanted in primary motor cortex (M1)—symmetrically, 16 electrodes per hemisphere. This was used to control a robotic arm, which the rat used to press levers. Meanwhile the Critic component is implemented as a computer agent that adapts via the Reinforcement Learning paradigm based on the rewards the rat user receives, and the rat user is learning to modulate its neural activation modifying the directional tuning of the units in M1. An extension to this approach involves extracting the goal success signal directly from the subject. By recording from the Nucleus Accumbens in the ventral striatum of rats, an area believed to associate sensory perception with motor tasks, (Mahmoudi and Sanchez, 2011) were able to use the rat subject's internal representation of goal success as the evaluative feedback signal to the Critic component.

PID Feedback Control

The Proportional-Integral-Derivative (PID) controller is an extremely common and widely deployed controller in closed-loop systems. The three terms—proportional, integral, and derivative are calculated from the plant's response to the input and are summed to generate the error signal (Åström and Wittenmark, 1990). Chaos control approaches, such as delayed feedback control, utilize the dynamics of the system to modify the control input. By taking advantage of the chaotic system sensitivity to perturbation, system state can be changed with minimal cost. In Vlachos et al. (2016) the use of delayed feedback control enables closed loop control of a seizure model (a spiking neural network) and the recovery of the non-seizure dynamics, while in Slutzky et al. (2003) seizure activity induced in rat hippocampal slice preparations was moderately controlled.

Control Policies with Classifiers

Classifiers don't need a model of the system instead they attempt to determine a relationship between a set of measurements and a given state. Some classifiers can be sensitive to changes in the data they use to determine the classes (Lotte et al., 2007), such as Artificial Neural Networks whereas Linear Discriminant Analysis is more robust in the face of changes to data used to train the classifier.

Linear Discriminant Analysis

Linear discriminant analysis (LDA), and other related techniques, are statistical methods that find the features in the measurement of a signal that indicate the probability that it belongs to a given class (Mika et al., 1999). The assignment to a class can be used to trigger a neuroprosthetic intervention, such as the detection via EEG of a motor command and the subsequent activation of an ankle exoskeleton (Xu et al., 2014).

Artificial Neural Network

The Artificial Neural Network is a data driven approach to classification that in contrast to LDA and other statistical methods does not rely on the assumption of the underlying probability distribution of the system (Zhang, 2000). ANNs are organized in layers, with nodes or neurons connected typically in an input, hidden and output layer structure (**Figure 4**). There are numerous topologies, but among the most popular is the Multi Layer Perceptron (MLP), a three layer feedforward network. ANNs are trained with the presentation of input data that has been identified as belonging to an output class, and a learning rule is applied to adjust the weights on the connections between the nodes, of which back propagation is the most well-known.

ANNs have been used to predict end-point gait parameters from the EMG recorded from the neuromuscular activation of subjects with Spina Bifida (SB; Chang et al., 2009), and to achieve realtime dexterous control of a myoelectric prosthetic hand from cortical recordings of rhesus monkeys (Aggarwal et al., 2008). Echostate Neural Networks are a Recurrent Neural Network (Sussillo et al., 2012) that have been used in non-human primates for a motor BMI, and have been able to outperform the Kalman Filter.

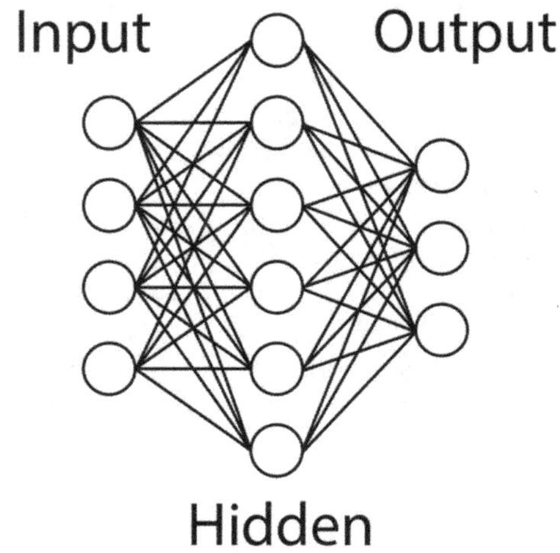

FIGURE 4 | Artificial Neural Network. An illustration of a typical ANN topology. An input layer projects to a single hidden layer, which connects to the output layer. Common variations include additional hidden layers and recurrent connections.

Support Vector Machines

The Support Vector Machine (SVM) is a supervised machine learning approach that can perform classification or regression. The SVM identifies a hyperplane that separates classes within the data, by non-linearly projecting data points into a higher dimensional space (Tapson et al., 2013).

Linear Solutions to Higher Dimensional Interlayers

Linear Solutions of Higher Dimensional Interlayers (LSHDI) are a class of networks that have some similarity in architecture to ANNs, with an input, hidden, and output layer. They are distinct due to the much larger hidden layer, the random generation of the weights on between the input and the hidden layer, and the linear response of the output layer (Tapson et al., 2013). The Neural Engineering Framework (NEF) builds systems out of networks that have LSHDI characteristics (Eliasmith and Anderson, 2004). The NEF has been used to design Spiking Neural Network that implements the Kalman Filter as part of a cortical motor BMI (Dethier et al., 2011). The Synaptic Kernel Inverse Method (SKIM) is an LSHDI network for spiking input (Tapson et al., 2013) that can perform both classification and regression.

FEEDBACK

There can be more than one feedback loop in the neuroprosthetic system (Broccard et al., 2014). Feedback can be the visual observation of the robotic effector as it is in many motor BMI allowing the operator to modulate their neural activity before it is decoded. Or in the case of a DBS neuroprosthetic the feedback signal may be acquired from recording electrodes implanted alongside the stimulating electrodes, in which case the feedback signal is returned directly to the device (Herron and Chizeck, 2014). Bidirectional interfaces, via the PNS or the CNS, enable the transformed signals of sensors on the robotic effector to be transmitted into the operators nervous system and interpreted as a sensory percept (Armiger et al., 2013). Feedback can also be from sensors on the robotic effector directly to the controller, bypassing the operator (Broccard et al., 2014; Markovic et al., 2014). And finally, reversing the direction of information, natural sensors can be used as a source of feedback for the controller (Holinski et al., 2013; Mendez et al., 2013; Wright et al., 2015) and the brain can be used as the source of the error signal (Mahmoudi and Sanchez, 2011).

DISCUSSION

We have reviewed the control policies employed by recent neuroprosthetic systems. For the purposes of this review we included motor BMIs, assistive devices, neuromodulatory systems, and other devices with an interface into a subject's nervous system. Many of the devices reported on in the literature are being developed in non-human primate or other animal models, only a subset have been tested in human subjects. There is a frequent conflation of detection and classification approaches with digital or Bang-Bang control within the literature.

Although closed-loop systems have been demonstrated experimentally there remain significant limits on our ability to describe the activity in the brain, and consequently develop control policies to respond to that activity. Simulation of cortical activity (Ehrens et al., 2015; Sandler et al., 2015; Vlachos et al., 2016), the use of experimental platforms (Keren and Marom, 2014), and the use of animal models has enabled the development of a wide range of neuroprosthetic systems. However, the appropriate method to transition these systems in human subjects is not clear. Among the difficulties is the body's response to chronic implantation of microelectrodes (Fernandez et al., 2014), the appropriate place to collect a signal (Krook-Magnuson et al., 2015), and the possibility that longterm attempts to control a cortical system may compromise some of the desirable behavior (Keren and Marom, 2014).

Comparisons of control policies across different modalities, interfaces and levels of invasiveness are difficult. Even within a given neuroprosthetic category it can be difficult to perform a comparison due to the wide variety of task designs, different subject training regimes and varying reported metrics; (Koyama et al., 2010; Sussillo et al., 2012) are rare exceptions. Examination of **Table 1** reveals that the motor BMI discipline appears to have explored the widest variety of control policies, and that the use of the Kalman Filter as part of a closed-loop system has broad support. Improvements to the traditional Kalman Filter to allow non-linear models of neural activity combined with its ability to be implemented in real-time continue to make it an attractive approach.

Closed-loop motor BMI systems have had significant success with closed-loop decoder adaption (CLDA; Shanechi and Carmena, 2013), supporting the use of closed-loop control. However, the CLDA approach has identified two distinct strategies in motor neuroprosthetics—decoding vs. learning. The decoding approach aims to read the natural motor plan whereas the learning approach monitors the changing neural activity as the brain learns to operate the prosthetic. It is not known at this stage if a similar duality of strategies will be applicable in other modalities. The difficulty in specifying a model for use in many of the control policies previously describes arises from our continued uncertainty about specific action of many of the components of the nervous system. It has been observed that users of Cochlear Implants have improved speech recognition performance after completing training with the device (Doucet et al., 2006), which may argue for a learning interpretation. An important caveat for the learning approach is that the neuroprosthetic system must be stable as regards the interface and transform of the input signal to the effector output, to allow the subject the opportunity to develop the "prosthetic motor memory" necessary for skillful operation (Carmena, 2013).

Neuroprosthetic development of closed-loop systems has been driven in part by the concern that the risks involved in highly invasive interfaces need to be mitigated by a strong case for the therapeutic benefit. Patient abandonment for upper limb prosthetics is high, with many wearers ceasing upper limb prosthetic use within 12 months of receipt of the device. Concerns cited by users are weight, appearance and difficulty of use (Biddiss and Chau, 2007). Extrapolating to more invasive systems, it may be difficult to argue the cost benefit if patient dissatisfaction is very high. Although these devices cannot be abandoned in the same manner as a detachable prosthetic limb, there is some suggestive research indicating an unwillingness to participate in experimental trials, which may suggest that the perceived benefit of neuroprosthetic systems by the target patient populations remains low (Illes et al., 2011). By improving control we can offer improved functionality and increased therapeutic benefit.

AUTHOR CONTRIBUTIONS

JW performed the review and drafted the manuscript. JT, AS, and VM revised the manuscript.

REFERENCES

gashe, H. A., and Contreras-Vidal, J. L. (2011). Reconstructing hand kinematics during reach to grasp movements from electroencephalographic signals. *Conf. Proc. IEEE Eng. Med. Biol. Soc.* 2011, 5444–5447. doi: 10.1109/iembs.2011.6091389

ggarwal, V., Kerr, M., Davidson, A. G., Davoodi, R., Loeb, G. E., Schieber, M. H., et al. (2011). "Cortical control of reach and grasp kinematics in a virtual environment using musculoskeletal modeling software," in *2011 5th International IEEE/EMBS Conference on Neural Engineering (NER)* (Cancún), 388–391. doi: 10.1109/NER.2011.5910568

Aggarwal, V., Singhal, G., He, J., Schieber, M. H., and Thakor, N. V. (2008). Towards closed-loop decoding of dexterous hand movements using a virtual integration environment. *Conf. Proc. IEEE Eng. Med. Biol. Soc.* 2008, 1703–1706. doi: 10.1109/iembs.2008.4649504

Ajemian, R., Green, A., Bullock, D., Sergio, L., Kalaska, J., and Grossberg, S. (2008). Assessing the function of motor cortex: single-neuron models of how neural response is modulated by limb biomechanics. *Neuron* 58, 414–428. doi: 10.1016/j.neuron.2008.02.033

Andersen, R. A., Hwang, E. J., and Mulliken, G. H. (2010). Cognitive neural prosthetics. *Annu. Rev. Psychol.* 61, 169–190, C161–C163. doi: 10.1146/annurev.psych.093008.100503

Åström, K. J., and Wittenmark, B. (1990). *Computer-Controlled Systems: Theory and Design.* Upper Saddle River, NJ: Prentice-Hall International.

Armiger, R. S., Tenore, F. V., Katyal, K. D., Johannes, M. S., Mahklin, A., Natter, M. L., et al. (2013). Enabling closed-loop control of the Modular Prosthetic Limb through haptic feedback. *Johns Hopkins APL Tech. Dig.* 31, 345–353.

Berger, T. W., Hampson, R. E., Song, D., Goonawardena, A., Marmarelis, V. Z., and Deadwyler, S. A. (2011). A cortical neural prosthesis for restoring and enhancing memory. *J. Neural Eng.* 8:046017. doi: 10.1088/1741-2560/8/4/046017

Biddiss, E. A., and Chau, T. T. (2007). Upper limb prosthesis use and abandonment: a survey of the last 25 years. *Prosthet. Orthot. Int.* 31, 236–257. doi: 10.1080/03093640600994581

Borton, D., Bonizzato, M., Beauparlant, J., DiGiovanna, J., Moraud, E. M., Wenger, N., et al. (2014). Corticospinal neuroprostheses to restore locomotion after spinal cord injury. *Neurosci. Res.* 78, 21–29. doi: 10.1016/j.neures.2013.10.001

Broccard, F. D., Mullen, T., Chi, Y. M., Peterson, D., Iversen, J. R., Arnold, M., et al. (2014). Closed-loop brain-machine-body interfaces for noninvasive rehabilitation of movement disorders. *Ann. Biomed. Eng.* 42, 1573–1593. doi: 10.1007/s10439-014-1032-6

Carmena, J. M. (2013). Advances in neuroprosthetic learning and control. *PLoS Biol.* 11:e1001561. doi: 10.1371/journal.pbio.1001561

Chang, C. L., Jin, Z., Chang, H. C., and Cheng, A. C. (2009). From neuromuscular activation to end-point locomotion: an artificial neural network-based technique for neural prostheses. *J. Biomech.* 42, 982–988. doi: 10.1016/j.jbiomech.2009.03.030

Chase, S. M., Schwartz, A. B., and Kass, R. E. (2009). Bias, optimal linear estimation, and the differences between open-loop simulation and closed-loop performance of spiking-based brain-computer interface algorithms. *Neural Netw.* 22, 1203–1213. doi: 10.1016/j.neunet.2009.05.005

Cisotto, G., Pupolin, S., Silvoni, S., Cavinato, M., Agostini, M., and Piccione, F. (2013). "Brain-computer interface in chronic stroke: an application of sensorimotor closed-loop and contingent force feedback," in *IEEE International Conference on Communications* (Budapest), 4379–4383. doi: 10.1109/ICC.2013.6655255

Corbett, E. A., Kording, K. P., and Perreault, E. J. (2013). Real-time evaluation of a noninvasive neuroprosthetic interface for control of reach. *IEEE Trans. Neural Syst. Rehabil. Eng.* 21, 674–683. doi: 10.1109/TNSRE.2013.2251664

Corbett, E. A., Kording, K. P., and Perreault, E. J. (2014). Dealing with target uncertainty in a reaching control interface. *PLoS ONE* 9:e86811. doi: 10.1371/journal.pone.0086811

Crago, P. E., Lan, N., Veltink, P. H., Abbas, J. J., and Kantor, C. (1996). New control strategies for neuroprosthetic systems. *J. Rehabil. Res. Dev.* 33, 158–172.

Cunningham, J. P., Nuyujukian, P., Gilja, V., Chestek, C. A., Ryu, S. I., and Shenoy, K. V. (2011). A closed-loop human simulator for investigating the role of feedback control in brain-machine interfaces. *J. Neurophysiol.* 105, 1932–1949. doi: 10.1152/jn.00503.2010

Dangi, S., Gowda, S., Héliot, R., and Carmena, J. M. (2011). "Adaptive Kalman filtering for closed-loop Brain-Machine Interface systems," in *2011 5th International IEEE/EMBS Conference on Neural Engineering (NER)* (Cancún), 609–612. doi: 10.1109/NER.2011.5910622

Dangi, S., Gowda, S., Moorman, H. G., Orsborn, A. L., So, K., Shanechi, M., et al. (2014). Continuous closed-loop decoder adaptation with a recursive maximum likelihood algorithm allows for rapid performance acquisition in brain-machine interfaces. *Neural Comput.* 26, 1811–1839. doi: 10.1162/NECO_a_00632

Danziger, Z. (2014). A reductionist approach to the analysis of learning in brain-computer interfaces. *Biol. Cybern.* 108, 183–201. doi: 10.1007/s00422-014-0589-3

Deisseroth, K. (2011). Optogenetics. *Nat. Methods* 8, 26–29. doi: 10.1038/nmeth.f.324

Dethier, J., Nuyujukian, P., Eliasmith, C., Stewart, T., Elassaad, S. A., Shenoy, K. V., et al. (2011). A brain-machine interface operating with a real-time spiking neural network control algorithm. *Adv. Neural Inf. Process. Syst.* 2011, 2213–2221.

Dethier, J., Nuyujukian, P., Ryu, S. I., Shenoy, K. V., and Boahen, K. (2013). Design and validation of a real-time spiking-neural-network decoder for brain-machine interfaces. *J. Neural Eng.* 10:036008. doi: 10.1088/1741-2560/10/3/036008

DiGiovanna, J., Mahmoudi, B., Fortes, J., Principe, J. C., and Sanchez, J. C. (2009). Coadaptive brain-machine interface via reinforcement learning. *IEEE Trans. Biomed. Eng.* 56, 54–64. doi: 10.1109/TBME.2008.926699

Dommel, N. B., Wong, Y. T., Lehmann, T., Dodds, C. W., Lovell, N. H., and Suaning, G. J. (2009). A CMOS retinal neurostimulator capable of focussed, simultaneous stimulation. *J. Neural Eng.* 6:035006. doi: 10.1088/1741-2560/6/3/035006

Doucet, M. E., Bergeron, F., Lassonde, M., Ferron, P., and Lepore, F. (2006). Cross-modal reorganization and speech perception in cochlear implant users. *Brain* 129, 3376–3383. doi: 10.1093/brain/awl264

Ehrens, D., Sritharan, D., and Sarma, S. V. (2015). Closed-loop control of a fragile network: application to seizure-like dynamics of an epilepsy model. *Front. Neurosci.* 9:58. doi: 10.3389/fnins.2015.00058

Eliasmith, C., and Anderson, C. H. (2004). *Neural Engineering: Computation, Representation, and Dynamics in Neurobiological Systems.* Cambridge, MA: MIT press.

Fernandez, E., Greger, B., House, P. A., Aranda, I., Botella, C., Albisua, J., et al. (2014). Acute human brain responses to intracortical microelectrode arrays: challenges and future prospects. *Front. Neuroeng.* 7:24. doi: 10.3389/fneng.2014.00024

García, C. E., Prett, D. M., and Morari, M. (1989). Model predictive control: theory and practice—A survey. *Automatica* 25, 335–348. doi: 10.1016/0005-1098(89)90002-2

Gilja, V., Nuyujukian, P., Chestek, C. A., Cunningham, J. P., Yu, B. M., Fan, J. M., et al. (2012). A high-performance neural prosthesis enabled by control algorithm design. *Nat. Neurosci.* 15, 1752–1757. doi: 10.1038/nn.3265

Golub, M. D., Yu, B. M., Schwartz, A. B., and Chase, S. M. (2014). Motor cortical control of movement speed with implications for brain-machine interface control. *J. Neurophysiol.* 112, 411–429. doi: 10.1152/jn.00391.2013

Gowda, S., Orsborn, A. L., and Carmena, J. M. (2012). Parameter estimation for maximizing controllability of linear brain-machine interfaces. *Conf. Proc. IEEE Eng. Med. Biol. Soc.* 2012, 1314–1317. doi: 10.1109/embc.2012.6346179

Grahn, P. J., Mallory, G. W., Khurram, O. U., Berry, B. M., Hachmann, J. T., Bieber, A. J., et al. (2014). A neurochemical closed-loop controller for deep brain stimulation: toward individualized smart neuromodulation therapies. *Front. Neurosci.* 8:169. doi: 10.3389/fnins.2014.00169

Green, A. M., and Kalaska, J. F. (2011). Learning to move machines with the mind. *Trends Neurosci.* 34, 61–75. doi: 10.1016/j.tins.2010.11.003

Grill, W. M., Norman, S. E., and Bellamkonda, R. V. (2009). Implanted neura interfaces: biochallenges and engineered solutions. *Annu. Rev. Biomed. Eng.* 11 1–24. doi: 10.1146/annurev-bioeng-061008-124927

Guggenmos, D. J., Azin, M., Barbay, S., Mahnken, J. D., Dunham, C., Mohseni P., et al. (2013). Restoration of function after brain damage using a neura prosthesis. *Proc. Natl. Acad. Sci. U.S.A.* 110, 21177–21182. doi: 10.1073 pnas.1316885110

Hatsopoulos, N., Mukand, J., Polykoff, G., Friehs, G., and Donoghue, J. (2005). Cortically controlled brain-machine interface. *Conf. Proc. IEEE Eng. Med. Bio Soc.* 7, 7660–7663. doi: 10.1109/iembs.2005.1616286

Helms Tillery, S. I., Taylor, D. M., and Schwartz, A. B. (2003). "Th general utility of a neuroprosthetic device under direct cortical control in *Engineering in Medicine and Biology Society, 2003. Proceedings of th 25th Annual International Conference of the IEEE* (Cancún), 2043–2046. do 10.1109/IEMBS.2003.1280137

Herron, J., and Chizeck, H. J. (2014). "Prototype closed-loop deep brai stimulation systems inspired by Norbert Wiener," in *2014 IEEE Conferenc on Norbert Wiener in the 21st Century (21CW)* (Boston, MA), 1–6. do 10.1109/NORBERT.2014.6893922

Hochberg, L. R., Bacher, D., Jarosiewicz, B., Masse, N. Y., Simeral, J. D Vogel, J., et al. (2012). Reach and grasp by people with tetraplegia using neurally controlled robotic arm. *Nature* 485, 372–375. doi: 10.1038/Natu 11076

Hogri, R., Bamford, S. A., Taub, A. H., Magal, A., Del Giudice, P., and Mintz, M. (2015). A neuro-inspired model-based closed-loop neuroprosthesis for the substitution of a cerebellar learning function in anesthetized rats. *Sci. Rep.* 5:8451. doi: 10.1038/srep08451

Holinski, B. J., Everaert, D. G., Mushahwar, V. K., and Stein, R. B. (2013). Real-time control of walking using recordings from dorsal root ganglia. *J. Neural Eng.* 10:056008. doi: 10.1088/1741-2560/10/5/056008

Horch, K., Meek, S., Taylor, T. G., and Hutchinson, D. T. (2011). Object discrimination with an artificial hand using electrical stimulation of peripheral tactile and proprioceptive pathways with intrafascicular electrodes. *IEEE Trans. Neural Syst. Rehabil. Eng.* 19, 483–489. doi: 10.1109/TNSRE.2011.2162635

Hosain, M. K., Kouzani, A., and Tye, S. (2014). Closed loop deep brain stimulation: an evolving technology. *Australas. Phys. Eng. Sci. Med.* 37, 619–634. doi: 10.1007/s13246-014-0297-2

Houk, J. C. (1988). Control strategies in physiological systems. *FASEB J.* 2, 97–107.

Hu, J., Si, J., Olson, B. P., Clement, R. S., and He, J. (2003). "Decoding motor cortical spike trains for brain machine interface applications," in *Engineering in Medicine and Biology Society, 2003. Proceedings of the 25th Annual International Conference of the IEEE*, 2071–2074. doi: 10.1109/IEMBS.2003.1280144

Illes, J., Reimer, J. C., and Kwon, B. K. (2011). Stem cell clinical trials for spinal cord injury: readiness, reluctance, redefinition. *Stem Cell Rev.* 7, 997–1005. doi: 10.1007/s12015-011-9259-1

Inmann, A., and Haugland, M. (2004). Functional evaluation of natural sensory feedback incorporated in a hand grasp neuroprosthesis. *Med. Eng. Phys.* 26, 439–447. doi: 10.1016/j.medengphy.2004.03.002

Iolov, A., Ditlevsen, S., and Longtin, A. (2014). Stochastic optimal control of single neuron spike trains. *J. Neural Eng.* 11:046004. doi: 10.1088/1741-2560/11/4/046004

Ionescu, C., and De Keyser, R. (2006). Activating paralyzed muscles using adaptive control and a neuroprosthetic technique. *Automat. Quality Test. Robotics 2006 IEEE Int. Conf.* 1, 43–47. doi: 10.1109/AQTR.2006.254494.

Iturrate, I., Grizou, J., Omedes, J., Oudeyer, P. Y., Lopes, M., and Montesano, L. (2015). Exploiting task constraints for self-calibrated brain-machine interface control using error-related potentials. *PLoS ONE* 10:e0131491. doi: 10.1371/journal.pone.0131491

Jarosiewicz, B., Masse, N. Y., Bacher, D., Cash, S. S., Eskandar, E., Friehs, G., et al. (2013). Advantages of closed-loop calibration in intracortical brain-computer interfaces for people with tetraplegia. *J. Neural Eng.* 10:046012. doi: 10.1088/1741-2560/10/4/046012

Kameneva, T., Abramian, M., Zarelli, D., Nesic, D., Burkitt, A. N., Meffin, H., et al. (2015). Spike history neural response model. *J. Comput. Neurosci.* 38, 463–481. doi: 10.1007/s10827-015-0549-5

Keren, H., and Marom, S. (2014). Controlling neural network responsiveness: tradeoffs and constraints. *Front. Neuroeng.* 7:11. doi: 10.3389/fneng.2014.00011

Kim, S. P., Simeral, J. D., Hochberg, L. R., Donoghue, J. P., and Black, M. J. (2008). Neural control of computer cursor velocity by decoding motor cortical spiking activity in humans with tetraplegia. *J. Neural Eng.* 5, 455–476. doi: 10.1088/1741-2560/5/4/010

Koyama, S., Chase, S. M., Whitford, A. S., Velliste, M., Schwartz, A. B., and Kass, R. E. (2010). Comparison of brain-computer interface decoding algorithms in open-loop and closed-loop control. *J. Comput. Neurosci.* 29, 73–87. doi: 10.1007/s10827-009-0196-9

Krook-Magnuson, E., Gelinas, J. N., Soltesz, I., and Buzsaki, G. (2015). Neuroelectronics and biooptics: closed-loop technologies in neurological disorders. *JAMA Neurol.* 72, 823–829. doi: 10.1001/jamaneurol.2015.0608

Kuiken, T. A., Li, G., Lock, B. A., Lipschutz, R. D., Miller, L. A., Stubblefield, K. A., et al. (2009). Targeted muscle reinnervation for real-time myoelectric control of multifunction artificial arms. *JAMA* 301, 619–628. doi: 10.1001/jama.2009.116

LeDuc, P. R., Messner, W. C., and Wikswo, J. P. (2011). How do control-based approaches enter into biology? *Annu. Rev. Biomed. Eng.* 13, 369–396. doi: 10.1146/annurev-bioeng-071910-124651

Li, Z., O'Doherty, J. E., Hanson, T. L., Lebedev, M. A., Henriquez, C. S., and Nicolelis, M. A. (2009). Unscented Kalman filter for brain-machine interfaces. *PLoS ONE* 4:e6243. doi: 10.1371/journal.pone.0006243

Lotte, F., Congedo, M., Lecuyer, A., Lamarche, F., and Arnaldi, B. (2007). A review of classification algorithms for EEG-based brain-computer interfaces. *J. Neural Eng.* 4, R1–R13. doi: 10.1088/1741-2560/4/2/R01

Mahmoudi, B., Digiovanna, J., Principe, J. C., and Sanchez, J. C. (2008). Neuronal tuning in a brain-machine interface during Reinforcement Learning. *Conf. Proc. IEEE Eng. Med. Biol. Soc.* 2008, 4491–4494. doi: 10.1109/iembs.2008.4650210

Mahmoudi, B., Pohlmeyer, E. A., Prins, N. W., Geng, S., and Sanchez, J. C. (2013). Towards autonomous neuroprosthetic control using Hebbian reinforcement learning. *J. Neural Eng.* 10:066005. doi: 10.1088/1741-2560/10/6/066005

Mahmoudi, B., and Sanchez, J. C. (2011). A symbiotic brain-machine interface through value-based decision making. *PLoS ONE* 6:e14760. doi: 10.1371/journal.pone.0014760

Marathe, A. R., and Taylor, D. M. (2013). Decoding continuous limb movements from high-density epidural electrode arrays using custom spatial filters. *J. Neural Eng.* 10:036015. doi: 10.1088/1741-2560/10/3/036015

Markovic, M., Dosen, S., Cipriani, C., Popovic, D., and Farina, D. (2014). Stereovision and augmented reality for closed-loop control of grasping in hand prostheses. *J. Neural Eng.* 11:046001. doi: 10.1088/1741-2560/11/4/046001

Marzullo, T. C., Lehmkuhle, M. J., Gage, G. J., and Kipke, D. R. (2010). Development of closed-loop neural interface technology in a rat model: combining motor cortex operant conditioning with visual cortex microstimulation. *IEEE Trans. Neural Syst. Rehabil. Eng.* 18, 117–126. doi: 10.1109/TNSRE.2010.2041363

Matlack, C., Haddock, A., Moritz, C. T., and Chizeck, H. J. (2014). Motor cortical decoding performance depends on controlled system order. *Conf. Proc. IEEE Eng. Med. Biol. Soc.* 2014, 2553–2556. doi: 10.1109/embc.2014.6944143

McCreadie, K. A., Coyle, D. H., and Prasad, G. (2014). Is sensorimotor BCI performance influenced differently by mono, stereo, or 3-D auditory feedback? *IEEE Trans. Neural Syst. Rehabil. Eng.* 22, 431–440. doi: 10.1109/TNSRE.2014.2312270

McFarland, D. J., Krusienski, D. J., and Wolpaw, J. R. (2006). Brain–computer interface signal processing at the Wadsworth Center: mu and sensorimotor beta rhythms. *Prog. Brain Res.* 159, 411–419. doi: 10.1016/s0079-6123(06)59026-0

Mendez, A., Sawan, M., Minagawa, T., and Wyndaele, J. J. (2013). Estimation of bladder volume from afferent neural activity. *IEEE Trans. Neural Syst. Rehabil. Eng.* 21, 704–715. doi: 10.1109/TNSRE.2013.2266899

Micera, S., Carpaneto, J., and Raspopovic, S. (2010). Control of hand prostheses using peripheral information. *IEEE Rev. Biomed. Eng.* 3, 48–68. doi: 10.1109/RBME.2010.2085429

Mika, S., Rätsch, G., Weston, J., Schölkopf, B., and Müllers, K.-R. (1999). "Fisher discriminant analysis with kernels," in *Neural Network Signal Processing IX* (Madison, WI), 41–48.

Morimoto, J., and Kawato, M. (2015). Creating the brain and interacting with the brain: an integrated approach to understanding the brain. *J. R. Soc. Interface* 12:20141250. doi: 10.1098/rsif.2014.1250

Nagasako, J. M., Fenwick, C. M., Kennedy, I. L., Marion, K. R., Zizzi, M. G., Riofrio, J. A., et al. (2015). "Closed-loop electromyography controller for augmented hand exoskeleton gripping," in *41st Annual Northeast Biomedical Engineering Conference (NEBEC)* (Troy, NY), 1–2. doi: 10.1109/NEBEC.2015.7117233

Navarro, X., Krueger, T. B., Lago, N., Micera, S., Stieglitz, T., and Dario, P. (2005). A critical review of interfaces with the peripheral nervous system for the control of neuroprostheses and hybrid bionic systems. *J. Peripher. Nerv. Syst.* 10, 229–258. doi: 10.1111/j.1085-9489.2005.10303.x

Olson, B. P., Si, J., Hu, J., and He, J. (2005). Closed-loop cortical control of direction using support vector machines. *IEEE Trans. Neural Syst. Rehabil. Eng.* 13, 72–80. doi: 10.1109/TNSRE.2004.843174

Olson, B., and Si, J. (2010). Evidence of a mechanism of neural adaptation in the closed loop control of directions. *Int. J. Intelligent Comput. Cybernetics* 3, 5–23. doi: 10.1108/17563781011028523

Orsborn, A. L., Dangi, S., Moorman, H. G., and Carmena, J. M. (2012). Closed-loop decoder adaptation on intermediate time-scales facilitates rapid BMI performance improvements independent of decoder initialization conditions. *IEEE Trans. Neural Syst. Rehabil. Eng.* 20, 468–477. doi: 10.1109/TNSRE.2012.2185066

Orsborn, A. L., Moorman, H. G., Overduin, S. A., Shanechi, M. M., Dimitrov, D. F., and Carmena, J. M. (2014). Closed-loop decoder adaptation shapes neural plasticity for skillful neuroprosthetic control. *Neuron* 82, 1380–1393. doi: 10.1016/j.neuron.2014.04.048

Ortiz-Catalan, M., Branemark, R., Hakansson, B., and Delbeke, J. (2012). On the viability of implantable electrodes for the natural control of artificial limbs: review and discussion. *Biomed. Eng. Online* 11:33. doi: 10.1186/1475-925X-11-33

Pan, H., Ding, B., Zhong, W., Kumar, G., and Kothare, M. V. (2015). "Designing closed-loop brain-machine interfaces with network of spiking neurons using MPC strategy," in *2015 American Control Conference (ACC)* (Chicago, IL), 2543–2548. doi: 10.1109/ACC.2015.7171117

Peters, T. E., Bhavaraju, N. C., Frei, M. G., and Osorio, I. (2001). Network system for automated seizure detection and contingent delivery of therapy. *J. Clin. Neurophysiol.* 18, 545–549. doi: 10.1097/00004691-200111000-00004

Raspopovic, S., Capogrosso, M., Petrini, F. M., Bonizzato, M., Rigosa, J., Di Pino, G., et al. (2014). Restoring natural sensory feedback in real-time bidirectional hand prostheses. *Sci. Transl. Med.* 6:222ra219. doi: 10.1126/scitranslmed.3006820

Sandler, R. A., Song, D., Hampson, R. E., Deadwyler, S. A., Berger, T. W., and Marmarelis, V. Z. (2015). Hippocampal closed-loop modeling and implications for seizure stimulation design. *J. Neural Eng.* 12:056017. doi: 10.1088/1741-2560/12/5/056017

Schwartz, A. B. (2004). Cortical neural prosthetics. *Annu. Rev. Neurosci.* 27, 487–507. doi: 10.1146/annurev.neuro.27.070203.144233

Shanechi, M. M., and Carmena, J. M. (2013). "Optimal feedback-controlled point process decoder for adaptation and assisted training in brain-machine Interfaces (Providence)," in *2013 6th International IEEE/EMBS Conference on Neural Engineering (NER)* (San Diego, CA), 653–656. doi: 10.1109/NER.2013.6696019

Shanechi, M. M., Chemali, J. J., Liberman, M., Solt, K., and Brown, E. N. (2013). A brain-machine interface for control of medically-induced coma. *PLoS Comput. Biol.* 9:e1003284. doi: 10.1371/journal.pcbi.1003284

Shanechi, M. M., Orsborn, A., Moorman, H., Gowda, S., and Carmena, J. M. (2014). High-performance brain-machine interface enabled by an adaptive optimal feedback-controlled point process decoder. *Conf. Proc. IEEE Eng. Med. Biol. Soc.* 2014, 6493–6496. doi: 10.1109/embc.2014.6945115

Shpigelman, L., Lalazar, H., and Vaadia, E. (2009). "Kernel-ARMA for hand tracking and brain-machine interfacing during 3D motor control," in *Advances in Neural Information Processing Systems* (Red Hook, NY: Curran Associates, Inc.), 1489–1496.

Slutzky, M. W., Cvitanovic, P., and Mogul, D. J. (2003). Manipulating epileptiform bursting in the rat hippocampus using chaos control and adaptive techniques. *IEEE Trans. Biomed. Eng.* 50, 559–570. doi: 10.1109/TBME.2003.810701

So, K., Dangi, S., Orsborn, A. L., Gastpar, M. C., and Carmena, J. M. (2014). Subject-specific modulation of local field potential spectral power during brain-machine interface control in primates. *J. Neural Eng.* 11:026002. doi: 10.1088/1741-2560/11/2/026002

Sun, F. T., and Morrell, M. J. (2014). Closed-loop neurostimulation: the clinical experience. *Neurotherapeutics* 11, 553–563. doi: 10.1007/s13311-014-0280-3

Sussillo, D., Nuyujukian, P., Fan, J. M., Kao, J. C., Stavisky, S. D., Ryu, S., et al. (2012). A recurrent neural network for closed-loop intracortical brain-machine interface decoders. *J. Neural Eng.* 9:026027. doi: 10.1088/1741-2560/9/2/026027

Tan, D. W., Schiefer, M. A., Keith, M. W., Anderson, J. R., Tyler, J., and Tyler, D. J. (2014). A neural interface provides long-term stable natural touch perception. *Sci. Transl. Med.* 6:257ra138. doi: 10.1126/scitranslmed.3008669

Tapson, J. C., Cohen, G. K., Afshar, S., Stiefel, K. M., Buskila, Y., Wang, R. M., et al. (2013). Synthesis of neural networks for spatio-temporal spike pattern recognition and processing. *Front. Neurosci.* 7:153. doi: 10.3389/fnins.2013.00153

Vlachos, I., Deniz, T., Aertsen, A., and Kumar, A. (2016). Recovery of dynamics and function in spiking neural networks with closed-loop control. *PLoS Comput. Biol.* 12:e1004720. doi: 10.1371/journal.pcbi.1004720

Vogelstein, R. J., Tenore, F., Guevremont, L., Etienne-Cummings, R., and Mushahwar, V. K. (2008). A silicon central pattern generator controls locomotion *in vivo*. *IEEE Trans. Biomed. Circuits Syst.* 2, 212–222. doi: 10.1109/TBCAS.2008.2001867

Wilder, A. M., Hiatt, S. D., Dowden, B. R., Brown, N. A., Normann, R. A., and Clark, G. A. (2009). Automated stimulus-response mapping of high-electrode-count neural implants. *IEEE Trans. Neural Syst. Rehabil. Eng.* 17, 504–511. doi: 10.1109/TNSRE.2009.2029494

Williams, J. J., Rouse, A. G., Thongpang, S., Williams, J. C., and Moran, D. W. (2013). Differentiating closed-loop cortical intention from rest: building an asynchronous electrocorticographic BCI. *J. Neural Eng.* 10:046001. doi: 10.1088/1741-2560/10/4/046001

Wodlinger, B., Downey, J. E., Tyler-Kabara, E. C., Schwartz, A. B., Boninger, M. L., and Collinger, J. L. (2015). Ten-dimensional anthropomorphic arm control in a human brain-machine interface: difficulties, solutions, and limitations. *J. Neural Eng.* 12:016011. doi: 10.1088/1741-2560/12/1/016011

Wright, J., Macefield, V. G., van Schaik, A., and Tapson, J. (2015). "Decoding force from multiunit recordings from the median nerve," in *2015 IEEE International Conference on Rehabilitation Robotics (ICORR)* (Singapore), 956–960. doi: 10.1109/ICORR.2015.7281327

Xu, R., Jiang, N., Mrachacz-Kersting, N., Lin, C., Asin Prieto, G., Moreno, J. C., et al. (2014). A closed-loop brain-computer interface triggering an active ankle-foot orthosis for inducing cortical neural plasticity. *IEEE Trans. Biomed. Eng.* 61, 2092–2101. doi: 10.1109/TBME.2014.2313867

Xu, Z., Guan, C., So, R. Q., Ang, K. K., and Toe, K. K. (2015). "Motor cortical adaptation induced by closed-loop BCI," in *2015 7th International IEEE/EMBS Conference on Neural Engineering (NER)* (Montpellier), 21–24. doi: 10.1109/NER.2015.7146550

Yanagisawa, T., Hirata, M., Saitoh, Y., Goto, T., Kishima, H., Fukuma, R., et al. (2011). Real-time control of a prosthetic hand using human electrocorticography signals. *J. Neurosurg.* 114, 1715–1722. doi: 10.3171/2011.1.JNS101421

Yeom, H. G., Kim, J. S., and Chung, C. K. (2014). High-accuracy brain-machine interfaces using feedback information. *PLoS ONE* 9:e103539. doi: 10.1371/journal.pone.0103539

Zhang, G. P. (2000). Neural networks for classification: a survey. *IEEE Trans. Syst. Man Cybernet. Part C (Applications and Reviews)* 30, 451–462. doi: 10.1109/5326.897072

Zhang, Y., Schwartz, A. B., Chase, S. M., and Kass, R. E. (2012). Bayesian learning in assisted brain-computer interface tasks. *Conf. Proc. IEEE Eng. Med. Biol. Soc.* 2012, 2740–2743. doi: 10.1109/EMBC.2012.6346531

18

A Rodent Model of Dynamic Facial Reanimation Using Functional Electrical Stimulation

Mark A. Attiah, Julius de Vries, Andrew G. Richardson and Timothy H. Lucas *

Department of Neurosurgery, Center for Neuroengineering and Therapeutics, Perelman School of Medicine, University of Pennsylvania, Philadelphia, PA, USA

Edited by:
Paolo Bonifazi,
Tel Aviv University, Israel

Reviewed by:
Andrew Joseph Fuglevand,
University of Arizona, USA
George C. McConnell,
Stevens Institute of Technology, USA

***Correspondence:**
Timothy H. Lucas
timothy.lucas@uphs.upenn.edu

Facial paralysis can be a devastating condition, causing disfiguring facial droop, slurred speech, eye dryness, scarring and blindness. This study investigated the utility of closed-loop functional electric stimulation (FES) for reanimating paralyzed facial muscles in a quantitative rodent model. The right buccal and marginal mandibular branches of the rat facial nerve were transected for selective, unilateral paralysis of whisker muscles. Microwire electrodes were implanted bilaterally into the facial musculature for FES and electromyographic (EMG) recording. With the rats awake and head-fixed, whisker trajectories were tracked bilaterally with optical micrometers. First, the relationship between EMG and volitional whisker movement was quantified on the intact side of the face. Second, the effect of FES on whisker trajectories was quantified on the paralyzed side. Third, closed-loop experiments were performed in which the EMG signal on the intact side triggered FES on the paralyzed side to restore symmetric whisking. The results demonstrate a novel *in vivo* platform for developing control strategies for neuromuscular facial prostheses.

Keywords: paralysis, facial nerve, functional electrical stimulation, electromyography, rodent

INTRODUCTION

Facial paralysis is a disfiguring condition affecting 127,000 individuals annually (Bleicher et al., 1996). Beyond cosmetic disfigurement, facial paralysis can lead to permanent disability. Blindness may occur if the cascade of corneal dryness, conjunctivitis, and ulceration develops (Otto et al., 1986). Nasal obstruction and mouth leakage result from an inability to keep nasal passages patent and mouth closed, respectively (May et al., 1977). Finally, dysarthria and distorted facial expressions hinder both spoken and nonverbal communication (Coulson et al., 2004), resulting in awkward and strained social interactions.

The ultimate goal of facial reanimation is to enable independent control of paralyzed facial muscles. This goal has proven elusive. Development of effective treatment options is confounded by the wide range of causes that result in a shared facial palsy phenotype, namely, trauma, infection, neoplasm, iatrogenic insults and idiopathic etiologies (Melvin and Limb, 2008). Current treatments palliate the condition by partially restoring muscle tone or by attempting to prevent catastrophic consequences, like blindness. These procedures all have significant drawbacks. Sacrifice of the hypoglossal nerve for nerve transfer results in ipsilateral tongue paralysis. Cross-facial nerve grafts route contralateral facial branches to the paralyzed side, but this procedure places the healthy nerves at risk (Hontanilla et al., 2013). Dynamic procedures routinely take 9–18 months to become effective and require rigorous rehabilitation (Spector et al., 1991; Robey and Snyder, 2011).

Spontaneous movement or emotional expression is rarely achieved and the functional status is often compromised by synkinesis. To improve outcomes researchers are developing several new treatments (Hadlock and Cheney, 2008), including the use of functional electrical stimulation (FES) to reanimate paralyzed facial muscles (Griffin and Kim, 2011).

The effectiveness of FES in activating paralyzed facial muscles, in particular the orbicularis oculi to restore eye blink, has been demonstrated in rabbits and dogs (Rothstein and Berlinger, 1986; Salerno et al., 1991; Otto, 1997; Somia et al., 2001; Sachs et al., 2007; Jie et al., 2016). Since many facial movements including eye blink are symmetric, a natural closed-loop FES control signal in unilateral facial paralysis can be derived from the intact side of the face. In particular, electromyographic (EMG) recordings from a facial muscle contralateral to the injury can be used to trigger FES of the homologous paralyzed muscle. A similar, bilateral, closed-loop approach has been used to rehabilitate hand movements after stroke (Knutson et al., 2012, 2016). In the context of facial paralysis, this closed-loop strategy has been demonstrated in rabbits, dogs, and humans (Zealear and Dedo, 1977; Tobey and Sutton, 1978; Broniatowski et al., 1987, 1989, 1991; Cao et al., 2009; McDonnall et al., 2009; Kurita et al., 2010; Frigerio and Cavallari, 2012; Yi et al., 2013). Most of these studies focused on restoration of eye blink and utilized largely qualitative measures of FES performance.

In the present work, we sought to develop a new, quantitative animal model of FES-controlled facial reanimation. Quantitative tracking of bilateral facial movements is typically done with video cameras and feature recognition software (Sachs et al., 2007). But this strategy is error-prone and has low temporal resolution. An alternative strategy is to track a more conspicuous facial feature present on some animals: facial vibrissae (whiskers). Rodent whiskers are controlled by muscles innervated by the facial nerve (Berg and Kleinfeld, 2003), typically exhibit bilateral symmetric motion (Gao et al., 2001), and can be readily tracked with high spatiotemporal resolution (Bermejo et al., 1998). Thus, we hypothesized that a rodent model of unilateral facial paralysis could provide an improved assessment of FES performance for dynamic facial reanimation. A similar approach with rats was developed previously for the study of facial nerve function (Heaton et al., 2008). In the present study we quantified, for the first time, the effects of open- and closed-loop FES on whisker motion. The results suggest this new approach could be useful for designing improved FES control policies for a facial prosthesis.

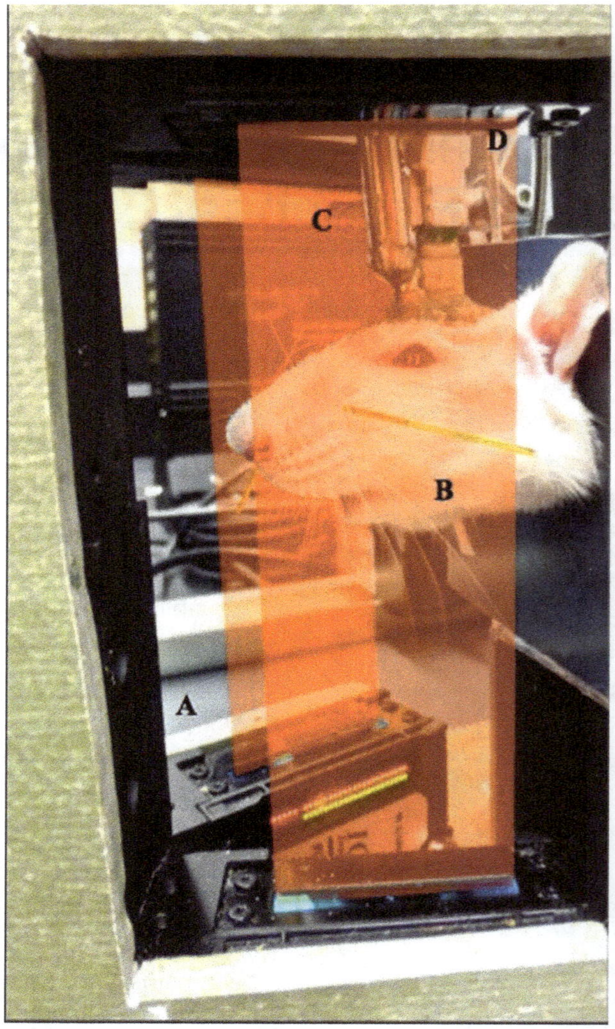

FIGURE 1 | Experimental setup. (A) Laser micrometers positioned on either side of the face were used to monitor whisker movement. **(B)** Polyimide tubes were placed on selected whiskers and micrometer sensitivity was adjusted such that only the motion of one pair of whiskers was detected. **(C)** Head restraint was achieved using magnetic implant and a repositionable rod. **(D)** Microwire electrodes implanted in facial muscles were accessed via a connector anchored to the skull.

METHODS

All procedures were approved by the University of Pennsylvania Institutional Animal Care and Use Committee. Four female Sprague-Dawley rats were used for these experiments.

Training and Experimental Apparatus

Prior to surgery, all animals were habituated to the laboratory environment and the experimental apparatus. The apparatus (**Figure 1**) consisted of (1) a half-pipe with hook-and-loop strap to restrain the rat's body, (2) neck plates at the front of the pipe to restrain forward or backward head motion (3) a metal rod with magnet that mated with a head mounted magnet to further restrain the head, and (4) two commercial laser micrometers in a V-configuration such that they approximated both sides of the face (see details below). The half pipe could be moved to adjust the position of the rat relative to the micrometers. A Faraday cage, which enclosed the entire apparatus, was assembled with copper mesh and red translucent acrylic in order to shield recordings from ambient electromagnetic interference and to provide an enclosed environment that minimized the stress of the animals. Rats were placed in the restraints each day until they were able to be calm for at least 1 h.

Implant

For each rat, a custom microwire array was constructed to interface with the facial musculature. Seventeen insulated stainless steel wires (50 μm, A-M Systems) were soldered to a printed circuit board (PCB, 6.68 × 7.05 × 1.59 mm) and routed to a miniature connector on the board (A79042-001, Omnetics Corp). Sixteen of the wires served as working electrodes in facial muscles (eight on each side) and one as a reference electrode. An uninsulated silver wire (127 μm, A-M Systems) was also soldered to the PCB to serve as the ground. Wires were impedance tested to ensure the integrity of the electrical connections. The PCB was covered with an epoxy to insulate and stabilize the solder connections and traces. The distal 2 mm of the stainless steel wires was stripped of insulation. Before surgery the implant was cold sterilized in chlorhexidine (0.1%).

Surgical Procedure

Our development of the rodent model proceeded in two sequential phases: (1) establish the techniques for bilateral recording of facial EMG and whisking motion (animals 1 and 2) and (2) paralyze and implement open- and closed-loop FES (animals 3 and 4). As such, the facial nerve transection portion of the surgical procedure applied only to animals 3 and 4.

Each rat was anesthetized with intraperitoneal administration of ketamine (60 mg/kg) and dexmedetomidine (0.25 mg/kg). The animal was kept on a heating pad and the respiratory rate, palpebral reflex, and pedal pinch reflex were monitored periodically throughout the procedure to track depth of anesthesia. Once a surgical plane of anesthesia was reached, the head and right side of the face posterior to the whisker pad were shaved and cleaned with povidone-iodine. Lidocaine was administered subcutaneously at the incision sites for further analgesia.

The buccal and marginal mandibular branches of the facial nerve, the only branches supplying motor input to the whisker pad (Semba and Egger, 1986), were exposed through a single vertical skin incision on the right side of the face. Nerve identity was confirmed with bipolar stimulation, which elicited movement from the whisker pad. A 3 mm section of each nerve was transected. Functional denervation was confirmed again with bipolar stimulation to the proximal and distal stumps. The incision was closed with 6-0 nylon suture.

The animal was then placed in a stereotaxic frame. An incision was made on the midline of the scalp and skin, soft tissue, and periosteum were retracted laterally to expose the frontal and parietal bones. Six burr holes were made on the skull bilaterally and six screws (00-90 × 1/8″) were inserted. The implant PCB was positioned in the middle of the skull screws and the silver ground wire was wrapped around the screws. To aid head fixation, a high-strength cylindrical neodymium magnet (D34-52, K&J Magnetics Inc.) was placed rostral to the PCB. Dental acrylic was then poured over the PCB, screws, and around the magnet to secure them to the skull.

The stainless steel microwires were then inserted into the muscles of the whisker pad in pairs. The hooked ends of each pair of wires were placed in a 23-gauge hypodermic needle that was used to drive them into the targeted muscle (Carvell et al., 1991). The targets initially included both intrinsic and extrinsic muscles of the whisker pad, which protract and retract the whiskers, respectively (Dörfl, 1982). However, in preliminary studies we found that actively controlling the retractor muscles, nasolabialis and maxillolabialis, introduced significant complexity (see Section Discussion). Whisker retractions can occur passively, due to the viscoelastic properties of the facial connective tissue (Bermejo et al., 1998). Accordingly, the intrinsic muscles were targeted preferentially. Intramuscular placement was confirmed with bipolar stimulation that evoked whisker protraction. The stainless steel reference wire was placed subcutaneously on the dorsal aspect of the nasal bone. The midline incision was closed with 6-0 nylon sutures.

Anesthesia was reversed with atipamezole (5 mg/kg). For 3 days postoperatively, animals were maintained on an analgesic regimen of ketoprofen (5 mg/kg, once daily) and buprenorphine (0.05 mg/kg, twice daily), administered subcutaneously. To prevent infection, gentamicin sulfate drops (0.3%, once daily) were applied around the implant.

Whisker Monitoring

After surgery, the rats were further acclimated to the experimental apparatus via training sessions in which their heads were held stationary by the magnetic attachment (**Figure 1**). Horizontal whisker motion was monitored bilaterally by two laser micrometers (IG-028, Keyence Corp) mounted in front of the body restraint apparatus. The micrometers had a measurement range of 28 mm, a spatial resolution of 5 μm, and a temporal resolution of 490 μs. One bilateral homologous pair of whiskers was selected for monitoring. Selection was based on (1) the ability to fully capture the whisking motion on the micrometer array and (2) the ability to actuate the whisker on the paralyzed side with FES. A small polyimide tube (0.36 mm diameter) was placed on the selected pair of whiskers to facilitate its detection by the micrometer arrays (Heaton et al., 2008). The spatial sensitivity settings of the micrometers were adjusted such that they only detected the whisker in the tube and not the other whiskers.

Data Acquisition and FES

The laser micrometer output and EMG signals from the implanted microwires were simultaneously recorded at 3052 samples/s (PZ2 preamplifer, RZ2 processor, Tucker-Davis Technologies). EMG signals were recorded differentially with respect to the subcutaneous reference wire. Pairs of digitized EMG channels were then subtracted to yield the bipolar EMG signal used in offline analyses and online stimulus triggering. Electrical stimulation delivered to the microwires consisted of trains of charge-balanced, biphasic square pulses (IZ2H stimulator, Tucker-Davis Technologies). Pulse amplitude, pulse width, number of pulses, and pulse frequency were the adjustable stimulation parameters used to achieve different whisker motions. For closed-loop, EMG-triggered FES, the digital signal processors of the RZ2 were programmed for real-time EMG signal conditioning (bipolar subtraction, rectification, and 10–1,000 Hz bandpass filtering). Stimuli were then triggered when the conditioned signal amplitude reached an experimentally defined threshold, determined by trial and error at the beginning of the closed-loop sessions. A trigger lockout period starting with the first pulse and ending 20 ms after the end of the pulse train was imposed to prevent stimulus artifacts from triggering the stimulator.

Data Analysis

In offline analyses, the EMG envelope was estimated by bandpass filtering (5–100 Hz passband), rectifying, and then lowpass filtering (10 Hz cutoff) the raw bipolar signal. Power spectra of both the whisking signal and EMG envelope were computed using Welch's averaging method on 1-s, Hamming-windowed data segments with 50% overlap. Time delays between local peaks in the EMG envelope and whisking were used to assess the lag between these signals. Pearson's correlation coefficient was used to assess the linear relationship between peak whisking and EMG envelope amplitudes. For comparison of FES effects across animals, we identified the stimulus intensity required to evoke a 2 ± 0.2 mm whisker protraction, where protraction amplitude was defined as the peak positive displacement after subtracting the baseline mean. Closed-loop stimulation effects were summarized by stimulus-triggered average displacement of both paralyzed and intact whiskers, with 95% confidence intervals based on the t-distribution. The onset and duration of the post-stimulus protraction were defined by the first and last occurrences of positive displacement (i.e., lower confidence bound >0) in these averages, averaged across animals.

RESULTS

We developed a rodent model for studying FES-based facial reanimation. Optical micrometers (**Figure 1A**) were used to track a pair of whiskers bilaterally (**Figure 1B**) in head-fixed rats (**Figure 1C**). The facial musculature of the rats was implanted with microwires to allow both EMG recording and FES of facial muscles (**Figure 1D**). This system allowed us to study, at high spatiotemporal resolution, facial movements resulting from either volitional or artificial (i.e., FES) commands.

Whisking and EMG activity

The head-fixed rats engaged in bouts of volitional, rhythmic whisking behavior (**Figure 2A**). This behavior could be produced spontaneously but often needed prompting by delivering scents near the nose. Rhythmic activity in the EMG of the whisker-protracting muscles corresponded with rhythmic motion of the tracked whisker on the intact side of the face (**Figure 2A**). To quantify the EMG-whisking relationship, the envelope of the EMG signal was computed using a zero-phase low pass filter. The dominant frequency of whisking and of the EMG envelope oscillation was 6 Hz in all four rats (**Figure 2B**). The EMG envelope led the whisker motion by an average of 28.7, 24.9, 24.7

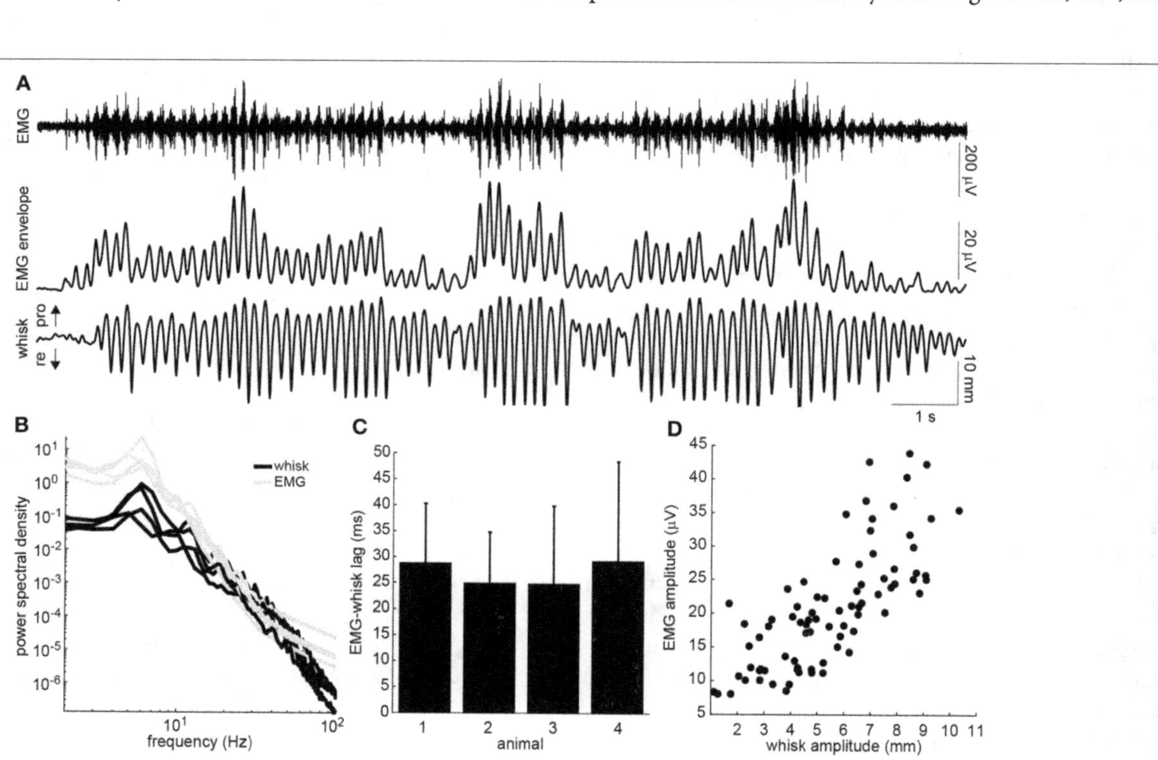

FIGURE 2 | Relationship of intrinsic muscle EMG to ipsilateral whisking. (A) Example raw EMG recorded from the intrinsic muscle (top), envelope of the EMG signal (middle), and whisker motion (bottom). Directions of whisker protraction (pro) and retraction (re) are indicated. **(B)** Power spectra of the measured whisker (black) and EMG envelope (gray) signals for four rats. Note the prominent peak around 6 Hz. **(C)** Lag between the peaks of the EMG envelope and the corresponding protraction peaks of the whisker displacement (mean + standard deviation). **(D)** Relationship between the peak protraction amplitude and the peak EMG amplitude for the data shown in A ($r = 0.75$).

and 29.2 ms in each of these animals, respectively (**Figure 2C**). Thus, the timing of each of cycle of the whisker motion could be accurately determined from the EMG. In one case, amplitude of the whisker motion could also be inferred from the EMG. The best observed correlation between peak whisk amplitude and peak EMG envelope amplitude was 0.75 (**Figure 2D**). However, in the other animals the whisk amplitude estimate was less reliable, with whisk-EMG correlations of 0.35, 0.32, 0.24, likely due to suboptimal electrode placement.

A unilateral transection of the buccal and marginal mandibular branches of the facial nerve was performed in two of the four rats (**Figure 3A**). This procedure was effective in focally paralyzing the whisker pad. Rhythmic whisking was completely absent on the paralyzed side (**Figure 3B**). Only miscellaneous fibrillations up to 0.5 mm were present in the de-efferented whiskers. For over a month after the lesion, the rats maintained proper weight and eating habits and exhibited no self-injurious behavior.

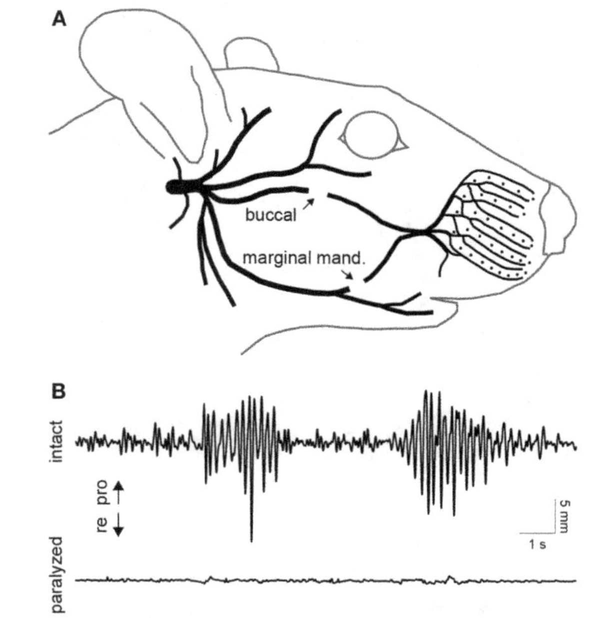

FIGURE 3 | Facial nerve transection and paralysis. (A) Illustration of the peripheral branches of the facial nerve distal to the stylomastoid foramen. The two sites of transection are indicated by arrows. **(B)** Typical whisking behavior recorded simultaneously on the intact (top) and paralyzed (bottom) side. Whisker movements were recorded 10 days after transection of the buccal and marginal mandibular branches of the facial nerve on the paralyzed side.

FES of Intrinsic Muscles

Next, electrical stimuli were delivered to the paralyzed intrinsic muscles to reanimate the whiskers. Trains of current-controlled square pulses were delivered between the pair of electrodes that produced whisker motion at lowest current amplitude. Across four testing sessions, the current to produce a 2-mm protraction was 43 ± 6 μA (animal 3) and 98 ± 13 μA (animal 4), when using 0.3-ms pulse widths, 10 pulses, and 200-Hz pulse frequencies. We characterized how variations in these stimulus parameters changed the evoked whisker motion. Increases in whisker displacement could be produced by increasing pulse width (**Figure 4A**), number of pulses (**Figure 4B**), or pulse frequency (**Figure 4C**). However, only pulse width affected amplitude without also changing the shape or timing of the motion. Increasing the number of pulses increased the amplitude and duration of the motion (**Figure 4B**). For both animals the duration, measured as time to peak amplitude, increased linearly, with a mean slope of 2.7 ± 0.37 ms/pulse when stimulating at 200 Hz. Increasing pulse frequency increased the amplitude and the velocity of the protraction (**Figure 4C**). The relationship between pulse frequency and whisker velocity, measured as the slope of the initial protraction for each frequency, was steeper in one animal and more graded in the other (**Figure 4D**). The results demonstrate that the amplitude and shape of the whisker motion can be controlled by stimulus pulse trains.

Contralaterally-Triggered FES

Finally, in the unilaterally paralyzed rats, we used EMG activity recorded on the intact side to trigger stimulation of the paralyzed intrinsic muscles. The EMG was bandpass filtered and thresholded in real-time to generate stimulus triggers (**Figure 5A**). A train of stimulus pulses with fixed parameters was delivered immediately after each trigger. The stimulus parameters were chosen to achieve a whisker motion comparable to that observed on the intact side. A typical example of the EMG-triggered stimulation is shown in **Figure 5A**. The system was able to accurately deliver stimuli during each protraction of the intact whisker, as expected based on the preceding analyses. However, the overall symmetry between the intact and paralyzed whiskers was limited by several factors, including the inability to actively control retraction. To summarize the results, we computed the stimulus-triggered average motion of the paralyzed and intact whiskers in both animals (**Figure 5B**). The mean evoked motion on the paralyzed side had a peak amplitude and timing that was very similar to the mean intact-side protraction. Average onset of the post-stimulus protraction was 27 ms (paralyzed) and 24 ms (intact). The duration of post-stimulus motion was 150 ms (paralyzed) and 156 ms (intact). The average whisker motion of both sides was triphasic, although the intact motion was more variable being drive volitionally (**Figure 5B**).

DISCUSSION

In this study, we developed and tested a rodent model of closed-loop FES-based facial reanimation in the setting of unilateral facial paralysis. A primary strength of the model was the ability to track the relevant facial feature (i.e., whiskers) with high spatiotemporal resolution. The documented whisking behavior confirmed earlier findings. Prior studies have observed 5–6 Hz whisking frequencies in head-fixed rats (Gao et al., 2001). This is in contrast to the significantly higher, 6–12 Hz whisking frequencies seen in unrestrained rats (Hill et al., 2008). Also, the observed 24–29 ms lag between intrinsic muscle EMG and whisker protraction is nearly equivalent to a prior report (Berg and Kleinfeld, 2003). This lag can be attributed to the

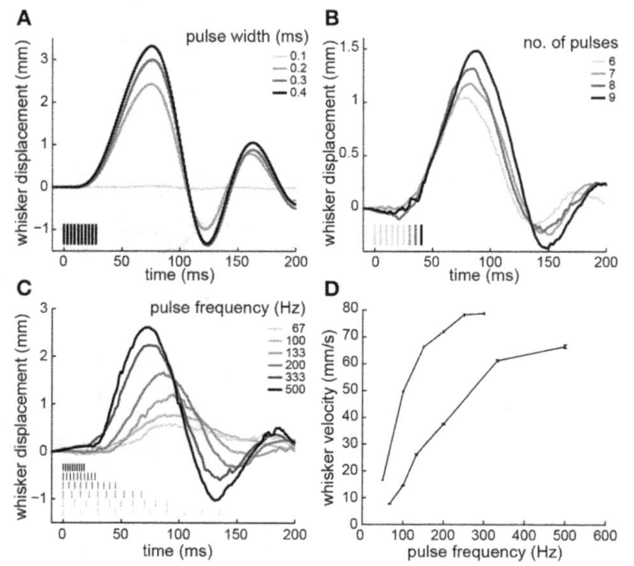

FIGURE 4 | Whisker motion resulting from electrical stimulation of paralyzed intrinsic muscles. (A) Displacements produced by varying pulse widths (10 pulses at 333-Hz; animal 3). **(B)** Varying number of pulses (200-Hz frequency, 0.3-ms width; animal 4). **(C)** Varying pulse frequency (10 pulses, 0.3-ms width; animal 4). **(D)** Whisker velocity as a function of pulse frequency (10 pulses, 0.3-ms width; animals 3 and 4). Error bars are 95% confidence intervals on the slope of the initial protraction. Pulse amplitudes were 45 μA in animal 3 and 85 μA in animal 4. In **(A–C)**, time 0 is the start of the stimulus train. Stimulus pulses are indicated by vertical lines. Positive and negative displacements correspond to whisker protraction and retraction, respectively.

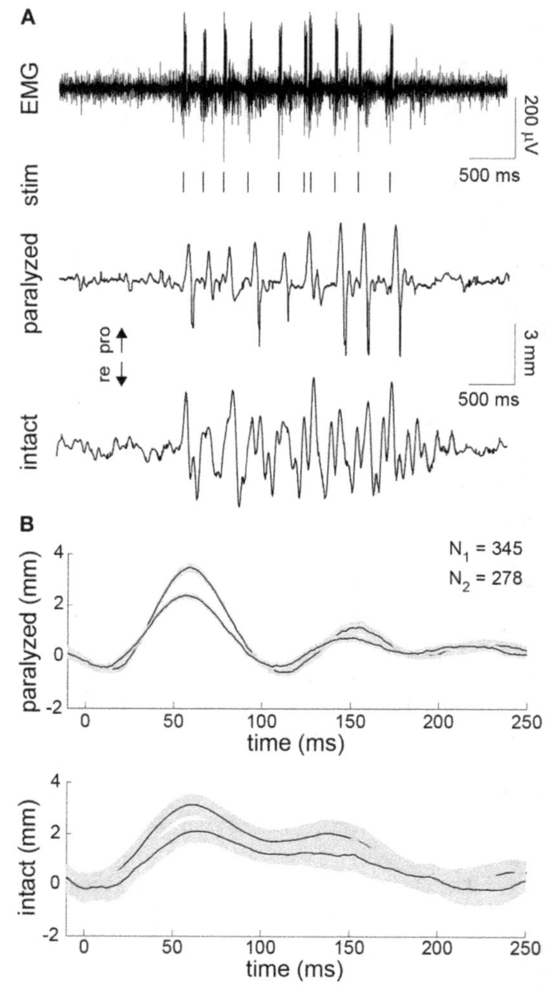

FIGURE 5 | Contralaterally-triggered electrical stimulation to restore symmetric whisking. (A) Typical result during one burst of exploratory whisking. EMG was recorded on the intact side (top). The EMG was bandpass filtered and thresholded in real-time to produce stimulus triggers (vertical lines under EMG). The series of stimulus trains (10 pulses/train delivered at 200 Hz with 0.3-ms pulse width and 45-μA (animal 3) or 95-μA (animal 4) pulse amplitude) produced whisker motion on the paralyzed side (middle) that approximated the motion seen on the intact side (bottom). **(B)** Stimulus-triggered average of whisker displacements on the paralyzed (top) and intact (bottom) side for animals 3 and 4 compiled from all 345 and 278 stimulus trains delivered during the closed-loop experiment, respectively. Ninety-five percent confidence intervals on the mean are shown in gray.

viscoelastic properties of the whisker pad. Electrical stimulation of the intrinsic muscles has previously been shown to protract the whiskers (Hill et al., 2008). However, here for the first time we documented how protraction varied with stimulation parameters. The velocity, peak amplitude, and duration of the protraction could largely be controlled through the number of stimulus pulses and pulse frequency. Finally, we demonstrated a closed-loop, contralaterally-triggered FES strategy that has been proposed for dynamic facial reanimation in humans (Cao et al., 2008; Griffin and Kim, 2011).

A limitation of the animal model is the difficult in durable placement of electrodes in the intrinsic muscles. These small, sling-like muscles around the base of each whisker cannot be directly visualized during implantation. As a result the electrode placement, and thus the recording and stimulation effects, can vary. This likely explains variability in the results, include the relationship between EMG amplitude and protraction amplitude and the relationship between whisker velocity and stimulus pulse frequency. A second limitation, which impacted the ability to restore symmetric whisking, is not actively controlling retraction. Whisker retraction is controlled by the nasolabialis and maxillolabialis muscles (Berg and Kleinfeld, 2003). However, these muscles pull the whiskers out of the horizontal plane along dorsal-posterior and ventral-posterior trajectories, respectively (Hill et al., 2008). The vertical components of these motions could not be captured by our micrometers, but could be monitored if the setup was extended to including two orthogonal micrometers on each side of the face (Hill et al., 2008). Alternatively, simultaneous stimulation of both retracting muscles can produce a mostly in-plane, posterior movement (Hill et al., 2008). Initial experiments found it quite difficult to get the concurrent electrode placement in all four muscles bilaterally. Thus, we relied on the passive retraction that occurs following active protraction (Berg and Kleinfeld, 2003).

Another potential limitation involves the FES strategy itself. Most etiologies of unilateral facial paralysis leave facial sensation intact, as the trigeminal nerve is not affected. Therefore

FES has the potential to activate sensory axons associated with nociceptors, evoking painful percepts. However, several lines of evidence suggest this issue does not completely undermine the strategy. No signs of pain (flinching, blinking, or vocalizing) were observed in our experiments. A prior study observed that rabbits initially flinched in response to orbicularis oculi stimulation, but signs of pain diminished over time (Otto, 1997). There is evidence that FES paradigms including interferential stimulation (McDonnall et al., 2009) and low-intensity multichannel stimulation (Somia et al., 2001) render facial muscle stimulation functional but not painful. Finally, facial FES has been achieved in humans reporting only mild pain (McDonnall et al., 2009; Frigerio et al., 2015).

An issue that was not studied, but should be considered, in this model of chronic facial paralysis is the time-dependent effects of denervation and the modulation of these effects by FES. Denervation is associated with muscle atrophy, which in the rat can result in a 50% loss of muscle weight after 2 weeks (Ohira, 1989). Importantly for FES, denervation also causes a transient increase in excitability, due in part to increased sensitivity to acetylcholine, followed after a few days by decreased excitability due to Wallerian degeneration of the axons distal to the injury (Sunderland, 1978). Nevertheless, prior animal studies of facial FES have elicited functional movement (e.g., complete eyelid closure) for several months after paralysis (Salerno et al., 1991; Otto, 1997; Sachs et al., 2007). This may be explained in part by demonstrations that FES can prevent and even reverse the effects of denervation, both in facial muscles (Salerno et al., 1991) and non-facial muscles (Eberstein and Eberstein, 1996). Reinnervation, potentially from motor axons in surrounding, non-denervated muscles, may also play a role (Sachs et al., 2007). Our rodent model of facial paralysis provides another means to explicitly study the interaction of muscle denervation and FES, with the benefit of precise quantification of muscle activation through whisker monitoring.

Previous research on contralaterally-triggered facial FES has been done in larger animal models and humans over the course of several decades (Zealear and Dedo, 1977; Tobey and Sutton, 1978; Broniatowski et al., 1987, 1989, 1991; Cao et al., 2009; McDonnall et al., 2009; Kurita et al., 2010; Frigerio and Cavallari, 2012). However, the therapy has not advanced beyond proof of concept. Our motivation for developing a less expensive, more quantifiable animal model for this therapy was to move toward clinical translation by improving performance through advanced closed-loop controllers. In the present study, as in all previous work, the closed-loop controller was simple: deliver hand-tuned, fixed-parameter stimuli to the paralyzed muscle when triggered by thresholded EMG activity of the homologous intact muscle. Myriad strategies, including iterative learning control (Bristow et al., 2006), adaptive feedforward control (Abbas and Triolo, 1997), and supervised learning with a distal teacher (Jordan and Rumelhart, 1992), could be used to automatically tune a mapping between EMG activity and stimulation parameters based on measured facial asymmetries to yield superior performance. The animal model developed here provides an improved platform with which to test these advanced controllers. We believe this is a necessary step to develop a therapy that could improve the quality of life of thousands of patients with facial paralysis.

ETHICS STATEMENT

This study was carried out in accordance with the recommendations of the National Institutes of Health guidelines on the use of animals. The protocol was approved by the University of Pennsylvania Institutional Animal Care and Use Committee.

AUTHOR CONTRIBUTIONS

AR and TL designed the study. MA, Jd, and AR conducted the experiments and analyzed the results. All authors contributed to writing the manuscript.

ACKNOWLEDGMENTS

The authors thank Pauline Weigand, Erica Von Stein, and Nathan Kidambi for experimental assistance and helpful discussions.

REFERENCES

Abbas, J. J., and Triolo, R. J. (1997). Experimental evaluation of an adaptive feedforward controller for use in functional neuromuscular stimulation systems. *IEEE Trans. Rehabil. Eng.* 5, 12–22. doi: 10.1109/86.559345

Berg, R. W., and Kleinfeld, D. (2003). Rhythmic whisking by rat: retraction as well as protraction of the vibrissae is under active muscular control. *J. Neurophysiol.* 89, 104–117. doi: 10.1152/jn.00600.2002

Bermejo, R., Houben, D., and Zeigler, H. P. (1998). Optoelectronic monitoring of individual whisker movements in rats. *J. Neurosci. Methods* 83, 89–96. doi: 10.1016/S0165-0270(98)00050-8

Bleicher, J. N., Hamiel, S., Gengler, J. S., and Antimarino, J. (1996). A survey of facial paralysis: etiology and incidence. *Ear Nose Throat J.* 75, 355–358.

Bristow, D. A., Tharayil, M., and Alleyne, A. G. (2006). A survey of iterative learning control. *IEEE Control Syst. Mag.* 26, 96–114. doi: 10.1109/MCS.2006.1636313

Broniatowski, M., Grundfest-Broniatowski, S., Davies, C. R., Jacobs, G. B., Tucker, H. M., and Nose, Y. (1991). Dynamic rehabilitation of the paralyzed face: III: balanced coupling of oral and ocular musculature from the intact side in the canine. *Otolaryngol. Head Neck Surg.* 105, 727–733.

Broniatowski, M., Ilyes, L. A., Jacobs, G. B., Rosenthal, D. I., Maniglia, A. J., Tucker, H. M., et al. (1987). Dynamic rehabilitation of the paralyzed face: I. Electronic control of reinnervated muscles from intact facial musculature in the rabbit. *Otolaryngol. Head Neck Surg.* 97, 441–445. doi: 10.1177/019459988709700502

Broniatowski, M., Ilyes, L. A., Jacobs, G., Nosé, Y., and Tucker, H. M. (1989). Dynamic rehabilitation of the paralyzed face–II. Electronic control of the reinnervated facial musculature from the contralateral side in the rabbit. *Otolaryngol. Head Neck Surg.* 101, 309–313.

Cao, J., Li, L., Tong, K., Lu, B., Chu, C., Li, H., et al. (2009). FNS therapy for the functional restoration of the paralysed eyelid. *J. Plast. Reconstr. Aesthet. Surg.* 62, e622–e624. doi: 10.1016/j.bjps.2008.10.018

Cao, J., Lu, B., Li, L., Tong, K., and Wang, W. (2008). Implanted FNS system in closed-circle may become a way for the restoration of eye blinking and closing function for facial paralysis patient. *Med. Hypotheses* 70, 1068–1069. doi: 10.1016/j.mehy.2007.11.008

Carvell, G. E., Simons, D. J., Lichtenstein, S. H., and Bryant, P. (1991). Electromyographic activity of mystacial pad musculature during whisking behavior in the rat. *Somatosens. Mot. Res.* 8, 159–164. doi: 10.3109/08990229109144740

Coulson, S. E., O'Dwyer, N. J., Adams, R. D., and Croxson, G. R. (2004). Expression of emotion and quality of life after facial nerve paralysis. *Otol. Neurotol.* 25, 1014–1019. doi: 10.1097/00129492-200411000-00026

Dörfl, J. (1982). The musculature of the mystacial vibrissae of the white mouse. *J. Anat.* 135(Pt 1), 147–154.

Eberstein, A., and Eberstein, S. (1996). Electrical stimulation of denervated muscle: is it worthwhile? *Med. Sci. Sports Exerc.* 28, 1463–1469.

Frigerio, A., and Cavallari, P. (2012). A closed-loop stimulation system supplemented with motoneurone dynamic sensitivity replicates natural eye blinks. *Otolaryngol. Head Neck Surg.* 146, 230–233. doi: 10.1177/0194599811427255

Frigerio, A., Heaton, J. T., Cavallari, P., Knox, C., Hohman, M. H., and Hadlock, T. A. (2015). Electrical stimulation of eye blink in individuals with acute facial palsy: progress toward a bionic blink. *Plast. Reconstr. Surg.* 136, 515e–523e. doi: 10.1097/PRS.0000000000001639

Gao, P., Bermejo, R., and Zeigler, H. P. (2001). Whisker deafferentation and rodent whisking patterns: behavioral evidence for a central pattern generator. *J. Neurosci.* 21, 5374–5380. Available online at: http://www.jneurosci.org/content/21/14/5374

Griffin, G. R., and Kim, J. C. (2011). Potential of an electric prosthesis for dynamic facial reanimation. *Otolaryngol. Head Neck Surg.* 145, 365–368. doi: 10.1177/0194599811406065

Hadlock, T., and Cheney, M. L. (2008). Facial reanimation: an invited review and commentary. *Arch. Facial Plast. Surg.* 10, 413–417. doi: 10.1001/archfaci.10.6.413

Heaton, J. T., Kowaleski, J. M., Bermejo, R., Zeigler, H. P., Ahlgren, D. J., and Hadlock, T. A. (2008). A system for studying facial nerve function in rats through simultaneous bilateral monitoring of eyelid and whisker movements. *J. Neurosci. Methods* 171, 197–206. doi: 10.1016/j.jneumeth.2008.02.023

Hill, D. N., Bermejo, R., Zeigler, H. P., and Kleinfeld, D. (2008). Biomechanics of the vibrissa motor plant in rat: rhythmic whisking consists of triphasic neuromuscular activity. *J. Neurosci.* 28, 3438–3455. doi: 10.1523/JNEUROSCI.5008-07.2008

Hontanilla, B., Marre, D., and Cabello, A. (2013). Facial reanimation with gracilis muscle transfer neurotized to cross-facial nerve graft versus masseteric nerve: a comparative study using the FACIAL CLIMA evaluating system. *Plast. Reconstr. Surg.* 131, 1241–1252. doi: 10.1097/PRS.0b013e31828bd4da

Jie, T., Zhiqiang, G., Guodong, F., Yubin, X., Xiuyong, D., Tingting, C., et al. (2016). The effective stimulating pulse for restoration of blink function in unilateral facial nerve paralysis rabbits, verified by a simple FES system. *Eur. Arch. Otorhinolaryngol.* 273, 2959–2964. doi: 10.1007/s00405-015-3884-2

Jordan, M. I., and Rumelhart, D. E. (1992). Forward models: supervised learning with a distal teacher. *Cogn. Sci.* 16, 307–354. doi: 10.1207/s15516709cog1603_1

Knutson, J. S., Gunzler, D. D., Wilson, R. D., and Chae, J. (2016). Contralaterally controlled functional electrical stimulation improves hand dexterity in chronic hemiparesis: a randomized trial. *Stroke* 47, 2596–2602. doi: 10.1161/STROKEAHA.116.013791

Knutson, J. S., Harley, M. Y., Hisel, T. Z., Hogan, S. D., Maloney, M. M., and Chae, J. (2012). Contralaterally controlled functional electrical stimulation for upper extremity hemiplegia: an early-phase randomized clinical trial in subacute stroke patients. *Neurorehabil. Neural Repair* 26, 239–246. doi: 10.1177/1545968311419301

Kurita, M., Takushima, A., Muraoka, Y., Shiraishi, T., and Harii, K. (2010). Feasibility of bionic reanimation of a paralyzed face: a preliminary study of functional electrical stimulation of a paralyzed facial muscle controlled with the electromyography of the contralateral healthy hemiface. *Plast. Reconstr. Surg.* 126, 81e–83e. doi: 10.1097/PRS.0b013e3181df6ff3

May, M., West, J. W., and Hinderer, K. H. (1977). Nasal obstruction from facial palsy. *Arch. Otolaryngol.* 103, 389–391. doi: 10.1001/archotol.1977.00780240047005

McDonnall, D., Guillory, K. S., and Gossman, M. D. (2009). "Restoration of blink in facial paralysis patients using FES," in *Proceedings of the 4th Int IEEE EMBS Conference Neural Engineering* (Antalya).

Melvin, T. A., and Limb, C. J. (2008). Overview of facial paralysis: current concepts. *Facial Plast. Surg.* 24, 155–163. doi: 10.1055/s-2008-1075830

Ohira, Y. (1989). Effects of denervation and deafferentation on mass and enzyme activity in rat skeletal muscles. *Jpn. J. Physiol.* 39, 21–31. doi: 10.2170/jjphysiol.39.21

Otto, R. A. (1997). Restoration of function in the paralyzed rabbit orbicularis oculi muscle by direct functional electrical stimulation. *Laryngoscope* 107, 101–111. doi: 10.1097/00005537-199701000-00020

Otto, R. A., Gaughan, R. N., Templer, J. W., and Davis, W. E. (1986). Electrical restoration of the blink reflex in experimentally induced facial paralysis. *Ear Nose Throat J.* 65, 37.

Robey, A. B., and Snyder, M. C. (2011). Reconstruction of the paralyzed face. *Ear Nose Throat J.* 90, 267–275.

Rothstein, J., and Berlinger, N. T. (1986). Electronic reanimation of facial paralysis–a feasibility study. *Otolaryngol. Head Neck Surg.* 94, 82–85. doi: 10.1177/019459988609400114

Sachs, N. A., Chang, E. L., Vyas, N., Sorensen, B. N., and Weiland, J. D. (2007). Electrical stimulation of the paralyzed orbicularis oculi in rabbit. *IEEE Trans. Neural Syst. Rehabil. Eng.* 15, 67–75. doi: 10.1109/TNSRE.2007.891372

Salerno, G. M., McClellan, G. A., Bleicher, J. N., Stromberg, B. V., and Cheng, S. C. (1991). Electrical stimulation treatment of dog's denervated orbicularis oculi muscle. *Ann. Plast. Surg.* 26, 431–440. doi: 10.1097/00000637-199105000-00004

Semba, K., and Egger, M. D. (1986). The facial "motor" nerve of the rat: control of vibrissal movement and examination of motor and sensory components. *J. Comp. Neurol.* 247, 144–158. doi: 10.1002/cne.902470203

Somia, N. N., Zonnevijlle, E. D., Stremel, R. W., Maldonado, C., Gossman, M. D., and Barker, J. H. (2001). Multi-channel orbicularis oculi stimulation to restore eye-blink function in facial paralysis. *Microsurgery* 21, 264–270. doi: 10.1002/micr.1050

Spector, J. G., Lee, P., Peterein, J., and Roufa, D. (1991). Facial nerve regeneration through autologous nerve grafts: a clinical and experimental study. *Laryngoscope* 101, 537–554. doi: 10.1288/00005537-199105000-00017

Sunderland, S. (1978). *Nerves and Nerve Injuries*. New York, NY: Churchill Livingstone.

Tobey, D. N., and Sutton, D. (1978). Contralaterally elicited electrical stimulation of paralyzed facial muscles. *Otolaryngology* 86, 812–818 doi: 10.1177/019459987808600528

Yi, X., Jia, J., Deng, S., Shen, S. G., Xie, Q., and Wang, G. (2013). A blink restoration system with contralateral EMG triggered stimulation and real-time artifact blanking. *IEEE Trans. Biomed. Circuits Syst.* 7, 140–148 doi: 10.1109/TBCAS.2013.2255051

Zealear, D. L., and Dedo, H. H. (1977). Control of paralyzed axial muscle by electrical stimulation. *Trans. Sect. Otolaryngol. Am. Acad. Ophthalmol. Otolaryngol.* 84, 310.

19

Bio-Inspired Controller on an FPGA Applied to Closed-Loop Diaphragmatic Stimulation

Adeline Zbrzeski[1,2]*, *Yannick Bornat*[1,2], *Brian Hillen*[3], *Ricardo Siu*[3], *James Abbas*[4], *Ranu Jung*[3] *and Sylvie Renaud*[1,2]

[1] *Bordeaux INP, IMS, UMR 5218, Talence, France,* [2] *Univ. Bordeaux, IMS, UMR 5218, Talence, France,* [3] *Department of Biomedical Engineering, Florida International University, Miami, FL, USA,* [4] *School of Biological and Health Systems Engineering, Arizona State University, Tempe, AZ, USA*

Edited by:
Eberhard E. Fetz, University of Washington, USA

Reviewed by:
Jan-Marino Ramirez, University of Washington, USA
Andrew Joseph Fuglevand, University of Arizona, USA

***Correspondence:**
Adeline Zbrzeski
adelinezbrz@gmail.com

Cervical spinal cord injury can disrupt connections between the brain respiratory network and the respiratory muscles which can lead to partial or complete loss of ventilatory control and require ventilatory assistance. Unlike current open-loop technology, a closed-loop diaphragmatic pacing system could overcome the drawbacks of manual titration as well as respond to changing ventilation requirements. We present an original bio-inspired assistive technology for real-time ventilation assistance, implemented in a digital configurable Field Programmable Gate Array (FPGA). The bio-inspired controller, which is a spiking neural network (SNN) inspired by the medullary respiratory network, is as robust as a classic controller while having a flexible, low-power and low-cost hardware design. The system was simulated in MATLAB with FPGA-specific constraints and tested with a computational model of rat breathing; the model reproduced experimentally collected respiratory data in eupneic animals. The open-loop version of the bio-inspired controller was implemented on the FPGA. Electrical test bench characterizations confirmed the system functionality. Open and closed-loop paradigm simulations were simulated to test the FPGA system real-time behavior using the rat computational model. The closed-loop system monitors breathing and changes in respiratory demands to drive diaphragmatic stimulation. The simulated results inform future acute animal experiments and constitute the first step toward the development of a neuromorphic, adaptive, compact, low-power, implantable device. The bio-inspired hardware design optimizes the FPGA resource and time costs while harnessing the computational power of spike-based neuromorphic hardware. Its real-time feature makes it suitable for *in vivo* applications.

Keywords: bio-inspired controller, spiking neural network (SNN), closed-loop paradigm, ventilatory control system, metabolic demands, spinal-cord injury (SCI), field programmable gate array (FPGA), assisted ventilation

INTRODUCTION

Approximately 282,000 Americans (~0.1% of the US population) have traumatic spinal cord injury (SCI), with approximately 17,000 new injuries being reported each year (National Spinal Cord Injury Statistical Center—NSCISC, 2016). The cervical cord is the most common site of injury (54% of all cases). An individual with high-level cervical SCI at or above the fifth cervical level may experience partial or complete loss of ventilatory control (Warren et al., 2014) because the motor fibers of the phrenic nerve, which innervates the diaphragm, originate from the 3rd to 5th cervical level. Respiratory diseases and failure are the leading cause of death after SCI (67.4% of these were cases of pneumonia) (NSCISC, 2016). Ventilatory insufficiency is often managed with positive pressure mechanical ventilation, but such treatment is associated with significant discomfort, diaphragmatic atrophy, atelectasis and barotrauma (DiMarco, 2005). Most mechanical ventilators act in an open-loop manner, but some systems for partial ventilatory support offer dynamical control of the mechanical ventilation through proportional assist ventilation or neurally adjusted ventilatory assist (Yonis et al., 2015). These systems aim to amplify the patient's native intrinsic respiratory effort. The practicality of these designs is limited by the need for non-invasive and reliable measures of the mechanical characteristics of the respiratory system and need for a reliable positioning of an instrumented transtracheal catheter to obtain reliable measure of the diaphragm electrical activity (Navalesi and Costa, 2003; Terzi et al., 2012).

An alternative approach to mechanical ventilation uses trains of electrical pulses to elicit contractions of the paralyzed (or paretic) ventilatory musculature (DiMarco, 2009; Madsen, 2012; Ho et al., 2014). In many individuals, this approach has been used to achieve suitable ventilation, but the performance of existing assistive ventilatory control system technology is limited. Open-loop ventilatory control systems require iterative manual tuning by a practitioner of parameters of a fixed stimulation pattern. Open-loop systems do not have the ability to adjust these parameters if manual tuning does not produce a stimulation pattern that adequately meets metabolic demands. Furthermore, muscle fatigue and changes in electrode response properties can alter the degree of ventilation produced by an open-loop stimulation, which can also result in an unmet respiratory need. In other systems that use electrical stimulation of paralyzed muscles, traditional feedback controllers (e.g., Abbas and Chizeck, 1991; Schearer et al., 2014) and adaptive approaches (e.g., Abbas and Chizeck, 1995; Riess and Abbas, 2001; Fairchild et al., 2010) have been able to achieve high quality control of limb movements. For ventilatory assistance, a closed-loop adaptive control system that uses electrical stimulation could overcome the drawbacks of open-loop control and offer improved quality of life to individuals with paralysis that impairs ventilation.

Neural networks in the brain modulate the drive to the respiratory muscles to meet metabolic demands under diverse conditions. The spatially distributed pontine–medullary respiratory network activates the spinal motor neurons that innervate the respiratory muscles (Richter, 1996; Smith et al., 2009). The activity of the respiratory network is continually adjusted by two major types of feedback: mechanical feedback (lung volume mechanoreceptors) and chemical feedback (levels of CO_2 and O_2 in the blood and brain tissue chemical receptors). This activity can be modulated by higher brain centers (voluntary control, posture, emotion, etc.). Therefore, the respiratory network activity is sensitive to various stimuli to drive breathing and non-breathing behaviors (vocalization, eating, straining, airway protection reflexes, e.g., coughing, sneezing, or swallowing, etc.). The respiratory network has a robust yet highly flexible network organization that can permit multiple state-dependent modes of operation (Smith et al., 2009). The neural network can be computationally modeled as a network of spiking neurons. Spiking neural network (SNN) paradigms have gained significant attention in the past decades (Maass, 1997) and have inspired many hardware control systems used for robot control algorithms (Arena et al., 2010; Ayers et al., 2010; Nichols et al., 2013), classifier devices (Hsieh and Tang, 2012), new algorithms (Lagorce et al., 2015), or assistive devices for therapy or rehabilitation (Jung et al., 2001; Vogelstein et al., 2008; Sun et al., 2011; Ambroise et al., 2013). Some closed-loop ventilatory control systems have been proposed (Sharshar et al., 2003; Beck et al., 2007) but none have used a bio-inspired SNN control system.

In this paper, we address the need for an adaptive ventilatory control system with a new concept: a bio-inspired SNN controller (**Figure 1**). If the native diaphragmatic drive is totally or partially interrupted by SCI, then ventilation may not be sufficient. A closed-loop system can provide stimulation that adapts in response to measures of physiological variables. Our innovative closed-loop architecture for ventilation assistance is inspired by the pontine–medullary respiratory network to benefit from its robustness and flexibility. The neural network controller is implemented on an FPGA (Field Programmable Gate Array), which is a general approach that has been used since the early 1990s (Cox and Blanz, 1992). It is a fully reconfigurable digital integrated circuit that has low demands on power and computational resources. To achieve high computational efficiency, our controller uses fixed-point computation and implements low computational cost neuron and synapse models. Our design is inspired by the biological circuits but it is not intended to emulate a precise model at the network or cellular level. Our multidisciplinary collaboration has produced a hardware-in-the-loop real-time (HL) simulation platform that uses a computational model of rat ventilation and a fixed-point SNN controller model. The HL simulation was used to validate the bio-inspired SNN controller prior to its implementation in hardware and use in animal experiments.

We first assess the feasibility of implementing a bio-inspired SNN controller in digital hardware. Then, we develop a design methodology for a closed-loop ventilatory control system using our HL computational model and its FPGA implementation. We describe the models (both mathematical and animal) as well as their implementation and use in a HL simulated experiment. Finally, we provide proof-of-concept HL computational results that illustrate ability of the system to adapt the stimulation parameters to meet metabolic demands.

MATERIALS AND METHODS

Bio-Inspired Controller Architectures

The neural networks underlying respiratory rhythm and pattern generation and control of ventilation have been studied extensively. Based on these investigations a pontine–medullary respiratory network model has been proposed for control of ventilation (Smith et al., 2000, 2009) that includes a tonic drive network in the pons, the retrotrapezoid nucleus/parafacial respiratory group, and in raphe nuclei; a respiratory rhythm

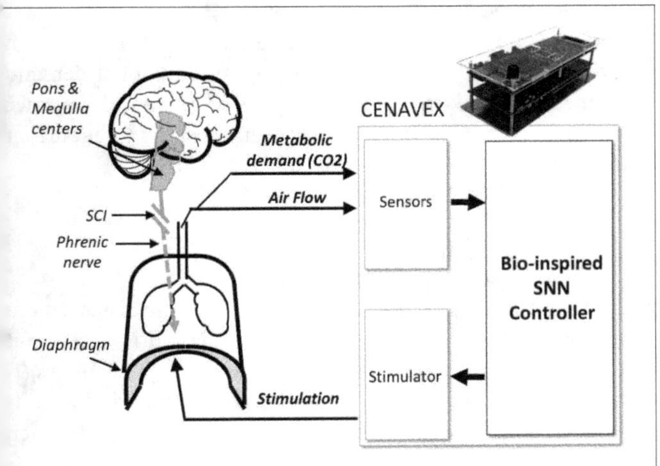

FIGURE 1 | Closed-loop injured respiratory system with the system Computation-Enabled Adaptive Ventilatory Control System (CENAVEX). In the context of spinal cord injury (SCI) or any disruption between the brain and the respiratory muscles, a hardware closed-loop system could provide a complimentary stimulation to the main respiratory muscles (e.g., the diaphragm) for efficient ventilation. A new bio-inspired spiking neural network (SNN) controller drives electric stimulation according to the metabolic status and demands through various physiological feedback signals (air flow, metabolic demand as measured by CO_2 amount).

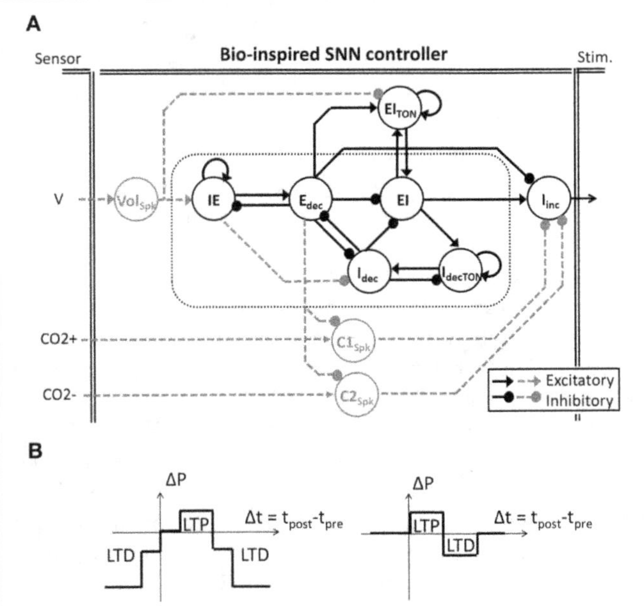

FIGURE 2 | Bio-inspired Spiking Neural Network (SNN) for ventilatory control systems. (A) The bio-inpired controller is used in open and closed-loop paradigms (solely black architecture and black and dashed-gray architecture, respectively). Follower I_{inc} neuronal activity triggers and shapes the electrical stimulation accordingly with the core activities (in doted box). In the closed-loop system, gray tonic neurons activities modulate the core behavior accordingly with the sensor measures (Volume V, CO_2 increase and decrease CO_{2+} and CO_{2-}). Tonic neuron EI_{TON} is used in both open and closed-loop paradigms to modulate the EI core neuron. **(B)** Two modulations of SNN connection strength (ΔP) rely on SNN learning rules (left and right, respectively). Simplified spike-timing-dependent plasticity includes Long-Term Potentiation (LTP) and Long-Term Depression (LTD).

nitiating and generating core in the Bötzinger and Pre-ötzinger regions of the medulla; and follower rostral and audal ventral respiratory neural network groups. In this model, he core network generates the respiratory rhythm and shapes nspiratory and expiratory motor patterns of the follower ventral espiratory group neurons. The latter contain the pre-motor eurons projecting to the phrenic motoneurons and bulbospinal xpiratory neurons for the control of respiratory muscles. The espiratory neural populations are identified by their spiking ischarge patterns and by their possible main contribution in entilatory control (Richter, 1996; Nuding et al., 2009; Smith t al., 2009; Mellen and Thoby-Brisson, 2012; Richter and Smith, 014). Computational scientists have proposed network models mimic both the neural population activity patterns and specific nodulation of the respiratory network (Lindsey et al., 2012; Iolkov et al., 2014; Toporikova et al., 2015).

The bio-inspired SNN controller is based on experimental euroscience and computational studies of the pontine–edullary respiratory network at a high level (i.e., the rchitecture) as well as at a low level (i.e., the population ctivity). We have developed two generations of architecture: n open-loop system (solely black architecture in **Figure 2A**) nd a closed-loop system (both black and gray architecture in **igure 2A**). In the network, each SNN controller neuron is spired by the behavior of one population of the respiratory etwork. The basic organization includes three sub-networks: e FPGA core network defines the stimulation dynamics for ch breath, the FPGA tonic network controls the core network, nd the FPGA follower network converts the core network iking activity into a stimulation signal to the diaphragm. The N controller's core and follower neurons are used in both open and closed-loop architectures. Neuron names in the SNN refer to their discharge pattern (*dec* for decreasing, *inc* for increasing) during a respiratory phase (E for expiration, I for inspiration): decreasing activity pattern expiration (E_{dec} neuron), spiking activity during the inspiration-expiration transition (IE neuron), decreasing activity pattern inspiration (I_{dec} neuron), spiking activity during the expiration-inspiration transition (EI neuron), and increasing pattern inspiration (I_{inc} neuron). Other neurons enable reproduction of specific features of the dynamics of the biological network (e.g., additional triggering neurons such as I_{decTON} and EI_{TON} implement excitatory neuron's dynamics). Finally, additional neurons modulate in real-time the bio-inspired SNN controller behavior using sensor information: Vol_{Spk} directly influences volume; $C1_{Spk}$ and $C2_{Spk}$ increase and decrease CO_2, respectively. CO_2 was chosen as the primary chemical controller for metabolic demand as end-tidal CO_2 which reflects the partial pressure of arterial CO_2 is measureable *in vivo* and provides a very strong influence to respiratory drive.

The bio-inspired SNN controller architecture reflects the respiratory rhythm and pattern generation network architectures presented by Richter and Smith (Richter, 1996; Smith et al., 2009) while being adapted to high density and low power consumption constraints of implanted technology. The Richter and Smith architectures mostly describe the same populations with little variation, such as the core population late-I in Richter (1996) is not explicitly represented in Smith et al. (2009). One common description is the network formed by reciprocal inhibitory connections between two neurons—called the primary inhibitory oscillator. The coupled I_{dec} and E_{dec} neurons mimic the so-called early-I and post-inspiration populations (or PI or post-I).

It should be noted that the SNN architecture does not possess intrinsic pacemakers as in the biological network. The FPGA controller uses a self-excitation connection to mimic intrinsic rhythmogenic capability: the I_{decTON} neuron triggers the I_{dec}; the IE neuron triggers the E_{dec} neuron; and the EI_{TON} triggers the EI neuron. Another example is the connections between the core and follower populations. The follower population could either be inhibited by most of the core population (Richter, 1996) or excited by one core population (pre-I/I in Smith et al., 2009) but in both cases it is an excitatory follower population. In the FPGA controller, a self-excitatory connection on the follower I_{inc} neuron is implemented. This self-excitatory connection was already presented in Richter (1996). The EI neuron triggers I_{inc}, as suggested by the short activation of the pre-I population prior to the follower activity in Richter (1996). Similarly, the E_{dec} neuron inhibits the follower neuron I_{inc} as suggested by the inhibition of PI neuron on the follower neuron in Richter (1996).

The closed-loop architecture adds three tonic neurons to the open-loop architecture: Vol_{spk}, $C1_{spk}$, and $C2_{spk}$ (gray in **Figure 2A**). Tonic neurons encode signals measured by sensors into spike patterns. The tonic neuron activities can update the strength of specific connections in the bio-inspired SNN controller at each computation step. There is scarce information on the network architecture and the activity of biological tonic populations., Spike-timing-dependent plasticity (STDP) as a Hebbian synaptic learning rule has been identified in biological neurons (Markram et al., 1997; Bi and Poo, 1998). It has been demonstrated in various neural circuits over a wide spectrum of species, from insects to humans (Caporale and Dan, 2008), and various types of STDP have been identified (Abbott and Nelson, 2000). We chose to use simplified STDP learning rules (**Figure 2B**) to modulate connections according to breathing rate and depth as well as for injury level and metabolic demands: P(f), P(a), and P(inj). While the open-loop controller is triggered by an external excitatory stimulation (not shown in **Figure 2A**), the closed-loop controller is triggered by the tonic neuron Vol_{spk} activity.

The electrical drive pattern reflects the follower neuron I_{inc} on-going activity. Neuroscience and computational studies usually refer to the neuronal population activity as integrated population activity (population spike frequency histograms) or cycle-triggered histograms (average firing rates of the neurons during the respiratory cycle) reported as spikes per second per neuron (Nuding et al., 2009; Smith et al., 2009). The stimulation ratio is the number of spikes out of 20 measured over the last 20 computation steps (i.e., 10 ms). It represents the activity of each neuron from the bio-inspired SNN. The stimulation ratio is the proportion of maximum activation (stimulus) of the respiratory muscle, 0–1 (in this case, 0 spikes = 0, 10 spikes = 0.5, and 20 spikes = 1, etc.).

Spiking Neural Network Model

The low complexity leaky integrate-and-fire (LIF) neuron formalism was chosen for its minimal computational demand while maintaining key timing properties of biological neurons. The neuron is modeled as a leaky integrator of its total current from all synapses $I_{tot}(t)$, defined in Equation (1):

$$\tau_m \frac{dv_m(t)}{dt} = -v_m(t) + R_m I_{tot}(t) \quad (1)$$

where τ_m is the membrane time constant, $v_m(t)$ the displacement of neuron voltage from the resting potential, and R_m the input resistance. The LIF neuron fires a spike when the variable $v_m(t)$ reaches a fixed threshold. An absolute refractory period forbids the neuron to fire a spike within a fixed period of time after each spike.

The kinetic model for SNN connectivity is an adaptation of the alpha model presented by Destexhe et al. (Destexhe et al., 1994). This kinetic model requires a single multiplier component. It eases the implementation of various kinetics and it "accounts for saturation and summation of multiple synaptic events, obviating the need for event queuing" (Destexhe et al., 1994). The kinetic model is based on a fraction of bound receptors $r(t)$. Destexhe et al. approximate kinetics by two expressions, described in Equations (2) and (3):

1. During a Spike (t0 < t =< t1):

$$r(t - t0) = r_\infty + (r(t0) - r_\infty)\exp(-\frac{t - t0}{\tau_r})$$
$$\text{with } r_\infty = \frac{\alpha}{\alpha + \beta} \& \tau_r = \frac{1}{\alpha + \beta} \quad (2)$$

2. After a Spike (t > t1):

$$r(t - t1) = r(t1)\exp(-\beta(t - t1)) \quad (3)$$

where r_∞ is the maximum fraction of bound receptors, τ_r and $1/\beta$ are time constants of the two phases of $r(t)$ (i.e., during and after spike), and α and β are the forward and backward rate constants for transmitter binding (i.e., how fast or slow the kinetic model is). Unlike the Hodgkin and Huxley conductance model (Hodgkin and Huxley, 1952), α and β in this model are not time-dependent.

The total current from all synapses $I_{tot}(t)$ is the sum of synaptic currents $I_S(t)$. Each synaptic current is taken to be proportional to the fraction of bound receptors $r(t)$, defined in Equation (4):

$$I_S(t) = A_{SE}\, r(t) \quad (4)$$

where A_{SE} is the absolute synaptic strength, which can be exhibited only by activating all bound receptors. Nichols et al. (2013) used a similar approach to compute synaptic current to simulate a biologically inspired SNN for robot motion control. They used an alternative kinetic model with three interdependent derivative equations (Tsodyks et al., 1998). Although their system was easily implemented in software for simulation, it was no implemented in hardware. The R_m $I_{tot}(t)$ variable, equivalent to the Total Post-synaptic Potential (TPP), is defined in Equation (5):

$$R_m I_{tot}(t) = \sum_i P_i \, r_i(t) \quad (5)$$

where P is the absolute synaptic strength potential as determined by the multiplication of A_{SE} by R_m—the input resistance of the neuron. The input resistance R_m is fixed in this model; A_{SE} could be modified by plasticity rules. Combining both variables into one, P, avoids the use of a multiplier component. Finally, absolute synaptic strength potential is used as the connection strength in the bio-inspired SNN network.

To summarize, the neural network model is defined by three processes. The "Kinetic" process updates the fraction of bound receptors *r(t)* according to defined kinetic model. The "TPP" process computes each neuron R_m $I_{tot}(t)$ variable. The "V_m & Spike" process updates the $V_m(t)$ variable, the refractory period status, and may fire a new spike according to the defined LIF neuron model.

FPGA Implementation (Open-Loop)

The bio-inspired SNN controller was described in Very High Speed Integrated Circuits Hardware Description Language (VHDL) to define how to use and connect the hardware components available on the FPGA. The SNN controller was implemented on a Xilinx Spartan-6 FPGA (XC6SLX150: 4 Mbit full speed block RAM, 180 embedded multipliers, 92 k 6-input look-up tables and 184 kb distributed memory), hosted on a custom board, presented elsewhere (Zbrzeski et al., 2015). We used UART communication for storage and display of real-time variable data from the SNN.

A sequencer coordinates two computing phases of the SNN that update and share two dynamical variables, *r(t)* and $V_m(t)$ (**Figures 3A,B**). Both computing phases rely on the previously defined models, taking advantage of their simplicity and their computational efficiency. Then, the sequencer controls a third idle phase to refresh the variables at a defined frequency (in order to achieve biological real-time). In this application, real-time is defined by the controller's ability to elicit diaphragm contraction with on-going real-time updates of the stimulation parameters. The stimulation frequency range is between 75 Hz (typical) and 500 Hz in open-loop stimulation on a rat phrenic nerve or diaphragm (injured or not) (Mantilla et al., 2010; Kowalski et al., 2013). Stimulation frequency is lower for larger animals (e.g., dog, 10–50 Hz) (Walter et al., 2011). The bio-inspired controller updates the SNN behavior and variables at kHz, i.e., the computation time-step *dt* is 0.5 ms. It does not depend on the number of neurons and it ensures accurate control of stimulation pattern.

The first phase is the Kinetic computing. The "Kinetic" process is the conversion over discrete *dt* time-steps of the fraction of bound receptors *r(t)* from the model defined in Equations (6)–(8) using forward Euler integration.

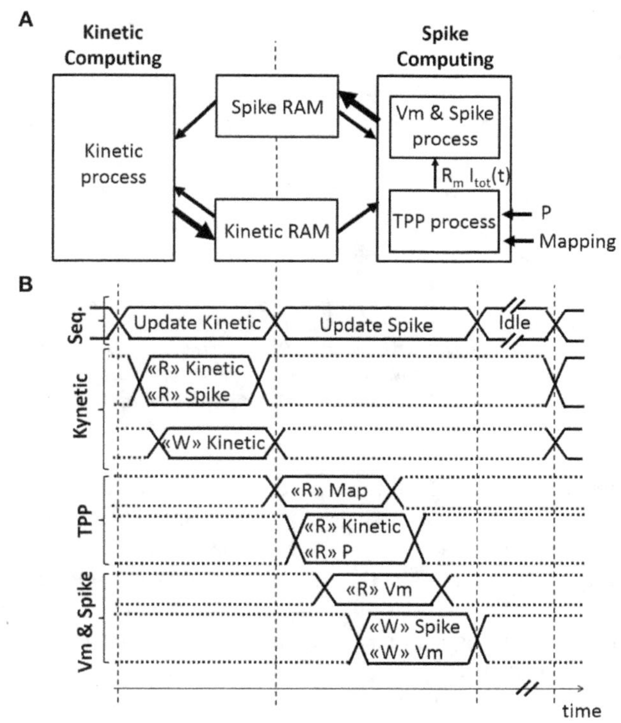

FIGURE 3 | Architecture of the Spiking Neural Network (SNN) implemented on an FPGA. (A) Spatial and **(B)** temporal SNN representations, with *r(t)* the fraction of bound receptors stored in the Kinetic RAM, *P* the absolute synaptic strength potential, R_m $I_{tot}(t)$ the Total Post-synaptic Potential (TPP), and *Vm* the displacement of neuron voltage from the resting potential stored in the Spike RAM as well as the spiking activity of the associated neuron. Small or bold arrows represent, respectively, a computing process reading "R" or writing "W" in a Random-Access Memory (RAM). The SNN sequencer (Seq.) manages two computing phases, followed by an idle phase. The first computing phase updates each kinetic variable *r(t)* associated with one pre-neuron. The second computing phase updates the spike status for each neuron by computing R_m $I_{tot}(t)$ variable with the TPP process, followed by computing *Vm*, the refractory period, and the spike status with the "Vm & Spike." The SNN connectivity is stored in mapping RAM.

1. During a spike (t0 < t = < t1)

$$r[t+1] = A\, r[t] + B \quad (6)$$

2. After a spike (t > t1)

$$r[t+1] = C\, r[t] \quad (7)$$

where A, B, C are constants defined as.

$$A = dt\,\alpha \quad B = 1 - dt\,(\alpha + \beta) \quad C = 1 - (\beta/dt) \quad (8)$$

Table 1 presents five sets of kinetic parameters associated with one neuron. Each set consists of 4 parameters: the maximum fraction of bound receptors (r_∞), the rising exponential time constant (τ_r), and the forward (α) and backward (β) rate constants for transmitter binding. Each kinetic parameter set determines the values of constants (A, B, and C) that are

TABLE 1 | Available kinetics parameter sets.

Kinetic set #	r_∞	τ_r (ms)	α (ms^{-1})	β (ms^{-1})	A	B	C
5	0.90	1.0	900	100	0.4500	0.5000	0.9500
4	0.90	2.0	450	50	0.2250	0.7500	0.9750
3	0.92	4.0	230	20	0.1150	0.8750	0.9900
2	0.92	8.0	115	10	0.0575	0.9375	0.9950
1	0.92	15.9	58	5	0.0290	0.9685	0.9975

Each row presents a pre-defined parameter set that is available for selection when implementing the controller. The α and β are the forward and backward rate constants for transmitter binding. r_8 is the maximum fraction of bound receptors. τ_r is the time constant of the increasing exponential characterizing the r(t) behavior during a spike. A, B, C are the unsigned 14-bit constants used for implementation on the FPGA.

implemented using 14-bit unsigned integers to streamline real-time computation. A 3-stage pipeline is used to update all five kinetic parameters connected to one neuron output. One multiplier is used per kinetic parameter. It takes 519 clock cycles to update 512*5 fractions of bound receptors *r(t)*, saved in block RAM as 0.18 unsigned vectors (i.e., rational values between 0 and 1 coded on 18 bits).

The second phase consists of computing spikes. It is the conversion over discrete *dt* time-steps of the LIF model using forward Euler integration, defined in Equation (9). After a spike, a neuron has a minimum refractory time of one time-step during which membrane potential is set at its resting potential (in this case, −70 mV).

$$v_m[t+1] = v_m[t] + \frac{dt}{\tau_m}(v_{rest} - v_m[t] + R_m I_{tot}[t])$$
$$\text{with } R_m I_{tot}[t] = \sum P\, r[t] \quad (9)$$

The ratio dt/τ_m is set at 8 to use a shift operation instead of a multiplication. The "TPP" process updates the $R_m\, I_{tot}[t]$ signal, as illustrated in **Figures 3A,B**. The $R_m\, I_{tot}[t]$ signal is connected to the "V_m & Spike" process. The implemented architecture does not include the plasticity mechanism, but the block RAM accesses are already available for such a mechanism. The "TPP" and "V_m & Spike" processes each use a 3-stage pipeline to update all neurons. Four multipliers are used in the "TPP" process. It takes 1036 clock cycles to update 512 neurons during this second phase.

The SNN architecture can construct up to an 8-to-all 512-neuron network. Each connection is modeled by 1 among the 5 possible kinetic connections of **Table 1**. The implemented network has a low connectivity density. The implemented SNN controller uses the open-loop architecture (**Figure 2A**). **Table 2** presents the open-loop SNN synaptic parameters.

Hardware-in-the-Loop Real-Time Computational Model

The bio-inspired SNN controller can provide complementary diaphragmatic electrical stimulation to the native phrenic stimulation. The closed-loop version of the SNN controller adapts the stimulation (timing, amplitude) to meet the metabolic demands by adapting the depth and frequency of breathing.

As a precursor to animal experiments, the SNN controller was evaluated in a computational model. **Figure 4A** illustrates a hardware-in-the-loop real-time (HL) computational model using a rat computational model and a fixed-point FPGA SNN controller model. The HL model maintains real-time processing capability (0.5 ms).

The computational model of rat ventilation is a real-time dynamical model with the ability to simulate rat ventilation for various breathing states. The bio-computational model includes a native drive model, an activation model (a linear summation of native and stimulated activation, a simplified first approximation), a musculoskeletal model, and a metabolism model. The model was developed to reproduce the phrenic native drive of an injured/non-injured animal, the combined muscle activation drive, eupneic respiratory volume, and a residual CO_2 quantity in the model.

The musculoskeletal model was scaled to fit the eupneic respiratory output of a non-injured rat. This model was developed from a human computational model in Simulink/SimMechanics implementing the physiologically realistic muscle model from MSMS (Hillen and Jung, 2014). Proportional muscle activation (0–1, proportion of spikes out of 20) as provided by the SNN was transformed into motor unit activation using the intramuscular functional electrical stimulation model from Virtual Muscle (Song et al., 2008) as implemented in MSMS which uses a single motor unit of each type where firing frequency is specified for stimulus intensity using a recruitment order from Singh et al. (2000) for intramuscular stimulation. The lung volume displacement was assumed linearly related to the diaphragm displacement, as illustrated in Richter (1996). This approximation was determined to be acceptable, especially when considering the system in eupneic conditions and when focusing on the volume shape during inspiration phase. Ventilatory compliance was modeled as a damped spring with non-linear stiffness. The non-linear stiffness values for the rat thorax/diaphragm were chosen from experimental data (Young et al., 1992). Damped spring and activation amplitude from the human musculoskeleta model were adjusted such that the rat musculoskeletal mode produced lung volume trajectories similar to experimenta collected rat data (10 experimental data recordings, as presente in **Figure 4B**). Native activation was represented as a space sawtooth function and defined the pattern of the native model.

Experimental data from one male Sprague Dawley rat ($n = 1$ 360 g) (Siu et al., 2015) was used to determine the desired lung volume waveforms that were then used by the control system in the simulation studies. Data was collected with the approva of the Institutional Animal Care and Use Committee of Florid International University. The rat was maintained under eupnei conditions (21% O_2, 0% CO_2, balance N_2) through the us of a gas mixer (GSM-3, CWE Inc.). The rat was anesthetize via IP delivery of pentobarbital (45 mg/kg) with supplementa isoflurane (0.5–1%). A pulse oximeter monitored SpO_2, whil end-tidal CO_2 was monitored via a CO_2 analyzer (Capstar 100, CWE Inc.) throughout the study to monitor and asses animal health. A pneumotachometer (8420A, Hans-Rudolph collected air flow, which was then processed through a hardwar

TABLE 2 | Connectivity between the tonic and core populations of the open-loop SNN controller implemented on the FPGA.

	Post-I		Early-I		PreI/I		-
	$Edec_{TON}$ $K_{i,1}; P_{i,1}$	$Edec_{OUT}$ $K_{i,2}; P_{i,2}$	$Idec_{TON}$ $K_{i,3}; P_{i,3}$	$Idec_{OUT}$ $K_{i,4}; P_{i,4}$	EI_{TON} $K_{i,5}; P_{i,5}$	EI_{OUT} $K_{i,6}; P_{i,6}$	ON $K_{i,7}; P_{i,7}$
1: $Edec_{TON}$	3; +600	1; +5000	–	–	–	–	–
2: $Edec_{OUT}$	1; −2200	–	–	4; −250	4; +8000	4; −500	–
3: $Idec_{TON}$	–	–	3; +40	4; +500	–	–	–
4: $Idec_{OUT}$	–	1; −1500	3; −5000	–	–	4; −350	–
5: EI_{TON}	–	–	–	–	3; +40	2; +400	–
6: EI_{OUT}	–	–	2; +200	–	2; +1280	–	–
7: ON	4; +1280	–	–	–	–	–	–

Each row corresponds to a pre-synaptic neuron i; each column corresponds to a post-synaptic neuron, j. For each pair of connected neurons, the first value indicates the kinetic connection $K_{i,j}$ between neurons i and j; the second value indicates the absolute synaptic strength potential $P_{i,j}$. Note that the ON neuron is used to automatically start the SNN controller after its initializations when used in open-loop mode.

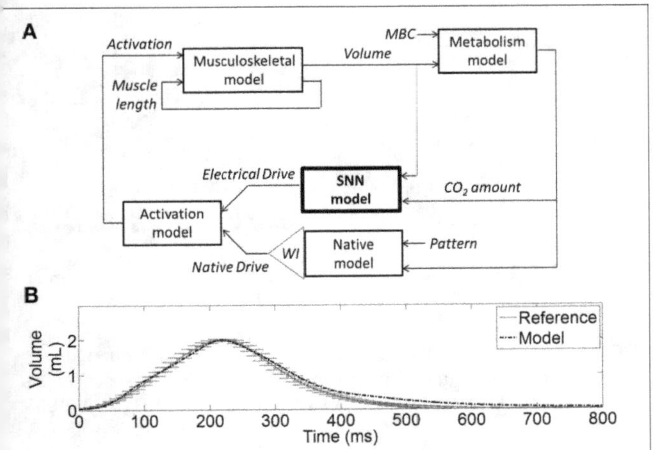

FIGURE 4 | Hardware-in-the-loop (HL) real-time computational model. **(A)** Diagram of the HL computational model including the SNN controller model (bold) and the rat computational model. The SNN controller model (electrical stimulation) and the native model drives (phrenic nerve) are combined in an activation signal (normalized) to stimulate the muscle model. The musculoskeletal model provides the dynamic volume. The metabolism model provides the CO_2 amount in the body, considering a fixed reference CO_2 production (or metabolic demands parameter MBC). The weighted injury factor WI can attenuate the native drive to reflect the impact of spinal cord injury on ventilation. The native drive pattern was defined to mimic experimental data (see **B**). The native model includes a dynamical respiratory rate mechanism: it modulates the native drive pace to reach a constant CO_2 amount on a breath-by-breath basis. **(B)** The non-injured native activation elicits a volume (Model) that is similar to experimental rat volume (Reference).

integrator (PI-1000, CWE Inc.) to obtain breath volume. Bipolar stainless steel barb electrodes were inserted into the diaphragm to record electromyography. Flow, volume, end tidal CO_2, and electromyography measurements were collected at 6 kHz.

The metabolism model was created to dynamically represent the quantity of CO_2 in the computational model. The metabolism model describes generation of CO_2 (by mass) in the body and the exhalation of CO_2 with each breath (as determined by breath volume/rate). Baseline CO_2 production (MBC0) was set for net-zero increase in CO_2 in the body during tidal breathing/eupnea. Increases in metabolic demand are represented by increases in CO_2 production rate. The eupneic computational condition was defined for a respiratory rate (RR) of 56 breaths per minute and a tidal volume of 2 mL. The CO_2 amount is constant on a breath-by-breath basis. If there is an increased metabolic demand while the rat computational model RR and/or volume are not altered, then the CO_2 amount will increase on a breath-by-breath basis.

The native model output is the native drive (e.g., phrenic drive) with a fixed amplitude, and fixed or variable respiratory rate. In a biological rat, RR and tidal volume would increase to keep the CO_2 amount constant. A linear regression defines the relationship between RRs and MBC parameters to provide constant CO_2 amount. It defines the dynamical RR mechanism. Increased metabolic demand conditions of +11% and +17% are called MBC11 and MBC17. These two increased metabolic demands lead to a RR of 62.31 and 65.75 breaths per minute in the non-injured rat model to maintain constant average CO_2. Also, the native model was varied to roughly mimic the effect of an incomplete spinal cord injury on ventilation by attenuation of the native drive through a weighted injury factor. In experimental studies, at 1 day post-injury and in the eupneic condition, rat tidal volumes were reported to be between 70 and 90% of the non-injured tidal volumes (Fuller et al., 2006; Navarrete-Opazo et al., 2015). For use in these simulations, we defined 6 pairs of injury level and metabolic demand conditions: 90%-MBC11, 90%-MBC17, 80%-MBC11, 80%-MBC17, 75%-MBC11, 75%-MBC17.

The SNN controller provides a simulated electrical drive. The SNN network was simulated using the computing phases, computing algorithms and pipeline implementations, and hardware limitations (fixed-point dynamic and accuracy), detailed in section FPGA Implementation (Open-Loop). The HL computational model predicts the behavior of the FPGA implementation of the SNN controller.

Computational results for both open and closed-loop SNN controllers are presented. The open-loop SNN controller was simulated with parameters that represent a complete injured rat computational model (native drive: 0%) with normal metabolic demands (MBC0). The closed-loop SNN controller was simulated with parameters that represent an incomplete injured rat computational model (native drive: 90, 80, 75%) with normal and increased metabolic demands (MBC0, MBC11, MBC17). The coefficient of variation (CV) of RR was computed over the last 10 breathing cycles to assess the variation of the RR over time. Constant RR was defined as breathing that exhibited a coefficient of variation of RR less than 4%.

The same SNN architecture was used for all models. The strength synaptic potentials *P(inj)* were set to optimize the efficiency of the bio-inspired controller for each pair of injury level and metabolic demand. *P(a)* and *P(f)* were set only in open-loop configuration, and were adapted by the controller in the closed-loop configuration. Breathing conditions are characterized with respiratory rate using the 10 last breathing cycles, and the related coefficient of variation.

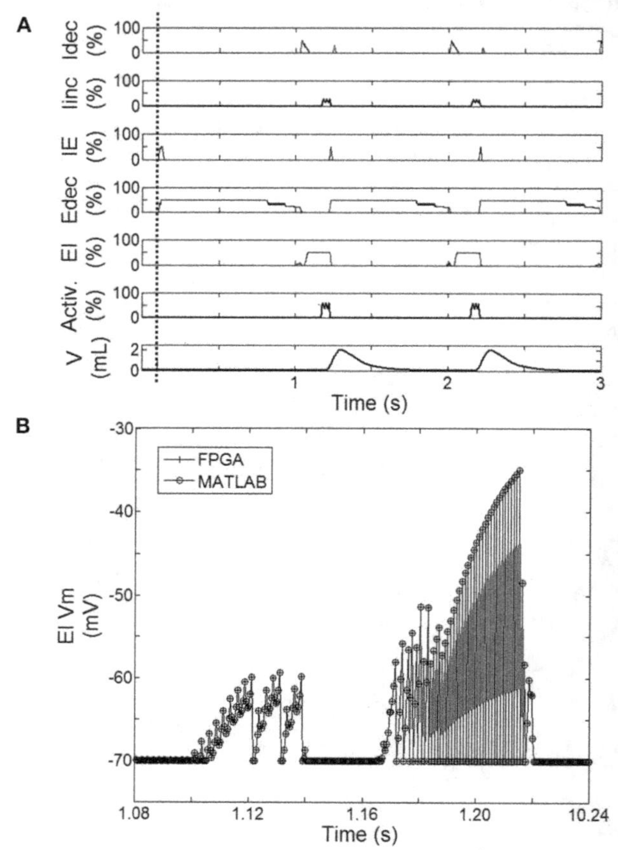

FIGURE 5 | Behavior of the spiking neural network (SNN) when the system is turned ON (after dashed line). (A) Averaged spike count on the last 20 computation steps for each SNN neuron (I_{dec}, I_{inc}, IE, E_{dec}, EI). 100% means the neuron has spiked 20 times over the last 20 computation steps. Results are computed using the hardware-in-the-loop (HL) real-time computational model. SNN model uses the first architecture presented **Figure 2A** with a complete injured model (native drive 0%). Activation drive Activ. and Volume V are reported. **(B)** Illustration of the exact match between FPGA measure and HL computation. Example using the displacement of neuron voltage from the resting potential (Vm) for EI neuron.

RESULTS

Complete Injury Experiment with Open-Loop Controller

The bio-inspired controller described in Section Materials and Methods was used with the complete lesion model (native drive: 0%): diaphragm activation was specified as described in Section Bio-Inspired Controller Architectures. The electrical drive mimics the activity of the follower neuron I_{inc} (**Figure 5A**). Both frequency and amplitude of the electrical drive are fixed in the open-loop paradigm. The open-loop bio-inspired SNN controller uses 7 neurons and 17 connections with low computational power (e.g., neuron and kinetic simplified behavioral models). Device utilization after synthesis of the SNN controller for the open-loop system is listed in **Table 3**. The design operates at 124 MHz. Mixed pipeline, parallel structure and shift operations were used to design a network with optimized hardware resource costs.

The activity of this bio-inspired network is similar to experimental reports (Richter, 1996), as reflected in activity patterns of individual populations and in temporal sequencing and coordination across the network (**Figure 5A**). The coordinated pattern of observed activity is as follows: the I_{dec} activity increases quickly before slightly decreasing, this is followed by a slight then a fast increase of I_{inc} activity; the I_{inc} activity decreases abruptly when the IE activity quickly increases; this triggers E_{dec} activity (and IE activity goes off); then E_{dec} activity increases first quickly then slowly, which turns on EI activity to briefly activate I_{dec} activity; and the activation sequence is repeated. The Matlab SNN computational model was designed to emulate the high level dynamic behavior as well as the exact data processing dynamics of the FPGA component. The HL computational delay is the computation time-step itself; there is no buffering effect at the network level. The MATLAB implementation was used to develop the FPGA implementation, which runs in real-time with sub-microsecond precision. Dynamic behaviors and values are strictly the same between the computational model running on Matlab and its FPGA implementation from the network to intrinsic neuron variables as illustrated in **Figure 5B**. This observation was verified for all SNN variables: membranes voltages, spike states and fractions c bound receptors of the kinetic model (not shown).

The relationship between the accuracy of the fractions c bound receptors and the system's ability to drive a wide rang of stimulated respiratory rates is presented in **Figure 6**. W evaluated the impact of *r(t)* accuracy (number of bits) on th SNN output resolution. The HL computational tool facilitat the identification of the most sensitive absolute synaptic strengt potentials, P(f), to the modulation of electrical drive frequenc (i.e., the node between pre-neuron IE and post-neuron Ed neurons). The HL computational tool helps to find appropria tradeoffs between technology resources and application functio in a varied respiratory context. All SNN variable accuracies a fixed except for the *r(t)* accuracy (kinetic model). The maximu RR variation between bio-inspired controller with the highe simulated *r(t)* accuracy (32-bit) and lower accuracies (under, and above 18-bit) are, respectively 4, 2, and 1 Br.min^{-1}. Anoth

TABLE 3 | Device utilization (Xilinx Spartan XC6SLX150) for the implementation of the open-loop SNN controller on FPGA.

Resource	Used	Percent utilization (%)
Slice LUTs	4502	4
LUT-FF pairs	2124	36
Slice registers	3427	1
18Kb RAM/FIFO	19	7
Mults (18 × 18)	9	5

Results obtained using XST synthesis software from Xilinx Inc. with standard optimization effort on timing, under the ISE 14.7 development environment.

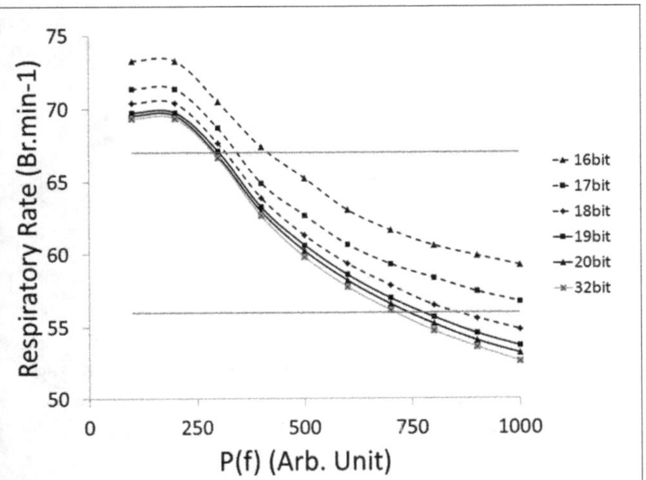

FIGURE 6 | Computational Respiratory rate (RR) vs. tuned open-loop bio-inspired controller. The absolute synaptic strength potential between pre-neuron IE and post-neuron E_{dec} is P(f), identified in **Figure 2A**. Fractions of bound receptors of the kinetic model can have an accuracy ranging from 16 bit to 32 bit. Native drive is 0 to mimic a complete injured model. Horizontal lines identify RR at 56 and 67 $Br.min^{-1}$, targeting range of rat eupneic RR.

comparison is set by targeting a range of rat eupneic RRs (e.g., between 56 and 67 $Br.min^{-1}$). The associated range of absolute synaptic strength potentials P with high accuracy (32 bit) is from 300 to 700. The bio-inspired controller with $r(t)$ accuracy above 18-bit approximately shares the same lower range, and can vary up to 100 with the lowest accuracy. The $r(t)$ accuracy has a stronger impact on the higher range, e.g., from 700 (32-bit) to 850 (18-bit). Therefore, using low accuracy could potentially limit the ability of the system to deliver stimulation at a high frequency. Finally, we used 18-bit accuracy for the fractions of bound receptors $r(t)$ in the bio-inspired controller: it has shown to be closely equivalent to a 32-bit structure and it minimizes the number of multipliers (limited in this technology to a 18-bit accuracy).

Incomplete Injury Experiment with Closed-Loop Controller

The closed-loop architecture of bio-inspired SNN controller was designed, developed, and modeled for HL computation. It can dynamically synchronize its electrical drive with the native drive. The electrical drive can modify simulated animal breathing depth as well as respiratory rate. **Figure 7** shows the effect of activating the bio-inspired controller in an incomplete injury model (native drive: 90%). Breathing was not optimal prior to activation of the bio-inspired controller; depth of breathing was lower than in the non-injured model. The metabolism model sets a slightly higher breathing rate in the injured than in the non-injured model to keep equivalent minute ventilation: respiration depth was higher in the injured model with bio-inspired controller as compared to the non-injured model. The CV of RR reaches a peak of approximately 5% at cycle #11. The stabilization of the amplitude and frequency of respiration occurs in the 16th breath cycle, about 15 s after activation of the bio-controller while the CV of the respiratory rate parameter drops below the 4% mark. The activation pattern after $t = 15$ s was consistent. The stabilization of P(f) (sensitive to electrical stimulation frequency) has a faster timescale of 4 cycles ($t = 6$ s). The absolute synaptic strength potential, P(a), did not vary much upon activation of the bio-inspired controller (not shown).

The closed-loop system demonstrated robust performance when tested on 3 types of incomplete injury (native drive: 90, 80, 75%) with perturbations induced by activating the bio-inspired controller and by alterations in the rat model (sudden increases in metabolism of 11 and 17%). The bio-inspired controller performed well in all cases by responding to the perturbation. The bio-inspired controller demonstrated adaptability by modifying the electrical drive to assist the incomplete injured model to reach equivalent breath depth and rate as in a non-injured model. The HL computational results with respect to a non-injured model are presented in **Figure 8** for all pairs of injury level and metabolic demand and for all perturbations. The absolute synaptic strength potentials P(inj) are more sensitive to the injury level than the metabolic demand increase except for one of them (P between Vol_{spk} and IE neurons, not shown). Data quantifying the effectiveness of the bio-inspired controller are presented in **Table 4**. First, the breath depth and rate were evaluated when the bio-controller was turned ON (**Figure 8A**). Initially, with the bio-controller OFF, the respiratory rates were all higher when the level of injury was large: respiratory rate increased from 11 to 31% from a non-injured model. Respiratory rate was reduced in all cases when the bio-controller was turned ON: a 4–10% error was measured when compared to the non-injured model but with a 5–23% improvement when compared to incomplete injured models with the bio-inspired controller OFF. The stabilization of the synchronized bio-inspired controller was reached in 14 breathing cycles with high injury models (80 and 75%) vs. 17 cycles with the lowest injury model (90%). The performance after activation of the bio-inspired controller was independent of network parameters for each injury level: e.g., injury at 90% has both a synchronization time and stabilization time of 17 breathing cycles.

Bio-inspired controller behavior as a function of metabolic demand is shown in **Figures 8B,C**. All but one condition was stable between 10 and 15 cycles after a metabolic perturbation. In the particular case of 80%-MBC17, the I_{inc} neuron behavior is slower than other SNNs. At cycle #100, bio-inspired controllers

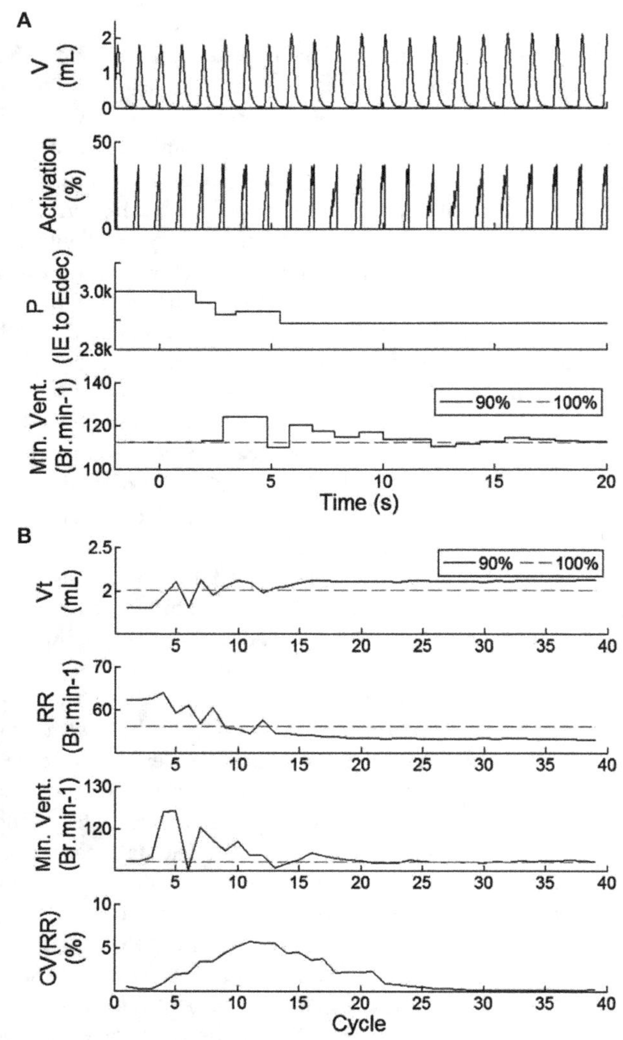

FIGURE 7 | Effect of the SNN electrical stimulation on the ventilation of an incomplete injured rat illustrated by hardware-in-the-loop real-time computational model in eupnea. (A) Electrical drive effect on the rat computational breathing over time when the SNN controller was turned ON (at $t = 0$ s). Volume V, Activation drive to the musculoskeletal model, and absolute synaptic strength potential P between the IE and Edec population are presented for incomplete injured model. Minute ventilation (Min.Vent.) is compared between incomplete injured and non-injured models. Associated native drives are 90% and 100%. **(B)** Evolution of respiratory parameters vs. breathing cycle. The SNN controller was turned ON at cycle #1. Tidal volume (Vt), respiratory rate (RR), minute ventilation (Min.Vent.), and coefficient of variation of the RR parameter (over the last 10 cycles) are presented for both incomplete injured and non-injured models.

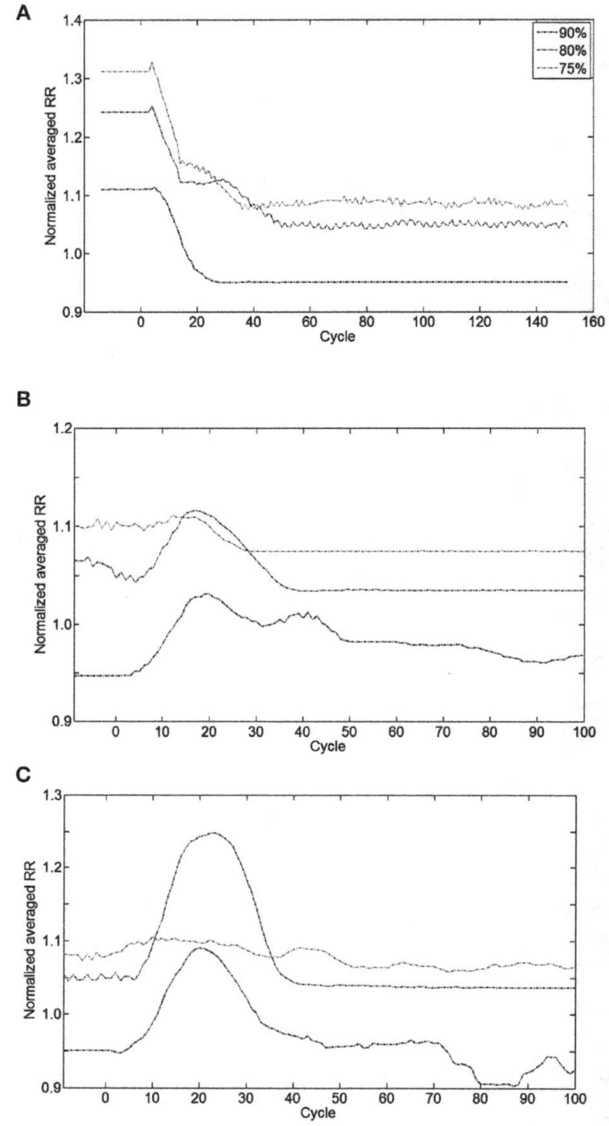

FIGURE 8 | Effect of bio-inspired controller electrical stimulation on breathing using injured model (native drive: 90, 80, 75%) vs. non-injured model (native drive: 100%). The normalized averaged respiratory rate (RR) is the ratio of averaged RR over the last 10 breathing cycles between injured and non-injured models. Normalized averaged RR of 1.0 means the averaged RR is equal between injured and non-injured models. Perturbations start at cycle #0. **(A)** The bio-inspired controller was turned ON at cycle #0 using initialization parameters set for a future metabolic demand increase of 17%. Results of the bio-inspired controller set for a future metabolic demand increase of 11% are not shown for readability. **(B)** Metabolic demand increased from eupneic to +11%, or **(C)** to +17% at cycle #0. Controller was turned ON at cycle #0 in **(B,C)**. At cycle #0, the non-injured RR was set at the final metabolic demand non-injured RR is 56.0, 62.2, 65.7 Br.min^{-1} in, respectively, **(A–C)** results.

are synchronized and lead to a difference in respiratory rate of 3–8% when compared to non-injured models in the same metabolic demand condition. All results are stable at least for 300 s after controller activation and 180 s after metabolic perturbation.

DISCUSSION

This work demonstrates the potential benefit of using bio-inspired SNN controllers to restore impaired functions, e.g., impaired breathing ability with incomplete spinal cord injury. In addition, this work shows exploitation of hardware-in-the-loop (HL) real-time computation to facilitate efficient design and development of a closed-loop system in a multidisciplinary research environment.

TABLE 4 | Delay of the bio-inspired controller to adapt to various perturbations expressed in breathing cycles.

Network vs. perturbation	OFF/ON	+MBC
90%–MBC11	17 cycles (1.11–0.94)	13 cycles (0.94–0.96)
90%–MBC11	17 cycles (1.11–0.95)	15 cycles (0.95–0.92)
80%–MBC11	14 cycles (1.24–1.06)	13 cycles (1.04–1.03)
80%–MBC17	14 cycles (1.24–1.04)	17 cycles (1.04–1.03)
75%–MBC11	14 cycles (1.31–1.10)	10 cycles (1.10–1.07)
75%–MBC17	14 cycles (1.31–1.08)	13 cycles (1.07–1.06)

Perturbation is either when the controller is turned ON (OFF/ON) or when the metabolic demand increases (from eupneic to +11% or +17%) while the controller is ON. Injury level is defined by the native drive percentage (90, 80, 75%). One spiking neural network architecture was set with 6 slight variations of few absolute synaptic strength potentials to optimize the efficiency of the bio-inspired controller for each pair of injury level/metabolic demand increase. The number of breathing cycles where the coefficient of variation of the respiratory rate was less than 4% is reported. Also, normalized averaged respiratory rate at cycle #0 and #100 are reported between brackets.

The FPGA development of a closed-loop system benefits from the bio-inspired architecture. This has been demonstrated by the fact that an all-to-all connectivity pattern is not mandatory to achieve suitable performance. This bio-inspired controller is functional in open and closed-loop configurations with a connection density of 30.3 and 30.7%, respectively. The summary presented in **Table 5** indicates that connection and neuron numbers vary widely across architectures. The biologically-based half-center or pattern generator architectures (Jung et al., 2001; Vogelstein et al., 2008; Molkov et al., 2014) have larger all-to-all density than those with feedforward architecture (Arena et al., 2010; Ayers et al., 2010), which are inspired by artificial neural network paradigms. We observe similar connection densities (29.9 ± 7.6%) to the biologically-based architectures when using 8-to-all connectivity. With our architecture, up to 1660 neurons can be implemented with the same multiplier resources and computation time-step by increasing the Spike computing phase and decreasing the idle phase. If hardware implementations used densities comparable to the computational network, then increasing the maximum number of connection per neuron to MaxC would result in a very large network. The networks presented in **Table 5** have different ratios between the maximum numbers of connection C per neuron N. Therefore, a better understanding of the biological neural networks upon which we base our controllers may be as important as our ability to increase both neurons and MaxC resources to significantly improve closed-loop system functionality. The bio-inspired SNN controller functions appropriately with limited resources, as demonstrated in both open and closed-loop paradigms with perturbations (**Figures 6–8**). **Table 3** reports the device utilization where only 5 multipliers and 19 18 kb-RAM-blocks are required. As mentioned earlier, the implemented system can extend its number of neurons up to hundreds without requiring additional resources. Moreover, the architecture presented in **Figure 3** is easily scalable.

This bio-inspired ventilatory controller simultaneously adapts and coordinates the breathing rate and pattern of the electrical drive over long timescales (breaths) with high computational power using short timescales (spikes). The intrinsic activity of the bio-inspired SNN controller is similar to respiratory networks (compare **Figure 5A** to results reported in Richter, 1996). The primary inhibitory oscillator is described as a coupled population of early-I and post-inspiration (or PI or post-I) neurons; these neurons are equivalent to the I_{dec} and E_{dec} neurons of the bio-inspired controller.

Surprisingly, a 10-neuron bio-inspired SNN also exhibits secondary behavior that is similar to that of the biological system: the double peak activity of the EI neuron. Yet, using a population instead of a single neuron could potentially improve the activity of others, such as Idec neuron. Indeed, the short duration of I_{dec} activity affects the duration of the EI second peak activity (longer than experimental measures). The functionality of the spike-based bio-inspired approach has been illustrated with various conditions. Bio-inspired controller activities were computed over an equivalent relatively long time (from 3 to 5 min) while showing good stability (coefficient of variation of respiratory rate remains under 5%). In addition, SNNs are known to be robust to noise or artifacts (Navalesi and Costa, 2003; Terzi et al., 2012). The capacity for stable regulation and dynamic properties of the biological system (Warren et al., 2014) are reproduced by the bio-inspired SNN controller, as shown in **Figures 7, 8**. These results demonstrate smooth synchronization with native breathing activity and robust responses to perturbations (turning ON the bio-inspired controller or sudden metabolic demand increase, for 3 examples of incomplete injury). In contrast with existing ventilatory assist systems that use electrical stimulation, the controller does not impose a fixed breathing rate. Also, the contribution of the electrical stimulation was appropriate and sufficient enough to improve respiratory rate despite disruptions in 3 injury models, reproducing the original desired breathing pattern.

One important aspect of this work is the hardware-in-the-loop (HL) real-time computational model. The spectrum of rehabilitation applications is wide, especially considering all possible contexts, but few HL models have been presented: epilepsy and Parkinson's disease (Detorakis et al., 2015; Ehrens et al., 2015). Experimental and clinical studies will always ultimately be required to validate the safety and functionality of closed-loop rehabilitation systems, but computational studies can be utilized as intermediary steps. Regulatory agencies are increasingly recognizing the potential contributions of simulation studies throughout the device development and evaluation process. One of the highest priorities for 2016 of the Center for Devices and Radiological Health of the US Food and Drug Administration is to develop computational modeling technologies to support regulatory decision making. Computational model results could be used as evidence to reduce the size of some clinical trials.

One important asset of the HL model is that it enables efficient investigation of controller performance under a wide range of conditions (physiological parameters and controller parameters). For example, we identified one of the main sensitive nodes in the bio-inspired SNN to regulate and synchronize

TABLE 5 | Literature review of connection densities for various spiking neural networks used in neuroscience or applicable controller research.

		C (* w/inputs)	N	MaxC	All-to-all density (%)	MaxC-to-all density (%)	8-to-all density (%)	C/N
Open-loop	This work	17	7	3	34.6	80.9	30.3	2.4
	Richter, 1996	16	6	4	44.4	66.6	33.3	2.6
	Ambroise et al., 2013	12	8	2	18.7	75.0	18.7	1.5
Closed-loop	This work	24 (*27)	10	4	24.0	60.0	30.0	2.4
	Molkov et al., 2014	30 (*33)	13	6	17.7	38.4	28.8	2.3
	Jung et al., 2001	12 (*18)	6	3	33.3	66.6	25.0	2.0
	Vogelstein et al., 2008	14 (*16)	4	4	87.5	87.5	43.7	3.5
	Ayers et al., 2010	31 (*44)	27	2	4.2	57.4	14.3	1.1
	Arena et al., 2010	32 (*46)	20	10	8.0	16.0	20.0	1.6
	Average (std)	20.8 ± 8.3	11.2 ± 7.6	4.2 ± 2.4	30.2 ± 25.02	60.9 ± 22.0	27.1 ± 8.8	2.1 ± 0.7

MaxC is the maximum number of connections C per neuron N in the network. All MaxC and 8-to-all densities were computed using the number of connections in the network vs., respectively, all-to-all neurons, MaxC-to-all and 8-to-all connections. Connections from external signals in closed-loop network were not included in the computation but are reported in brackets.

the electrical drive with the native drive (**Figures 6, 7A**) prior to any animal experiment. HL results highlight strengths and weakness in the network architecture. Another example is the identification of the importance of adapting I_{inc} absolute synaptic strength potentials for the control of the electrical drive pattern: the I_{inc} related plasticity can improve the electrical drive behavior with sufficient resolution in real-time. However, the proposed closed-loop architecture does not provide high enough accuracy in this respect (**Figure 7**). The HL results advocate turning the single I_{inc} neuron into a sub-network, or population. The HL tool allows such development without compromising the other closed-loop functions. A third example is the independent implementation of active expiratory drive. The presented bio-controller does not include expiratory neurons identified in the literature (Richter, 1996; Molkov et al., 2014) but it still provides significant ventilatory assistance. Finally, the HL results call for further examination and development of learning rules. Learning rules in this work assist the breath depth and rate. Six similar sets of absolute synaptic strength potentials *P(inj)* were set to optimize the efficiency of the bio-inspired controller for each couple of injury level/metabolic demand increase (**Figure 8**). This HL computational study shows the need for a third learning rule related to the customization between the patient condition (injury level/ metabolic demand) and absolute synaptic strength potentials using a single SNN controller architecture. This third learning rule could be seen as equivalent to meta-plasticity in neuroscience. Learning rules could be easily implemented on the FPGA due to its scalable and modular structure at no additional time cost: updating all absolute synaptic strength potentials will be done during the kinetic phase, described in **Figure 3B**. Implementation of that third rule is the next step of this study combined with upcoming *in vivo* rat experiments.

In this study, we developed a rat computational model along with the accurate hardware implementation model to evaluate the feasibility of a bio-inspired controller for ventilation assistance in spinal cord injury applications. Each component of this model could be improved to more closely match experimental results. For example, the activation could include results reported from investigations of mechanisms of nerve electrical stimulation. Also, the metabolism model has a limited sensitivity: respiratory rate CV should not be higher than 0 at any time to represent breathing variability (**Figure 8**). Increasing the sensor diversity and number of sensors could improve the performance and versatility of the closed-loop system. Further insight from studies investigating the primary and secondary roles of various chemoreceptors (Ballantyne and Scheid, 2001; Huckstepp and Dale, 2011) could drive further enhancements to the bio-inspired system. For eventual implementation in humans, sensors will be required to gather reliable measures in a manner that minimizes inconvenience and limitations on activities such as speech. To measure the variables used in the simulation studies presented here, a small tube placed in or near the mouth or nose could be used to sample expired CO_2; chest expansion sensors could be used to monitor volume. Further developments of sensor technologies would greatly facilitate clinical translation of adaptive ventilatory control systems.

CONCLUSION

This innovative controller is inspired by neuroscientific investigations and computational models of the respiratory neural network. Its SNN architecture has been designed to be functional and resource- efficient when implemented on an FPGA device while using neuron and kinetic models with low demands on computational resources. The closed-loop architecture takes advantages of the SNN structure to adapt the ventilatory control system with potentially numerous and varied types of feedback signals as illustrated by our custom hardware-in-the-loop real-time platform simulations. This work helps to design cross-disciplinary research experiments that pave the way to the design of the next generation of ventilation control systems.

AUTHOR CONTRIBUTIONS

AZ developed the bio-inspired controller architecture and the SNN model. AZ and YB developed and tested the FPGA hardware. AZ and BH developed the HL models. RS prepared experimental materials and provided processed experimental data. AZ and SR analyzed simulated results. All authors contributed to the closed-loop concept for ventilatory assistance. SR, RJ, and JA supervised all aspects of the work. All authors discussed the results and commented on the manuscript.

ACKNOWLEDGMENTS

The authors would like to acknowledge the technical support of Ashwin MANGALORE and Gilles N'KAOUA. The authors would like to thank Dr. Jennifer HASLER for valuable discussions. This work was supported by the US-French Collaborative Research in Computational Neuroscience program: Agence Nationale pour la Recherche (ANR-13-NEUC-0001) and National Institutes of Health (R01-NS086088).

REFERENCES

Abbas, J. J., and Chizeck, H. J. (1991). Feedback control of coronal plane hip angle in paraplegic subjects using functional neuromuscular stimulation. *IEEE Trans. Biomed. Eng.* 38, 687–698. doi: 10.1109/10.83570

Abbas, J. J., and Chizeck, H. J. (1995). Neural network control of functional neuromuscular stimulation systems: computer simulation studies. *IEEE Trans. Biomed. Eng.* 42, 1117–1127. doi: 10.1109/10.469379

Abbott, L. F., and Nelson, S. B. (2000). Synaptic plasticity: taming the beast. *Nat. Neurosci.* 3(suppl), 1178–1183. doi: 10.1038/81453

Ambroise, M., Levim, T., Joucla, S., Yvert, B., Saïghi, S. (2013). Real-time biomimetic central pattern generators in an FPGA for hybrid experiments. *Front. Neurosci.* 7:215. doi: 10.3389/fnins.2013.00215

Arena, P., De Fiore, S., Patané, L., Pollino M., and Ventura C. (2010). Insect inspired unsupervised learning for tactic and phobic behavior enhancement in a hybrid robot. *Int. Joint Conf. Neural Netw.* 1–8. doi: 10.1109/ijcnn.2010.5596542

Ayers, J., Rulkov, N., Knudsen, D., Kim, Y.-B., Volkovski, A., and Selverston, A. (2010). Controlling underwater robots with electronic nervous systems. *Appl. Bionics Biomech.* 7, 57–67. doi: 10.1080/11762320903244843

Ballantyne, D., and Scheid, P. (2001). Central chemosensitivity of respiration: a brief overview. *Respir. Physiol.* 129, 5–12. doi: 10.1016/S0034-5687(01)00297-3

Beck, J., Campoccia, F., Allo, J. C., Brander, L., Brunet, F., Slutsky, A. S., et al. (2007). Improved synchrony and respiratory unloading by neurally adjusted ventilatory assist (NAVA) in lung-injured rabbits. *Pediatr. Res.* 61, 289–294. doi: 10.1203/01.pdr.0000257324.22406.93

Bi, G.-Q., and Poo, M.-M. (1998). Synaptic modifications in cultured hippocampal neurons: dependence on spike timing, synaptic strength, and postsynaptic cell type. *J. Neurosci.* 18, 10464–10472.

Caporale, N., and Dan, Y. (2008). Spike timing-dependent plasticity: a Hebbian learning rule. *Annu. Rev. Neurosci.* 31, 25–46. doi: 10.1146/annurev.neuro.31.060407.125639

Cox, C. E., and Blanz, E. (1992). GangLion – a fast field-programmable gate array implementation of a connectionist classifier. *IEEE J. Solid S. Circuits* 28, 288–299.

Destexhe, A., Mainen, Z. F., and Sejnowski, T. J. (1994). An efficient method for computing synaptic conductances based on a kinetic model of receptor binding. *Neural. Comp.* 6, 14–18. doi: 10.1162/neco.1994.6.1.14

Detorakis, G. I., Chaillet, A., Palfi, S., and Senova, S. (2015). Closed-loop stimulation of a delayed neural fields model of parkinsonian STN-GPe network: a theoretical and computational study. *Front. Neurosci.* 9:237. doi: 10.3389/fnins.2015.00237

DiMarco, A. F. (2005). Restoration of respiratory muscle function following spinal cord injury: review of electrical and magnetic stimulation techniques. *Respir. Physiol. Neurobiol.* 147, 273–287. doi: 10.1016/j.resp.2005.03.007

DiMarco, A. F. (2009). Phrenic nerve stimulation in patients with spinal cord injury. *Respir. Physiol. Neurobiol.* 169, 200–209. doi: 10.1016/j.resp.2009.09.008

Ehrens, D., Sritharanand, D., and Sarma, S. V. (2015). Closed-loop control of a fragile network: application to seizure-like dynamics of an epilepsy model. *Front. Neurosci.* 9:58. doi: 10.3389/fnins.2015.00058

Fairchild, M. D., Kim, S. J., Iarkov, A., Abbas, J. J., and Jung, R. (2010). Repetetive hindlimb movement using intermittent adaptive neuromuscular electrical stimulation in an incomplete spinal cord injury rodent model. *Exp. Neurol.* 223, 623–633. doi: 10.1016/j.expneurol.2010.02.011

Fuller, D. D., Golder, F. J., Olson, E. B. Jr., and Mitchell, G. S. (2006). Recovery of phrenic activity and ventilation after cervical spinal hemisection in rats. *J. Appl. Physiol.* 100, 800–806. doi: 10.1152/japplphysiol.00960.2005

Hillen, B. K., and Jung, R. (2014). Computational model of human ventilation for electrical stimulation following cervical spinal cord injury. *BMC Neurosci.* 15(suppl. 1):133. doi: 10.1186/1471-2202-15-S1-P133

Ho, C. H., Triolo, R. J., Elias, A. L., Kilgore, K. L., DiMarco, A. F., Bogie, K., et al. (2014). Functional electrical stimulation and spinal cord injury. *Phys. Med. Rehabil. Clin. N. Am.* 25, 631–654. doi: 10.1016/j.pmr.2014.05.001

Hodgkin, A. L., and Huxley, A. F. (1952). A quantitative description of membrane current and its application to conduction and excitation in nerve. *J. Physiol.* 117, 500–544. doi: 10.1113/jphysiol.1952.sp004764

Hsieh, H.-Y., and Tang, K.-T. (2012). VLSI implementation of a bio-inspired olfactory spiking neural network. *IEEE Trans. Neural. Netw. Learn. Syst.* 23, 1065–1073. doi: 10.1109/TNNLS.2012.2195329

Huckstepp, R. T., and Dale, N. (2011). Redefining the components of central CO_2 chemosensitivity-towards a better understanding of mechanism. *J. Physiol.* 589, 5561–5579. doi: 10.1113/jphysiol.2011.214759

Jung, R., Brauer, E. J., and Abbas, J. J. (2001). Real-time interaction between a neuromorphic electronic circuit and the spinal cord. *IEEE Trans. Neural Syst. Rehabil. Eng.* 9, 319–326. doi: 10.1109/7333.948461

Kowalski, K. E., Hsieh, Y. H., Dick, T. E., and DiMarco, A. F. (2013). Diaphragm activation via high frequency spinal cord stimulation in a rodent model of spinal cord injury. *Exp. Neurol.* 247, 689–693. doi: 10.1016/j.expneurol.2013.03.006

Lagorce, X., Stromatias, E., Galluppi, F., Plana, L. A., Liu, S.-C., Furber, S. B., et al. (2015). Breaking the millisecond barrier on SpiNNaker: implementing asynchronous event-based plastic models with microsecond resolution. *Front. Neurosci.* 9:206. doi: 10.3389/fnins.2015.00206

Lindsey, B. G., Rybak, I. A., and Smith, J. C. (2012). Computational models and emergent properties of respiratory neural networks. *Compr. Physiol.* 2, 1619–1670. doi: 10.1002/cphy.c110016

Maass, W. (1997). Networks of spiking neurons: the third generation of neural network models. *Neural Netw.* 10, 1659–1671. doi: 10.1016/S0893-6080(97)00011-7

Madsen, A. (2012). A closer look: diaphragm pacing system. *MDA/ALS Newsmagazine.* 17, 1. Available online at: http://alsn.mda.org/article/closer-look-diaphragm-pacingsystem (Accessed November 10, 2014).

Mantilla, C. B., Seven, Y. B., Zhan, W. Z., and Sieck, G. C. (2010). Diaphragm motor unit recruitment in rats. *Respir. Physiol. Neurobiol.* 173, 101–106. doi: 10.1016/j.resp.2010.07.001

Markram, H., Lübke, J., Frotscher, M., and Sakmann, B. (1997). Regulation of synaptic efficacy by coincidence of postsynaptic APs and EPSPs. *Science* 275, 213–215. doi: 10.1126/science.275.5297.213

Mellen, N. M., and Thoby-Brisson, M. (2012). Respiratory circuits: development, function and models. *Curr. Opin. Neurobiol.* 22, 676–685. doi: 10.1016/j.conb.2012.01.001

Molkov, Y. I., Shevtsova, N. A., Park, C., Ben-Tal, A., Smith, J. C., Rubin, J. E., et al. (2014). A closed-loop model of the respiratory system: focus on hypercapnia and active expiration. *PLoS ONE* 9:e109894. doi: 10.1371/journal.pone.0109894

National Spinal Cord Injury Statistical Center (NSCISC) (2016). *Facts and Figures at a Glance*. Birmingham, AL: University of Alabama at Birmingham.

Navalesi, P., and Costa, R. (2003). New modes of mechanical ventilation: proportional assist ventilation, neurally adjusted ventilatory assist, and fractal ventilation. *Curr. Opin. Crit. Care* 9, 51–58. doi: 10.1097/00075198-200302000-00010

Navarrete-Opazo, A., Vinit, S., Dougherty, B. J., and Mitchell, G. S. (2015). Daily acute intermittent hypoxia elicits functional recovery of diaphragm and inspiratory intercostal muscle activity after acute cervical spinal injury. *Exp. Neurol.* 266, 1–10. doi: 10.1016/j.expneurol.2015.02.007

Nichols, E., McDaid, L. J., and Siddique, N. (2013). Biologically inspired SNN for robot control. *IEEE Trans. Cyb.* 43, 115–128. doi: 10.1109/TSMCB.2012.2200674

Nuding, S. C., Segers, L. S., Baekey, D. M., Dick, T. E., Solomon, I. C., Shannon, R., et al. (2009). Pontine–ventral respiratory column interactions through raphé circuits detected using multi-array spike train recordings. *J. Neurophysiol.* 101, 2943–2960. doi: 10.1152/jn.91305.2008

Richter, D. W. (1996). "Neural regulation of respiration: rhythmogenesis and afferent control," in *Comprehensive Human Physiology: From Cellular Mechanisms to Integration*, eds R. Greger and U. Windhorst (Berlin; Heidelberg: Springer), 2079–2095.

Richter, D. W., and Smith, J. C. (2014). Respiratory rhythm generation *in vivo*. *Physiology* 29, 58–71. doi: 10.1152/physiol.00035.2013

Riess, J., and Abbas, J. J. (2001). Adaptive control of cyclic movements as muscles fatigue using functional neuromuscular stimulation. *IEEE Trans. Neural Syst. Rehabil. Eng.* 9, 326–330. doi: 10.1109/7333.948462

Schearer, E. M., Liao, Y. W., Perreault, E. J., Tresch, M. C., Memberg, W. D., Kirsch, R. F., et al. (2014). Multi-muscle FES force control of the human arm for arbitrary goals. *IEEE Trans. Neural Syst. Rehabil. Eng.* 22, 654–663. doi: 10.1109/TNSRE.2013.2282903

Sharshar, T., Desmarais, G., Louis, B., Macadou, G., Porcher, R., Harf, A., et al. (2003). Transdiaphragmatic pressure control of airway pressure support in healthy subjects. *Am. J. Respir. Crit. Care Med.* 168, 760–769. doi: 10.1164/rccm.200203-241OC

Singh, K., Richmond, F. J., and Loeb, G. E. (2000). Recruitment properties of intramuscular and nerve-trunk stimulating electrodes. *IEEE Trans. Rehabil. Eng.* 8, 276–285. doi: 10.1109/86.867869

Siu, R., Hillen, B. K., Abbas, J. J., Renaud, S., and Jung, R. (2015). "Neuromuscular stimulation of respiratory muscles for respiratory pacing in the rat model. Program No. 430.02." in *Neuroscience Meeting Planner* (Chicago, IL: Society for Neuroscience).

Smith, J. C., Abdala, A. P. L., Rybak, I. A., and Paton, J. F. R. (2009). Structural and functional architecture of respiratory networks in the mammalian brainstem. *Philos. Trans. R. Soc. Lond. B. Biol. Sci.* 364, 2577–2587. doi: 10.1098/rstb.2009.0081

Smith, J. C., Butera, R. J., Koshiya, N., Del Negro, C., Wilson, C. G., and Johnson, S. M. (2000). Respiratory rhythm generation in neonatal and adult mammals: the hybrid pacemaker-network model. *Respir. Physiol.* 122, 131–147. doi: 10.1016/S0034-5687(00)00155-9

Song, D., Raphael, G., Lan, N., and Loeb, G. E. (2008). Computationally efficient models of neuromuscular recruitment and mechanics. *J. Neural Eng.* 5, 175–184. doi: 10.1088/1741-2560/5/2/008

Sun, Q., Schwartz, F., Michel, J., Herve, Y., and Dalmolin, R. (2011). Implementation study of an analog spiking neural network for assisting cardiac delay prediction in a cardiac resynchronization therapy device. *IEEE Trans Neur Netw.* 2, 858–869. doi: 10.1109/TNN.2011.2125986

Terzi, N., Piquilloud, L., Rozé, H., Mercat, A., Lofaso, F., Delisle, S., et al. (2012). Clinical review: update on neurally adjusted ventilatory assist - report of a round-table conference. *Crit. Care* 16, 225. doi: 10.1186/cc11297

Toporikova, N., Chevalier, M., and Thoby-Brisson, M. (2015). Sigh and eupnea rhythmogenesis involve distinct interconnected subpopulations: a combined computational and experimental study(1,2,3). *eNeuro* 2. doi: 10.1523/ENEURO.0074-14.2015

Tsodyks, M. V., Pawelzik, K., and Markram, H. (1998). Neural networks with dynamic synapses. *Neural Comput.* 10, 821–835. doi: 10.1162/089976698300017502

Vogelstein, R. J., Tenore, F., Guevremont, L., Etienne-Cummings, R., and Mushahwar, V. K. (2008). A silicon central pattern generator controls locomotion *in vivo*. *IEEE Trans. Biomed. Circuits Syst.* 2, 212–222. doi: 10.1109/TBCAS.2008.2001867

Walter, J. S., Wurster, R. D., Zhu, Q., and Laghi, F. (2011). Respiratory muscle pacing with chronically implanted intramuscular Permaloc electrodes: a feasibility study. *J. Rehabil. Res. Dev.* 48, 103–114. doi: 10.1682/JRRD.2010.05.0086

Warren, P. M., Awad, B. I., and Alilain, W. J. (2014). Reprint of drawing breath without the command of effectors: the control of respiration following spinal cord injury. *Respir. Physiol. Neurobiol.* 204, 120–130. doi: 10.1016/j.resp.2014.09.018

Yonis, H., Crognier, L., Conil, J.-M., Serres, I., Rouget, A., Virtos, M., et al. (2015). Patient-ventilator synchrony in Neurally Adjusted Ventilatory Assist (NAVA) and Pressure Support Ventilation (PSV): a prospective observational study. *BMC Anesthesiol.* 15:117. doi: 10.1186/s12871-015-0091-z

Young, I. S., Warren, R. D., and Altringham, J. D. (1992). Some properties of the mammalian locomotory and respiratory systems in relation to body mass. *J. Exp. Biol.* 164, 283–294.

Zbrzeski, A. M., Siu, R., Bornat, Y., Hillen, B. K., Jung, R., and Renaud, S. (2015). A versatile fast-development platform applied to closed-loop diaphragmatic pacing. *IEEE Proc. Neur. Eng.* 781–984. doi: 10.1109/ner.2015.7146742

Permissions

All chapters in this book were first published in CLSNGN, by Frontiers; hereby published with permission under the Creative Commons Attribution License or equivalent. Every chapter published in this book has been scrutinized by our experts. Their significance has been extensively debated. The topics covered herein carry significant findings which will fuel the growth of the discipline. They may even be implemented as practical applications or may be referred to as a beginning point for another development.

The contributors of this book come from diverse backgrounds, making this book a truly international effort. This book will bring forth new frontiers with its revolutionizing research information and detailed analysis of the nascent developments around the world.

We would like to thank all the contributing authors for lending their expertise to make the book truly unique. They have played a crucial role in the development of this book. Without their invaluable contributions this book wouldn't have been possible. They have made vital efforts to compile up to date information on the varied aspects of this subject to make this book a valuable addition to the collection of many professionals and students.

This book was conceptualized with the vision of imparting up-to-date information and advanced data in this field. To ensure the same, a matchless editorial board was set up. Every individual on the board went through rigorous rounds of assessment to prove their worth. After which they invested a large part of their time researching and compiling the most relevant data for our readers.

The editorial board has been involved in producing this book since its inception. They have spent rigorous hours researching and exploring the diverse topics which have resulted in the successful publishing of this book. They have passed on their knowledge of decades through this book. To expedite this challenging task, the publisher supported the team at every step. A small team of assistant editors was also appointed to further simplify the editing procedure and attain best results for the readers.

Apart from the editorial board, the designing team has also invested a significant amount of their time in understanding the subject and creating the most relevant covers. They scrutinized every image to scout for the most suitable representation of the subject and create an appropriate cover for the book.

The publishing team has been an ardent support to the editorial, designing and production team. Their endless efforts to recruit the best for this project, has resulted in the accomplishment of this book. They are a veteran in the field of academics and their pool of knowledge is as vast as their experience in printing. Their expertise and guidance has proved useful at every step. Their uncompromising quality standards have made this book an exceptional effort. Their encouragement from time to time has been an inspiration for everyone.

The publisher and the editorial board hope that this book will prove to be a valuable piece of knowledge for researchers, students, practitioners and scholars across the globe.

List of Contributors

Eduardo López-Larraz and Luis Montesano
Departamento de Informática e Ingeniería de Sistemas, University of Zaragoza, Zaragoza, Spain
Instituto de Investigación en Ingeniería de Aragón (I3A), Zaragoza, Spain

Fernando Trincado-Alonso, Soraya Pérez-Nombela, Antonio J. del-Ama and Angel Gil-Agudo
Biomechanics and Technical Aids Unit, National Hospital for Spinal Cord Injury, Toledo, Spain

Vijaykumar Rajasekaran
Institute for Bioengineering of Catalunya, Universitat Politécnica de Catalunya, Barcelona, Spain

Javier Minguez
Departamento de Informática e Ingeniería de Sistemas, University of Zaragoza, Zaragoza, Spain
Instituto de Investigación en Ingeniería de Aragón (I3A), Zaragoza, Spain
Bit & Brain Technologies, Zaragoza, Spain

Simin Li, Jie Li and Zheng Li
State Key Laboratory of Cognitive Neuroscience and Learning and IDG/McGovern Institute for Brain Research, Beijing Normal University, Beijing, China
Center for Collaboration and Innovation in Brain and Learning Sciences, Beijing Normal University, Beijing, China

Shih-Hung Yang and Thanh Dat Phan
Department of Mechanical and Computer Aided Engineering, Feng Chia University, Taichung, Taiwan

You-Yin Chen, Ching-Fu Wang and Po-Chuan Chen
Department of Biomedical Engineering, National Yang Ming University, Taipei, Taiwan

Sheng-Huang Lin
Institute of Biomedical Engineering, College of Medicine, National Taiwan University, Taipei, Taiwan
Department of Neurology, Tzu Chi General Hospital, Tzu Chi University

Lun-De Liao
Institute of Biomedical Engineering and Nanomedicine, National Health Research Institutes, ZhunanTownship, Taiwan
Singapore Institute for Neurotechnology, National University of Singapore, Singapore, Singapore

Henry Horng-Shing Lu
Institute of Statistics, National Chiao Tung University, Hsinchu, Taiwan

Yu-Chun Lo
The Ph.D. Program for Neural Regenerative Medicine, College of Medical Science and Technology, Taipei Medical University, Taipei, Taiwan

Hsiang-Ya Chao
Department of Electrical Engineering, National Taiwan University, Taipei, Taiwan

Hui-Ching Lin
Department and Institute of Physiology, School of Medicine, National Yang Ming University, Taipei, Taiwan

Hsin-Yi Lai
Interdisciplinary Institute of Neuroscience and Technology, Qiushi Academy for Advanced Studies, Zhejiang University, Hangzhou, China

Wei-Chen Huang
Department of Materials Science and Engineering, Carnegie Mellon University Pittsburgh, PA, USA

Danilo Pani, Paolo Meloni, Giuseppe Tuveri and Luigi Raffo
EOLab - Microelectronics and Bioengineering Lab, Department of Electrical and Electronic Engineering, University of Cagliari, Cagliari, Italy

Francesca Palumbo
Information Engineering Unit, PolComIng Department, University of Sassari, Sassari, Italy

Paolo Massobrio
Neuroengineering and Bio-nano Technology Lab, Dibris, University of Genova, Genova

Kevin Kern, Georgios Naros and Alireza Gharabaghi
Division of Functional and Restorative Neurosurgery and Centre for Integrative Neuroscience, Eberhard Karls University Tuebingen, Tuebingen, Germany

Christoph Braun
Magnetoencephalography Center, Eberhard Karls University Tuebingen, Tuebingen,Germany
Center for Mind/Brain Sciences (CIMeC), University of Trento, Italy

Daniel Weiss
Department for Neurodegenerative Diseases and Hertie Institute for Clinical Brain Research and German Centre of Neurodegenerative Diseases (DZNE), Eberhard Karls University Tuebingen, Tuebingen, Germany

Ilknur Telkes and Nuri F. Ince
Clinical Neural Engineering Lab., Biomedical Engineering Department, University of Houston, Houston, TX, USA

Joohi Jimenez-Shahed
Department of Neurology, Baylor College of Medicine, Houston, TX, USA

Ashwin Viswanathan
Department of Neurosurgery, Baylor College of Medicine, Houston, TX, USA

Aviva Abosch
Department of Neurosurgery, University of Colorado, Aurora, CO, USA

Fatemeh Karimi, Jonathan Kofman and Ning Jiang
Department of Systems Design Engineering, Faculty of Engineering, University of Waterloo, Waterloo, ON, Canada

Natalie Mrachacz-Kersting
Department of Health Science and Technology, Aalborg University, Aalborg, Denmark

Dario Farina
Neurorehabilitation Engineering Department of Bioengineering, Imperial College London, London, United Kingdom

Tim Mullen and John R. Iversen
Swartz Center for Computational Neuroscience, University of California, San Diego, San Diego, CA, United States

Hristos Courellis
Swartz Center for Computational Neuroscience, University of California, San Diego, San Diego, CA, United States

Gert Cauwenberghs
Department of Bioengineering, University of California, San Diego, San Diego, CA, United States
Institute for NeuralComputation, University of California, San Diego, San Diego, CA, United States

Howard Poizner
Institute for NeuralComputation, University of California, San Diego, San Diego, CA, United States

Dario Farina
Department of Neurorehabilitation Engineering, Bernstein Center for Computational Neuroscience, University Medical Center, Göttingen, Germany
Institute of Computer Science, Faculty of Mathematics and Computer Secience, Georg-August University, Göttingen, Germany
Department of Systems Design Engineering, University of Waterloo, Waterloo, ON, Canada
Center for Sensory-Motor Interaction, Department of Health Science and Technology, Aalborg University, Aalborg, Denmark

Ren Xu
Department of Neurorehabilitation Engineering, Bernstein Center for Computational Neuroscience, University Medical Center, Göttingen, Germany
Institute of Computer Science, Faculty of Mathematics and Computer Secience, Georg-August University, Göttingen, Germany

Ning Jiang
Department of Systems Design Engineering, University of Waterloo, Waterloo, ON, Canada

Natalie Mrachacz-Kersting and Kim Dremstrup
Center for Sensory-Motor Interaction, Department of Health Science and Technology, Aalborg University, Aalborg, Denmark

Sébastien Joucla, Thierry Lafon and Philippe Chauvet
Centre National de la Recherche Scientifique, Institute for Cognitive and Integrative Neuroscience (INCIA), UMR 5287, Talence, France
Institute for Cognitive and Integrative Neuroscience (INCIA), UMR 5287, University of Bordeaux, Talence, France

Sylvain Saïghi, Noëlle Lewis, Matthieu Ambroise and Timothée Levi
Laboratoire de l'Intégration du Matériau au Système, UMR 5218, University of Bordeaux, Talence, France
CentreNational de la Recherche Scientifique, Laboratoire de l'Intégration du Matériau au Système, UMR 5218, Talence, France

Sylvie Renaud and Yannick Bornat
Laboratoire de l'Intégration du Matériau au Système, UMR 5218, University of Bordeaux, Talence, France
Bordeaux INP, Laboratoire de l'Intégration du Matériau au Système, UMR 5218, Talence, France

Linda Wilson
Formerly affiliated with the International Technology Roadmap for Semiconductors (ITRS), Washington, USA

Blaise Yvert
Centre National de la Recherche Scientifique, Institute for Cognitive and Integrative Neuroscience (INCIA), UMR 5287, Talence, France
Bordeaux INP, Laboratoire de l'Intégration du Matériau au Système, UMR 5218, Talence, France, ZInstitut National de la Santé et de la Recherche Médicale, Clinatec-Lab, U1205, Grenoble, France
Université Grenoble Alpes, Clinatec-Lab,U1205, Grenoble, France

P. Justin Rossi, Aysegul Gunduz, Jack Judy, Daniel Martinez-Ramirez, Rene Molina, Enrico Opri, Kevin J. Otto, Karim G. Oweiss, Aparna Shukla, Jonathan Shute, Kelly D. Foote and Michael S. Okun
Department of Neuroscience, Center for Movement Disorders and Neurorestoration, University of Florida, Gainesville, FL, USA

Andre Machado
Neurological Institute Cleveland Clinic, Cleveland, OH, USA

James J.Giordano
Neuroethics Studies Program, Department of Neurology, Georgetown University Medical Center, Washington, DC, USA

W. Jeff Elias
Neurological Surgery and Neurology, Stereotactic and Functional Neurosurgery, Department of Neurosurgery, University of Virginia Health Science Center, Charlottesville, VA, USA

Marvin A. Rossi, Leopoldo Cendejas-Zaragoza and Leonard Verhagen
Department of Neurology, Rush University Medical Center, Chicago, IL, USA

Christopher L. Butson
Scientific Computing and Imaging Institute,University of Utah, Salt Lake City, UT, USA

Michael D. Fox, Ron L. Alterman and Ludy C. Shih
Beth Israel Deaconess Medical Center, Harvard Medical School, Boston, MA,USA

Cameron C. McIntyre
Department of Biomedical Engineering, School of Medicine, Case Western Reserve University, Cleveland, OH, USA

Nader Pouratian
Department of Neurosurgery, University of California, Los Angeles, Los Angeles, CA, USA

Nicole C. Swann and Coralie de Hemptinne
University of California, San Francisco, San Francisco, CA, USA

Robert E. Gross
The Emory Clinic, Emory University, Atlanta, GA, USA

Howard J. Chizeck and Jeffrey Herron
Department of Electrical Engineering, University of Washington, Seattle, WA, USA

Michele Tagliati
Movement Disorders Program, Department of Neurology, Cedars-Sinai Medical Center, Los Angeles, CA, USA

Andres M. Lozano and Anthony E. Lang
Department of Neurosurgery, University of Toronto, Toronto, ON, Canada

Wayne Goodman and Brian H. Kopell
The Icahn School of Medicine at Mount Sinai, New York, NY, USA

Jean-Philippe Langevin
Greater Los Angeles Veterans AffairsHealthcare System, Los Angeles, CA, USA

Umer Akbar
Department of Neurology, Alpert Medical School, Brown University,Providence, RI, USA

Greg A. Gerhardt and Craig van Horne
University of Kentucky Medical Center, Lexington, KY, USA

Warren M. Grill
Department of Biomedical Engineering,Duke University, Durham, NC, USA

Mark Hallett, Codrin Lungu and Kareem A. Zaghloul
National Institute of Neurological Disorders and Stroke, National Institutes of Health,Bethesda, MD, USA

Todd Herrington
Massachusetts General Hospital, Harvard Medical School, Boston, MA, USA

Alon Y. Mogilner
Department of Neurosurgery-Center for Neuromodulation, NYU Langone Medical Center, New York, NY, USA

Yagna Pathak, Sameer A. Sheth and Nora Vanegas
Neurological Institute,Columbia University Medical Center, New York, NY, USA

G. Karl Steinke
25 Boston Scientific Neuromodulation, Valencia, CA, USA

Alexander I. Tröster
Department of Clinical Neuropsychology, Barrow Neurological Institute, Phoenix, AZ, USA

Nora Vanegas
Department of Clinical Neuropsychology, Barrow Neurological Institute, Phoenix, AZ, USA

Kareem A. Zaghloul
National Institute of Neurological Disorders and Stroke, National Institutes of Health, Bethesda, MD, USA

Leopoldo Cendejas-Zaragoza and Leonard Verhagen
Department of Neurology, Rush University Medical Center, Chicago, IL, USA

Kelly D. Foote and Michael S. Okun
Department of Neuroscience, Center for Movement Disorders and Neurorestoration, University of Florida, Gainesville, FL, USA

Alycia Gailey and Marco Santello
School of Biological and Health Systems Engineering, Tempe, AZ, USA

Panagiotis Artemiadis
School for Engineering of Matter, Transport, and Energy, Arizona State University, Tempe, AZ, USA

Takashi Kohno and Kazuyuki Aihara
Institute of Industrial Science, University of Tokyo, Tokyo, Japan

Munehisa Sekikawa
Department of Mechanical and Intelligent Engineering, Utsunomiya University, Utsunomiya, Japan

Jing Li
College of Electronic Engineering, Xi'an Shiyou University, Xi'an, China

Takuya Nanami
Department of Electrical Engineering and Information Systems, University of Tokyo, Tokyo, Japan

Fabio Boi, Vito De Feo and Alessandro Vato
Computation Laboratory, Istituto Italiano di Tecnologia, Rovereto, Italy

Timoleon Moraitis and Giacomo Indiveri
Institute of Neuroinformatics, University of Zurich and ETH Zurich, Zurich, Switzerland

Francesco Diotalevi
Brain and Cognitive Sciences, Istituto Italiano di Tecnologia, Genova, Italy

Chiara Bartolozzi
iCub Facility, Istituto Italiano di Tecnologia, Genova, Italy

Simona Ferrante, Noelia Chia Bejarano, Giancarlo Ferrigno and Alessandra Pedrocchi
Neuroengineering and Medical Robotics Laboratory, Department of Electronics, Information and Bioengineering, Politecnico di Milano, Milan, Italy

Emilia Ambrosini
Neuroengineering and Medical Robotics Laboratory, Department of Electronics, Information and Bioengineering, Politecnico di Milano, Milan, Italy
Medicine and Rehabilitation Unit, Scientific Institute of Lissone, Fondazione Salvatore Maugeri (IRCCS), Lissone, Monza Brianza, Italy

Antonio Nardone and Anna M. Turcato
and Movement Laboratory, Division of Physical Medicine and Rehabilitation, Scientific Institute of Veruno, Fondazione Salvatore Maugeri (IRCCS), Veruno, Novara, Italy
Department of Translational Medicine, University of Eastern Piedmont, Novara, Italy

Marco Monticone
Medicine and Rehabilitation Unit, Scientific Institute of Lissone, Fondazione Salvatore Maugeri (IRCCS), Lissone, Monza Brianza, Italy
Department of Pubilc Health, Clinical Medicine, University of Cagliari, Cagliari, Italy

Mitsuhiro Hayashibe
Institut National de Recherche en Informatique et en Automatique (INRIA), University of Montpellier, Montpellier, France

James Wright, André van Schaik and Jonathan C. Tapson
Biomedical Engineering and Neuroscience, The MARCS Institute, University of Western Sydney, NSW, Australia

James Abbas
School of Biological and Health System Engineering, Arizona State University, Tempe, AZ. USA

Mark A. Attiah, Julius de Vries, Andrew G. Richardson and Timothy H. Lucas
Department of Neurosurgery, Center for Neuroengineering and Therapeutics, Perelman School of Medicine, University of Pennsylvania, Philadelphia, PA, USA

Vaughan G. Macefield
Biomedical Engineering and Neuroscience, The MARCS Institute, University of Western Sydney, Sydney, NSW, Australia
School of Medicine, University of Western Sydney, Sydney, NSW, Australia
Neuroscience Research Australia, Sydney, NSW, Australia

Mark A. Attiah, Julius de Vries, Andrew G. Richardson and Timothy H. Lucas
Department of Neurosurgery, Center for Neuroengineering and Therapeutics, Perelman School of Medicine, University of Pennsylvania, Philadelphia, PA, USA

Adeline Zbrzeski, Yannick Bornat and Sylvie Renaud
Bordeux INR, IMS, UMR 5218, Talence, France
Univ. Bordeaux, IMS, UMR 5218, Talence, France

Brian Hillen, Ricardo Siu and Ranu Jung
Department of Biomedical Engineering, Florida International University, Miami, FL,USA

Index

R

S

T

V